Drug			
Amikacin	Peak: 3 ... Trough: ... dose		mcg/mL
Chloram-phenicol	Peak 1.5 hr after infusion Trough: just prior to next dose	30 min	Peak: 15–25 mcg/mL
Digoxin	Trough: just prior to next dose (or at least 6 hr after dose)	≥ 5 min	0.9–2.0 ng/mL
Gentamicin	Peak: 30 min after infusion Trough: <0.5 hr prior to next dose	30 min	Peak: 4–8 mcg/mL Trough: 0.5–2 mcg/mL
Lidocaine	Steady state levels usually achieved after 6–12 hr	—	1.50–5.0 mcg/mL
Pheno-barbital	Trough: just prior to next dose	60 mg/min Peds: 30 mg/min	10–30 mcg/mL
Phenytoin	Trough: just prior to next dose	50 mg/min	10–20 mcg/mL
Free Pheny-toin	May be drawn at same time as total level		1–2 mcg/mL
Procaina-mide	Trough: just prior to next dose Infusion: 6–12 hrs after start Combined PA and NAPA	50 mg/min	PA: 4–10 mcg/mL NAPA: 10–20 mcg/mL PA+NAPA: < 30 mcg/mL
Theophyl-line	30 mins after loading dose 24 hrs after start of infusion or dosage change	—	10–20 mcg/mL
Tobramy-cin	Peak: 30 min after infusion Trough: <0.5 hr prior to next dose	30 min	Peak: 4–8 mcg/mL Trough: 0.5–2 mcg/mL
Vancomy-cin	Peak: 1 hr after 1 hr infusion Trough: <0.5 hr prior to next dose	0.5–1 hr	Peak: 20–40 mcg/mL Trough: 5–10 mcg/mL

ᵃVaries depending on laboratory assay

Nurses' IV Drug Manual

Jacqueline Derolf Sutton, PharmD
Assistant Director
Clinical Services/Pharmacy Development
Cooper Hospital/University Medical Center
Camden, New Jersey

Donna Whyte Thalken, RN, MSN, CCRN
Clinical Nurse Specialist
Medical/Respiratory Intensive Care Unit
Thomas Jefferson University Hospital
Philadelphia, Pennsylvania

Maryann C. Powell, RN, BSN, CCRN
Nurse Manager
Medical-Surgical ICU, Cardiothoracic ICU, Intermediate ICU
Cooper Hospital/University Medical Center
Camden, New Jersey

APPLETON & LANGE
Norwalk, Connecticut

Copyright © 1993 by Appleton & Lange
Simon & Schuster Business and Professional Group

All rights reserved. This book, or any parts thereof, may not be used or reproduced in any manner without written permission. For information, address Appleton & Lange, 25 Van Zant Street, East Norwalk, Connecticut 06855.

93 94 95 96 97 / 10 9 8 7 6 5 4 3 2 1

Prentice Hall International (UK) Limited, *London*
Prentice Hall of Australia Pty. Limited, *Sydney*
Prentice Hall Canada, Inc., *Toronto*
Prentice Hall Hispanoamericana, S.A., *Mexico*
Prentice Hall of India Private Limited, *New Delhi*
Prentice Hall of Japan, Inc., *Tokyo*
Simon & Schuster Asia Pte. Ltd., *Singapore*
Editora Prentice Hall do Brasil Ltda., *Rio de Janeiro*
Prentice Hall, *Englewood Cliffs, New Jersey*

Library of Congress Cataloging-in-Publication Data
Sutton, Jacqueline Derolf.
    Nurses' IV drug manual / Jacqueline Derolf Sutton, Donna Whyte Thalken, Maryann C. Powell.
        p.   cm.
    Includes bibliographical references and index.

    1. Intravenous therapy—Handbooks, manuals, etc.   2. Nursing—Handbooks, manuals, etc.   I. Thalken, Donna Whyte.   II. Powell, Maryann C.   III. Title.
    [DNLM: 1. Drugs—administration & dosage—handbooks. 2. Drugs—administration & dosage—nurses' instruction.   3. Infusions, Intravenous—Handbooks.   4. Infusions, Intravenous—nurses' instruction.   QV 39 S967n]
    RM170.S88   1993
    615.5'8—dc20
    DNLM/DLC   92-49638
    for Library of Congress   CIP

Editor in Chief: Barbara Ellen Norwitz
Production Editor: Elizabeth Ryan
Cover: Michael J. Kelly

PRINTED IN THE UNITED STATES OF AMERICA

CONTENTS

PREFACE

The primary purpose of the *Nurses' IV Drug Manual* is to provide students and practitioners with a quick and comprehensive guide for the safe and knowledgeable administration of intravenous medications.

Since safe and accurate medication administration are primary nursing responsibilities, knowledge of a drug's pharmacologic activity is essential. To foster the concept of quality care and patient safety, this IV drug manual was developed to provide easy access to information for professionals.

The initial concept for this IV drug manual evolved from the nursing staff at Cooper Hospital/UMC. The need for a concise but comprehensive guide for intravenous drug administration was identified. In an effort to support our nursing colleagues, this book was developed, and is dedicated to nurses who, in their patients' best interests, never hesitate to ask the what, when, where, and why of drug administration.

Jacqueline Derolf Sutton
Donna Whyte Thalken
Maryann C. Powell

HOW TO USE NURSES' IV DRUG MANUAL

The *Nurses' IV Drug Manual* is arranged in a two column format to facilitate access to information necessary for the administration of intravenous medications.

The following describes how and where to retrieve information from the drug monograph:

Generic Name: The generic name of the active component(s) of the preparation is listed. If a common standard chemical name is also available, it will be listed in parentheses.

Pronunciation Key: A phonetic pronunciation key is available with the syllable to be emphasized with a stress mark.

Trade Name(s): The most commonly used trade names are listed alphabetically. If a trade name is only used in Canada, a maple leaf symbol (♦) will be designated after the name. If a product is only referred to by its generic/chemical name, a trade name will not be listed.

Classification(s): The most common classifications of uses of the drug are listed alphabetically.

Pregnancy Category: The FDA assigned pregnancy risk category (as defined in Appendix A) is included, if available; otherwise, a designation of Unknown is used. This category identifies the risk to the fetus as determined by animal and/or human data. Since most drugs have limited or no safety data from controlled trials, a risk versus benefit assessment should occur prior to administration.

Controlled Substance Schedule: This DEA designation (as defined in Appendix B) indicates the abuse potential associated with use of the identified agent.

PHARMACODYNAMICS/KINETICS

Pharmacodynamics describes the mechanism of action and the expected therapeutic effect. Pharmacokinetics describes the parameters associated with the drug following absorption, distribution, metabolism and elimination. If specific data is unavailable, poorly defined or unknown, it will not be listed.

Mechanism of Action: Briefly describes the activity, at a cellular level and at the primary site of action, that results in the anticipated therapeutic effect.

Onset of Action: Describes the time when pharmacologic effect occurs.

Peak Effect: Describes the time when pharmacologic effect is at its maximum.

Peak serum level: Describes the time required to reach a maximal serum concentration (usually immediately following intravenous administration).

Duration of Action: Describes the time over which the pharmacologic effect persists.

Therapeutic Serum Levels: Refers to the accepted therapeutic serum levels for monitoring purposes. Since all drugs are not able to be routinely assayed, data will be included for those for which it is available (values will vary according to each institution or laboratory).

Distribution: Drugs distribute to various body fluids and tissues, and ultimately to the primary site of activity. Data regarding transfer across the placental barrier or into breast milk will be noted under the pregnancy "precautions" section. Drugs bind to tissues and proteins to varying degrees as noted. If a drug is extensively protein bound (>90%), displacement from the binding site may occur through drug interactions or a reduction in the binding protein, i.e., albumin. If this occurs, the increased free drug may result in toxic side effects.

Metabolism/Elimination: Describes the extent, if any, of metabolic activation/inactivation and the primary route of elimination. If the drug is primarily eliminated by the kidneys, the impact of hemodialysis and/or peritoneal dialysis will be noted if available.

Half-Life: Describes the terminal elimination half-life ($t_{1/2}$) with normal end organ function. This refers to the time by which the serum drug concentration declines by 50%. This value assists in estimating when pharmacologic effect will begin to occur (usually at steady state in 4 to 5 half-lives) or decline. Impairment of the primary organ of elimination and its effect on half-life will also be noted.

INDICATIONS/DOSAGE

All FDA labeled indications and usual dosage ranges will be listed for adult, pediatric, and neonatal patients, as they apply to the respective populations. Modified dosage/intervals may be necessary based on individual patient situations. When literature supports unlabeled indications or use in specific patient populations, dosage guidelines will be presented. Additional information following publication of this manual may modify guidelines. Recommendations for dosage/interval adjustments based on clinical parameters especially in elderly and changing end organ function, specifically creatinine clearance (CrCl), will be made when applicable; refer to product literature or reference sources for specific adjustments. Pediatric dosages are usually based on "mg/kg" body weight or "mg/m^2" body surface area; doses should not exceed adult guidelines unless specifically indicated.

Contraindications/Precautions Describes the situations or patient populations requiring careful consideration and/or administration.

Contraindicated in: As identified by the manufacturer, patients, or conditions in which the drug should not be administered. In certain circumstances, the physician may determine that a relative (rather than absolute) risk versus benefit exists.

Use Cautiously in: Patients or conditions requiring careful monitoring with use; alternative regimens may need to be considered.

Pregnancy/Lactation: Most drugs have no well-controlled trials to establish safety in pregnancy/lactation; however, the FDA has assigned designated safety categories for risk versus benefit assessment. If teratogenic data clearly is available, a recommendation not to administer the drug will be included. Specific information regarding drug passage across placenta or into breast milk will also be noted.

Pediatrics: If there is no or limited safety and efficacy data, this will be noted. If organ immaturity or patient sensitivity is an issue, cautionary statements will be included.

PREPARATION
Describes the details involved in preparing the drug for administration. All agents should be prepared using aseptic technique and have no evidence of particulate matter.

Availability: The most commonly available strengths/concentrations, dosage form and packaging size; additional information such as sodium or benzyl alcohol content are noted.

Reconstitution: If the product is available in a lyophilized/powder for injection, the diluent and volume required to prepare the initial constitution is listed.

Syringe/Infusion: If further dilution of the drug is required prior to administration, as an IV push or infusion, the volumes and compatible diluents/solutions are noted.

STABILITY/STORAGE
Manufacturer specified storage requirements (ie, refrigeration) of the intact vial/ampule and subsequent diluted product are noted. Manufacturer sta-

bility is indicated by the expiration date if stored as specified. Stability of the products in the various dilutions are listed. If a preparation does not contain a preservative, use within 24 hours is suggested unless otherwise specified.

ADMINISTRATION

General information is provided, which includes infusion device requirements, test dose use, trained personnel/ventilatory support requirements, and extravasation/treatment information. Additionally, IV sites should be rotated to avoid phlebitis development especially with frequent IV administration. If the agent has cytotoxic potential, recommendations to handle as per institutional guidelines is included (see Appendix C) for preparation and administration. If spills occur, specific information will be provided if available.

IV Push: Specific rates of administration are identified if available. If recommended to give slowly, a specific rate is not given since institutional policy varies; however, 1 to 5 minutes is acceptable depending on the volume to be given. If small volumes are to be given, further dilution may be considered to increase the accuracy of administration.

Intermittent/Continuous Infusion: Intermittent infusion includes infusion over 0.5 to 12 hours; continuous infusion over 12 to 24 hours as per physician specified order.

COMPATIBILITY/INCOMPATIBILITY

Only information documented for concurrent administration is included. The composition of individual solutions must be identified to ensure complete compatibility. Consider flushing between medications with compatible solution. Products may vary by manufacturer in composition; assess IV tubing and site frequently with initial administrations. Consult the pharmacy department and/or additional reference resources to determine the feasibility of administration of multiple or unlisted agents.

Solution: Unless specifically indicated, dextrose solutions include dextrose 5% and 10%; sodium chloride solutions include 0.2%, 0.3%, 0.45%, and 0.9%; or a combination of dextrose–sodium chloride if compatible in either.

Syringe: Data available for drugs drawn up in same syringe just prior to administration.

Y-Site: Data available for drugs administered through y-site connection.

Additive: Data included only if the need for admixture in the same IV bag is considered necessary.

ADVERSE, EFFECTS

Underline indicates most frequently reported effects; CAPITAL indicates life threatening effects. If a particular effect is important from a safety perspective, this will be listed first in the description. The following abbreviations describe the body systems in a head-to-toe order:

CNS: Central nervous system
Ophtho: Ophthalmic
CV: Cardiovascular

Resp: Respiratory
GI: Gastrointestinal
GU: Genitourinary
Renal: Renal
MS: Musculoskeletal
Derm: Dermatologic
Endo: Endocrine
Fld/Lytes: Fluid and electrolytes
Heme: Hematologic. A nadir is noted when applicable.
Hypersens: Hypersensitivity
Metab: Metabolic
Other: Includes uncategorized effects and effects at the site of administration

TOXICITY/OVERDOSE

This describes the signs/symptoms associated with excessive dosage and/or drug accumulation. Specific treatment, other than symptomatic and supportive measures, is noted if available. If a specific antidote is recognized, this is mentioned. In all cases, a physician should be notified for specific patient management. Anaphylactic reactions are not included; however, additional toxicity treatment measures may be used.

DRUG INTERACTIONS

Includes an alphabetical listing of the agents commonly known to interact with the identified agent, noting the type of drug-drug interaction and/or pharmacologic effect. Drug-food interactions are included if available.

NURSING CONSIDERATIONS

Assessment: Evaluate information in this section prior to and during therapy to assess therapeutic effect and/or toxicity development.
General: Information to be assessed includes vital signs, daily weights, intake/output ratios, hypersensitivity, and infectious disease status determined by the specific agent.
Physical: Information to be assessed includes various body/organ systems.
Lab Alterations: Data to be assessed includes laboratory values requiring baseline and/or periodic monitoring. Also noted will be drug-lab interactions or false positive/negative effects on particular lab tests, if known.
Intervention/Rationale: Describes the reasons for assessment and the particular interventions that may be necessary during evaluation of the patient.
Patient/Family Education: Describes instructions for the patient and/or family regarding the expected adverse and/or therapeutic effects of therapy. This section will aid in targeting those issues pertinent to the patient's understanding. Information may be included to assist the patient in day-to-day activities with minimal interference. In most circumstances, the patient should be aware of the reasons for therapy and what the expected therapeutic outcome/goals should be. Education should include adverse effects and drug interactions relative to the patient and point in therapy.

Alphabetical Listing
of Drugs

ACETAZOLAMIDE

(a-set-a-zole'-a-mide)
Trade Name(s): Diamox
Classification(s): Carbonic
anhydrase inhibitor
Pregnancy Category: C

PHARMACODYNAMICS/KINETICS

Mechanism of Action: Inhibits carbonic anhydrase resulting in decreased rate of aqueous humor formation and intraocular pressure. Causes inhibition of renal tubule hydrogen ion secretion and alkaline diuresis. Results in metabolic acidosis. **Onset of Action:** 2 min. **Peak Effect:** 15 min. **Duration of Action:** 4–5 hr. **Distribution:** Distributed throughout body tissues with high concentration in erythrocytes, plasma and kidneys. **Metabolism/Elimination:** Eliminated unchanged by the kidneys

INDICATIONS/DOSAGE

Diuresis in CHF/Drug Induced Edema

Adult: 250–375 mg once daily in morning. Alternate day therapy may be useful in refractory patients. *Pediatric:* 5 mg/kg/dose or 150 mg/m² once daily in morning. Alternate day therapy may be useful in refractory patients.

Treatment of Acute Closed Angle Glaucoma (*Change to oral therapy when possible*).

Adult: 500 mg followed by 125–250 mg in 2–4 hr and every 4–6 hr as needed. *Pediatric:* 5–10 mg/kg every 6 hr as needed.

Epilepsy

Adult: 8–30 mg/kg/day in divided doses. Usual dosage range 375–1000 mg. *Pediatric:* 8–30 mg/kg/day in divided doses every 6–8 hr. Maximum dose 1 g/day.

Hydrocephalus

Pediatric/Neonate: 25 mg/kg/day in 3 divided doses. Increase by 25 mg/kg/day to a maximum of 100 mg/kg/day (up to 2 g/day).

CONTRAINDICATIONS/PRECAUTIONS

Contraindicated in: Adrenocortical insufficiency, hepatic/renal failure, hyperchloremic acidosis, hypersensitivity to sulfa-related agents, severe pulmonary obstruction, significant hypokalemia/hyponatremia. **Use cautiously in:** Emphysema, pulmonary obstruction, respiratory acidosis. **Pregnancy/Lactation:** No well-controlled trial to establish safety. Benefits must outweigh risks. Animal studies demonstrate teratogenic effects at high doses. Crosses placenta.

PREPARATION

Availability: 500 mg vials; 2.05 mEq of sodium/500 mg. **Reconstitution:** Dilute 500 mg vial with at least 5 mL sterile water for injection to yield a solution containing not more than 100 mg/mL. **Infusion:** Prepare just prior to administration. Add to volume large enough to infuse over 4–8 hr.

STABILITY/STORAGE

Vial: Stable 1 week refrigerated. Use within 24 hr (contains no preservative). **Infusion:** Stable for 24 hr.

In the Adverse Effects section, underline indicates most frequent;
CAPS indicates life threatening.

ADMINISTRATION
General: Direct IV administration is preferred due to alkaline pH. **IV Push:** Administer at a rate of 100–500 mg/min. **Intermittent Infusion:** Infuse over 4–8 hr.

COMPATIBILITY
Solution: Dextrose solutions, lactated Ringer's, sodium chloride solutions.

ADVERSE EFFECTS
CNS: Ataxia, confusion, convulsions, depression, dizziness, headache, malaise, paralysis, paresthesia of extremities/mucocutaneous areas, sedation, tremor. **Ophtho:** Transient myopia. **GI:** Anorexia, constipation, hepatic insufficiency, melena, nausea, vomiting. **GU:** Crystalluria, glycosuria, hematuria, polyuria. **Renal:** Renal calculi/colic. **Derm:** Photosensitivity. **Endo:** Hyperglycemia. **Fld/Lytes:** Hyperchloremic acidosis, hypokalemia. **Heme:** AGRANULOCYTOSIS, bone marrow depression, hemolytic anemia, leukopenia, pancytopenia, thrombocytopenia. **Hypersens:** Rash, urticaria, pruritus. **Other:** Fever, weight loss.

TOXICITY/OVERDOSE
Signs/Symptoms: Extension of adverse effects. **Treatment:** Symptomatic and supportive treatment.

DRUG INTERACTIONS
Amphetamines, ephedrine, flecainide, pseudoephedrine, quinidine: Enhanced pharmacologic effect. **Digitalis:** Increased potential for digitalis toxicity secondary to diuresis-induced hypokalemia. **Methenamine:** Decreased efficacy of acetazolamide. **Salicylates:** Increased potential for salicylate toxicity secondary to diuresis-induced acidosis. Decreased acetazolamide clearance.

NURSING CONSIDERATIONS

Assessment
General:
Intake/output ratio, baseline/daily weights, vital signs.
Physical:
Musculoskeletal system, hypersensitivity reactions.
Lab Alterations:
Monitor electrolytes (serum potassium daily), serum glucose, CBC with differential and platelet count (baseline and regularly during therapy). Measurement of urinary protein levels may result in false positive results secondary to urine alkalinization.

Intervention/Rationale
Assess for signs/symptoms of dehydration. Drug may lead to water/electrolyte depletion. Drug may cause muscle weakness and cramps due to hypokalemia. ● Assess patients receiving digitalis glycosides for signs/symptoms of toxicity (nausea/vomiting, anorexia, visual disturbances, confusion, cardiac dysrhythmias), especially when hypokalemia is present. ● Monitor patient for hematologic effects similar to sulfa drug reactions. ● Diuresis failures may result from overdosage or too frequent administration; consider alternate day or every 2 day use.

Patient/Family Education
May cause drowsiness (avoid activities requiring alertness). Seek as-

In the Adverse Effects section, underline indicates most frequent; CAPS indicates life threatening.

3

sistance with ambulatory activities. Notify physician/nurse of sore throat, fever, unusual bleeding/bruising, tingling or tremors of feet/hands, flank pain, rash. Note any signs of dehydration (decreased urination, loss of skin turgor, excessive thirst and leg cramps). Avoid excess exposure to sunlight.

ACYCLOVIR
(ay-sye′-kloe-veer)
Trade Name(s): Zovirax
Classification(s): Antiviral
Pregnancy Category: C

PHARMACODYNAMICS/KINETICS
Mechanism of Action: Inhibits viral DNA replication. **Peak Serum Level:** 1.5–2 hr. **Distribution:** Widely distributed in tissues/body fluids. 9%–33% protein bound. **Metabolism/Elimination:** Eliminated primarily as unchanged drug (62%–91%) by the kidneys. Removed by hemodialysis. **Half-Life:** 2.5–3.0 hr. Anuria 19 hr.

INDICATIONS/DOSAGE

Treatment of Herpes Simplex Encephalitis
Adult: 10 mg/kg every 8 hr for 10 days. *Pediatric:* 500 mg/m² every 8 hr for 10 days.

Mucosal/Cutaneous Herpes Simplex Virus (HSV) Infection in Immunocompromised States
Adult: 5 mg/kg every 8 hr for 7 days. *Pediatric:* 250 mg/m² every 8 hr for 7 days.

Varicella/Zoster Infections in Immunocompromised States
Adult: 10 mg/kg every 8 hr for 7 days. *Pediatric:* 500 mg/m² every 8 hr for 7 days.

Treatment of HSV Infections in Patients Receiving Hemodialysis
Adult/Pediatric: 5 mg/kg daily after each dialysis or 2.5 mg/kg every 24 hr, with an additional 2.5 mg/kg after each dialysis.

CONTRAINDICATIONS/PRECAUTIONS
Contraindicated in: Hypersensitivity to acyclovir or ganciclovir. **Pregnancy/Lactation:** No well-controlled trials to establish safety. Benefits must outweigh risks. Animal studies demonstrate maternal and fetal anomalies. Distributed in breast milk.

PREPARATION
Availability: 500 mg or 1000 mg vials; 2.1 mEq sodium/500 mg. **Reconstitution:** Dilute each 500 mg with 10 mL sterile water for injection to a final concentration of 50 mg/mL. **Infusion:** Further dilute each 500 mg vial with at least 50–100 mL compatible IV solution. Maximum final concentration 7–10 mg/mL.

STABILITY/STORAGE
Vial: Use reconstituted vial within 12 hr. Do not refrigerate. Crystals will redissolve at room temperature without affecting drug strength. **Infusion:** Store at room temperature. Use within 24 hr.

ADMINISTRATION
General: Avoid rapid bolus. Administer dose after hemodialysis. Infusion times shorter than 1 hr may

In the Adverse Effects section, <u>underline</u> indicates most frequent;
CAPS indicates life threatening.

4

cause increased risk of renal toxicity. **Intermittent Infusion:** Infuse over at least 1 hr via infusion pump.

COMPATIBILITY

Solution: Dextrose solutions, lactated Ringer's, sodium chloride solutions. **Y-site:** Amikacin, ampicillin, cefazolin, cefotaxime, ceftazidime, ceftizoxime, ceftriaxone, cefuroxime, chloramphenicol, cimetidine, clindamycin, dexamethasone, diphenhydramine, doxycycline, erythromycin, gentamicin, heparin, hydrocortisone, hydromorphone, imipenem, lorazepam, magnesium sulfate, meperidine, methylprednisolone, metronidazole, morphine, multivitamins, nafcillin, oxacillin, penicillin, piperacillin, potassium chloride, ranitidine, sodium bicarbonate, theophylline, ticarcillin, tobramycin, trimethoprim/sulfa, vancomycin, zidovudine.

INCOMPATIBILITY

Solution: Bacteriostatic water. **Y-site:** Dobutamine, dopamine, foscarnet, ondansetron.

ADVERSE EFFECTS

CNS: <u>Headache,</u> confusion, hallucinations, lethargy, lightheadedness, seizures, tremor. **CV:** Chest pain, PULMONARY EDEMA WITH TAMPONADE, edema, hypotension. **GI:** Abdominal pain, anorexia, nausea, increased ALT (SGPT)/AST (SGOT), thirst, vomiting. **GU:** Anuria, hematuria, pain on urination. **Renal:** Transient increases in serum creatinine/BUN. **Fld/Lytes:** Hypokalemia. **Heme:** Anemia, NEUTROPENIA, THROMBOCYTOPENIA. **Hypersens:** Rash, urticaria. **Other:** Phlebitis, fever.

TOXICITY/OVERDOSE

Signs/Symptoms: Crystal precipitation in renal tubules may occur with bolus injections and poor hydration status.

Treatment: Hemodialysis for 6 hr provides 60% decrease in plasma concentrations. In acute renal failure/anuria, hemodialysis may be beneficial until renal function is restored. Peritoneal dialysis is less effective.

DRUG INTERACTIONS

Interferon, Intrathecal methotrexate: Potentiates acyclovir adverse effects. **Probenecid:** Decreased acyclovir urinary excretion. **Zidovudine:** Increased drowsiness and lethargy.

NURSING CONSIDERATIONS

Assessment
General:
Intake/output ratio, hydration status.
Physical:
Neurologic/mental status, cardiopulmonary status, integumentary system.
Lab Alterations:
Monitor BUN, serum creatinine, CBC with differential and platelet count.

Intervention/Rationale
Adequate hydration should be administered concurrently to enhance renal elimination and prevent renal toxicity. ● Assess skin and mucosa lesions for improvement/change.

Patient/Family Education
Maintain good oral fluid intake/hydration. Avoid persons with known infections and crowds. Use condoms (HIV virus may be dormant

---

In the Adverse Effects section, <u>underline</u> indicates most frequent;
CAPS indicates life threatening.

and can be transmitted to sexual partner). Inform physician/nurse of signs/symptoms of bleeding, increased bruising, fever, infection.

ADENOSINE
(a-den'-oh-seen)
Trade Name(s): Adenocard
Classification(s): Antiarrhythmic agent
Pregnancy Category: C

PHARMACODYNAMICS/KINETICS
Mechanism of Action: Slows atrioventricular (AV) conduction and interrupts reentry pathways. **Onset of Action:** Immediate. **Duration of Action:** 0.5–1.0 min. **Distribution:** Distributes rapidly in circulation. Taken up by erythrocytes and vascular endothelial cells. Exhibits direct effect on myocardial tissue. **Metabolism/Elimination:** Primarily metabolized to inosine and adenosine monophosphate (AMP). **Half-Life:** < 10 sec.

INDICATIONS/DOSAGE

Paroxysmal Supraventricular Tachycardia (Including Accessory Bypass Tracts)
Adult: Initial dose 6 mg. Give 12 mg after 1–2 min and may repeat once if needed. Doses > 12 mg are not recommended.

CONTRAINDICATIONS/ PRECAUTIONS
Contraindicated in: Hypersensitivity, atrial flutter/fibrillation, second/ third degree AV block or sick sinus syndrome (except with functional pacemaker), ventricular tachycar-

dia. **Use cautiously in:** Asthma, first degree heart block. **Pregnancy/Lactation:** No well-controlled trials to establish safety. Benefits must outweigh risks. Adenosine is endogenous material and no fetal effects are expected. **Pediatrics:** Safety and efficacy not established.

PREPARATION
Availability: 6 mg/2 mL vial.

STABILITY/STORAGE
Vial: Do not refrigerate. Discard unused portion.

ADMINISTRATION
General: Administer directly into vein or in as proximal an IV line as possible to assure drug reaches systemic circulation. Flush line with saline following administration. **IV Push:** Rapid bolus over 1–2 sec.

COMPATIBILITY
Solution: Dextrose solutions, sodium chloride solutions.

ADVERSE EFFECTS
CNS: Dizziness, lightheadedness, burning sensation, extremity tingling, numbness, headache. **Ophtho:** Blurred vision. **CV:** <u>Bradycardia,</u> chest pain, hypotension (especially with large doses), palpitations. **Resp:** Chest pressure, hyperventilation, shortness of breath. **GI:** Metallic taste, nausea, throat tightness. **GU:** Groin pressure. **Other:** <u>Facial flushing,</u> sweating.

TOXICITY/OVERDOSE
Signs/Symptoms: Rapidly self-limiting. **Treatment:** Symptomatic treatment of prolonged effects.

DRUG INTERACTIONS
Carbamazepine: Concomitant use may increase degree of heart block.

In the Adverse Effects section, <u>underline</u> indicates most frequent; CAPS indicates life threatening.

Dipyridamole: Increased adenosine effects. **Methylxanthines** (caffeine, theophylline): Antagonizes adenosine effects. Increased doses may be necessary.

NURSING CONSIDERATIONS

Assessment
General:
Vital signs, continuous ECG monitoring
Physical:
Cardiac status.

Intervention/Rationale
Emergency equipment, pacemaker, and defibrillator must be readily available. Continuous ECG monitoring required during administration. Rapid treatment of extrasystoles and AV block may be required. During conversion, new, transient rhythms may appear (e.g., premature ventricular contraction (PVC), premature atrial contraction (PAC), sinus bradycardia/tachycardia) and resolve spontaneously in few seconds. May cause severe but transient bradycardia (ventricular response rates may be as low as 30).

Patient/Family Education
Educate regarding expected therapeutic outcome and side effects. Seek assistance with ambulatory activities.

ALBUMIN, NORMAL HUMAN SERUM
(al-byoo'-min)
Trade Name(s): Albuminar, Albutein, Buminate, Plasbumin

Classification(s): Blood derivative, volume expander
Pregnancy Category: C

PHARMACODYNAMICS/KINETICS
Mechanism of Action: Expands blood volume by increasing intravascular oncotic pressure. Causes shift of fluid from interstitial spaces into the circulation. **Onset of Action:** Within 15 min. **Duration of Action:** Several hours. **Distribution:** Distributes throughout intra/extravascular spaces. **Half-Life:** 16 hr.

INDICATIONS/DOSAGE

Shock
Adult: 500 mL (5%). May repeat in 30 min. Dose not to exceed 125 g/24 hr. *Pediatric:* 50 mL (5%). May repeat in 30 min. *Neonate:* 10–20 mL/kg (5%). May repeat in 30 min.

Burns
Adult/Pediatric: Varies according to severity of condition. Optimum regimen not established. Maintain serum albumin at 2–3 g/100 mL or total serum protein 5.2 g/100 mL. Subsequent doses determined by patient's condition. Dose not to exceed 125 g/24 hr.

Acute Hypoproteinemia
Adult: 50–75 g of 5% solution daily or 25–100 g of 25% solution daily. Subsequent doses determined by patient's condition. Dose not to exceed 125 g/24 hr. *Neonate:* 1.4–1.8 mL/kg of 25% albumin (350–450 mg/kg).

In the Adverse Effects section, underline indicates most frequent;
CAPS indicates life threatening.

7

Hyperbilirubinemia, Erythroblastosis Fetalis

Neonate: 4 mL/kg or 1 g/kg (30 g/m²) of 25% solution 1–2 hr before exchange transfusion.

Pump Prime Solution in Cardiopulmonary Bypass Procedures

Adult/Pediatric/Neonate: Dosage dependent on patient needs.

CONTRAINDICATIONS/ PRECAUTIONS

Contraindicated in: Cardiac failure, hypersensitivity, normal or increased intravascular volume, renal insufficiency, severe anemia. **Use cautiously in:** Hepatic/renal failure, lack of albumin deficiency, poor cardiac reserve, sodium restriction. **Pregnancy/Lactation:** No well-controlled trials to establish safety. Benefits must outweigh risks.

PREPARATION

Availability: 5%–50, 250, 500, and 1000 mL vials. 25%–20, 50, and 100 mL vials. Contains 130–160 mEq/L of sodium. **Infusion:** No further dilution required. Sterile water for injection may be used for dilution. Consider toxicity if dilution is substantial (i.e., < 90 mEq sodium/L).

STABILITY/STORAGE

Vial: Store at room temperature. **Infusion:** Use within 4 hr after opening vial. Contains no preservatives.

ADMINISTRATION

Intermittent/Continuous Infusion:
Shock: 5% solution should not exceed 2–4 mL/min and 25% solution should not exceed 1 mL/min. Rate for children is one quarter to one half adult rate. **Hypoproteinemia:** 5% solution should not exceed 5–10 mL/min and 25% should not exceed 2–3 mL/min.

COMPATIBILITY

Solution: Dextrose solutions, lactated Ringer's, Ringer's injection, sodium chloride solutions.

INCOMPATIBILITY

Y-site: Verapamil.

ADVERSE EFFECTS

CNS: Headache. **CV:** Cardiac failure, fluid/volume overload, hypotension, pulmonary edema. **GI:** Increased salivation, nausea. **Hypersens:** Chills, rash, urticaria. **Other:** Fever.

NURSING CONSIDERATIONS

Assessment
General:
Vital signs, baseline/daily weight, intake/output ratio, hypersensitivity reactions.
Physical:
Cardiopulmonary status.
Lab Alterations:
Monitor serum electrolytes frequently, especially in patients prone to pulmonary edema and/or congestive heart failure (due to high sodium content.) Monitor for decreased hemoglobin/hematocrit (dilutional).

Intervention/Rationale
Observe vital signs regularly. ● Monitor daily weights in patients on long-term replacement. ● Monitor for circulatory overload; assessment includes CVP, intake/output ratio, adventitious breath sounds

In the Adverse Effects section, <u>underline</u> indicates most frequent; CAPS indicates life threatening.

and presence of jugular venous distention. ● Antihistamines may be required to treat serum reactions. Consider red blood cell and plasma transfusions if received more than 250 g of albumin in 24 hr.

Patient/Family Education
Inform physician/nurse of signs/ symptoms of allergic reactions/side effects.

ALFENTANIL

(al-fen′-ta-nil)
Trade Name(s): Alfenta
Classification(s): Narcotic analgesic
Pregnancy Category: C
Controlled Substance Schedule: II

PHARMACODYNAMICS/KINETICS

Mechanism of Action: CNS depression. **Onset of Action:** Within 2 min. **Duration of Action:** 10 min (bolus); 0.5–3.0 hr (infusion). **Distribution:** 82%–95% bound to plasma proteins. **Metabolism/Elimination:** Primarily metabolized by the liver. Inactive metabolites excreted by the kidneys. **Half-Life:** 1–2 hr.

INDICATIONS/DOSAGE

Analgesic Adjunct in Anesthesia

Adult: Individualized dosage. Use ideal body weight for obese patients.
■ Incremental injection (for anesthesia < 30 min): 8–20 mcg/kg followed by 3–5 mcg/kg or 0.5–1.0 mcg/kg/min, up to a total dose of 8–40 mcg/kg.

■ Incremental injection (for anesthesia 30–60 minutes): 20–50 mcg/kg followed by 5–15 mcg/kg, up to a total dose of 75 mcg/kg.

Anesthetic Induction

Adult: For anesthesia > 45 min: 130–245 mcg/kg followed by 0.5–1.5 mcg/kg/min. Total dose depends on duration of procedure. Individualize dosage. Use ideal body weight for obese patients.

Anesthesia Adjunct: Continuous Infusion

Adult: For anesthesia > 45 min: 50–75 mcg/kg followed by 0.5–3.0 mcg/kg/min. Total dose depends on duration of procedure. Individualize dosage. Use ideal body weight for obese patients.

CONTRAINDICATIONS/ PRECAUTIONS

Contraindicated in: Acute bronchial asthma, narcotic hypersensitivity, upper airway obstruction. **Use cautiously in:** Addison's disease, cardiovascular disease, convulsive disorders, decreased respiratory reserve, elderly, gallbladder disease, recent GI/GU surgery, hypothyroidism, increased intraocular pressure, myxedema, prostatic hypertrophy, ulcerative colitis. **Pregnancy/Lactation:** No well-controlled trials to establish safety. Animal data demonstrates embryocidal effects. Crosses placenta. Benefits must outweigh risks. Distributed into breast milk. Use with caution with breastfeeding. **Pediatrics:** Not recommended for use in children < 12 yr old. Neonates with respiratory distress may develop hypotension.

In the Adverse Effects section, underline indicates most frequent; CAPS indicates life threatening.

9

PREPARATION
Availability: 500 mcg/mL in 2, 5, 10, and 20 mL ampules. **Infusion:** Dilute in compatible solution to a final concentration of 25–80 mcg/mL.

STABILITY/STORAGE
Vial: Store at room temperature. **Infusion:** Use immediately after preparation.

ADMINISTRATION
IV Push: For small doses, use tuberculin syringe or equivalent. **Infusion:** Discontinue 10–15 min prior to surgery completion.

COMPATIBILITY
Solution: Dextrose solutions, lactated Ringer's, sodium chloride solutions.

ADVERSE EFFECTS
CNS: <u>Sedation,</u> agitation, postoperative confusion, anxiety, dizziness, dysphoria, euphoria, faintness, fear, hallucination, headache, insomnia, lightheadedness, tremor. **Ophtho:** Blurred vision, miosis, visual disturbances. **CV:** CARDIAC ARREST, bradycardia, circulatory depression, dysrhythmias, hypertension, palpitations, peripheral circulatory collapse, shock, tachycardia. **Resp:** APNEA, RESPIRATORY ARREST, respiratory depression, BRONCHOSPASM, depressed cough reflex, hypercarbia, hypercapnia. **GI:** Abdominal pain, anorexia, constipation, cramping, diarrhea, dry mouth, nausea, vomiting. **GU:** Oliguria, ureteral spasm, urine retention. **Hypersens:** LARYNGOSPASM, diaphoresis, edema, pruritus, rash, urticaria. **Other:** Shivering, sweating, chills, flushing.

TOXICITY/OVERDOSE
Signs/Symptoms: Apnea, CNS depression, circulatory collapse, convulsions, miosis, respiratory depression. **Treatment:** Maintain airway and supportive measures. **Antidote(s):** Naloxone reverses respiratory and cardiovascular depression.

DRUG INTERACTIONS
Barbiturate anesthetics: Increased respiratory/CNS depression. **Chlorpromazine:** Increased analgesic/toxic effects. **Cimetidine:** Increased CNS toxicity. **Diazepam:** Cardiovascular depression. **MAO inhibitors:** Avoid administration 14 days prior to use. Severe cardiovascular and respiratory effects may occur.

NURSING CONSIDERATIONS

Assessment
General:
Vital signs prior to, during, and after administration.
Physical:
Pulmonary assessment, especially airway; neurologic status.
Lab Alterations:
Increased levels of amylase or lipase up to 24 hr after administration may occur.

Intervention/Rationale
Assure patent/protected airway, as drug is used primarily as adjunct to anesthesia. Use should be restricted to trained personnel with adequate ventilation ability.

Patient/Family Education
Change positions slowly and gradually following administration to minimize orthostatic changes.

In the Adverse Effects section, <u>underline</u> indicates most frequent; CAPS indicates life threatening.

Avoid alcohol and CNS depressants after administration.

ALPHA-1 PROTEINASE INHIBITOR

(alfa one pro′-tin-ace in-hib′-i-toor)
Trade Name(s): Prolastin
Classification(s): Alpha-1 Proteinase (alpha-1-P_1) inhibitor
Pregnancy Category: C

PHARMACODYNAMICS/KINETICS
Mechanism of Action: Replacement therapy of enzyme deficiency producing panacinar emphysema. **Distribution:** Distributes to epithelial lining of lower respiratory tract. **Metabolism/Elimination:** Catabolized in intravascular space. **Half-Life:** 4.5 days.

INDICATIONS/DOSAGE

Congenital Alpha-1 Antitrypsin Deficiency with Panacinar Emphysema
Adult: 60 mg/kg weekly to increase and maintain level of functional alpha-1-P_1.

CONTRAINDICATIONS/ PRECAUTIONS
Contraindicated in: None known. **Use cautiously in:** Patients at risk of circulatory overload. **Pregnancy/Lactation:** No well-controlled trials to establish safety. Benefits must outweigh risks. **Pediatrics:** Safety and efficacy not established.

PREPARATION
Availability: Approximately 500 mg and 1000 mg of activity per vial. **Reconstitution:** Dilute each 500 mg activity with 20 mL sterile water for injection to yield > 20 mg alpha-1-P_1/mL.

STABILITY/STORAGE
Vial: Use within 3 hr of reconstitution. Do not refrigerate.

ADMINISTRATION
General: Infuse at > 0.8 mL/kg/min (refer to specific manufacturer's instructions).

COMPATIBILITY
Solution: Sodium chloride solutions.

ADVERSE EFFECTS
CNS: Dizziness, lightheadedness. **Heme:** Mild leukocytosis (hours after infusion). **Hypersens:** Delayed (up to 12 hr) fever (resolves over 24 hr).

NURSING CONSIDERATIONS

Assessment
General:
Vital signs, observe for delayed fever
Physical:
Cardiopulmonary (signs/symptoms of circulatory overload: auscultate lung sounds, assess for jugular venous distention, peripheral edema, changes in vital signs, and weight gain). Signs and symptoms of hypersensitivity reactions.
Lab Alterations:
Monitor serum alpha-1-P_1 levels (normal 80 mg/dL)

Intervention/Rationale
Hepatitis B vaccine prophylaxis is needed prior to administration (if time does not allow, concurrent hepatitis B immune globulin is needed since this product is pre-

In the Adverse Effects section, underline indicates most frequent; CAPS indicates life threatening.

11

pared from large pools of human plasma). Risk of transmission of HIV/hepatitis B is present; however, advances in screening techniques reduce risks. ● Delayed fever may occur up to 12 hr after administration.

Patient/Family Education

Observe for fever up to 12 hr following administration. Small risk of HIV/hepatitis B transmission exists.

ALPROSTADIL

(al-pros′-ta-dill)
Trade Name(s): Prostin VR Pediatric
Classification(s): Prostaglandin E1 (PGE_1)

PHARMACODYNAMICS/KINETICS

Mechanism of Action: Produces vasodilation, platelet aggregation inhibition, and stimulation of intestinal and uterine smooth muscle. **Distribution:** Weakly bound to albumin. **Metabolism/Elimination:** Rapidly metabolized by the lungs. Metabolites excreted via kidneys within 24 hr. **Half-Life:** 5–10 minutes.

INDICATIONS/DOSAGE

Temporary Palliative Maintenance of Ductus Arteriosus Patency

Neonate: 0.05–0.1 mcg/kg/min. After therapeutic response, reduce rate to lowest dosage (0.1 to 0.05 to 0.025 to 0.01 mcg/kg/min). Doses greater than 0.1 mcg/kg/min have not been associated with increased efficacy.

CONTRAINDICATIONS/PRECAUTIONS

Contraindicated in: None known. **Use cautiously in:** Bleeding tendencies, respiratory distress syndrome.

PREPARATION

Availability: 500 mcg/mL in dehydrated alcohol (1 mL ampule). **Infusion:** Dilute 500 mcg/mL to 25–250 mL volume to yield 20–2 mcg/mL, respectively (refer to package insert for chart).

STABILITY/STORAGE

Vial: Store vial in refrigerator. **Infusion:** Stable for 24 hr after preparation.

ADMINISTRATION

General: Administer only by trained personnel in facilities that provide pediatric intensive care. Administer via large vein or umbilical artery catheter at ductal opening. **Continuous Infusion:** Infuse for the shortest time and at the lowest dose to achieve desired effect. See package insert for dilution/infusion rate chart as per manufacturer.

COMPATIBILITY

Solution: Dextrose solutions, sodium chloride solutions.

ADVERSE EFFECTS

CNS: Cerebral bleed, seizures, hyperirritability, hypothermia, lethargy. **CV:** CARDIAC ARREST, congestive heart failure, bradycardia, hypotension, second degree heart block, shock, supraventricular tachycardia, tachycardia, edema. **Resp:** APNEA, respiratory depression, respiratory distress, bradypnea, bronchial wheezing, hyper-

In the Adverse Effects section, underline indicates most frequent; CAPS indicates life threatening.

capnia. **GI:** Diarrhea, gastric regurgitation, hyperbilirubinemia, peritonitis. **Renal:** Anuria, hematuria. **MS:** Cortical proliferation of long bones, stiffness. **Endo:** Hypoglycemia **Heme:** Disseminated intravascular coagulation, thrombocytopenia, anemia, bleeding. **Other:** Sepsis, fever, flushing.

TOXICITY/OVERDOSE

Signs/Symptoms: Apnea, bradycardia, flushing, hypotension, pyrexia. **Treatment:** Discontinue infusion and begin symptomatic treatment for bradycardia/apnea. Use caution upon restarting. Reduce rate to decrease symptoms of pyrexia and bradycardia.

NURSING CONSIDERATIONS

Assessment
General:
Arterial pressure (by umbilical artery catheter, auscultation or doppler).
Physical:
Cardiopulmonary.

Intervention/Rationale
Monitor respiratory status during treatment, especially in neonates < 2 kg, and during the first hour of infusion because of potential changes in pulmonary blood flow. In infants with restricted pulmonary blood flow, measure efficacy of drug by monitoring blood oxygenation. In infants with restricted systemic blood flow, measure systemic blood pressure and blood pH. ● If cutaneous flushing occurs, reposition intra-arterial catheter. ● Decrease infusion rate immediately if significant fall in arterial pressure occurs. ● Extravasation may cause

tissue sloughing and necrosis due to high osmolality. ● Administer only by trained personnel in facilities that provide pediatric intensive care.

Patient/Family Education
Explain purpose of drug and expected therapeutic outcome to parents/family.

ALTEPLASE, RECOMBINANT

(al'-te-place)
Trade Name(s): Activase
Classification(s): Thrombolytic agent, tissue plasminogen activator
Pregnancy Category: C

PHARMACODYNAMICS/KINETICS

Mechanism of Action: Derived from recombinant DNA. Promotes thrombolysis by binding to fibrin in a thrombus. Converts entrapped plasminogen to plasmin, which initiates local fibrinolysis. **Peak Serum Level:** 30–90 min. **Duration of Action:** 4–6 hr following infusion. **Distribution:** Rapidly cleared from circulating plasma by the liver. **Metabolism/Elimination:** Primarily metabolized by the liver. Metabolites excreted by the kidneys. **Half-Life:** 30 min (inversely proportional to body weight).

INDICATIONS/DOSAGE

Thrombolytic Agent in Evolving Transmural Myocardial Infarction (MI)

Adult: Usual total dose 100 mg (58 million IU) over 3 hr. For patients

< 65 kg, 1.25 mg/kg over 3 hr. Maximum dose 150 mg.

Lysis of Acute Pulmonary Embolism

Adult: 40–100 mg over 2–7 hr as IV infusion. Alternately, 30–50 mg IV via pulmonary artery over 1.5–2.0 hr. Use with or without concomitant heparin therapy.

Reduction of Reocculsion Rate after Thrombolysis (*unlabeled use*)

Adult: 3.3 mcg/kg/min for 4 hr concomitantly with heparin (1000 units/hr) immediately after initial thrombolytic infusion.

CONTRAINDICATIONS/ PRECAUTIONS

Contraindicated in: Active internal bleeding; arteriovenous malformation; history of cerebrovascular accident; intracranial neoplasm, aneurysm, or recent intracranial or intraspinal surgery or trauma (within 2 months); known bleeding diathesis; severe uncontrolled hypertension. **Use cautiously in:** Acute pericarditis; cerebrovascular disease; concurrent oral anticoagulant administration; diabetic hemorrhagic retinopathy; geriatric patients older than 75; hemostatic defects; hypertension (systolic BP > 180 mm Hg, diastolic BP > 110 mm Hg); obstetric delivery, organ biopsy, previous puncture of noncompressible vessels; mitral stenosis with atrial fibrillation; profound left ventricular dyskinesia; recent GI or GU bleeding, major surgery, trauma (within 10 days); septic thrombophlebitis; subacute bacterial endocarditis; substantial liver dysfunction. **Pregnancy/Lactation:** No well-controlled trials to establish safety. Benefits must outweigh risks. **Pediatrics:** Safety and efficacy not established.

PREPARATION

Availability: Lyophilized powder for injection in 20 and 50 mg (11.6 and 29 million IU) per vial with diluent (20 and 50 mL sterile water for injection). **Reconstitution:** Add 20 or 50 mL sterile water for injection without preservatives to 20 or 50 mg vial, respectively. Use large-bore needle (18-gauge) and direct the stream of diluent into the lyophilized plug of powder. Resultant solution 1 mg/mL. Allow vial to remain undisturbed for several minutes if foaming occurs during reconstitution. **Infusion:** Use as is after initial reconstitution or further dilute with dextrose or sodium chloride to a concentration of no less than 0.5 mg/mL. More dilute concentrations may precipitate. Do not excessively agitate when diluting (gently swirl or slowly invert).

STABILITY/STORAGE

Vial: Store at room temperature or refrigerate. Use immediately after reconstitution. Discard unused portions. **Infusion:** Stable for 8 hr at room temperature.

ADMINISTRATION

General: Initiate therapy as soon as possible after MI, preferably within 6 hr. Potential clinical benefit diminishes as time interval to treatment increases. Administer via infusion device. **Intermittent Infusion:** *> 65 kg:* Give initial 60 mg (35.8 million IU) as lytic dose in the first hour. Rapidly infuse or bolus 6–10 mg of lytic dose over 1–2 min and give remainder as maintenance

In the Adverse Effects section, underline indicates most frequent;
CAPS indicates life threatening.

infusion of 20 mg/hr (11.6 million IU) for the next 2 hr. **< 65 kg:** Give initial 0.75 mg/kg as lytic dose in the first hour. Rapidly infuse or bolus 0.075–0.125 mg/kg of lytic dose over 1–2 min and give remainder as maintenance infusion of 0.25 mg/kg for the next 2 hr.

COMPATIBILITY
Solution: Dextrose solutions, sodium chloride solutions. **Y-site:** Lidocaine.

INCOMPATIBILITY
Solution: Bacteriostatic water for injection. **Y-site:** Dobutamine, dopamine, heparin, nitroglycerin.

ADVERSE EFFECTS
CV: Dysrhythmias (reperfusion), hypotension. **GI:** Nausea, vomiting. **Heme:** <u>Bleeding</u>—internal bleeding (GI tract, retroperitoneal, intracranial), superficial bleeding (arterial or venous puncture sites, recent surgical sites). **Hypersens:** Urticaria. **Other:** Fever.

TOXICITY/OVERDOSE
Signs/Symptoms: Extension of pharmacologic and adverse effects, primarily affecting hemostasis. **Treatment:** Discontinue therapy. Replace extensive blood loss with packed red blood cells and volume expanders other than dextran. Antifibrinolytic agents (aminocaproic acid, tranexamic acid) may be beneficial in cases of life-threatening hemorrhage (efficacy not established).

DRUG INTERACTIONS
Aspirin, dipyridamole, heparin, warfarin: Increased risk of bleeding.

NURSING CONSIDERATIONS
Assessment
General:
Continuous ECG monitoring/rhythm interpretation, blood pressure, potential bleeding sites.
Lab Alterations:
Monitor hemoglobin/hematocrit, platelet count, thrombin time, activated partial thromboplastin time, prothrombin time and fibrinogen prior to therapy and every 4 hr throughout administration of the drug.

Intervention/Rationale
Reperfusion-related atrial and/or ventricular dysrhythmias may occur during therapy. ● Hematoma formation and bleeding may occur (occurs most at vascular access sites). Avoid IM injections and nonessential handling of patient. Avoid arterial punctures unless absolutely necessary (use brachial or radial artery) and if done, apply pressure for at least 30 minutes, followed by application of pressure dressing and frequent inspection of site.

Patient/Family Education
Explain purpose of drug and expected therapeutic outcome.

AMIKACIN
(am-i-kay'-sin)
Trade Name(s): Amikin
Classification(s): Aminoglycoside antibiotic
Pregnancy Category: D

PHARMACODYNAMICS/KINETICS
Mechanism of Action: Bactericidal, blocks bacterial protein synthesis,

In the Adverse Effects section, <u>underline</u> indicates most frequent; CAPS indicates life threatening.

15

exhibits some neuromuscular blocking action. **Peak Serum Level:** Within 30 min of infusion completion. **Therapeutic Serum Levels:** Peak 8–16 mcg/mL. Trough < 5 mcg/mL. **Distribution:** Widely distributed in extracellular fluids. Lower serum concentrations result with expanded extracellular fluid volume. **Metabolism/Elimination:** Excreted unchanged via glomerular filtration in kidneys. **Half-Life:** 2–3 hr, extended in renal failure (up to 24–60 hr).

INDICATIONS/DOSAGE

Treatment of Gram Negative Organisms/Combination Therapy in Severe Immunocompromised Patients:

Dosage interval may need to be adjusted in renal impairment. Adjust dosage based on serum levels.

Adult: 15 mg/kg/day in divided doses every 8–12 hr. Not to exceed 1.5 g/day). *Pediatric:* 15 mg/kg/day in divided doses every 8–12 hr. Not to exceed 1.5 g/day. *Neonate:* 15 mg/kg/day in divided doses every 12 hr.

CONTRAINDICATIONS/ PRECAUTIONS

Contraindicated in: Known hypersensitivity. **Use cautiously in:** Neuromuscular disorders (myasthenia gravis, Parkinson's disease, infant botulism), newborns of mothers receiving high doses of magnesium sulfate, concurrent administration of neuromuscular blocking agents. **Pregnancy/Lactation:** No well-controlled trials to establish safety. Benefits must outweigh risks. Crosses placenta. **Pediatrics:** Caution in premature infants/neonates due

to renal immaturity and prolonged half-life.

PREPARATION
Availability: 50 mg/mL (in 2 mL vial), 250 mg/mL (in 2 and 4 mL vials). **Infusion:** Not to exceed 5 mg/mL. **Adults:** Further dilute in 50–200 mL of compatible IV solution. **Pediatrics:** Further dilute in compatible solution to a volume sufficient to infuse over 20–30 minutes.

STABILITY/STORAGE
Vial: Store at room temperature. **Infusion:** Stable for 30 days refrigerated, 24 hr room temperature.

ADMINISTRATION
General: Avoid rapid bolus administration. Schedule first maintenance dose at a dosing interval apart from loading dose. Administer additional dose after hemodialysis. Schedule dosing of penicillins and aminoglycosides as far apart as possible to prevent inactivation of aminoglycosides. **Intermittent Infusion:** Infuse over at least 30–60 min.

COMPATIBILITY
Solution: Dextrose solutions, lactated Ringer's, sodium chloride solutions. **Syringe:** Clindamycin. **Y-site:** Acyclovir, cyclophosphamide, enalaprilat, esmolol, foscarnet, furosemide, labetalol, magnesium sulfate, morphine, ondansetron, zidovudine.

INCOMPATIBILITY
Syringe: Heparin. **Y-site:** Hetastarch.

ADVERSE EFFECTS
CNS: Confusion, convulsions, disorientation, neuromuscular blockade, lethargy, depression, headache, numbness, nystagmus,

In the Adverse Effects section, <u>underline</u> indicates most frequent; CAPS indicates life threatening.

pseudotumor cerebri. **CV:** Hypertension, hypotension, palpitations. **Resp:** Respiratory depression, pulmonary fibrosis. **GI:** Anorexia, hepatic necrosis, hepatomegaly, increased bilirubin/lactic dehydrogenase (LDH)/serum transaminases, nausea, salivation, stomatitis, vomiting. **GU:** Casts, hematuria. **Renal:** Azotemia, increased BUN/serum creatinine, oliguria, proteinuria. **MS:** Arthralgia. **Fld/Lytes:** Hyperkalemia, hypomagnesemia. **Heme:** Agranulocytosis (transient), anemia (transient), eosinophilia, leukocytosis, leukopenia, pancytopenia, reticulocyte count alterations, thrombocytopenia. **Hypersens:** Angioneurotic edema, exfoliative dermatitis, purpura, rash, urticaria. **Other:** Fever, ototoxicity (deafness, dizziness, tinnitus, vertigo).

TOXICITY/OVERDOSE

Signs/Symptoms: Increased serum levels with associated nephrotoxicity and ototoxicity (tinnitus, high frequency hearing loss). **Treatment:** Removed by peritoneal/hemodialysis. Hemodialysis is more efficient. Exchange transfusions may be used in neonates. **Antidote(s):** Ticarcillin (12–20 g/day) may be given to promote complex formation with aminoglycosides to lower elevated serum levels.

DRUG INTERACTIONS

Amphotericin B, bacitracin, cephalothin, cisplatin, methoxyflurane, potent diuretics, vancomycin: Increased potential for nephrotoxicity, neurotoxicity, ototoxicity. **Anesthetics, anticholinesterase agents, citrate anticoagulated blood, metocurine, neuromuscular blocking agents, pancuronium, succinyl-** **choline, tubocurarine:** Increased neuromuscular blockade/respiratory paralysis. **Beta lactam antibiotics (penicillins, cephalosporins) especially ticarcillin:** Inactivation of aminoglycosides. **Cephalosporins, penicillins:** Synergism against gram negatives and enterococci.

NURSING CONSIDERATIONS

Assessment
General:
Maintain adequate hydration, superinfection.
Physical:
CN VIII evaluation, renal function.
Lab Alterations:
Measure peak/trough levels. Beta lactam antibiotic (penicillins, cephalosporins) may cause in vitro inactivation of amikacin.

Intervention/Rationale
Antibiotic use may cause overgrowth of resistant organisms; observe for fever, change in vital signs, increased WBC, vaginal infection/discharge. Draw peak serum levels 30 min after the infusion is complete and trough 30 min prior to the next dose. ● Assess BUN and serum creatinine/creatinine clearance to determine presence of renal toxicity. Adequate hydration recommended to prevent renal toxicity. ● CN VIII evaluation important to assess presence of ototoxicity.

Patient/Family Education
Increase oral fluid intake in order to minimize chemical irritation of kidneys. Notify physician/nurse if tinnitus, vertigo, or hearing loss is noted.

In the Adverse Effects section, underline indicates most frequent;
CAPS indicates life threatening.

17

AMINOCAPROIC ACID

(a-mee-noe-ka-proe'-ik)
Trade Name(s): Amicar
Classification(s): Systemic
hemostatic
Pregnancy Category: C

PHARMACODYNAMICS/KINETICS

Mechanism of Action: Inhibits fibrin-olysis via inhibition of plasminogen activator and antiplasmin activity. **Onset of Action:** 1 hr. **Peak Serum Level:** 2 hr. **Duration of Action:** < 3 hr. **Distribution:** Prolonged administration distributes to extra/intravascular compartments. **Metabolism/Elimination:** Primarily excreted unchanged by the kidneys. Removed by peritoneal and hemodialysis. **Half-Life:** 1–2 hr.

INDICATIONS/DOSAGE

Treatment of Excessive Bleeding from Systemic Hyperfibrinolysis or Urinary Fibrinolysis

Adult: 5 g initially followed by 1.0–1.25 g every hour to achieve 0.13 mg/mL plasma level. Continue for 8 hr or until bleeding controlled. Not recommended to exceed 30 g/24 hr. *Pediatric:* 100 mg/kg or 3 g/m² first hour followed by 33.3 mg/kg/hr or 1 g/m²/hr. Do not exceed 18 g/m²/hr.

Prevent Recurrence Subarachnoid Hemorrhage (*unlabeled use*)

Adult: 36 g/day in divided doses.

Amegakaryocytic Thrombocytopenia (*unlabeled use*)

Adult: 8–24 g/day in divided doses.

CONTRAINDICATIONS/PRECAUTIONS

Contraindicated in: Disseminated intravascular coagulopathy, intravascular clotting process evidence. **Use cautiously in:** Cardiac, hepatic, renal disease; hematuria of upper urinary tract origin. **Pregnancy/Lactation:** No well-controlled trials to establish safety. Animal data demonstrates teratogenicity. Benefits must outweigh risks. **Pediatrics:** Do not use in newborns due to benzyl alcohol content.

PREPARATION

Availability: 250 mg/mL, 20, 96, and 100 mL vials. Contains 0.9% benzyl alcohol. **Infusion:** Dilute 4–5 g in 250 mL for first hour, then dilute 1.0–1.25 g/hr in 50 mL.

STABILITY/STORAGE

Vial: Store at room temperature. **Infusion:** Prepare just prior to administration. Stable for 7 days refrigerated in sterile water for injection.

ADMINISTRATION

General: Undiluted rapid injection not recommended. **Intermittent/Continuous Infusion:** Infuse at 1.0–1.25 g/hr.

COMPATIBILITY

Solution: Dextrose solutions, Ringer's solutions, sodium chloride solutions, sterile water for injection.

ADVERSE EFFECTS

CNS: Cerebral ischemia, hydrocephalus, vasospasm (in subarachnoid hemorrhage); delirium; dizziness; hallucinations; headache; seizures; tinnitus; weakness. **Ophtho:** Conjunctival suffusion. **CV:** Hypotension: **GI:** Cramps, diarrhea,

---

In the Adverse Effects section, <u>underline</u> indicates most frequent; CAPS indicates life threatening.

nausea. **GU:** Transient dry ejaculate. **Renal:** Reversible acute renal failure. **MS:** Fatigue, increased creatine phosphokinase, malaise, myopathy with weakness. **Derm:** Rash. **Fld/Lytes:** Serum potassium elevation especially in renal impairment. **Other:** Nasal stuffiness, thrombophlebitis.

DRUG INTERACTIONS
Oral contraceptives/estrogens: Increased clotting factors/tendencies.

NURSING CONSIDERATIONS
Assessment
General:
Vital signs (decreases in blood pressure or rapid/irregular pulse), fever, dark urine.
Physical:
Neurological status, muscle weakness, diaphoresis.
Lab Findings:
Monitor coagulation profile (fibrinogen, fibrin degradation products, PT/PTT).

Intervention/Rationale
Monitor coagulation profile to assess for drug efficacy/dosage.

Patient/Family Education
Explain purpose of drug and therapeutic outcome.

AMINOPHYLLINE
(am-in-off´-i-lin)
Classification(s): Bronchodilator
Pregnancy Category: C

PHARMACODYNAMICS/KINETICS
Mechanism of Action: Directly relaxes smooth muscle of respiratory tract, central respiratory stimulation. **Onset of Action:** Within minutes. **Peak**

Effect: 30 minutes. **Therapeutic Serum Levels:** 10–20 mcg/mL. **Distribution:** Readily distributed throughout extracellular fluids and body tissue. Does not distribute into fatty tissue. 60% protein bound. **Metabolism/Elimination:** Metabolized by the liver. Approximately 80% excreted by the kidneys as metabolites and 15% excreted unchanged. Removed by hemodialysis. **Half-Life:** Adult non-smokers: 7–9 hr; adult smokers: 4–5 hr; children: 3–5 hr; neonates: 20–30 hr.

INDICATIONS/DOSAGE

Symptomatic Treatment of Asthma, Reversible Bronchospasm Associated with Bronchitis or Emphysema, Status Asthmaticus Refractory to Epinephrine

Adult: Dosages based on lean body weight. Smokers may need higher doses.
Loading dose: 6 mg/kg.
Maintenance infusion:
- Healthy, nonsmokers: 0.5–0.7 mg/kg/hr in first 12 hr, then 0.1–0.5 mg/kg/hr thereafter.
- Elderly/cor pulmonale: 0.6 mg/kg/hr in first 12 hr, then 0.3 mg/kg/hr thereafter.
- CHF/liver disease: 0.5 mg/kg/hr in first 12 hr, then 0.1–0.2 mg/kg/hr thereafter.

Pediatric: Dosages based on lean body weight.
Loading dose: 6 mg/kg. Not recommended for infants under 6 months.
Maintenance infusion:
- 6 mo–9 yr: 1.2 mg/kg/hr in first 12 hr, then 1.0 mg/kg/hr thereafter.
- 9–16 yr: 1.0 mg/kg/hr in first 12 hr, then 0.8 mg/kg/hr thereafter.

In the Adverse Effects section, underline indicates most frequent; CAPS indicates life threatening.

19

Neonate (unlabeled use): Dosages based on lean body weight.
Loading dose: 6 mg/kg. Not recommended for infants under 6 months.
Maintenance infusion: 0.2 mg/kg/hr.

Periodic Apnea in Cheyne-Stokes Respiration (*unlabeled use*)

Adult: 253–506 mg (aminophylline equivalent dose of theophylline).

Apnea and Bradycardia of Prematurity (*unlabeled use*)

Neonate: 1 mg/kg for each 2 mcg/mL serum theophylline level desired, to maintain serum concentrations between 3–5 mcg/mL.

Cystic Fibrosis (*unlabeled use*)

Pediatric: 12.6–15.2 mg/kg as daily maintenance dose (aminophylline equivalent dose of theophylline).

CONTRAINDICATIONS/ PRECAUTIONS

Contraindicated in: Hypersensitivity to ethylenediamine or xanthine, uncontrolled seizure disorder. **Use cautiously in:** Acute MI, CHF (may have prolonged half-life), cor pulmonale, elderly, hyperthyroidism, neonates, peptic ulcer, renal or hepatic disease, severe cardiac disease, severe hypertension, severe hypoxemia. **Pregnancy/Lactation:** No well-controlled trials to establish safety. Crosses placenta. Benefits must outweigh risks. Readily distributes into breast milk. **Pediatrics:** Use cautiously in children under the age of 6 months.

PREPARATION

Availability: 25 mg/mL, 10 and 20 mL vials, amps, and syringes. **Infusion:**

Further dilute loading dose in 25–100 mL and maintenance dose in 250–1000 mL compatible solution.

STABILITY/STORAGE

Vial: Store at room temperature. **Infusion:** Stable for 24 hr at room temperature.

ADMINISTRATION

General: Slow administration—not to exceed 25 mg/min. Administer via infusion device to monitor accuracy of dosage. **Intermittent Infusion:** Infuse over at least 15–30 min. **Continuous Infusion:** Infuse at physician specified rate.

COMPATIBILITY

Solution: Amino acids 4.25%/dextrose 25%, dextrose solutions, lactated Ringer's, Ringer's solutions, sodium chloride solutions. **Syringe:** Heparin, metoclopramide, pentobarbital, thiopental. **Y-site:** Amrinone, atracurium, cimetidine, enalaprilat, esmolol, famotidine, foscarnet, heparin, hydrocortisone, labetalol, morphine, netilmicin, pancuronium, potassium chloride, ranitidine, tolazoline, vecuronium, vitamin B complex with C.

INCOMPATIBILITY

Syringe: Doxapram. **Y-site:** Amiodarone, dobutamine, hydralazine, ondansetron.

ADVERSE EFFECTS

CNS: Seizures, dizziness, headache, insomnia, <u>irritability</u>, reflex hyperexcitability, <u>restlessness</u>, severe depression. **CV:** CIRCULATORY FAILURE, VENTRICULAR DYSRHYTHMIAS, extrasystoles, hypotension, <u>palpitations</u>, <u>sinus tachycardia</u>. **GI:** <u>Abdominal cramps</u>, <u>anorexia</u>, diarrhea, <u>epigastric pain</u>,

In the Adverse Effects section, <u>underline</u> indicates most frequent; CAPS indicates life threatening.

hematemesis, increased AST (SGOT), <u>nausea</u>, <u>vomiting</u>. **GU:** Urinary retention (in males with prostate enlargement). **Renal:** Deyhdration, diuresis, proteinuria. **Derm:** Rash. **Endo:** Hyperglycemia. **Hypersens:** Exfoliative dermatitis. **Other:** Flushing.

TOXICITY/OVERDOSE

Signs/Symptoms: Agitation, anorexia, cardiac arrest, headache, insomnia, irritability, muscle fasciculations, nausea, nervousness, tachycardias, tachypnea, ventricular dysrhythmias, vomiting. Tonic/clonic seizures may occur without other preceding symptoms. Toxicity may occur with serum levels > 20 mcg/mL. May result in death. **Treatment:** Overall treatment is supportive. Mild symptoms—drug may be continued at reduced rate of administration. Discontinue drug for more serious symptoms. Maintain adequate hydration and electrolyte balance. Seizures may be refractory to anticonvulsants. Hemodialysis or charcoal hemoperfusion may be beneficial.

DRUG INTERACTIONS

Aminoglutethimide, barbiturates, carbamazepine, charcoal, cigarettes/marijuana, hydantoins, isoniazid, ketoconazole, loop diuretics, rifampin, sulfinpyrazone, sympathomimetics: Decreased aminophylline levels. **Allopurinol, beta blockers, calcium channel blockers, carbamazepine, cimetidine, corticosteroids, disulfiram, ephedrine, influenza vaccine, interferon, isoniazid, loop diuretics, mexiletine, oral contraceptives, quinolones, ranitidine, thiabendazole, thyroid hormone:** Increased aminophylline levels. **Digitalis:** Enhanced digitalis sensitivity

and toxicity. **Halothane:** Cardiac dysrhythmias. **Ketamine:** Seizures (toxicity). **Lithium carbonate:** Increased lithium excretion and reduction of lithium effect. **Nondepolarizing muscle relaxants:** Resistance to or reversal of neuromuscular blockade. **Propofol:** Aminophylline antagonizes sedative effects.

NURSING CONSIDERATIONS

Assessment
General:
Vital signs (every 15 min for first hour), intake/output ratio, serum theophylline levels.
Physical:
Lung sounds.
Lab Alterations:
False-positive elevations of serum uric acid may occur.

Intervention/Rationale
Monitor intake/output ratios for an increase in diuresis or fluid volume overload. ● Elevated/toxic levels may cause excessive nausea, vomiting, tremors, palpitations. ● Monitor ABGs and electrolytes (when given for Cheyne-Stokes respiration).

Patient/Family Education
Notify physician/nurse if side effects develop or if condition worsens during therapy. Avoid smoking. Minimize intake of xanthine-containing foods or beverages (colas, coffee, chocolate).

AMMONIUM CHLORIDE
(ah-moe'-nee-um klo'-ride)
Classification(s): Acidifying agent, electrolyte
Pregnancy Category: B

In the Adverse Effects section, <u>underline</u> indicates most frequent; CAPS indicates life threatening.

21

PHARMACODYNAMICS/KINETICS

Mechanism of Action: Acidifying agent that causes hydrogen and chloride ion liberation resulting in decreased pH. **Distribution:** Distributes to muscle and plasma. **Metabolism/Elimination:** Metabolized in the liver, eliminated by the kidneys.

INDICATIONS/DOSAGE

Treatment of Hypochloremic States and Metabolic Alkalosis

Adult: Dose dependent on severity of alkalosis and patient tolerance. Dose calculated on basis of chloride deficit-formula: mEq of chloride ion = (chloride deficit in mEq/L × 0.2 × body weight in kg). Administer one half calculated volume and recheck pH and bicarbonate.

CONTRAINDICATIONS/PRECAUTIONS

Contraindicated in: High total carbon dioxide, primary respiratory acidosis, severe hepatic dysfunction, severe renal disease. **Use cautiously in:** CHF, pulmonary insufficiency. **Pregnancy/Lactation:** No well-controlled trials to establish safety. Benefits must outweigh risks. **Pediatrics:** Safety and efficacy not established.

PREPARATION

Availability: 26.75% (5 mEq/mL), 20 mL (100 mEq) vials, 18.7 mEq is equal to 1 g of ammonium chloride. **Infusion:** Add 100–200 mEq of ammonium chloride (20–40 mL of the 26.75% injection) to 500–1000 mL of 0.9% sodium chloride. Do not exceed final concentration of 1–2% ammonium chloride.

STABILITY/STORAGE

Vial: Store at room temperature. **Infusion:** Highly concentrated solutions may crystallize when exposed to low temperatures, warm to room temperature in water bath if crystallization occurs.

ADMINISTRATION

General: Rapid IV injection may increase the likelihood of ammonia toxicity. Administer via infusion device. **Continuous Infusion/Intermittent Infusion:** Rate not to exceed 5 mL/min.

COMPATIBILITY

Solution: Dextrose solutions, lactated Ringer's, Ringer's injection, sodium chloride solutions.

ADVERSE EFFECTS

CNS: EEG abnormalities, excitement alternating with coma, headache, hyperreflexia, mental confusion, progressive drowsiness, tetany. **CV:** Bradycardia. **Resp:** Hyperventilation. **Renal:** Glycosuria. **Derm:** Rash. **Endo:** Hyperglycemia. **Fld/Lytes:** <u>Metabolic acidosis</u>, potassium depletion. **Other:** Pain and irritation at injection site.

TOXICITY/OVERDOSE

Signs/Symptoms: Acidosis, bradycardia, cardiac dysrhythmias, coma, death, disorientation, headache, hyperventilation, hypokalemia, local and general twitching, progressive drowsiness, mental confusion, nausea, pallor, sweating, thirst, tonic convulsions, vomiting. **Treatment:** Administer sodium bicarbonate or sodium lactate. Give potassium chloride for potassium depletion.

NURSING CONSIDERATIONS

Assessment
General:
Signs/symptoms of toxicity (asterixis, bradycardia, cardiac dysrhythmias, coma, irregular breathing, generalized twitching, pallor, sweating, tonic seizures, vomiting).
Lab Alterations:
Monitor blood pH.

Intervention/Rationale
Monitor for toxic symptoms and signs of metabolic acidosis.

Patient/Family Education
Notify physician/nurse of side effects.

AMOBARBITAL
(ah-mo-bar'-bi-tal)
Trade Name(s): Amytal Sodium
Classification(s): Barbiturate, sedative/hypnotic
Pregnancy Category: D
Controlled Substance Schedule: II

PHARMACODYNAMICS/KINETICS
Mechanism of Action: CNS depressant, mechanism not completely known. **Onset of Action:** 1–5 min. **Peak Effect:** 30 min. **Duration of Action:** 3–6 hr. **Distribution:** Rapidly distributed to all fluids with high concentrations in brain and liver. Bound to tissue and plasma proteins. **Metabolism/Elimination:** Metabolized to inactive metabolites by the liver, excreted by the kidneys. **Half-Life:** 14–42 hr.

INDICATIONS/DOSAGE

Management of Acute Episodes of Agitated Behavior in Psychoses (Catatonic, Negativistic or Manic Reactions). Management of Seizures Resulting from Meningitis, Poisons, Eclampsia, Tetanus or Chorea

Adult: 65–500 mg. Maximum dose 1000 mg. Dose should be individualized to patient response. *Pediatric:* Age 6–12: 2–3 mg/kg/dose (range 65–500 mg). Maximum dose 1000 mg. Children can tolerate comparatively higher doses because of their higher metabolic rate.

CONTRAINDICATIONS/ PRECAUTIONS
Contraindicated in: Bronchopneumonia, known hypersensitivity to any barbiturate, severe pulmonary insufficiency. **Use cautiously in:** Cardiovascular disease, history of drug abuse, hypertension, hypotension, mental depression, nephritis, renal insufficiency. **Pregnancy/Lactation:** Known teratogenic effects, may cause fetal damage/abnormalities, small amounts distributed into breast milk, drowsiness in infants reported. **Pediatrics:** May produce irritability, excitability, and aggression. Hyperkinetic states may be induced/aggravated.

PREPARATION
Availability: 500 mg vials. **Reconstitution:** Use sterile water only, dilute to 100 mg/mL concentration (10% solution) by adding 5 mL diluent. Rotate but do not shake vial after adding diluent. Do not use any solution that has not become completely clear within 5 min of mixing. Use within 30 min after reconstituting.

In the Adverse Effects section, <u>underline</u> indicates most frequent; CAPS indicates life threatening.

STABILITY/STORAGE
Vial: Store at room temperature. Stable for 30 min after reconstitution.

ADMINISTRATION
IV Push:
Adults: Do not exceed rate of 100 mg/min. **Children:** Do not exceed rate of 60mg/m²/min.

COMPATIBILITY
Solution: Dextrose solutions, lactated Ringer's, sodium chloride solutions.

ADVERSE EFFECTS
CNS: **Children:** Exacerbation of existing hyperactivity, paradoxical excitement, drowsiness. **Elderly:** Confusion, depression, excitement, headache, impaired judgment/motor skills, lethargy, severe CNS depression, neuralgia, vertigo. **Ophtho:** Photosensitivity. **CV:** Hypotension, vasodilation. **Resp:** APNEA, LARYNGOSPASM, SEVERE RESPIRATORY DEPRESSION, BRONCHOSPASM, coughing. **GI:** Constipation, diarrhea, nausea, vomiting. **MS:** Arthralgia, myalgia. **Derm:** Skin eruptions, stomatitis. **Heme:** AGRANULOCYTOSIS, MEGALOBLASTIC ANEMIA, THROMBOCYTOPENIC PURPURA. **Hypersens:** Angioedema, erythema multiforme (Stevens-Johnson syndrome), rash, urticaria. **Other:** Thrombophlebitis, tissue necrosis with extravasation, high fever, pain at injection site.

TOXICITY/OVERDOSE
Signs/Symptoms: Areflexia, cardiac dysrhythmias, CNS depression (sleep to profound coma), cold/clammy skin, cyanosis, CHF, hypothermia (early), hyperthermia (late), hypotension, oliguria, respiratory depression, shock, tachycardia, urinary tract infections. **Treatment:** Mainly supportive—maintain airway, treat shock.

DRUG INTERACTIONS
Acetaminophen, beta blockers, corticosteroids, digoxin, doxycycline, estrogens, metronidazole, oral anticoagulants, oral contraceptives, quinidine, rifampin, theophylline, tricyclic antidepressants: Amobrabital decreases effects of these agents. **Antihistamines, alcohol, chloramphenicol, CNS depressants, monoamine oxidase inhibitors, tranquilizers, valproic acid:** Enhanced pharmacologic and depressant effects. **Phenytoin:** Unpredictable effect on both drugs.

NURSING CONSIDERATIONS

Assessment
General:
Vital signs, signs/symptoms of hypersensitivity, history of chemical dependency.
Physical:
Mental status (especially children/elderly), pulmonary status (respiratory depression/barbiturate toxicity—coma, pupillary constriction, cyanosis, clammy skin, hypotension).
Lab Alterations:
Monitor hematologic profile.

Intervention/Rationale
Respiratory depression can precede potentially fatal reactions requiring discontinuation. ● Prolonged use may result in physical dependency—do not withdraw abruptly. ● Assure patient safety secondary to possible mental status

In the Adverse Effects section, <u>underline</u> indicates most frequent; CAPS indicates life threatening.

changes (side rails raised, help with ambulation).

Patient/Family Education
Increased dreaming may be experienced when drug is discontinued. Avoid activities requiring mental alertness. Change positions gradually. Call for help with ambulation activities.

AMPHOTERICIN B
(am-foe-ter'-i-sin B)
Trade Name(s): Fungizone
Classification(s): Antifungal
Pregnancy Category: B

PHARMACODYNAMICS/KINETICS
Mechanism of Action: Binds to fungal cell membranes. Is not active against bacteria, rickettsiae, or viruses. **Onset of Action:** 1 hr. **Peak Serum Level:** Immediately following infusion. **Duration of Action:** 20 hr. **Distribution:** Highly protein bound, poorly dialyzable. **Metabolism/Elimination:** Metabolism unknown, excreted by the kidneys. **Half-Life:** Biphasic-initial 24–48 hr, terminal 15 days.

INDICATIONS/DOSAGE

Treatment of progressive/potentially fatal fungal infections: aspergillosis, candida, cryptococcosis, blastomycosis, coccidioidomycosis, histoplasmosis, moniliasis, mucormycosis, sporotrichosis.

Individualize dosage. Duration of therapy varies with type and severity of infection.

Adult:
Test dose: 1 mg. **Maintenance dose:** 0.25 mg/kg and gradually increase dosage by 0.125–0.25 mg/kg/day at 1–2 day intervals as tolerance permits. Total dose range up to 1 mg/kg/day or 1.5 mg/kg/day on alternate days. Do not exceed a total daily dose of 1.5 mg/kg. Cumulative dose should not exceed 1–3 g over 4–10 weeks.

Pediatric:
Test dose: 0.05–0.1 mg/kg (up to 1 mg). **Maintenance dose:** 0.25–0.5 mg/kg/day and gradually increase dosage by 0.25–0.5 mg/kg/day at 1–2 day intervals as tolerance permits. Total dose range up to 0.5–1.0 mg/kg/day or 1.5 mg/kg/day on alternate days. Do not exceed a total daily dose of 1.5 mg/kg. Cumulative dose should not exceed 15–30 mg/kg or 1.5–2.0 g over 4–10 weeks.

Intrathecal or intraventricular injection for fungal meningitis (*unlabeled use*)

Adult: Doses range from 0.05 mg initially. Increase gradually up to 0.5–1.0 mg per dose daily or every other day.

CONTRAINDICATIONS/ PRECAUTIONS
Contraindicated in: Known amphotericin B hypersensitivity or pregnancy unless life-threatening condition exists that is only amenable to amphotericin B therapy. **Use cautiously in:** Cardiac disease, renal failure. **Pregnancy/Lactation:** Fungal infections have been treated successfully without harm to fetus. No well-controlled trials to establish safety. Benefits must outweigh

In the Adverse Effects section, underline indicates most frequent; CAPS indicates life threatening.

25

risks. Distribution into breast milk unknown. Discontinue breastfeeding while receiving drug. **Pediatrics:** Safety and efficacy not established in children.

PREPARATION

Availability: 50 mg vials. **Reconstitution:** Dilute each vial with 10 mL sterile water without preservatives only (final concentration 5 mg/mL). **Infusion:** Further dilute specified dose in D$_5$W. Not to exceed a concentration of 0.1 mg/mL. **Intrathecal/Intraventricular:** Dilute 0.1 mL of 0.25 mg/mL solution with 10–20 mL sterile water for injection (no preservative).

STABILITY/STORAGE

Vial: Refrigerate intact vials. Reconstituted solution stable for 24 hr at room temperature and 1 week refrigerated. Protect reconstituted solution from light. **Infusion:** Use diluted solutions promptly. Stable for 24 hr at room temperature. Loss of drug is negligible when exposed to light for 8–24 hr; may infuse unprotected from light.

ADMINISTRATION

General: Can be administered with inline filter. Use only filter with pore size not less than 1.0 micron. Adding a small amount of heparin (1 unit/mL of solution), rotating sites, removing needle after infusion, and administering through a large central or distal vein may lessen incidence of thrombophlebitis. Extravasation may cause chemical irritation.

Continuous Infusion: Adult/Pediatric: Test dose: Infuse slowly over 20–30 minutes or 2–4 hr. Observe for at least 4 hr prior to giving first maintenance dose. Maintenance: Infuse over 2–6 hr at concentration < 0.1 mg/mL.

COMPATIBILITY

Solution: D$_5$W, D$_5$0.2 NSS. **Syringe:** Heparin. **Y-site:** Zidovudine.

INCOMPATIBILITY

Solution: Amino acids 4.25%/dextrose 25%, D$_5$ NSS, lactated Ringer's, Ringer's injection, sodium chloride solutions. **Y-site:** Foscarnet, ondansetron.

ADVERSE EFFECTS

CNS: Convulsions, headache, hearing loss, peripheral neuropathy, tinnitus, transient vertigo. **Ophtho:** Blurred vision, diplopia. **CV:** CARDIAC ARREST, VENTRICULAR FIBRILLATION, dysrhythmias, hypertension, hypotension. **Resp:** Acute dyspnea, hypoxemia, interstitial infiltrates (most common in neutropenic patients receiving leukocyte transfusions). **GI:** Acute liver failure, hemorrhagic gastroenteritis, anorexia, cramping, diarrhea, dyspepsia, epigastric pain, melena, nausea, vomiting. **Renal:** Anuria, azotemia, hyposthenuria, oliguria, nephrocalcinosis, permanent kidney damage (related to cumulative doses > 5 g), renal tubular acidosis. **MS:** Joint pain, muscle pain. **Fld/Lytes:** Hypokalemia. **Heme:** Anemia, agranulocytosis, coagulation defects, eosinophilia, leukocytosis, leukopenia. **Hypersens:** Anaphylactoid reactions, maculopapular rash, pruritus. **Other:** Fever (sometimes with shaking chills), generalized pain, malaise, thrombophlebitis/phlebitis, venous pain at injection site, weight loss, flushing.

In the Adverse Effects section, underline indicates most frequent; CAPS indicates life threatening.

TOXICITY/OVERDOSE
Signs/Symptoms: Kidney damage—BUN > 40 mg/100 mL, serum creatinine > 3 mg/100 mL. **Treatment:** Discontinue drug or reduce dosage until renal function improves.

DRUG INTERACTIONS
Aminoglycosides, cyclosporine, diuretics, nephrotoxic agents, vancomycin: Increased nephrotoxicity. **Corticosteroids:** Potential for increased hypokalemia. **Digitalis glycosides, neuromuscular blocking agents:** Amphotericin may increase effects of these drugs. **Flucytosine:** Synergism with amphotericin B.

NURSING CONSIDERATIONS
Assessment
General:
Vital signs (during test dose check vital signs every 30 minutes for 4 hr), intake/output ratio.
Lab Alterations:
Monitor weekly electrolytes, BUN, creatinine, and liver function.

Intervention/Rationale
Fever may appear 1–2 hr after the start of infusion and should subside within 4 hr of discontinuation. ● Corticosteroids may be added to decrease the incidence and severity of febrile reactions. ● Hypotension and tachycardia may occur during test dose/subsequent infusion. ● Administration on alternate days may decrease the incidence of side effects. ● Treat/prevent side effects with acetaminophen, diphenhydramine, hydroxyzine, and/or meperidine. ● Monitor renal function (80% of patients develop some degree of renal impairment). Urinary alkalinizers may minimize the incidence of renal tubular acidosis.

Patient/Family Education
Explain purpose of drug and potential therapeutic outcome.

AMPICILLIN
(am-pi-sill'-in)
Trade Name(s): Ampicin ✿ , Ampilean ✿ , Omnipen-N, Penbritin ✿ , Polycillin-N, Totacillin-N
Classification(s): Antibiotic, broad spectrum
Pregnancy Category: B

PHARMACODYNAMICS/KINETICS
Mechanism of Action: Semisynthetic penicillin, bactericidal. **Onset of Action:** Rapid. **Peak Serum Level:** 15 min. **Distribution:** Distributed into bile and CSF in high concentrations. **Metabolism/Elimination:** Partially metabolized in the liver, excreted by the kidneys. Removed by hemodialysis. **Half-Life:** 1 hr, increased in renal impairment.

INDICATIONS/DOSAGE

Treatment of infections caused by susceptible gram-negative bacteria and gram-positive bacteria
Adult: 1–12 g daily in divided doses every 6 hr. *Pediatric:* 50–200 mg/kg/day in divided doses every 6 hr. *Neonate:* Over 7 days and > 2 kg: 100 mg/kg/day in divided doses every 6 hr; for meningitis 200 mg/kg/day. Over 7 days and < 2 kg: 75 mg/kg/day in divided doses every 8 hr; for meningitis 150 mg/kg/day. Under 7 days and > 2 kg: 75 mg/kg/day in divided doses every 8 hr; for meningitis

In the Adverse Effects section, underline indicates most frequent; CAPS indicates life threatening.

27

150 mg/kg/day. Under 7 days and < 2 kg: 50 mg/kg/day in divided doses every 12 hr; for meningitis 100 mg/kg/day.

Prophylaxis of bacterial endocarditis in GI, biliary, or genitourinary surgery or instrumentation

Adult/Pediatric: (> 27 kg): 2 g 0.5–1.0 hr prior to procedure. May repeat 8 hr later. *Pediatric:* (< 27 kg): 50 mg/kg 0.5–1.0 hr prior to procedure. May repeat 8 hr later.

CONTRAINDICATIONS/ PRECAUTIONS

Contraindicated in: Hypersensitivity to penicillin or cephalosporins. **Use cautiously in:** Hepatic and renal disease. **Pregnancy/Lactation:** No well-controlled trials to establish safety. Benefits must outweigh risks. Distributed into breast milk in low concentrations. Use during breastfeeding may cause diarrhea, candidiasis, or allergic reaction in infant. **Pediatraics:** Elimination rate markedly decreased in neonates.

PREPARATION

Availability: 125 mg, 250 mg, 500 mg, 1 g, and 2 g vials, 2.9–3.1 mEq of sodium/g. **Reconstitution:** Dilute each vial of < 1 g with 5 mL and 1 or 2 g vials with 10 mL sterile water for injection or bacteriostatic water. **Infusion:** Further dilute reconstituted vial with 50 or 100 mL compatible solution.

STABILITY/STORAGE

Vial: Store at room temperature. Use within 1 hr after reconstitution. **Infusion:** Stability is concentration dependent. Stability decreased significantly in dextrose. Stable for 48 hr if final concentration < 30 mg/mL or 72 hr if < 20 mg/mL in 0.9% sodium chloride.

ADMINISTRATION

General: Rapid administration may result in seizures. If concurrently given with aminoglycosides, administer in separate infusions as far apart as possible. **IV Push:** Administer slowly over 3–5 min for doses < 500 mg and over 10–15 min for larger doses. Do not exceed 100 mg/min. **Intermittent Infusion:** Infuse over 15–30 min. Do not exceed 100 mg/min.

COMPATIBILITY

Solution: Sodium chloride solutions. **Syringe:** Chloramphenicol, heparin, procaine. **Y-site:** Acyclovir, cyclophosphamide, enalaprilat, esmolol, famotidine, foscarnet, heparin, hydromorphone, labetalol, magnesium sulfate, meperidine, morphine, perphenazine, phytonadione, potassium chloride, tolazoline, vitamin B complex with C.

INCOMPATIBILITY

Solution: Amino acids 4.25%/dextrose 25%, fat emulsion, hetastarch, lactated Ringer's. **Syringe:** Erythromycin lactobionate, gentamicin, kanamycin, metoclopromide, streptomycin. **Y-site:** Epinephrine, hydralazine, ondansetron, verapamil.

ADVERSE EFFECTS

GI: <u>Diarrhea</u>. **Derm:** <u>Rash</u> (associated with viral infections). **Heme:** Thrombocytopenia, leukopenia, anemia. **Hypersens:** ANAPHYLAXIS, exfoliative dermatitis, rash, urticaria. **Other:** Thrombophlebitis (with long-term use).

In the Adverse Effects section, <u>underline</u> indicates most frequent; CAPS indicates life threatening.

DRUG INTERACTIONS
Allopurinol: Increased skin rash. **Probenecid:** Prolongs ampicillin blood levels. **Bacteriostatic antibiotics:** Diminished "cidal" effects. **Oral Contraceptives:** Possible oral contraceptive failure.

NURSING CONSIDERATIONS
Assessment
General:
Determine history of allergic or hypersensitivity reactions to penicillins/cephalosporins. Obtain specimens for culture and sensitivity before therapy is initiated (first dose may be given while awaiting results). Signs/symptoms of infection (prior to, during, and at completion of therapy). Signs/symptoms of superinfection/bacterial/fungal overgrowth (especially in elderly, debilitated, or immunosuppressed).
Physical:
Signs/symptoms of anaphylaxis.
Lab Alterations:
Periodically evaluate renal, hepatic, and hematologic systems. False-positive reaction with copper-sulfate urine glucose tests (Clinitest).

Intervention/Rationale
Hypersensitivity reactions may be immediate and severe in penicillin-sensitive patients with a history of allergy, asthma, hay fever, or urticaria. Patients with infectious mononucleosis or lymphatic leukemia may exhibit increased incidence of rash, unrelated to hypersensitivity.

Patient/Family Education
Notify physician/nurse if skin rash, itching, hives, severe diarrhea, or signs of superinfection occurs. Drug may interfere with action of oral contraceptives (advise possible alternate birth control method during course of therapy).

AMPICILLIN-SULBACTAM
(am-pi-sill′-in sul-bak′-tam)
Trade Name(s): Unasyn
Classification(s): Antibiotic, broad spectrum
Pregnancy Category: C

PHARMACODYNAMICS/KINETICS
Mechanism of Action: Semisynthetic penicillin, bactericidal, addition of sulbactam improves ampicillin's bactericidal activity against B-lactamase-producing strains resistant to penicillins. **Onset of Action:** Rapid. **Peak Serum Level:** 15 min. **Distribution:** Distributed into bile and CSF in high concentrations. **Metabolism/Elimination:** Partially metabolized in the liver, excreted by the kidneys. Removed by hemodialysis. **Half-Life:** 1 hr, increased in renal impairment.

INDICATIONS/DOSAGE

Treatment of infections caused by susceptible gram-negative bacteria and gram-positive bacteria, specifically effective against B-lactamase producing strains
Adult: 1.5 g (1 g ampicillin plus 0.5 g sulbactam) to 3 g (2 g ampicillin plus 1 g sulbactam) every 6 hr. Do not exceed 4 g/day sulbactam.

In the Adverse Effects section, underline indicates most frequent; CAPS indicates life threatening.

29

CONTRAINDICATIONS/ PRECAUTIONS

Contraindicated in: Hypersensitivity to penicillins, cephalosporins, or sulbactam. **Use cautiously in:** Hepatic and renal disease. **Pregnancy/Lactation:** No well-controlled trials to establish safety. Benefits must outweigh risks. **Pediatrics:** Safety and efficacy not established in children < 12 yr.

PREPARATION

Availability: 1.5 g (1 g ampicillin and 0.5 g sulbactam) and 3 g (2 g ampicillin and 1 g sulbactam) vials and piggyback vials. **Reconstitution:** Dilute each 1.5 g with 3.2 mL sterile water for injection for a final concentration of 375 mg/mL. **Infusion:** Further dilute reconstituted vial in 50–100 mL compatible solution to a final concentration of 3–45 mg/mL.

STABILITY/STORAGE

Vial: Store at room temperature. Use within 1 hr after reconstitution. **Infusion:** Stability is concentration dependent. Stability decreased significantly in dextrose. Stable for 48 hr if final concentration < 45 mg/mL or 72 hr if < 30 mg/mL in 0.9% sodium chloride.

ADMINISTRATION

General: Rapid administration may result in seizures. **IV Push:** Administer slowly over 10–15 min. **Intermittent Infusion:** Infuse over 15–30 min.

COMPATIBILITY

Solution: Lactated Ringer's, sodium chloride solutions, sterile water for injection. **Syringe:** Famotidine. **Y-site:** Enalaprilat, famotidine, meperidine, morphine.

INCOMPATIBILITY

Y-site: Ondansetron.

ADVERSE EFFECTS

CV: Substernal pain. **GI:** Abdominal distention, <u>diarrhea</u>, flatulence, nausea, vomiting. **GU:** Dysuria, urinary retention. **Derm:** <u>Rash</u> (associated with viral infections). **Heme:** Thrombocytopenia, leukopenia, anemia, epistaxis, mucosal bleeding. **Hypersens:** ANAPHYLAXIS, exfoliative dermatitis, chills, erythema, facial swelling, tightness in throat, rash, urticaria. **Other:** Thrombophlebitis (with long-term use), candidiasis, fatigue, malaise.

TOXICITY/OVERDOSE

Signs and Symptoms: Neurological reactions, including convulsions. **Treatment:** Overall treatment is symptomatic. Hemodialysis may be beneficial.

DRUG INTERACTIONS

Allopurinol: Increased skin rash. **Probenecid:** Prolongs ampicillin blood levels. **Bacteriostatic antibiotics:** Diminished "cidal" effects. **Oral contraceptives:** Possible oral contraceptive failure.

NURSING CONSIDERATIONS

Assessment
General:

Determine history of allergic or hypersensitivity reactions to penicillins/cephalosporins. Obtain specimens for culture and sensitivity before therapy is initiated (first dose may be given while awaiting results). Signs/symptoms of infection (prior to, during, and at completion of therapy). Signs/symp-

In the Adverse Effects section, <u>underline</u> indicates most frequent; CAPS indicates life threatening.

toms of superinfection/bacterial/ fungal overgrowth (especially in elderly, debilitated, or immunosuppressed).

Physical:
Signs/symptoms of anaphylaxis, neurological system (convulsions in patients receiving high doses), hematologic system.

Lab Alterations:
Periodically evaluate renal, hepatic, hematologic systems. False-positive reaction with copper-sulfate urine glucose tests (Clinitest).

Intervention/Rationale
Hypersensitivity reactions may be immediate and severe in penicillin-sensitive patients with a history of allergy, asthma, hay fever, or urticaria. Patients with infectious mononucleosis or lymphatic leukemia may exhibit increased incidence of rash, unrelated to hypersensitivity. ● Patients receiving high doses may develop convulsions.

Patient/Family Education
Notify physician/nurse if skin rash, itching, hives, severe diarrhea, signs of superinfection occurs. Drug may interfere with action of oral contraceptives (advise possible alternate birth control method during course of therapy).

AMRINONE
(am'-ri-none)
Trade Name(s): Inocor
Classification(s): Inotropic agent
Pregnancy Category: C

PHARMACODYNAMICS/KINETICS
Mechanism of Action: Inotropic agent (increases cellular levels of cyclic adenosine monophosphate), vasodilator (directly relaxes vascular smooth muscle). **Onset of Action:** 2–5 min. **Peak Effect:** 10 min. **Duration of Action:** 0.5–2.0 hr. **Distribution:** 10%–49% protein bound. **Metabolism/ Elimination:** Metabolized in the liver, excreted by the kidneys. **Half-Life:** 3–4 hr, prolonged in CHF.

INDICATIONS/DOSAGE

Short-term management of CHF

(Use should be reserved for patients who have not adequately responded to digitalis, diuretics, or vasodilators).

Adult: Initial bolus 0.75 mg/kg. Maintenance infusion 5–10 mcg/ kg/min, additional bolus of 0.75 mg/kg may be given 30 minutes after initiation of therapy. Total cumulative dosage should not exceed 10 mg/kg/day.

CONTRAINDICATIONS/ PRECAUTIONS
Contraindicated in: Hypersensitivity to amrinone or bisulfites, postmyocardial infarction (acute phase), severe aortic or pulmonic valvular disease in lieu of surgical relief of obstruction. **Use cautiously in:** Hypertrophic subaortic stenosis. **Pregnancy/Lactation:** No well-controlled trials to establish safety. Benefits must outweigh risks. **Pediatrics:** Safety and efficacy not established in children under 18 yr.

PREPARATION
Availability: 5 mg/mL in 20 mL amps.
Infusion: Dilute in 0.9% or

In the Adverse Effects section, underline indicates most frequent;
CAPS indicates life threatening.

31

0.45% NS to a concentration of 1–3 mg/mL.

STABILITY/STORAGE
Vial: Store at room temperature, protect from light. Solution is clear yellow. **Infusion:** Stable for 24 hr at room temperature. Protection from light not required.

ADMINISTRATION
General: Adjust rate of administration and duration of therapy according to patient response. **IV Push:** Give bolus slowly over 2–3 min. **Continuous Infusion:** Infuse at 5–10 mcg/kg/min via infusion device.

COMPATIBILITY
Solution: Sodium chloride solutions. **Y-site:** Aminophylline, atropine, bretylium, calcium chloride, cimetidine, dextrose (may inject into Y-site or into tubing), dobutamine, dopamine, epinephrine, famotidine, hydrocortisone, isoproterenol, lidocaine, metaraminol, methylprednisolone, nitroglycerin, nitroprusside, norepinephrine, phenylephrine, potassium chloride, procainamide, verapamil.

INCOMPATIBILITY
Solution: Dextrose solutions. **Y-site:** Furosemide, sodium bicarbonate.

ADVERSE EFFECTS
CV: <u>DYSRHYTHMIAS</u>, <u>hypotension</u>, chest pain. **GI:** Abdominal pain, anorexia, hepatotoxicity, <u>nasuea</u>, <u>vomiting</u>. **Heme:** <u>Thrombocytopenia</u> (dose dependent). **Other:** Burning at injection site.

TOXICITY/OVERDOSE
Signs/Symptoms: Severe hypotension. **Treatment:** Decrease dose or discontinue infusion. Overall treatment is supportive.

DRUG INTERACTIONS
Cardiac glycosides (digoxin): Additive inotropic effects. **Disopyramide:** Excess hypotension.

NURSING CONSIDERATIONS
Assessment
General:
Vital signs, ECG.
Physical:
Cardiovascular parameters (pulmonary artery pressures, systemic vascular resistance, cardiac output, blood pressure, heart rate, urine output).
Lab Alterations:
Monitor electrolytes and platelet count.

Intervention/Rationale
Adjust dose according to clinical response. Slow or stop infusion and call physician for significant hypotension. ● Patients who have been vigorously diuresed may require additional fluid and electrolyte replacement. ● Decrease dosage for platelet count below 150,000 mm^3.

Patient/Family Education
Explain rationale of therapy. Change positions slowly to prevent postural hypotension.

ANISTREPLASE
(a-ni-strep'-lace)
Trade Name(s): Eminase
Classification(s): Thrombolytic enzyme
Pregnancy Category: C

In the Adverse Effects section, <u>underline</u> indicates most frequent; CAPS indicates life threatening.

PHARMACODYNAMICS/KINETICS
Mechanism of Action: In solution, a complex is formed that converts plasminogen to plasmin in the bloodstream or within the thrombus. **Onset of Action:** Immediate. **Duration of Action:** 4–6 hr. **Metabolism/Elimination:** Unknown, possible proteolytic enzyme activity in serum degrades drug. **Half-Life:** 2 hr, fibrinolytic activity 70–120 min.

INDICATIONS/DOSAGE

Acute MI/lysis of coronary artery thrombi

Adult: 30 units within 6 hr of onset of symptoms.

CONTRAINDICATIONS/PRECAUTIONS
Contraindicated in: Active internal bleeding, arteriorvenous malformation, bleeding diathesis, history of CVA, recent (within 2 months) intracranial/intraspinal trauma/surgery, intracranial neoplasm, severe allergic reaction to anistreplase or streptokinase, uncontrolled hypertension. **Use cautiously in:** Acute pericarditis, cerebrovascular disease, elderly > 75 yr old, hemorrhagic ophthalmic conditions, hemostatic defects, hypertension (systolic BP > 180, diastolic BP > 110), oral anticoagulation, pregnancy, recent GI/GU bleed, recent major surgery, recent trauma/CPR, subacute bacterial endocarditis. **Pregnancy/Lactation:** No well-controlled trials to establish safety. Benefits must outweigh risks. **Pediatrics:** Safety, efficacy not established.

PREPARATION
Availability: 30 units/vial. **Reconstitution:** Dilute vial with 5 mL sterile water for injection. Direct diluent against side of vial. Gently roll vial, do not shake. **Syringe:** Withdraw entire contents of vial. Do not further dilute. No other medications should be added to vial/syringe.

STABILITY/STORAGE
Vial: Store vial in refrigerator. Discard 30 min after reconstitution if not administered.

ADMINISTRATION
IV Push: Administer over 2–5 min into an IV line or vein.

COMPATIBILITY/INCOMPATIBILITY
Data not available.

ADVERSE EFFECTS
CNS: Intracranial hemorrhage, dizziness, headache, paresthesia, tremor, vertigo. **CV:** CARDIAC RUPTURE, <u>dysrhythmias</u>, <u>hypotension</u>, shock, chest pain, conduction disorders. **Resp:** Dyspnea, lung edema. **GI:** Elevated transaminases, nausea, vomiting. **GU:** Hematuria. **MS:** Arthralgia. **Derm:** Purpura. **Heme:** <u>Bleeding</u>, decreased plasminogen and fibrinogen; increased thrombin time, APTT, PT; thrombocytopenia. **Hypersens:** ANAPHYLAXIS, eosinophilia, rash, urticaria. **Other:** Chills, fever, flushing, sweating.

DRUG INTERACTIONS
Antiplatelet agents, aspirin, dipyridamole, heparin, warfarin: Increased bleeding complications.

In the Adverse Effects section, <u>underline</u> indicates most frequent; CAPS indicates life threatening.

33

NURSING CONSIDERATIONS

Assessment

General:
Vital signs, ECG.

Physical:
Potential bleeding sites.

Lab Alterations:
Monitor hemoglobin/hematocrit, platelet count, thrombin time, activated partial thromboplastin time, prothrombin time, and fibrinogen prior to therapy and every 4 hr throughout administration of the drug.

Intervention/Rationale

Monitor all potential bleeding sites for hematoma formation and bleeding (bleeding occurs most at vascular access sites). Avoid IM injections and nonessential handling of patient. Avoid arterial punctures unless absolutely necessary (use brachial or radial artery) and if done, apply pressure for at least 30 min, followed by application of pressure dressing and frequent inspection of site. ● Monitor ECG during therapy for reperfusion-related atrial and/or ventricular dysrhythmias. ● If between 5 days to 6 months after previous anistreplase or streptokinase administration or presence of streptococcal infection, there is an increased likelihood of resistance/hypersensitivity reactions to drug.

Patient/Family Education

Inform of reason for therapy and possible side effects. Use soft toothbrush for oral care.

ANTIHEMOPHILIC FACTOR (FACTOR VIII)

(an'-ti-heem-o-fil'-ik fak'-tor)

Trade Name(s): Hemofil M, Kryobulin VH ♣ , Koate, Monoclate.

Classification(s): Antihemophilic factor (AHF)

Pregnancy Category: C

PHARMACODYNAMICS/KINETICS

Mechanism of Action: Replacement of antihemophlic factor necessary for clot formation. **Onset of Action:** Instantaneous rise in coagulant level. **Duration of Action:** Rapid decrease in activity. **Distribution:** Intravascular and extravascular distribution. **Metabolism/Elimination:** Rapidly cleared from plasma. **Half-Life:** 9–15 hr

INDICATIONS/DOSAGE

Management of Factor VIII deficiency associated with Hemophilia A

Adult/Pediatric: Dose is individualized depending on patient's weight, severity of Factor VIII deficiency, severity of hemorrhage, presence of inhibitors, and Factor VIII level desired.

Treatment of joint hemorrhages: 8 units/kg just prior to aspiration of joint. May repeat at 8 hr intervals as necessary. If not aspirated 8–10 units/kg at 8–12 hr intervals or 5–8 units/kg as a single dose. *Treatment of minor extremity or trunk hemorrhages:* 8–10 units/kg every 24 hr for 2–3 days. *Treatment of serious hemorrhages in nonvital area muscles:* 8 units/kg every 12 hr for 2 days, then once daily for 2 more days.

Treatment of hemorrhages in muscles near vital organs: 15 units/kg followed by 8 units/kg every 8 hr for 48 hr, then 4 units/kg every 8 hr for > 2 days. **Treatment of overt bleeding:** 15–25 units/kg followed by 8–15 units/kg every 8–12 hr for 3–4 days. **Treatment of bleeding from massive wounds or vital regions:** 40–50 units/kg followed by 20–25 units/kg every 8–12 hr. **During major surgery:** 26–30 units/kg prior to surgery followed by 15 units/kg every 8 hr after surgery. **Prophylaxis with severe Factor VIII deficiency:** < 50 kg: 250 units daily every 1–2 days. > 50 kg: 500 units daily every 1–2 days.

CONTRAINDICATIONS/ PRECAUTIONS

Contraindicated in: Hypersensitivity to mouse protein (monoclonal antibody derived Factor VIII—Hemofil M, Monoclate). **Pregnancy/Lactation:** No well-controlled trials to establish safety. Benefits must outweigh risks.

PREPARATION

Availability: Actual number of AHF units indicated on vials with diluent. **Reconstitution:** Warm vial and diluent to room temperature and gently agitate. Use diluent provided. May take 5–10 min for complete dissolution. Drug must be completely dissolved before administration. **Infusion:** Add contents of reconstituted vial to empty sterile IV bag or buretrol device.

STABILITY/STORAGE

Vial: Refrigerate lyophilized powder, do not freeze. Reconstituted solution stable for 24 hr. Administer within 3 hr after reconstitution. Do not refrigerate reconstituted solution. **Infusion:** Use within 3 hr of reconstitution. Store at room temperature only.

ADMINISTRATION

General: Administer slowly via infusion device. Must be filtered prior to administration. Use single donor products in patients with mild hemophilia and those who have not received multiple blood product transfusions. **IV Push/Intermittent Infusion:** 2–4 mL/min. Do not exceed 10 mL/min.

COMPATIBILITY/INCOMPATIBILITY

Data not available.

ADVERSE EFFECTS

CNS: Headache, lethargy, loss of consciousness, paresthesias, somnolence. **Ophtho:** Visual disturbances. **CV:** Chest tightness, hypotension, tachycardia. **GI:** Nausea, vomiting. **MS:** Back pain. **Hypersens:** ANAPHYLAXIS, hypotension, fever, hives, mild chills, urticaria, wheezing. **Other:** Stinging at injection site, flushing.

NURSING CONSIDERATIONS

Assessment
General:
Heart rate.
Physical:
Signs/symptoms of hypersensitivity reactions.
Lab Alterations:
Monitor AHF levels.

Intervention/Rationale
Reduce flow rate or discontinue and notify physician if pulse rate significantly increases. ● Assess AHF levels to assure adequate levels are reached and maintained. If the AHF level fails to reach ex-

In the Adverse Effects section, underline indicates most frequent; CAPS indicates life threatening.

35

pected levels or bleeding is uncontrolled, inhibitors may be present (anti-inhibitors or additional AHF doses may be necessary).

Patient/Family Education
Observe for early signs of allergic reactions: hives, chest tightness, wheezing, difficulty breathing. Risk of transmission of HIV/hepatitis B is present (however, advances in screening techniques reduce risk). Notify nurse/physician if bleeding occurs from gums, stools, skin, or urine.

ANTI-INHIBITOR COAGULANT COMPLEX

(an'-ti-in-hib-i'-toor)
Trade Name(s): Autoplex T, Feiba VH Immuno
Classification(s): Antihemophilic Factor (AHF)
Pregnancy Category: C

PHARMACODYNAMICS/KINETICS
Mechanism of Action: Complexes with Factor VIII inhibitors.

INDICATIONS/DOSAGE

Patients with Factor VIII inhibitors who are bleeding or undergoing surgery
Adult/Pediatric: 25–100 Factor VIII correctional units/kg, depending on the severity of hemorrhage. Dose can be repeated if no hemostatic improvement is observed within 6 hr. Adjust subsequent doses and administration according to patient's clinical response. Maximum dose 200 units/kg/day.

CONTRAINDICATIONS/ PRECAUTIONS
Contraindicated in: Disseminated intravascular coagulation, fibrinolysis, patients with a normal coagulation mechanism. **Use cautiously in:** Impaired liver function. **Pregnancy/ Lactation:** No well-controlled trials to establish safety. Benefits must outweigh risks. **Pediatrics:** No data available on use in neonates.

PREPARATION
Availability: Actual number of AHF units indicated on vials with diluent. **Reconstitution:** Reconstitute with diluent provided. Do not refrigerate after reconstitution. **Infusion:** Add contents of reconstituted vial to empty sterile IV bag or buretrol device.

STABILITY/STORAGE
Vial: Refrigerate unreconstituted complex, avoid freezing, do not refrigerate after reconstitution.

ADMINISTRATION
General: Too rapid administration may cause headache, flushing, changes in pulse rate and blood pressure. **Infusion:** Complete administration within 1 hr (Autoplex) or 3 hr (Feiba) at rate up to 10 mL/min via infusion device unless headache, flushing, or changes in pulse rate and blood pressure appear. Stop infusion until symptoms disappear and reinitiate at 2 mL/min.

COMPATIBILITY/INCOMPATIBILITY
Data not available.

ADVERSE EFFECTS
CV: Hypotension, tachycardia. **Hypersens:** ANAPHYLACTOID REACTIONS (SEVERE), urticarial rash. **Other:** Chills, fever.

In the Adverse Effects section, <u>underline</u> indicates most frequent; CAPS indicates life threatening.

TOXICITY/OVERDOSE

Signs/Symptoms: Laboratory and clinical signs of disseminated intravascular coagulation (DIC) with high doses. **Treatment:** Monitor carefully, reduce dose, or discontinue.

NURSING CONSIDERATIONS

Assessment

Physical:
Signs/symptoms of hypersensitivity reactions, infectious disease status.
Lab Alterations:
Monitor fibrinogen levels (children).

Intervention/Rationale

Discontinue use and notify physician if hypersensitivity reactions occur. ● Individuals who have received multiple infusions of blood or plasma products are very likely to develop signs and symptoms of viral infections (non A, non B hepatitis).

Patient/Family Education

Inform of reason for administration and of potential side effects. Observe for early signs of allergic reactions (difficulty breathing, chills, chest tightness, hives, wheezing). Risk of transmission of HIV/hepatitis B is present (however, advances in screening techniques reduce risk).

ANTITHROMBIN III

(an-ti-throm′-bin)
Trade Name(s): ATnativ
Classification(s): Antithrombin
Pregnancy Category: C

PHARMACODYNAMICS/KINETICS

Mechanism of Action: Coagulation inhibitor, inactivates thrombin and the activated forms of IX, X, XI, XII. **Peak Serum Level:** 15–30 min (maximal increase in AT-III). **Duration of Action:** 50–70 hr. **Therapeutic Serum Levels:** Normal AT-III level 20–40 mg/dL or 1 unit/mL. **Metabolism/ Elimination:** Small amounts recovered unchanged in urine. **Half-Life:** 3 days.

INDICATIONS/DOSAGE

Treatment of hereditary antithrombin III (AT-III) deficiency in connection with surgical/obstetrical procedures or thromboembolism

Adult/Pediatric: Dose is individualized depending on patient's weight, degree of deficiency, and AT-III level desired. 1 unit/kg to raise AT-III level by 1%–2%. Subsequent doses should be modified based on the AT-III level achieved. Schedule dose once every 24 hr.

CONTRAINDICATIONS/ PRECAUTIONS

Contraindicated in: None known. **Use cautiously in:** Anticoagulated patients. **Pregnancy/Lactation:** No well-controlled trial to establish safety. Benefits must outweigh risks. Administration during third trimester has not shown adverse fetal effects. **Pediatrics:** Efficacy and safety not established.

PREPARATION

Availability: 500 IU/vial. 1 IU/1 mL of normal pooled human plasma (before reconstitution). **Reconstitution:** Add 10 mL sterile water for injection for a final concentration of

In the Adverse Effects section, underline indicates most frequent;
CAPS indicates life threatening.

37

50 IU/mL. Warm vial and diluent to room temperature and gently agitate. Do not shake. **Infusion:** May be further diluted with compatible IV solution.

STABILITY/STORAGE

Vial: Refrigerate. **Infusion:** Use within 3 hr of reconstitution. Store at room temperature.

ADMINISTRATION

Intermittent Infusion: May be infused over 5–10 min. Infuse at a rate of 50 IU/min. Not to exceed 100 IU/min.

COMPATIBILITY

Solution: Dextrose solutions, sodium chloride solutions, sterile water for injection.

ADVERSE EFFECTS

CV: Chest tightness. **Resp:** Shortness of breath. **GI:** Abdominal cramps, foul taste. **Heme:** Thrombocytopenia. **Other:** Drug fever.

DRUG INTERACTIONS

Heparin: Enhanced anticoagulation (reduce heparin dose).

NURSING CONSIDERATIONS

Assessment
General:
Vital signs.
Lab Alterations:
Monitor AT-III levels, assess baseline coagulation profile.

Intervention/Rationale
Monitor AT-III levels to assure desired levels are achieved (AT-III level should increase to 120% of normal after first dose, then maintain at > 80% above normal). Measure AT-III level at least twice daily

until stabilized, then once daily and always prior to next infusion.

Patient/Family Education
Inform of reason for administration and potential side effects. Drug is pooled from human serum and risk of transmission of HIV/hepatitis B is present (however, advances in screening techniques reduce risk).

ARGININE

(ar-ja′-neen)
Trade Name(s): R-GENE 10
Classification(s): Amino acid
Pregnancy Category: Unknown

PHARMACODYNAMICS/KINETICS

Mechanism of Action: Stimulates pituitary release of growth hormone and prolactin, as well as pancreatic release of glucagon and insulin. **Peak Effect:** 30 min to 1 hr. **Metabolism/Elimination:** Metabolized in the liver, eliminated by the kidneys via glomerular filtration.

INDICATIONS/DOSAGE

Pituitary stimulant for release of human growth hormone for diagnostic purposes

(Panhypopituitarism, pituitary dwarfism, adenoma, acromegaly, gigantism, growth problems.)

Adult: 300 mL as a single dose. *Pediatric:* 5 mL/kg.

Management of extreme metabolic alkalosis (*unlabeled use*)

Adult: Calculate dose by formula as follows: Dosage (grams) equals desired plasma bicarbonate de-

In the Adverse Effects section, underline indicates most frequent; CAPS indicates life threatening.

crease (mEq/L) multiplied by weight (kg) and divided by 9.6.

CONTRAINDICATIONS/ PRECAUTIONS
Contraindicated in: Hypersensitivity, severe electrolyte imbalance. **Use cautiously in:** Renal disease/anuria (hyperkalemia). **Pregnancy/Lactation:** No well-controlled trials to establish safety. Benefits must outweigh risks. Low concentrations of drug have been detected in the fetus.

PREPARATION
Availability: 10% solution (100 mg/mL), 500 mL bottles. 47.5 mEq chloride/100 mL.

STABILITY/STORAGE
Vial: Store at room temperature.

ADMINISTRATION
General: An interval of 24 hr is recommended prior to second administration. Confirm absolute patency of the vein, as infiltration can cause tissue necrosis. **Intermittent Infusion:** Distribute dose evenly over 30 minutes. Infuse within the 30 minute time period in order to ensure reliable test results.

COMPATIBILITY/INCOMPATIBILITY
Data not available.

ADVERSE EFFECTS
CNS: Headache, numbness. **CV:** Increased pulse rate, sweating. **Resp:** Choking, nasal discharge, nasal obstruction. **GI:** Nausea, vomiting. **Fld/Lytes:** Bicarbonate deficit, hyperkalemia. **Hypersens:** Macular rash. **Other:** Flushing, <u>local venous irritation</u>, tissue necrosis at infiltration site.

TOXICITY/OVERDOSE
Signs/Symptoms: Flushing, headache, local venous irritation. **Treatment:** Slow infusion rate to decrease side effects.

NURSING CONSIDERATIONS
Assessment
Physical:
Signs/symptoms of hypersensitivity (with particular emphasis on skin appearance to evaluate rash development).
Lab Alterations:
Monitor electrolytes prior to and following therapy.

Intervention/Rationale
Blood samples should be taken from arm opposite infusion site 30 minutes prior to and immediately before initiating infusion and at 30 min intervals for 2.5 hr after infusion completion.

Patient/Family Education
Growth hormone concentrations fluctuate spontaneously as a response to stress/exercise. Minimize apprehension and distress before and during testing procedures to avoid invalidation of test results. Frequent blood samples will be taken by venipuncture. Inform nurse/physician if pain or discomfort develops at site of infusion.

ASCORBIC ACID
Trade Name(s): Cenolate, Cevalin, Redoxon ♣
Classification(s): Water soluble vitamin
Pregnancy Category: C

In the Adverse Effects section, <u>underline</u> indicates most frequent; CAPS indicates life threatening.

PHARMACODYNAMICS/KINETICS

Mechanism of Action: Important in biological oxidations/reductions. Necessary for metabolic function, including cellular respiration. **Distribution:** Widely distributed in body tissues. 25% bound to plasma proteins. **Metabolism/Elimination:** Partially metabolized to inactive compounds that are eliminated by the kidneys. Removed by hemodialysis.

INDICATIONS/DOSAGE

Dietary supplementation, urinary acidifying agent, scurvy treatment.

Adult: 200 mg–2 g every 24 hr. May give up to 6 g every 24 hr. *Pediatric:* 100–300 mg/24 hr. *Neonate:* 75–100 mg/24 hr for premature infants.

CONTRAINDICATIONS/ PRECAUTIONS

Contraindicated in: Hypersensitivity. **Use cautiously in:** (avoid excess doses for prolonged periods) Diabetic patients; patients prone to recurrent renal calculi; glucose-6-phosphate dehydrogenase deficiency; patients undergoing stool occult blood tests; patients on sodium restricted diets; patients on anticoagulant therapy. **Pregnancy/Lactation:** No well-controlled trials to establish safety. Benefits must outweigh risks. Crosses placenta, distributed in breast milk.

PREPARATION

Availability: 100, 250, 500 mg ampules. 1 g sodium ascorbate contains 5 mEq sodium. **Infusion:** Dilute in compatible IV solution in physician specified volume.

STABILITY/STORAGE

Vial: Refrigeration is recommended. Gradually darkens with light exposure. Slight coloration does not interfere with therapeutic activity. Increased pressure may develop after prolonged storage at room temperature. **Infusion:** Stable for 24 hr refrigerated. Light protection not required.

ADMINISTRATION

General: Must be infused slowly. Rapid injection causes temporary dizziness. **IV Push:** Give 100 mg slowly over 1 min. **Intermittent/Continuous Infusion:** Infuse at physician specified rate.

COMPATIBILITY

Solution: Dextrose solutions, lactated Ringer's, Ringer's injection, sodium chloride solutions. **Syringe:** Metoclopramide.

INCOMPATIBILITY

Syringe: Cefazolin, doxapram.

ADVERSE EFFECTS

CNS: Dizziness, faintness, headache, insomnia, sleepiness. **CV:** Deep vein thrombosis. **GI:** Abdominal cramps, diarrhea, heartburn, nausea, vomiting. **GU:** Acidification of urine, precipitation of urate stones. **Other:** Flushing.

TOXICITY/OVERDOSE

Signs/Symptoms: Temporary dizziness, flushing, faintness. Diarrhea, renal calculi may occur with large doses of the drug. **Treatment:** Discontinue administration temporarily. Resume drug at a decreased rate. If signs and symptoms persist, notify physician and discontinue drug.

40

In the Adverse Effects section, underline indicates most frequent; CAPS indicates life threatening.

DRUG INTERACTIONS
Estrogens: Increased serum level of estrogens. **Iron:** Concurrent use increases iron absorption. **Salicylates:** Increased urinary excretion of ascorbic and decreased salicylate excretion. **Warfarin:** Decreased anticoagulant effect.

NURSING CONSIDERATIONS
Assessment
General:
Overall nutritional status.
Physical:
Observe for improvement in presenting symptoms, GI tract.
Lab Alterations:
False-negative urine glucose (with doses > 500 mg). False-negative stool for occult blood (if drug given within 48–72 hr).

Intervention/Rationale
Mild vitamin C deficiency symptoms may include faulty bone and tooth development, gingivitis, loosened teeth. ● May develop various gastrointestinal symptoms, including diarrhea and abdominal cramps. ● Assess calorie intake if necessary. ● Dietary consult.

Patient/Family Education
Increased Vitamin C requirements may be associated with pregnancy, lactation, hyperthyroidism, fever, stress, infection, trauma, burns, smoking, and cold exposure, as well as the use of certain drugs (i.e., estrogens, oral contraceptives, tetracyclines, salicylates).

ASPARAGINASE
(a-spare'-a-gin-ase)
Trade Name(s): Elspar, Kidrolase♣
Classification(s): Antineoplastic agent
Pregnancy Category: C

PHARMACODYNAMICS/KINETICS
Mechanism of Action: Catalyzes the conversion of the amino acid asparagine to aspartic acid and ammonia. Results in leukemic cell inability to synthesize asparagine for DNA synthesis. **Duration of Action:** Measurable plasma concentrations persist for up to 22 days. **Distribution:** Remains within intravascular space because of high molecular weight and poor capillary diffusion. **Metabolism/Elimination:** Metabolic fate unknown. Trace amounts appear in urine, minimal urinary and biliary excretion. **Half-Life:** 8–30 hr.

INDICATIONS/DOSAGE

Multiple agent induction regimen for acute lymphocytic leukemia in children
Pediatric: 1000 IU/kg/day for 10 successive days beginning on day 22. Dosage must be individualized based on the clinical response and tolerance of the patient in order to obtain optimum therapeutic results with minimum adverse effects.

Single agent induction therapy in acute lymphocytic leukemia
Adult/Pediatric: 200 IU/kg/day for 28 days.

In the Adverse Effects section, <u>underline</u> indicates most frequent; CAPS indicates life threatening.

CONTRAINDICATIONS/PRECAUTIONS

Contraindicated in: Hypersensitivity, pancreatitis or history of pancreatitis. **Use cautiously in:** Preexisting liver impairment. **Pregnancy/Lactation:** No well-controlled trials to establish safety. Benefits must outweigh risks. Laboratory animal studies show weight retardation of mothers and fetuses and has resulted in dose dependent embryotoxicity. Significant mutagenic potential.

PREPARATION

Availability: 10,000 IU/10 mL vial with 80 mg mannitol. **Reconstitution:** Reconstitute with 5 mL sterile water or sodium chloride to a final concentration of 2000 IU/mL. **Infusion:** Dilute reconstituted drug with compatible IV solution to physician specified volume.

STABILITY/STORAGE

Vial: Refrigerate vial before and after dilution. Stable for 48 hr at room temperature. Reconstituted vial stable for 8 hr refrigerated. **Infusion:** Stable for 8 hr refrigerated.

ADMINISTRATION

General: Handle drug with care and avoid inhalation and contact to skin, especially eyes. Adhere to institutional guidelines for handling of chemotherapeutic/cytotoxic agents. Filtration with a 5-micron filter is recommended. **Skin Test:** Required before initial dose of drug and whenever a 7 day lapse between doses occurs. Withdraw 0.1 mL from reconstituted solution (2000 IU/mL) and further dilute with 9.9 mL sodium chloride. Test dose of 0.1 mL of this 20 IU/mL solution is equivalent to a total of 2 IU and should be given intradermally. Observe patient closely for 1 hr for the appearance of a wheal or erythema. The risk of anaphylaxis is increased after repeated courses of therapy. Allergic reactions may occur even after initial administration, including direct skin testing. **Intermittent Infusion:** Administer infusion over not less than 30 minutes through the Y-site of an already infusing IV of compatible solution.

COMPATIBILITY

Solution: Dextrose solutions, sodium chloride solutions.

ADVERSE EFFECTS

CNS: EEG changes, depression, fatigue, lethargy, somnolence. **CV:** Hypotension. **GI:** Abdominal cramps, anorexia, nausea, vomiting, weight loss. **GU:** Uric acid nephropathy. **Renal:** Acute renal shutdown, azotemia, renal insufficiency. **Endo:** ACUTE HEMORRHAGIC PANCREATITIS, hepatotoxicity, pancreatitis. **Fld/Lytes:** Hyperglycemia, elevated uric acid. **Heme:** Bone marrow depression; decreased factor V, VIII; variable decrease in factor VII, IX; leukopenia; prolonged thrombin, prothrombin, and partial thromboplastin times. **Hypersens:** ANAPHYLAXIS, arthralgia, facial edema, rashes, respiratory distress, urticaria. **Other:** Hypothermia.

TOXICITY/OVERDOSE

Signs/Symptoms: Extension of adverse effects. **Treatment:** Symptomatic and supportive.

DRUG INTERACTIONS

Prednisone, vincristine: Administration of asparaginase before or con-

In the Adverse Effects section, underline indicates most frequent; CAPS indicates life threatening.

currently results in increased toxicity. **Methotrexate:** Decreased methotrexate cytotoxic effects.

NURSING CONSIDERATIONS

Assessment
General:
Signs/symptoms of hyperglycemia and hypersensitivity reactions, intake/output ratio, daily weights.
Physical:
Infectious disease status, GI tract, hematopoietic system.
Lab Alterations:
Monitor CBC with differential. May cause marked reduction in serum level of thyroxine binding globulin index.

Intervention/Rationale
Monitor blood and urine glucose before and during therapy. ● Severe hypersensitivity reactions, including respiratory distress and acute anaphylaxis have occurred, either as a first time dose or as part of repeat course of therapy. ● Assess daily for development of systemic infections (temperature, WBC). ● Hematest stools or vomitus for presence of occult blood.

Patient/Family Education
Observe closely for signs of infection (fever, sore throat, fatigue), evidence of bleeding (gums, nose bleeds, melena, easy bruising). Take and record oral temperatures daily and notify physician of hypothermia/hyperthermia. Notify physician immediately if fever or chills develop. Use consistent and reliable contraception throughout the duration of therapy due to potential teratogenic and mutagenic effects of drug.

ATENOLOL
(a-ten´-a-lol)
Trade Name(s): Tenormin
Classification(s): Beta-blocker
Pregnancy Category: C

PHARMACODYNAMICS/KINETICS
Mechanism of Action: Competitive beta-adrenergic blockade, primarily at beta-1 receptors at therapeutic doses. **Distribution:** Low lipid solubility with low blood–brain barrier penetration. **Metabolism/Elimination:** 50% excreted unchanged in feces. Removed by hemodialysis. **Half-Life:** 6–9 hr.

INDICATIONS/DOSAGE

Acute MI
Adult: 5 mg followed by 5 mg 10 minutes later. If total 10 mg dose is tolerated, oral dosage regimen may be initiated.

CONTRAINDICATIONS/ PRECAUTIONS
Contraindicated in: Cardiogenic shock, CHF (unless secondary to tachydysrhythmia responding to beta-blockers), hypersensitivity, overt cardiac failure, sinus bradycardia, second or third degree heart block. **Use cautiously in:** Nonallergic bronchospasm, peripheral vascular disease. **Pregnancy/Lactation:** No well-controlled trial to establish safety. Benefits must outweigh risks. Toxic effects seen in animal embryos at doses 5–50 times normal. Fetal beta-blocker effects seen

In the Adverse Effects section, underline indicates most frequent; CAPS indicates life threatening.

43

if administered during delivery. **Pediatrics:** Safety and efficacy not established.

PREPARATION

Availability: 5 mg/10 mL amp. **Infusion:** May be diluted in compatible solution to physician specified volume.

STABILITY/STORAGE

Vial: Store at room temperature. **Infusion:** Stable for 48 hr at room temperature.

ADMINISTRATION

General: Begin treatment as soon as possible on admission. **IV Push/Intermittent Infusion:** Give slowly over 5 min.

COMPATIBILITY

Solution: Dextrose solutions, sodium chloride solutions.

ADVERSE EFFECTS

CNS: Anxiety, depression, dizziness, fatigue, headache, insomina, lethargy, paresthesias. **Ophtho:** Conjunctivitis, visual disturbances. **CV:** Arterial/peripheral vascular insufficiency, bradycardia, cerebrovascular accident, chest pain, CHF, first/second degree heart block, hypotension, palpitations, peripheral ischemia, pulmonary edema, sinoatrial block, tachycardia. **Resp:** Bronchospasm, cough, dyspnea, rales, wheezing. **GI:** Abdominal discomfort, anorexia, constipation, diarrhea, dry mouth, elevated liver enzymes, nausea. **GU:** Dysuria, impotence, urinary retention/frequency. **MS:** Arthralgia, back pain, muscle cramps. **Derm:** Alopecia, pruritus. **Endo:** Hyperglycemia, hypoglycemia. **Heme:** AGRANULOCYTOSIS, nonthrombocyto-

penic/thrombocytopenic purpura. **Hypersens:** Rash. **Other:** Decreased exercise tolerance, weight gain/loss.

TOXICITY/OVERDOSE

Signs/Symptoms: Extension of adverse effects. **Treatment:** Treat heart block with isoproterenol and transvenous pacemaker, symptomatic and supportive, removed by hemodialysis.

DRUG INTERACTIONS

Nonsteroidal anti-inflammatory agents, salicylates: Decreased antihypertensive effects. **Dopamine, dobutamine, isoproterenol, norepinephrine:** Antagonizes beta-blocker effect, severe hypotension. **Lidocaine:** Increased lidocaine effects. **Verapamil:** Additive atrioventricular (AV) conduction and myocardial contractility depression. **Disopyramide:** Increased pharmacological effects of both drugs.

NURSING CONSIDERATIONS

Assessment

General:
Continuous ECG, blood pressure, and heart rate, serial chest x-rays.
Physical:
Lung sounds.
Lab Alterations:
Monitor serum glucose.

Intervention/Rationale

Follow serial chest x-rays to assess for development of CHF/pulmonary edema. ● Discontinue drug and call physician at first sign of rhythm change or impending cardiac failure. Have emergency equipment, including transvenous pacemaker, available. ● May mask

In the Adverse Effects section, <u>underline</u> indicates most frequent; CAPS indicates life threatening.

signs/symptoms of hypoglycemia and may potentiate insulin-induced hypoglycemia.

Patient/Family Education
Explain purpose of drug and potential therapeutic outcome.

ATRACURIUM
(a-tra-cure'-ee-um)
Trade Name(s): Tracrium
Classification(s):
Nondepolarizing neuromuscular blocking agent
Pregnancy Category: C

PHARMACODYNAMICS/KINETICS
Mechanism of Action: Causes partial paralysis by interfering with neural transmission at myoneural junction. Prevents acetylcholine from binding to receptors at muscle end plate. **Onset of Action:** 2.0–2.5 min, decreases with increasing doses. **Peak Effect:** 3–5 min. **Duration of Action:** 20–35 min, increases with increasing doses. **Distribution:** Distributes rapidly throughout the body. **Metabolism/Elimination:** Inactivated in plasma, excreted via bile and urine. **Half-Life:** 20 minutes.

INDICATIONS/DOSAGE

Intubation and maintenance of neuromuscular blockade
Adult: 0.4–0.5 mg/kg with maximum blockade achieved in 3–5 min. *Adult:* Significant cardiovascular disease and history suggestive of increased histamine release: Initially 0.3–0.4 mg/kg given slowly or in divided doses. *Pediatric:* 1

month to 2 years: Initial dose 0.3–0.4 mg/kg. More frequent maintenance doses can be expected.

Maintenance of neuromuscular blockade during prolonged operative procedures
Adult: 0.08–0.1 mg/kg 20–45 min after initial dose. Initial infusion rate of 9–10 mcg/kg/min may be required to rapidly counteract recovery of neuromuscular function. Dose range 2–15 mcg/kg/min. Dosage dependent on patient needs and response and is adjusted depending on previous drugs administered/length/degree of muscle relaxation required.

CONTRAINDICATIONS/PRECAUTIONS
Contraindicated in: Hypersensitivity. **Use cautiously in:** Bronchial asthma, myasthenia gravis, severe electrolyte disturbances. **Pregnancy/Lactation:** No well-controlled trials to establish safety. Benefits must outweigh risks. Unknown if drug has immediate/delayed adverse effects on fetus or need for resuscitative measures are increased. Potentially teratogenic in laboratory studies. Excreted in breast milk. **Pediatrics:** Safety and efficacy has not been established for children < 1 month old.

PREPARATION
Availability: 10 mg/mL in 5 mL amps and 10 mL vials. **Infusion:** Further dilute in compatible IV solution to physician specified volume. Usual final concentration 0.2 or 0.5 mg/mL.

In the Adverse Effects section, underline indicates most frequent; CAPS indicates life threatening.

STABILITY/STORAGE
Vial: Refrigerate. **Infusion:** Use within 24 hr of preparation. Solutions containing 0.2 or 0.5 mg/mL stable at room temperature or refrigerated for 24 hr.

ADMINISTRATION
General: Unconsciousness must be established prior to administration to prevent patient distress. Contains no analgesic properties. **IV Push:** Give initial bolus over 30–60 sec. **Continuous Infusion:** Give as per dosage guidelines.

COMPATIBILITY
Solution: Dextrose solutions, sodium chloride solutions. **Y-site:** Aminophylline, cefazolin, cefuroxime, cimetidine, dobutamine, dopamine, epinephrine, esmolol, fentanyl, gentamicin, heparin, hydrocortisone, isoproterenol, lorazepam, midazolam, nitroglycerin, ranitidine, sodium nitroprusside, trimethoprim-sulfamethoxazole, vancomycin.

INCOMPATIBILITY
Solution: Alkaline solutions, lactated Ringer's. **Y-site:** Diazepam.

ADVERSE EFFECTS
CV: Bradycardia, hypotension. **Resp:** Increased bronchial secretions, prolonged dose-related apnea, wheezing. **MS:** Inadequate blockade, prolonged neuromuscular blockade. **Derm:** Erythema. **Hypersens:** Allergic manifestations, pruritus, urticaria. **Other:** Flushing.

TOXICITY/OVERDOSE
Signs/Symptoms: Apnea, airway closure, hypersensitivity, including anaphylaxis, respiratory insufficiency. **Treatment:** Provide cardio-

vascular support. Assure patent airway and ventilation. Resuscitate as necessary. **Antidote(s):** Reverse blockade symptoms with anticholinesterase reversing agents (edrophonium, neostigmine, pyridostigmine) and anticholinergic agents (atropine, glycopyrrolate).

DRUG INTERACTIONS
Aminoglycosides, clindamycin, diuretics, general anesthetics (enflurane, isoflurane, halothane), lincomycin, lithium, magnesium sulfate, muscle relaxants, polypeptide antibiotics (bacitracin, polymyxin B), verapamil: Increased neuromuscular blockade. **Phenytoin, theophylline:** Resistance to or reversal of neuromuscular blockade. **Succinylcholine:** Increased onset and depth of neuromuscular blockade.

NURSING CONSIDERATIONS

Assessment
General:
Vital signs.
Physical:
Cardiopulmonary, neuromuscular.
Lab Alterations:
Monitor electrolytes.

Intervention/Rationale
Produces apnea (use cautiously in patients with cardiovascular disease, severe electrolyte disorders, bronchogenic cancer, neuromuscular disease). Maintain patent airway. ● Monitor response to drug during intraoperative period by use of a peripheral nerve stimulator. ● Assess postoperatively for presence of any residual muscle weakness. Evaluate hand grip, head lift, ability to cough in order to ascertain full recovery from residual effects of

In the Adverse Effects section, <u>underline</u> indicates most frequent;
CAPS indicates life threatening.

drug. ● Correct electrolyte deficiencies prior to surgery.

Patient/Family Education
Discuss the rationale for hand grip, head lift, cough demonstration in the immediate postoperative phase in order to assure patient cooperation.

ATROPINE SULFATE
(at'-ro-peen)
Trade Name(s): Atropine
Classification(s):
Anticholinergic, antimuscarinic, bronchodilator, cardiopulmonary resuscitant
Pregnancy Category: C

PHARMACODYNAMICS/KINETICS
Mechanism of Action: Anticholinergic and potent belladonna alkaloid, inhibits acetylcholine at parasympathetic junction, blocks vagal effect on sinoatrial node and increases conduction through atrioventricular node, thus increasing heart rate. **Onset of Action:** Immediate. **Peak Effect:** 2–4 min (peak increase in heart rate). **Distribution:** Well-distributed throughout body. Crosses blood–brain barrier. **Metabolism/Elimination:** Metabolized in the liver to several metabolites. 30%–50% of drug excreted by the kidneys. **Half-Life:** 2–3 hr.

INDICATIONS/DOSAGE

Antidote for anticholinesterase insecticide poisoning
Adult: 2–3 mg hourly until atropine intoxication symptoms ap-

pear. Severe cases may require up to 6 mg hourly. *Pediatric:* 0.05 mg/kg every 10–30 min as needed or until atropine intoxication symptoms appear.

Bradydysrhythmias, symptomatic bradycardia
Adult: 0.5–1.0 mg. Repeat every 5 min as needed to a maximum of 2 mg. *Pediatric:* 0.01–0.04 mg/kg. Repeat every 2–5 min as needed to a maximum of 1 mg (children) or 2 mg (adolescents).

Cardiac asystole, cardiopulmonary resuscitant
Adult: 1 mg. May be repeated at 0.5 mg increments up to a maximum of 2 mg.

Cardiovagal blockade, preoperative secretion inhibitor
Adult: Usual dose 0.5 mg (range of 0.4–0.6 mg) (usually given IM). May be given IV 45–60 min preanesthesia. *Pediatric:* 0.01 mg/kg/dose up to a maximum of 0.4 mg/dose. May be given IV 45–60 minutes preanesthesia.

CONTRAINDICATIONS/PRECAUTIONS
Contraindicated in: Acute glaucoma, acute hemorrhage with unstable cardiovascular status, asthma, hepatic disease, hypersensitivity, intestinal atony of elderly/debilitated, myasthenia gravis, myocardial ischemia, obstruction of GI/GU tracts, paralytic ileus, pyloric stenosis, renal disease, severe ulcerative colitis, tachycardia, toxic megacolon. **Use cautiously in:** Chronic lung disease, cyclopropane anesthesia, elderly/debilitated, prostatic hy-

In the Adverse Effects section, underline indicates most frequent; CAPS indicates life threatening.

47

pertrophy, urinary retention. **Pregnancy/Lactation:** No well-controlled trials to establish safety. Benefits must outweigh risks. Crosses placenta. Distributed in breast milk. **Pediatrics:** Safety for use in children has not clearly been established. Use for bradycardias/asystole in infants/children requires vagolytic doses. Smaller doses may cause a paradoxical bradycardia.

PREPARATION
Availability: 0.05 mg/mL in 5 mL syringes. 0.1 mg/mL in 5, 10 mL syringes. 0.3 mg/mL in 1 and 30 mL vials. 0.4 mg/mL in 1 mL amps, 1, 20, 30 mL vials. 0.8 mg/mL in 0.5, 1 mL amps and 0.5 mL syringes. 1 mg/mL in 1 mL amps/vials and 10 mL syringes. **IV Push:** May be given undiluted but desired dose may be diluted in 5–10 mL sterile water for injection. Not to be added to IV solutions.

STABILITY/STORAGE
Vial: Store at room temperature. Drug effloresces on exposure to air.

ADMINISTRATION
IV Push: Give 1.0 mg or less through Y-site or 3-way stopcock over a 1 minute period.

COMPATIBILITY
Solution: Dextrose solutions, lactated Ringer's, Ringer's injection, sodium chloride solutions. **Syringe:** Benzquinamide, butorphanol, chlorpromazine, cimetidine, diphenhydramine, droperidol, fentanyl, glycopyrrolate, heparin, hydromorphone, meperidine, metoclopramide, midazolam, morphine, nalbuphine, pentazocine, prochlor-

perazine, promethazine, ranitidine, scopolamine. **Y-site:** Amrinone, famotidine, heparin, hydrocortisone, nafcillin, potassium chloride, vitamin B complex with C.

ADVERSE EFFECTS
CNS: Coma, confusion, delirium, disorientation, dizziness, agitation, ataxia, excitement, hallucinations, headache, insomnia, restlessness. **Ophtho:** Dilated pupils, blurred vision, photophobia. **CV:** Palpitations, postural hypotension, tachycardia. **Resp:** Nasal congestion. **GI:** Constipation, dry mouth, gastroesophageal reflux, nausea, paralytic ileus, thirst, vomiting. **GU:** Impotence, urinary retention. **Derm:** Hot flushed skin. **Endo:** Suppression of lactation. **Heme:** Leukocytosis. **Other:** Decreased sweating.

TOXICITY/OVERDOSE
Signs/Symptoms:
Toxicity: Abdominal distention, dysphagia, dry mouth, nausea, neuromuscular blockade resulting in muscle weakness/paralysis, thirst, vomiting. **Overdose:** Coma, death, delirium, elevated blood pressure, fever, stupor, tachycardia. **Treatment:** Standard treatment to manage cardiac dysrhythmias, resuscitative and supportive efforts as required. Hemodialysis is ineffective for toxicity. **Antidote(s):** Physostigmine salicylate reverses most CV/CNS effects, may cause asystole, bradycardia, and seizures. Diazepam (short-acting barbiturate) or chloral hydrate may be used to relieve excitement caused by drug. Neostigmine methylsulfate 0.25–25 mg is an alternate antidote.

In the Adverse Effects section, underline indicates most frequent; CAPS indicates life threatening.

DRUG INTERACTIONS

Amantadine, tricyclic antidepressants: Increased anticholinergic side effects. **Atenolol, digoxin:** Increased pharmacologic effects by atropine. **Phenothiazines:** Decreased antipsychotic effects.

NURSING CONSIDERATIONS

Assessment

General:
Continuous ECG, blood pressure, intake/output ratio.
Physical:
Cardiac, GI tract.

Intervention/Rationale

Heart rate changes, paradoxical bradycardia, and tachydysrhythmias may occur. ● May cause urinary retention. ● Postural hypotension may develop. ● Assess abdomen for presence/absence of bowel sounds to evaluate development of paralytic ileus.

Patient/Family Education

Dry mouth may be due to medication. Seek assistance with ambulation/repositioning activities due to potential for postural hypotension. Notify nurse/physician with symptoms of difficulty in urination, constipation, abdominal bloating, increased sensitivity to light.

AZATHIOPRINE

(ay-za-thye′-oh-preen)
Trade Name(s): Imuran
Classification(s):
Immunosuppressant
Pregnancy Category: D

PHARMACODYNAMICS/KINETICS

Mechanism of Action: Purine antagonist, antimetabolite, suppresses T-cell mediated hypersensitivity. **Distribution:** 30% bound to plasma proteins. **Metabolism/Elimination:** Primarily metabolized to mercaptopurine. Inactivated by xanthine oxidase. Partially removed by hemodialysis. **Half-Life:** 5 hr.

INDICATIONS/DOSAGE

Renal transplantation

Adult/Pediatric: Initial dose 3–5 mg/kg daily beginning on the day of transplantation. Maintenance dose 1–3 mg/kg daily. May give 1–5 mg/kg/day for several days pre-transplant. Adjust dosing interval in renal failure.

Rheumatoid arthritis

Adult: 1 mg/kg (50–100 mg) as a single dose or twice daily. If unsatisfactory response after 6–8 weeks, increase dose by 0.5 mg/kg/day (up to a maximum of 2.5 mg/kg/day) at 4 week intervals.

CONTRAINDICATIONS/ PRECAUTIONS

Contraindicated in: Hypersensitivity, rheumatoid arthritis in pregnancy. **Use cautiously in:** Anuria, concomitant immunosuppressive agents, impaired liver function, severe organ rejection. **Pregnancy/Lactation:** No well-controlled trials to establish safety. Benefits must outweigh risks. Mutagenic and teratogenic potential exists. Safety for males/females capable of conception has not been established.

In the Adverse Effects section, <u>underline</u> indicates most frequent;
CAPS indicates life threatening.

PREPARATION

Availability: 100 mg vial. **Reconstitution:** Add 10 mL of sterile water for injection. **Infusion:** May be further diluted with compatible IV solution to minimum volume of 50 mL.

STABILITY/STORAGE

Vial: Use within 24 hr of reconstitution (contains no preservatives). Stable for 2 weeks after reconstitution at room temperature. **Infusion:** Prepare just prior to administration. Stable for 24 hr at room temperature.

ADMINISTRATION

General: IV administration reserved for patients unable to tolerate oral medications. Must be administered slowly due to alkaline pH. **IV Push/ Intermittent Infusion:** Infuse over 30–60 min. Infusion time ranges from 5 min to 8 hr for daily dose.

COMPATIBILITY

Solution: Dextrose solutions, sodium chloride solutions.

INCOMPATIBILITY

Solution: Alkaline solutions.

ADVERSE EFFECTS

CV: Hypotension, pulmonary edema. **GI:** Hepatotoxicity, esophagitis, anorexia, diarrhea, jaundice, <u>nausea</u>, steatorrhea, vomiting, biliary stasis. **MS:** Arthralgia, muscle wasting (long-term use). **Derm:** Alopecia. **Endo:** Pancreatitis. **Heme:** LEUKOPENIA, THROMBOCYTO-PENIA, bleeding. **Hypersens:** Rash. **Other:** Drug fever.

TOXICITY/OVERDOSE

Signs/Symptoms: Hematopoietic depression, serious infection. **Treatment:** Symptomatic and supportive treatment, consider temporary/permanent dosage reduction or discontinuation.

DRUG INTERACTIONS

Allopurinol: Potentiation of adverse effects. Must reduce dosage of azathioprine to ⅓ or ¼ usual dose. **Pancuronium, tubocurarine:** Reverses neuromuscular blockade.

NURSING CONSIDERATIONS

Assessment
Physical:
Bleeding tendencies, signs/symptoms of infection, rash, GI tract.
Lab Alterations:
Monitor CBC, platelets, and liver profile prior to, and at least weekly throughout therapy.

Intervention/Rationale
Administer antiemetic in accordance with symptoms of nausea.

Patient/Family Education
Report any signs of infection (even signs of mild infection such as fever and colds) since infections in immune compromised patients may be fatal. Observe for clay-colored stools, dark urine, pruritus, yellow skin, and sclera and notify physician immediately. Hair loss or thinning is possible. Avoid conception during therapy and up to 4 months after discontinuing drug due to potential mutagenic/teratogenic effects.

AZTREONAM
(az-tree'-o-nam)
Trade Name(s): Azactam
Classification(s): Synthetic

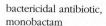

bactericidal antibiotic, monobactam
Pregnancy Category: B

PHARMACODYNAMICS/KINETICS

Mechanism of Action: Inhibits bacterial cell wall synthesis, causing destruction of cell wall, bactericidal. **Peak Serum Level:** 30 min. **Duration of Action:** 8 hr. **Distribution:** Serum protein binding averages 56% and is independent of dosage. **Metabolism/Elimination:** Primarily eliminated by the kidneys (60%–70%), 12% recovered in feces. Removed by hemodialysis. **Half-Life:** 1.7 hr.

INDICATIONS/DOSAGE

Treatment of susceptible gram-negative bacteria.

Treatment of urinary tract infection, moderately severe systemic infections, lower respiratory tract infections

Adult: 500 mg to 2 g every 8–12 hr.

Severe systemic or life-threatening infections, bacterial septicemia, localized parenchymal abscesses

Adult: 2 g every 6–8 hr.

CONTRAINDICATIONS/PRECAUTIONS

Contraindicated in: Hypersensitivity. **Use cautiously in:** Impaired hepatic/renal function. **Pregnancy/Lactation:** No well-controlled trials to establish safety. Benefits must outweigh risks. Crosses placenta. Excreted in breast milk. **Pediatrics:** Safety and efficacy not established.

PREPARATION

Availability: 500 mg, 1 g, 2 g in 15 mL vials and 100 mL infusion bottles. **Reconstitution:** Add compatible diluent to container and shake immediately and vigorously. For bolus injections add 6–10 mL sterile water for injection. Solution becomes light yellow in color and may become pink on standing. Color changes do not affect potency. **Infusion:** Further dilute 1–2 g in 50–100 mL (1 g/50 mL minimum volume) compatible IV solution.

STABILITY/STORAGE

Vial: Store at room temperature. **Infusion:** Stable up to 48 hr at room temperature or 7 days refrigerated.

ADMINISTRATION

General: Flush common IV tubing before/after administration. **IV Push:** Give slowly over 3–5 min. **Intermittent Infusion:** Infuse over 20–60 min.

COMPATIBILITY

Solution: Dextrose solutions, lactated Ringer's, Ringer's injection, sodium chloride solutions. **Syringe:** Clindamycin. **Y-site:** Ciprofloxacin, enalaprilat, foscarnet, ondansetron, zidovudine.

INCOMPATIBILITY

Y-site: Vancomycin.

ADVERSE EFFECTS

CNS: Seizures, confusion, dizziness, headache, tinnitus. **Ophtho:** Diplopia. **CV:** Hypotension, premature ventricular contractions, transient ventricular bigeminy. **GI:** Abdominal cramps, diarrhea related to C. difficile, nausea, vomiting. Elevated AST (SGOT), ALT (SGPT); hepatitis, increased alkaline phosphatase;

In the Adverse Effects section, <u>underline</u> indicates most frequent;
CAPS indicates life threatening.

jaundice. **GU:** Breast tenderness, vaginal candidiasis, vaginitis. **MS:** Muscular aches, weakness. **Heme:** Anemia, leukocytosis, neutropenia, pancytopenia, thrombocytopenia, thrombocytosis, increased prothrombin/partial thromboplastin times. **Hypersens:** ANAPHYLAXIS, allergic manifestations, rash. **Other:** Phlebitis/thrombophlebitis at injection site.

DRUG INTERACTIONS

Furosemide, probenecid: Minimal increases in aztreonam serum levels. **Beta-lactam antibiotics:** (cefoxitin, imipenem). May induce beta-lactamase, aztreonam antagonism.

NURSING CONSIDERATIONS

Assessment
General:
Vital signs, intake/output ratio.
Physical:
GI tract.
Lab Alterations:
Monitor coagulation profile.

Intervention/Rationale

Assess baseline laboratory values (including coagulation studies, platelets, and CBC) prior to initiating drug. ● Observe for irregular pulse rate or hypotension. ● Observe stools, consider culturing specimen if diarrhea develops.

Patient/Family Education

Persistent infection may require treatment for several weeks. Notify nurse/physician if any new signs of infection are noted. Notify nurse/physician with the onset of diarrhea.

BENZQUINAMIDE
(benz-kwin′-a-mide)
Trade Name(s): Emete-Con
Classification(s): Antiemetic, antihistamine, anticholinergic
Pregnancy Category: C

PHARMACODYNAMICS/KINETICS
Mechanism of Action: Depressive action on the chemoreceptor trigger zone associated with emesis. **Onset of Action:** 15 min. **Peak Effect:** 20–30 min. **Duration of Action:** 3–4 hr. **Distribution:** Rapidly and widely distributed throughout body, greatest distribution in liver and kidneys, 58% plasma bound. **Metabolism/Elimination:** Metabolized by the liver. Metabolites and 5%–10% unchanged drug excreted in the urine. **Half-Life:** 30–40 minutes.

INDICATIONS/DOSAGE

Prevention/treatment of nausea/vomiting associated with surgery and anesthesia

Adult: 25 mg (0.2–0.4mg/kg). Usual dose 25 mg with subsequent doses administered IM. Use lower doses in elderly, debilitated patients.

CONTRAINDICATIONS/PRECAUTIONS
Contraindicated in: Hypersensitivity. **Use cautiously in:** Cardiovascular disease, debilitated, elderly. **Pregnancy/Lactation:** No well-controlled trials to establish safety. Benefits must outweigh risks. **Pediatrics:** Safety and efficacy not established.

In the Adverse Effects section, <u>underline</u> indicates most frequent;
CAPS indicates life threatening.

PREPARATION
Availability: 50 mg/vial. **Reconstitution:** Initially reconstitute with 2.2 mL sterile water for injection or bacteriostatic water. Final concentration 25 mg/mL. Sodium chloride causes precipitation.

STABILITY/STORAGE
Vial: Store at room temperature. Reconstituted vial stable for 14 days at room temperature.

ADMINISTRATION
General: IV dosage should be restricted for use of patients without evidence of cardiovascular disease. **IV Push:** 25 mg (1 mL) over 30–60 seconds.

COMPATIBILITY
Syringe: Atropine, fentanyl with droperidol, glycopyrrolate, ketamine, meperidine, midazolam, morphine, naloxone, pentazocine, propranolol, scopolamine. **Y-site:** Foscarnet.

INCOMPATIBILITY
Solution: Sodium chloride. **Syringe:** Chlordiazepoxide, diazepam, pentobarbital, phenobarbital, secobarbital, thiopental.

ADVERSE EFFECTS
CNS: Dizziness, <u>drowsiness</u>, sedation, excitement, hiccups. **CV:** Atrial fibrillation, hypertension, hypotension, premature atrial contractions (PAC), premature ventricular contractions (PVC). **GI:** Abdominal cramps, anorexia, constipation, <u>dry mouth</u>, salivation, vomiting. **GU:** Urinary hesitancy. **MS:** Tremors, twitching, weakness. **Hypersens:** Allergic reactions, hives, rash. **Ophtho:** Blurred vision. **Other:** Chills, diaphoresis, fever, flushing, sweating.

TOXICITY/OVERDOSE
Signs/Symptoms: CNS stimulation and depressant effects. **Treatment:** Symptomatic and supportive. Atropine may be beneficial. Hemodialysis is not helpful due to high level plasma protein binding.

DRUG INTERACTIONS
Pressor agents: Potentiates hypotensive effects of benzquinamide. **Alcohol, antihistamines, narcotics, sedative/hypnotics:** Additive CNS depressive effects.

NURSING CONSIDERATIONS
Assessment
General:
Vital signs, ECG (if potential for ectopy is known or suspected), intake/output.
Physical:
GI tract.

Intervention/Rationale
Sudden hypertension, PVCs and PACs may occur following IV use. ● Evaluate bowel sounds/function daily and assess for abdominal distension and constipation. ● Severe nausea/vomiting may require IV hydration. ● Evaluate need for frequent oral hygiene as a comfort measure.

Patient/Family Education
Seek assistance with ambulatory/position changes in order to minimize significant orthostatic effects. Mouth may be very dry (frequent rinsing of mouth may be helpful). Avoid alcoholic beverages and other CNS depressants.

In the Adverse Effects section, <u>underline</u> indicates most frequent; CAPS indicates life threatening.

BENZTROPINE

(benz-troe'-peen)
Trade Name(s): Bensylate ♣,
Cogentin
Classification(s):
Anticholinergic, antiparkinson
Pregnancy Category: C

PHARMACODYNAMICS/KINETICS

Mechanism of Action: Anticholinergic, blocks central and dopaminergic receptors, inhibits acetylcholine at parasympathetic junction, assists with balancing cholinergic activity in the basal ganglia. **Onset of Action:** Several days. **Duration of Action:** Up to 24 hr.

INDICATIONS/DOSAGE

Acute dystonic reactions

Adult: 1–2 mg. Incremental increases 0.5 mg at 5–6 day intervals up to a maximum of 6 mg daily. Use least amount of drug necessary to manage symptoms.

Management of Parkinsonism

Adult: 1–2 mg/day. Range of 0.5–6.0 mg/day may be required for symptom control.

Drug-induced extrapyramidal disorders

Adult: 1–2 mg may relieve symptoms.

CONTRAINDICATIONS/ PRECAUTIONS

Contraindicated in: Achalasia, children < 3 years, hypersensitivity, megacolon, myasthenia gravis, narrow angle glaucoma, prostatic hypertrophy, pyloric or duodenal obstruction, stenosing peptic ulcers, tardive dyskinesia. **Use cautiously in:** Children > 3 years, elderly/debilitated (increased risks of adverse reactions). **Pregnancy/Lactation:** No well-controlled trial to establish safety. Benefits must outweigh risks. **Pediatrics:** Safety and efficacy not established.

PREPARATION

Availability: 1 mg/mL, 2 mL amp.

STABILITY/STORAGE

Vial: Store at room temperature.

ADMINISTRATION

General: Parenteral use should be solely restricted to acute situations requiring more immediate control or relief. Gradually taper drug when discontinuing therapy or withdrawal reaction may occur manifesting such signs as anxiety, insomnia, reappearance/worsening of parkinson/extrapyramidal reactions, or tachycardia. **IV Push:** Administer slowly at rate of 1 mg/min.

COMPATIBILITY

Solution: Sodium chloride. **Syringe:** Metoclopramide.

ADVERSE EFFECTS

CNS: Sedation, confusion, depression, dizziness, hallucinations, headache. **Ophtho:** Blurred vision, dry eyes, mydriasis. **CV:** Dysrhythmias, hypotension, palpitations, tachycardia. **GI:** Constipation. **GU:** Urinary hesitancy, urinary retention. **MS:** Weakness. **Other:** Decreased sweating.

In the Adverse Effects section, underline indicates most frequent; CAPS indicates life threatening.

TOXICITY/OVERDOSE
Signs/Symptoms:
Toxicity: Allergic reactions, blurred vision, constipation, depression, dizziness, dry mouth, listlessness, nausea, nervousness, numbness of digits, skin rash, vomiting.
Overdose: Anhidrosis, circulatory collapse, coma, dilation of pupils, dry mucous membranes, flushing, hyperpyrexia, glaucoma, paralytic ileus, respiratory depression, tachycardia, urinary retention.
Treatment: Notify physician immediately. Signs/symptoms of toxicity may be decreased/eliminated by discontinuing drug or decreasing dosage. Drug may be resumed if absolutely required but at a lower dosage. Overdose must be treated symptomatically and supported in accordance with manifestations. Resuscitation may be required. **Antidote:** Physostigmine 1–2 mg given at 1 mg/min. Reverses cardiovascular and CNS effects.

DRUG INTERACTIONS
Alcohol, amantadine, anticholinergic agents, antihistamines, barbiturates, disopyramide, haloperidol, narcotic analgesics, phenothiazines, tricyclic antidepressants: Additive anticholinergic effects. **Digoxin:** Increased oral digoxin serum levels. **Levodopa:** Reduced levodopa effect.

NURSING CONSIDERATIONS
Assessment
General:
Heart rate, blood pressure, intake/output ratio.
Physical:
Neurological/neuromuscular, GU system, GI tract.

Intervention/Rationale
Hypotension and/or ectopy may develop following administration. ● Evaluate baseline parkinson/extrapyramidal symptoms (note effectiveness of drug by improvement/worsening of symptoms in conjunction with drug schedule). ● Assess for signs of urinary retention (dysuria, overflow incontinence, voiding of small amounts at frequent intervals). ● Evaluate bowel sounds/function daily and assess for constipation, abdominal distention, evidence of ileus.

Patient/Family Education
Drug may cause drowsiness (seek help with ambulatory or repositioning activities). Notify physician with the development of any urinary hesitancy or urgency symptoms. Drug will cause dry mouth (frequent oral hygiene may be beneficial). Drug will cause a decrease in sweating that could cause hyperpyrexia, heat prostration, dehydration. Be aware of environmental temperatures and take proper precautions to prevent overheating.

BETAMETHASONE
(bay-ta-meth'-a-zone)
Trade Name(s): Celestone phosphate, Cel-U-Jec, Selestoject
Classification(s):
Anti-inflammatory, corticosteroid
Pregnancy Category: C

PHARMACODYNAMICS/KINETICS
Mechanism of Action: Stabilizes leukocyte lysosomal membranes, suppresses immune response, increases protein, fat, and carbo-

In the Adverse Effects section, underline indicates most frequent;
CAPS indicates life threatening.

55

hydrate production. **Peak Serum Level:** 10–36 min. **Distribution:** 64% protein bound. **Metabolism/Elimination:** Metabolized by the liver. Metabolites excreted by the kidneys and in bile. **Half-Life:** 5 hr (plasma), 36–54 hr (biological).

INDICATIONS/DOSAGE

Systemic and local anti-inflammatory agent, immunosuppressant

Adult: Dose is variable and dependent on condition. Must be individualized on the basis of need/response. Initial dose may range from 0.5–9.0 mg daily. Life-threatening situations may require extremely high doses.

CONTRAINDICATIONS/ PRECAUTIONS

Contraindicated in: Live virus vaccines with immunosuppressant doses, hypersensitivity, systemic fungal infections. **Use cautiously in:** Active/latent peptic ulcers, acute psychosis, acute/healed tuberculosis, diabetes mellitus, myasthenia gravis, septic shock. **Pregnancy/Lactation:** No well-controlled trials to establish safety. Benefits must outweigh risks.

PREPARATION

Availability: 4 mg/mL as phosphate, 5 mL vials.

STABILITY/STORAGE

Vial: Store at room temperature.

ADMINISTRATION

General: May be given without further dilution. **IV Push:** Give slowly over 1 min or less.

COMPATIBILITY

Solution: Dextrose solutions, lactated Ringer's, Ringer's injection, sodium chloride solutions. **Y-site:** Heparin, hydrocortisone, potassium chloride, vitamin B complex with C.

ADVERSE EFFECTS

CNS: Increased intracranial pressure with papilledema, convulsions, syncope, headache, vertigo. **Ophtho:** Exophthalmus, glaucoma. **CV:** CARDIAC ARREST, dysrhythmias, fat embolism, thromboembolism, thrombophlebitis. **GI:** Pancreatitis, abdominal distention, nausea, vomiting. **Derm:** Impaired wound healing. **Endo:** Cushingoid state. **Fld/Lytes:** Hypocalcemia, hypokalemia. **Heme:** Leukocytosis (without a left shift). **Hypersens:** Circulatory collapse, hypersensitivity reactions. **Metab:** Metabolic alkalosis.

TOXICITY/OVERDOSE

Signs/Symptoms: Symptoms of acute adrenal insufficiency as a result of too rapid withdrawal of drug after long-term use. Cushingoid changes (moonface, central obesity, hypertension, diabetes, fluid/electrolyte imbalance) may result from continuous use of large doses. **Treatment:** Supportive and symptomatic treatment, including fluid resuscitation, vasopressor therapy, and electrolyte replacement.

DRUG INTERACTIONS

Barbiturates, phenytoin, rifampin: Decreased corticosteroid effects. **Cyclosporine, theophylline:** Bethamethasone potentiates adverse effects. **Digoxin:** Increased potential for

---

In the Adverse Effects section, <u>underline</u> indicates most frequent; CAPS indicates life threatening.

56

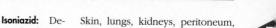

digoxin toxicity. **Isoniazid:** Decreased isoniazid concentration. **Salicylates:** Decreased salicylates levels and effect.

NURSING CONSIDERATIONS

Assessment
General:
Blood pressure, intake/output ratio.
Physical:
Infectious disease status.
Lab Alterations:
Altered serum glucose (especially in diabetics), electrolytes.

Intervention/Rationale
Drug may induce hypertension. ● Notify physician if unusual weight gain is noted or if swelling of lower extremities, muscle weakness, or facial puffiness is observed. ● Drug may increase insulin needs in diabetics. ● May mask signs/symptoms of infection (observe for fever, increased WBC, decreased wound healing).

Patient/Family Education
Wear/carry identification alerting emergency care givers of chronic steroid therapy. Avoid live virus vaccinations without physician approval.

BLEOMYCIN

(blee-oh-mye′-sin)
Trade Name(s): Blenoxane
Classification(s): Antineoplastic
Pregnancy Category: D

PHARMACODYNAMICS/KINETICS
Mechanism of Action: Inhibits synthesis of DNA and RNA. **Distribution:** Skin, lungs, kidneys, peritoneum, and lymphatics (in animal studies). **Metabolism/Elimination:** Metabolic fate unknown. Excreted 60%–70% unchanged by the kidneys. **Half-Life:** 2 hr, prolonged in renal impairment.

INDICATIONS/DOSAGE

Adjunct to surgery and radiation therapy in palliative treatment of selected neoplasms (as a single agent or in combination).

Squamous cell carcinoma, lymphosarcoma, reticulum cell sarcoma, testicular carcinoma

Adult: 0.25–0.50 units/kg (10–20 units/m^2) once or twice per week. Total dose should not exceed 400 units.

Hodgkin's disease

Adult: Test dose of 2 units or less for first two doses. If no reaction, initial dose 0.25–0.5 units/kg (10–20 units/m^2) once or twice per week. Maintenance dose 1 unit daily or 5 units weekly (after a 50% response). Total dose should not exceed 400 units.

CONTRAINDICATIONS/PRECAUTIONS
Contraindicated in: Hypersensitivity. **Use cautiously in:** Elderly (increased pulmonary toxicity in patients over age 70), renal or pulmonary impairment from nonmalignant disease. **Pregnancy/Lactation:** No well-controlled trials to establish safety. Benefits must outweigh risks.

PREPARATION
Availability: 15 units/vial. **Reconstitution:** Add a minimum of 5 mL dex-

---

In the Adverse Effects section, <u>underline</u> indicates most frequent; CAPS indicates life threatening.

B

trose or sodium chloride to provide solution containing not more than 3 units/mL. **Infusion:** Dilute in 50–100 mL dextrose or sodium chloride.

STABILITY/STORAGE
Vial: Refrigerate, reconstituted solution stable for 24 hr. **Infusion:** Stable for 24 hr at room temperature.

ADMINISTRATION
General: Handle drug with care and adhere to institutional guidelines for the handling of chemotherapeutic/cytotoxic agents. In the event of spills or leaks, use a 5% sodium hypochlorite (household bleach) solution to inactivate bleomycin. **IV Push:** Give slowly over 10 minutes.

COMPATIBILITY
Solution: Dextrose solutions, sodium chloride solutions. **Syringe:** Cisplatin, cyclophosphamide, doxorubicin, droperidol, fluorouracil. **Y-site:** Cisplatin, cyclophosphamide, doxorubicin, droperidol, fluorouracil, heparin, leucovorin, methotrexate, metoclopramide, mitomycin, ondansetron, vinblastine, vincristine.

INCOMPATIBILITY
Y-site: Amino acids, aminophylline, furosemide, riboflavin.

ADVERSE EFFECTS
CNS: Confusion. **Resp:** PULMONARY FIBROSIS, pneumonitis. **GI:** Anorexia, nausea, stomatitis, vomiting. **GU:** Cystitis, hematuria. **Derm:** Alopecia (reversible), erythematous swelling, hyperkeratosis, hyperpigmentation, mucocutaneous toxicity, ulcerations of lips and tongue. **Heme:** LEUKOPENIA, THROMBOCYTOPENIA. **Nadir:** 12 days. **Hypersens:** ANAPHYLACTOID REACTIONS, rash, urticaria. **Other:** Chills, fever, generalized weakness, pain at tumor site.

TOXICITY/OVERDOSE
Signs/Symptoms: Pulmonary toxicity is dose/age related and occurs most frequently in patients over age 70 and in those who have received a total dose of more than 400 units. Earliest signs are dyspnea and fine rales. Other signs are radiographic changes (nonspecific patchy opacities), microscopic tissue changes, abnormal pulmonary function tests, and pneumonitis progressing to pulmonary fibrosis. **Treatment:** Symptomatic and supportive.

DRUG INTERACTIONS
Digitalis glycosides: Decreased plasma digoxin levels and renal excretion. **Phenytoin:** Decreased phenytoin serum levels.

NURSING CONSIDERATIONS
Assessment
General:
Vital signs, anaphylactic reactions (during test dose administration).
Physical:
Pulmonary complications (onset of dyspnea, fine rales, mild chest pain, tachypnea), GI tract, infectious disease status.
Lab Alterations:
Monitor baseline and periodic renal/hepatic function and CBC.

Intervention/Rationale
Chest x-rays should be obtained every 1–2 weeks to monitor for pulmonary toxicity. If supplemental

In the Adverse Effects section, underline indicates most frequent; CAPS indicates life threatening.

oxygen or surgery is required, maintain oxygen concentrations as close to room air (21%) as possible (high oxygen concentration in conjunction with bleomycin therapy increases potential for pulmonary toxicity). ● Check for fever after administration, which can occur within 3–6 hr. ● Monitor for anaphylactoid reactions, particularly in lymphoma patients (hypotension, fever, chills, mental confusion, wheezing). ● Assess for presence of mucosal lesions, including mouth for stomatitis. Give gentle, thorough, and frequent mouth care with saline/chlorhexidine (do not use mouth rinses containing alcohol). ● Assess daily for development of systemic infections (temperature, WBC).

Patient/Family Education
Notify nurse/physician with onset of cough, shortness of breath, sores on mouth and lips. Perform thorough oral hygiene with a soft tooth brush or sponge brush in the morning and after each meal. Observe closely for signs of infection (fever, sore throat, fatigue), evidence of bleeding (gums, nose bleeds, melena, easy bruising). Avoid crowded environment and persons with known infections. Avoid consumption of fresh fruits and vegetables (during neutropenic periods). Hair loss may affect body image. Use consistent and reliable contraception throughout the duration of therapy due to potential teratogenic and mutagenic effects of drug. Smoking may worsen pulmonary toxicity.

BRETYLIUM
(bre-till'-ee-yum)
Trade Name(s): Bretylate Parenteral ♣, Bretylol
Classification(s): Antiarrhythmic (Type III)
Pregnancy Category: C

PHARMACODYNAMICS/KINETICS
Mechanism of Action: Inhibits norepinephrine release. **Onset of Action:** *Ventricular fibrillation:* 5–10 min. *Ventricular tachycardia:* 20–120 min. **Peak Effect:** 1 hr. **Duration of Action:** 6–24 hr. **Distribution:** Distributes to tissues with high adrenergic innervation (ex: heart, spleen). **Metabolism/Elimination:** Excreted 90% unchanged by kidneys. Removed by hemodialysis. **Half-Life:** 5–10 hr. Increased in renal impairment.

INDICATIONS/DOSAGE

Ventricular fibrillation or hemodynamically unstable ventricular tachycardia

(Resistant to lidocaine or other conventional antiarrhythmics.)

Adult: 5 mg/kg undiluted. If dysrhythmia persists, increase dose to 10 mg/kg, followed by 15 mg/kg every 15–30 min to a maximum of 30 mg/kg. Follow with constant infusion of 1–2 mg/min or intermittent infusion of 5–10 mg/kg every 6 hr. *Pediatric (unlabeled use):* 2.5–5.0 mg/kg. 10 mg/kg after 1–2 hr if necessary. Total dose not to exceed 40 mg/kg/day. Follow with constant infusion of 1–2 mg/min or intermittent infusion of 5–10 mg/kg every 6–8 hr.

In the Adverse Effects section, underline indicates most frequent; CAPS indicates life threatening.

B

CONTRAINDICATIONS/ PRECAUTIONS
Contraindicated in: Hypersensitivity. **Use cautiously in:** Aortic stenosis, conditions associated with reduced cardiac output, impaired renal function, pulmonary stenosis. **Pregnancy/Lactation:** No well-controlled trials to establish safety. Benefits must outweigh risks. May result in reduced uterine blood flow with fetal hypoxia/bradycardia.

PREPARATION
Availability: 50 mg/mL, 10 mL amp/vial. **Infusion:** Dilute 500 mg in at least 50 mL of compatible IV solution.

STABILITY/STORAGE
Vial: Store at room temperature. **Infusion:** Stable for 24 hr at room temperature.

ADMINISTRATION
General: For short-term use only. **IV Push:** Give rapidly over 1 min. **Intermittent Infusion:** Give over at least 8 minutes. Usual range 10–30 min. **Continuous Infusion:** Infuse at 1–2 mg/min. Maximum concentration 500 mg/50 mL. Administer via infusion pump.

COMPATIBILITY
Solution: Dextrose solutions, lactated Ringer's, sodium chloride solutions. **Y-site:** Amiodarone, amrinone, dobutamine, famotidine, isoproterenol, nitroglycerin, procainamide, ranitidine.

INCOMPATIBILITY
Syringe: Phenytoin.

ADVERSE EFFECTS
CNS: Dizziness, lightheadedness. **CV:** Angina, bradycardia, hypoten-sion (postural and supine), proarrhythmic effect, transient hypertension. **Resp:** Shortness of breath. **GI:** Diarrhea, nausea, vomiting. **Hypersens:** Erythematous macular rash. **Other:** Hyperthermia.

DRUG INTERACTIONS
Antiarrhythmics: Additive antiarrhythmic effects. **Digitalis:** Additive digoxin toxic effects.

NURSING CONSIDERATIONS
Assessment
General:
Continuous ECG, hourly blood pressure monitoring.
Physical:
GI tract.

Intervention/Rationale
IV infusion must be gradually reduced and tapered, depending on presence of ectopy. ● Patient should be recumbent to avoid postural hypotension. ● Assess for development of GI symptoms, especially nausea/vomiting.

Patient/Family Education
Change positions slowly to avoid orthostatic hypotension. Notify nurse/physician immediately if nausea, dizziness, or lightheadedness is noted.

BUMETANIDE
(byoo-met′-a-nide)
Trade Name(s): Bumex
Classification(s): Loop diuretic
Pregnancy Category: C

PHARMACODYNAMICS/KINETICS
Mechanism of Action: Inhibits sodium and chloride reabsorption in the as-

In the Adverse Effects section, underline indicates most frequent; CAPS indicates life threatening.

cending loop of Henle. Increases excretion of sodium, chloride, potassium, hydrogen, calcium, magnesium, ammonium, phosphate, and bicarbonate. Dilates renal vasculature and increases renal blood flow. **Onset of Action:** Within minutes. **Peak Effect:** 15–45 min. **Duration of Action:** 4–6 hr. **Distribution:** Highly protein bound. **Metabolism/Elimination:** Metabolized by the liver. Excreted largely unchanged by the kidneys. **Half-Life:** 1.0–1.5 hr.

INDICATIONS/DOSAGE

Edema associated with CHF, hepatic or renal disease; mild to moderate hypertension

Adult: 0.5–1 mg. May repeat every 2–3 hr. Not to exceed 10mg/day. Increase dose with impaired renal function (may require doses greater than 2 mg). 1 mg bumetanide is equivalent to 40 mg furosemide. IV dose should be reserved for patients with impaired GI absorption or in whom oral administration is not possible.

CONTRAINDICATIONS/ PRECAUTIONS

Contraindicated in: Anuria, hepatic coma, hypersensitivity, severe electrolyte imbalance. **Use cautiously in:** Allergy to sulfa drugs/furosemide, hypokalemia, hyperuricemia, increasing BUN and creatinine, volume and electrolyte depletion. **Pregnancy/Lactation:** No well-controlled trials to establish safety. Limited data have not revealed evidence of fetal harm. Benefits must outweigh risks. **Pediatrics:** Safety and efficacy not established.

PREPARATION

Availability: 0.25 mg/mL. 2 mL ampules and 2, 4, and 10 ml vials. **Infusion:** Dilute in compatible IV solution to physician specified volume.

STABILITY/STORAGE

Vial: Store at room temperature. Protect from light. Discolors when exposed to light. **Infusion:** Solution should be freshly prepared and used within 24 hr.

ADMINISTRATION

IV Push: Give slowly over 1–2 min. **Infusion:** Give per physician specified rate.

COMPATIBILITY

Solution: Dextrose solutions, lactated Ringer's, Ringer's injection, sodium chloride solutions. **Syringe:** Doxapram.

ADVERSE EFFECTS

CNS: Mood or mental status changes, dizziness, headache. **CV:** Chest pain, hypotension, irregular heartbeat. **GI:** Abdominal cramps, diarrhea, dry mouth, nausea, vomiting. **Endo:** Hyperglycemia. **Fld/Lytes:** Dehydration, electrolyte depletion (specifically hypokalemia, hypochloremia, hyponatremia), metabolic acidosis, hyperuricemia. **Heme:** Hyperuricemia. **Hypersens:** Pruritus, rash, urticaria. **Other:** Ototoxicity.

TOXICITY/OVERDOSE

Signs/Symptoms: Severe electrolyte depletion, circulatory collapse, thromboembolic episodes (caused by too vigorous diuresis, especially in the elderly). **Treatment:** Fluid/electrolyte replacement, supportive therapy.

In the Adverse Effects section, underline indicates most frequent; CAPS indicates life threatening.

B

DRUG INTERACTIONS
Aminoglycosides, amphotericin B, nephrotoxic agents: Increased risk of ototoxicity/nephrotoxicity. **Anticoagulants:** Decreased anticoagulant effect. **Antihypertensives:** Additive hypotensive effect. **Digitalis glycosides:** Increased potential for digitalis toxicity and hypokalemic-induced dysrhythmia. **Diuretics:** Concurrent use enhances volume depletion. **Dopamine:** Increased diuretic effect. **Lithium:** Decreased excretion, possible lithium toxicity. **Neuromuscular blocking agents:** Enhanced neuromuscular blockade.

NURSING CONSIDERATIONS

Assessment
General:
Blood pressure, ECG changes, intake/output ratio, daily weight.
Physical:
Hearing function, musculoskeletal system.
Lab Alterations:
Monitor electrolytes (serum potassium daily), hepatic and renal function tests, serum glucose and uric acid concentrations prior to and during therapy.

Intervention/Rationale
Assess for signs/symptoms of dehydration (skin turgor, mucous membranes, hypotension). Drug may lead to profound water/electrolyte depletion. Monitor urine output to assess therapeutic response. Drug may cause muscle weakness and cramps. ● Assess patients receiving cardiac glycosides for signs/symptoms of digitalis toxicity (nausea, vomiting, anorexia, visual disturbances, confusion, cardiac rhythm

disturbances), especially when hypokalemia is present.

Patient/Family Education
Change positions slowly to avoid orthostatic hypotension. Notify nurse/physician if muscle cramps/weakness occur.

BUPRENORPHINE
(byoo-pre-nor′-feen)
Trade Name(s): Buprenex
Classification(s): Narcotic agonist–antagonist analgesic
Pregnancy Category: C
Controlled Substance Schedule: V

PHARMACODYNAMICS/KINETICS
Mechanism of Action: Binds to CNS opiate receptors. **Onset of Action:** Within 15 min. **Peak Effect:** 1 hr. **Duration of Action:** 6 hr. **Distribution:** 96% protein bound. **Metabolism/Elimination:** Metabolized by the liver. Eliminated via feces. **Half-Life:** 2–3 hr.

INDICATIONS/DOSAGE

Management of moderate to severe pain
Adult: Initial dose 0.3 mg. Repeat once 30–60 min after initial dose, then every 6 hr as needed. Maximum dose 0.6 mg/dose. Dose dependent on severity of pain and patient response. 0.3 mg is equivalent to 10 mg morphine. Decrease dose by 50% in elderly, debilitated, and patients receiving CNS depressants.

Reversal of fentanyl-induced anesthesia (*unlabeled use*)

In the Adverse Effects section, <u>underline</u> indicates most frequent;
CAPS indicates life threatening.

Adult: 0.3–0.8 mg 1–4 hr after anesthesia induction and 30 min before surgery completion.

CONTRAINDICATIONS/ PRECAUTIONS
Contraindicated in: Hypersensitivity. **Use cautiously in:** Adrenal cortical insufficiency, acute alcoholism, compromised respiratory function, CNS depression/coma, concomitant use of other respiratory depressants, elderly/debilitated, head injury/ increased intracranial pressure, myxedema/hypothyroidism, narcotic drug dependence, prostatic hypertrophy, severe hepatic, pulmonary, or renal function, toxic psychoses, urethral stricture. **Pregnancy/Lactation:** No well-controlled trials to establish safety. Benefits must outweigh risks. Produced fetal death in animal studies. **Pediatrics:** Safety and efficacy not established for children under the age of 13.

PREPARATION
Availability: 0.3 mg/mL. 1 mL ampules. **Infusion (*unlabeled use*):** Dilute to final concentration of 15 mcg/mL in sodium chloride.

STABILITY/STORAGE
Vial: Store at room temperature. Protect from light.

ADMINISTRATION
General: Use extreme caution with administration, especially with initial dose. **IV Push:** May be given undiluted slowly over 1–2 minutes. **Infusion (*unlabeled use*):** 25–250 mcg/ hr. Give via infusion device.

COMPATIBILITY
Solution: Dextrose solution, lactated Ringer's, sodium chloride solutions.

Syringe: Droperidol, glycopyrrolate, haloperidol, midazolam, scopolamine.

ADVERSE EFFECTS
CNS: Coma, confusion, convulsions, agitation, <u>dizziness</u>, <u>sedation</u>, depression, dreaming, dysphoria, euphoria, fatigue, hallucinations, <u>headache</u>, malaise, nervousness, paresthesias, psychosis, slurred speech, tremors, <u>vertigo</u>, weakness. **Ophtho:** Blurred vision, conjunctivitis, diplopia, miosis (high doses). **CV:** <u>Hypotension</u>, second-degree heart block type I (Wenckebach), tachycardia, bradycardia, hypertension. **Resp:** APNEA, cyanosis, dyspnea, <u>hypoventilation</u>. **GI:** Anorexia, constipation, dry mouth, dyspepsia, flatulence, <u>nausea</u>, <u>vomiting</u>. **GU:** Urinary retention. **Hypersens:** Pruritus, rash. **Other:** Tinnitus, <u>sweating</u>.

TOXICITY/OVERDOSE
Signs/Symptoms: CNS and respiratory depression with large doses (over 6 mg). **Treatment:** Monitor cardiac and respiratory status. Maintain patent airway. Administer supplemental oxygen, ventilator support, IV fluids, vasopressors and other supportive measures. **Antidote(s):** Naloxone may partially reverse respiratory depression. Doxapram may be used as a respiratory stimulant.

DRUG INTERACTIONS
Benzodiazepines, diazepam: Enhanced respiratory and cardiovascular effects. **MAO inhibitors:** Additive CNS depression. **CNS depressants, general anesthetics, narcotic analgesics, phenothiazines, tran-**

In the Adverse Effects section, <u>underline</u> indicates most frequent; CAPS indicates life threatening.

63

quilizers, sedative hypnotics: Additive CNS depression.

NURSING CONSIDERATIONS

Assessment
General:
Pain assessment (assess type, location, severity, radiation, alleviating/aggravating factors before and after administration), vital signs.

Intervention/Rationale
Prolonged use may lead to physical and psychological dependence (potential low). Narcotic dependent patients may experience withdrawal symptoms up to 15 days after discontinuation because of the drug's antagonist effect. Lower narcotic doses may be required when nonnarcotics are concomitantly prescribed.

Patient/Family Education
Have patient request pain medication before pain becomes severe. Inform nurse if pain medication does not relieve pain. Medication may cause drowsiness or dizziness. Call for assistance with ambulation. Avoid alcohol/CNS depressant use during therapy. Cough, turn, and deep breathe to avoid atelectasis.

BUTORPHANOL
(byoo-tor′-fa-nole)
Trade Name(s): Stadol
Classification(s): Narcotic agonist–antagonist analgesic
Pregnancy Category: Unknown

PHARMACODYNAMICS/KINETICS
Mechanism of Action: Binds to CNS opiate receptors. May exert limbic system effect. **Onset of Action:** 1 min. **Peak Effect:** 4–5 min. **Duration of Action:** 2–4 hr. **Distribution:** Distributed throughout the body, especially in liver, kidneys, and intestines. **Metabolism/Elimination:** Metabolized by the liver. Inactive metabolites excreted by the kidneys. **Half-Life:** 2.5–3.5 hr.

INDICATIONS/DOSAGE

Relief of moderate to severe pain, preoperative sedation, relief of intrapartum pain
Adult: 0.5–2.0 mg every 3–4 hr as needed.

CONTRAINDICATIONS/PRECAUTIONS
Contraindicated in: Hypersensitivity, patients physically dependent on or currently receiving narcotics (may precipitate withdrawal). **Use cautiously in:** Bronchial asthma, head injury/increased intracranial pressure, MI (limit use to patients sensitive to morphine sulfate or meperidine), obstructive respiratory diseases (give lower dose), renal or hepatic impairment, respiratory depression, patients prone to drug abuse or who are emotionally unstable. **Pregnancy/Lactation:** Safe use in pregnancy prior to labor not established. May be used safely during labor. Not for use in women delivering premature infants. Distributes into breast milk. Not recommended for breastfeeding mothers. **Pediatrics:** Safety and efficacy not established.

PREPARATION
Availability: 1 mg/mL in 1 mL vial. 2 mg/mL in 1, 2, and 10 mL vials.

In the Adverse Effects section, <u>underline</u> indicates most frequent;
CAPS indicates life threatening.

STABILITY/STORAGE
Vial: Store at room temperature.

ADMINISTRATION
IV Push: May be given undiluted over 3–5 minutes.

COMPATIBILITY
Solution: Dextrose solutions. **Syringe:** Atropine, chlorpromazine, cimetidine, diphenhydramine, droperidol, fentanyl, hydroxyzine, meperidine, midazolam, morphine, pentazocine, perphenazine, prochlorperazine, promethazine, scopolamine. **Y-site:** Enalaprilat, esmolol, labetalol.

INCOMPATIBILITY
Syringe: Dimenhydrinate, pentobarbital.

ADVERSE EFFECTS
CNS: <u>Sedation</u>, <u>confusion</u>, <u>dizziness</u>, <u>lightheadedness</u>, <u>vertigo</u>, agitation, euphoria, <u>floating feeling</u>, hallucinations, <u>headache</u>, <u>lethargy</u>, unusual dreams. **Ophtho:** Blurred vision, diplopia. **CV:** Hypertension, hypotension, palpitations. **Resp:** Respiratory depression. **GI:** <u>Dry mouth</u>, <u>nausea</u>, vomiting. **Derm:** <u>Clamminess</u>. **Hypersens:** Hives, pruritus, rash. **Other:** <u>Sweating</u>.

TOXICITY/OVERDOSE
Signs/Symptoms: Respiratory depression, severe hypotension. **Treatment:** Supportive measures (IV fluids, supplemental oxygen, ventilatory support, vasopressors). **Antidote(s):** Naloxone.

DRUG INTERACTIONS
Barbiturate anesthetics, droperidol, MAO inhibitors, narcotic analgesics, phenothiazines, tranquilizers: Additive pharmacologic effects.

NURSING CONSIDERATIONS
Assessment
General:
Pain assessment (assess type, location, severity, radiation, alleviating/aggravating factors before and after administration), vital signs.

Intervention/Rationale
Narcotic dependent patients may experience withdrawal symptoms after discontinuation.

Patient/Family Education
Have patient request pain medication before pain becomes too severe. Inform nurse if pain medication does not relieve pain. Medication may cause drowsiness or dizziness. Avoid activities requiring mental alertness, call for assistance with ambulation. Avoid alcohol use. Cough, turn, and deep breathe to avoid atelectasis.

CALCIUM CHLORIDE
(kal'-see-um klor'-ide)
Classification(s): Calcium salt, electrolyte
Pregnancy Category: C

PHARMACODYNAMICS/KINETICS
Mechanism of Action: Precise mechanism unknown. Calcium is necessary for bone/clot formation, muscle contraction, and integrity of nervous system. **Onset of Action:** Immediate. **Therapeutic Serum Levels:** 8.5–10.0 mg/dL. **Distribution:** Primarily incorporated into bone. Small percentage distributed to intra/extracellular fluid. Moderately protein bound. **Metabolism/Elimination:** In-

In the Adverse Effects section, <u>underline</u> indicates most frequent;
CAPS indicates life threatening.

65

soluble salts eliminated 80% via feces and 20% in urine.

INDICATIONS/DOSAGE

Cardiac arrest

Adult: 6.8–13.6 mEq (0.5–1.0 g) per dose or 0.027–0.054 mEq (2–4 mg)/kg/dose. Use only if precipitated by hyperkalemia, hypocalcemia, or calcium channel blocker toxicity. *Pediatric:* 0.27–0.68 mEq (20–50 mg)/kg/dose every 10 minutes. Repeat in 10 min if indicated. Subsequent doses are based on calcium deficit. Maximum dose 13.6 mEq (1 g/dose)

Hyperkalemia with cardiac toxicity

Adult: 6.8–13.6 mEq (0.5–1.0 g). Dose should be adjusted according to ECG response.

Hypocalcemic tetany

Adult: 4.0–13.6 mEq (0.3–1.0 g). Repeat every 6–8 hr until response is seen. *Pediatric:* 0.5–0.68 mEq (36–50 mg)/kg/dose. Repeat every 6–8 hr until response is seen. *Neonate:* 2.4 mEq (175 mg)/kg/day. Repeat every 6–8 hr until response is seen.

Magnesium intoxication

Adult: 6.8 mEq (500 mg). Observe patient closely for signs of recovery before administering further doses.

Treatment of hypocalcemia, electrolyte replenishment

Adult: 6.8–13.2 mEq (0.5–1.0 g). May repeat every 1–3 days as needed, depending on patient response. *Pediatric:* 0.34 mEq (25 mg)/kg/dose.

CONTRAINDICATIONS/PRECAUTIONS

Contraindicated in: Digitalis toxicity risk, hypercalcemia, ventricular fibrillation. **Use cautiously in:** Cardiac disease, concomitant use of digitalis glycosides, impaired renal function, sarcoidosis. **Pregnancy/Lactation:** No well-controlled trials to establish safety. Crosses the placenta. Benefits must outweigh risks. Distributed into breast milk.

PREPARATION

Availability: 10% solution (100 mg/mL). 10 mL ampules, vials, and syringes. 1 g contains 270 mg (13.6 mEq) elemental calcium. **Infusion:** Dilute to a final concentration of 2%–10% in compatible diluent.

STABILITY/STORAGE

Vial: Store at room temperature. **Infusion:** Prepare just prior to administration. Stable for 24 hr at room temperature.

ADMINISTRATION

General: Too rapid administration may precipitate side effects. Do not allow extravasation (drug is irritating to tissues and will cause sloughing or necrosis). Recommend to physician to infiltrate area with 1% procaine and hyaluronidase to reduce venospasm and dilute calcium. Heat may be helpful. Assess IV site for patency. Administer through a small-bore needle into a large vein to prevent extravasation and the bolus effect on cardiac tissues. Emergency carts may contain calcium chloride/gluconate (note carefully—doses are not equivalent). **IV Push:** May be given undiluted by slow injection. Not to ex-

In the Adverse Effects section, <u>underline</u> indicates most frequent; CAPS indicates life threatening.

ceed 0.5–1.0 mL/min. **Intermittent Infusion:** Do not exceed 0.68 mEq (50 mg)/min via infusion device.

COMPATIBILITY
Solution: Dextrose solutions, sodium chloride solutions. **Y-site:** Amrinone, dobutamine, epinephrine, esmolol, morphine.

INCOMPATIBILITY
Solution: Fat emulsion. **Y-site:** Sodium bicarbonate.

ADVERSE EFFECTS
CNS: Tingling sensations, depression. **CV:** CARDIAC ARREST, bradycardia, irregular heartbeat, hypotension. **GI:** Anorexia, bitter taste in mouth, <u>constipation</u>, diarrhea, increased serum amylase, nausea, vomiting. **Fld/Lytes:** Hypercalcemia. **Other:** Burning at injection site, necrosis/sloughing at injection site, sweating.

TOXICITY/OVERDOSE
Signs/Symptoms: Hypercalcemia (confusion, somnolence). Total serum calcium concentration over 12 mg/dL may lead to cardiac arrest. **Treatment:** *Mild hypercalcemia:* Withhold additional calcium. *Moderate to severe hypercalcemia:* Calcitonin, chelating agents, corticosteroids, hydration, saline loop diuretics.

DRUG INTERACTIONS
Calcitonin: Antagonizes effects in treatment of hypercalcemia. **Calcium channel blockers:** Calcium may antagonize verapamil effects. **Calcium-containing medications, vitamin D:** Hypercalcemia (long-term therapy). **Digitalis glycosides, potassium supplements:** Precipitation of cardiac dysrhythmias. **Magnesium sulfate:** Neutralizes effects. **Tetracycline:** Tetracycline rendered inactive.

NURSING CONSIDERATIONS
Assessment
General:
Vital signs, continuous ECG.
Lab Alterations:
Monitor calcium levels, transient elevations in the first hour of serum II-hydroxycorticosteroid concentrations. False-negative results serum/urinary magnesium (Titan Yellow method).

Intervention/Rationale
Monitor calcium levels frequently to avoid hypercalcemia. Observe for signs of hypocalcemia (ECG changes, laryngospasm, muscle cramps, paresthesias, seizures, tetany). ● Patient should remain recumbent for ½ hour after administration to prevent orthostatic hypotension.

Patient/Family Education
Explain purpose of drug and theapeutic outcome. Inform physician/nurse of signs/symptoms of hypocalcemia/pain at injection site.

CALCIUM GLUCONATE
(kal′-see-um gloo′-koh-nate)
Classification(s): Calcium salt, electrolyte
Pregnancy Category: C

PHARMACODYNAMICS/KINETICS
Mechanism of Action: Precise mechanism unknown. Calcium is neces-

In the Adverse Effects section, <u>underline</u> indicates most frequent; CAPS indicates life threatening.

67

C

sary for bone/clot formation, muscle contraction, and integrity of nervous system. **Onset of Action:** Immediate. **Therapeutic Serum Levels:** 8.5–10.0 mg/dL. **Distribution:** Primarily incorporated into bone. Small percentage distributed to intra/extracellular fluid. Moderately protein bound. **Metabolism/Elimination:** Insoluble salts eliminated 80% via feces and 20% in urine.

INDICATIONS/DOSAGE

Emergency elevation of serum calcium

Adult: 7–14 mEq. Repeat every 1–3 days if needed. *Pediatric:* 1–7 mEq. Repeat every 1–3 days if needed. *Neonate:* < 1 mEq. Repeat every 1–3 days if needed. Dose not to exceed 1 mEq (200 mg).

Exchange transfusion

Adult: 1.35 mEq calcium/100 mL of citrated blood. *Pediatric:* 0.45 mEq/100 mL of exchanged citrated blood.

Hyperkalemia with cardiac toxicity

Adult: 2.25–15.0 mEq. Monitor ECG and repeat in 1–2 min if needed.

Magnesium intoxication

Adult: 0.5–9.0 mEq, subsequent doses based on patient response.

Treatment of hypocalcemia, electrolyte replacement

Adult: 2.3–9.2 mEq daily as needed. May require higher dosages. *Pediatric:* 2.3 mEq/kg/day in divided doses. May require higher dosages.

CONTRAINDICATIONS/ PRECAUTIONS

Contraindicated in: Digitalis toxicity risk, hypercalcemia, ventricular fibrillation. **Use cautiously in:** Cardiac disease, concomitant use of digitalis glycosides, impaired renal function, sarcoidosis. **Pregnancy/ Lactation:** No well-controlled trials to establish safety. Crosses the placenta. Benefits must outweigh risks. Distributed into breast milk.

PREPARATION

Availability: 10% solutions (100 mg/ mL). 10 mL amps, syringes, and vials. 50, 100, and 200 mL vials. 1 g contains 90 mg (4.6 mEq) elemental calcium. **Infusion:** Dilute to physician specified volume in compatible diluent.

STABILITY/STORAGE

Vial: Store at room temperature. **Infusion:** Prepare just prior to administration. Stable for 24 hr at room temperature.

ADMINISTRATION

General: May precipitate in vial. Warming may dissolve crystals. Assess IV site for patency. Administer through a small-bore needle into a large vein to prevent extravasation and the bolus effect on cardiac tissues. Recommend to physician to infiltrate area with 1% procaine and hyaluronidase to reduce venospasm and dilute calcium. Heat may be helpful. **IV Push:** Do not exceed 0.5 mL/min (side effects are frequently the result of too rapid administration). **Intermittent/Continuous Infusion:** Do not exceed 1 mEq (200 mg)/min.

In the Adverse Effects section, <u>underline</u> indicates most frequent; CAPS indicates life threatening.

COMPATIBILITY

Solution: Amino acids 4.25%/dextrose 25%, dextrose solutions, lactated Ringer's, sodium chloride solutions. **Y-site:** Cefazolin, dobutamine, enalaprilat, epinephrine, famotidine, heparin, hydrocortisone, labetalol, netilmicin, potassium chloride, tolazoline, vitamin B complex with C.

INCOMPATIBILITY

Solution: Fat emulsion. **Syringe:** Metoclopramide.

ADVERSE EFFECTS

CNS: Tingling sensation, depression. **CV:** CARDIAC ARREST, <u>bradycardia</u>, irregular heartbeat, hypotension. **GI:** Anorexia, bitter taste in mouth, <u>constipation</u>, diarrhea, nausea, vomiting. **Fld/Lytes:** Hypercalcemia. **Other:** <u>Burning at injection site</u>, necrosis/sloughing at injection site, sweating.

TOXICITY/OVERDOSE

Signs/Symptoms: Hypercalcemia (confusion, somnolence). Total serum calcium concentration over 12 mg/dL may lead to cardiac arrest. **Treatment:** *Mild hypercalcemia:* Withhold additional calcium. *Moderate to severe hypercalcemia:* Calcitonin, chelating agents, corticosteroids, hydration, saline loop diuretics.

DRUG INTERACTIONS

Calcitonin: Antagonizes effects in treatment of hypercalcemia. **Calcium channel blockers:** Calcium may antagonize verapamil effects. **Calcium-containing medications, vitamin D:** Hypercalcemia (long-term therapy). **Digitalis glycosides, potassium supplements:** Precipitation of cardiac dysrhythmias. **Magnesium sulfate:** Neutralizes effects. **Tetracycline:** Tetracycline rendered inactive.

NURSING CONSIDERATIONS

Assessment
General:
Vital signs, continuous ECG.
Lab Alterations:
Monitor calcium levels, transient elevations in the first hour of serum II-hydroxycorticosteroid concentrations, false-negative results serum/urinary magnesium (Titan Yellow method).

Intervention/Rationale
Monitor calcium levels frequently to avoid hypercalcemia. Observe for signs of hypocalcemia (ECG changes, laryngospasm, muscle cramps, paresthesias, seizures, tetany). ● Patient should remain recumbent for ½ hour after administration to prevent orthostatic hypotension.

Patient/Family Education
Explain purpose of drug and therapeutic outcome. Inform physician/nurse of signs/symptoms of hypocalcemia/pain at injection site.

CARBOPLATIN

(kar-bow-plat'-in)
Trade Name(s): Paraplatin
Classification(s): Antineoplastic
Pregnancy Category: D

PHARMACODYNAMICS/KINETICS

Mechanism of Action: Interferes with DNA synthesis. **Distribution:** Distrib-

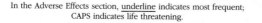

In the Adverse Effects section, <u>underline</u> indicates most frequent;
CAPS indicates life threatening.

69

uted in high concentrations in liver, kidneys, skin, and tumors. **Metabolism/Elimination:** Eliminated unchanged by the kidneys. **Half-Life:** Carboplatin: 2.6–5.9 hr. Protein bound platinum: 5 days.

INDICATIONS/DOSAGE

Treatment of recurrent ovarian carcinoma (palliative)

Adult: Single agent: 360 mg/m² IV every 4 weeks. Do not repeat dose until neutrophils are > 2000 mm³ and platelets are > 100,000 mm³. Reduce dose in renal impairment (200–250 mg/m²). Dosage adjustments are based on neutrophil/platelet counts and renal function.

CONTRAINDICATIONS/ PRECAUTIONS

Contraindicated in: Severe allergic reactions to cisplatin, other platinum, or mannitol, severe bone marrow depression/significant bleeding. **Use cautiously in:** Patients with concomitant aminoglycoside. **Pregnancy/Lactation:** No well-controlled trials to establish safety. Drug is teratogenic in rodents. Benefits must outweigh risks. Discontinue breast feeding during carboplatin treatment.

PREPARATION

Availability: 50, 150, and 450 mg vials. **Reconstitution:** Dilute each 50 mg with 5 mL sterile water for injection. Final concentration 10 mg/mL. **Infusion:** May further dilute to 0.5 mg/mL concentration with compatible solution.

STABILITY/STORAGE

Vial: Store at room temperature. Reconstituted vial stable for 8 hr at

room temperature. Protect from light. **Infusion:** Stable for up to 24 hr at room temperature.

ADMINISTRATION

General: Handle drug with care and adhere to institutional guidelines for the handling of chemotherapeutic/cytotoxic agents. Monitor IV to avoid extravasation (tissue necrosis may occur). No pretreatment or post-treatment hydration is required. Aluminum-containing IV needles or sets should not be used. **Intermittent Infusion:** Infuse over at least 15 min.

COMPATIBILITY

Solution: Dextrose solutions, sodium chloride solutions. **Y-site:** Ondansetron.

ADVERSE EFFECTS

CNS: Central neurotoxicity, peripheral neuropathies. **Ophtho:** Visual disturbances. **GI:** Diarrhea, constipation, elevated alkaline phosphatase / AST(SGOT) / bilirubin, nausea, vomiting. **Renal:** Elevated BUN/serum creatinine. **Derm:** Alopecia. **Fld/Lytes:** Hypocalcemia, hypokalemia, hypomagnesemia, hyponatremia. **Heme:** Thrombocytopenia, neutropenia, leukopenia, bleeding, anemia. **Nadir:** 21 days. **Hypersens:** ANAPHYLACTIC-LIKE REACTIONS, erythema, pruritus, rash, urticaria. **Other:** Ototoxicity.

TOXICITY/OVERDOSE

Signs/Symptoms: Complications and symptoms of overdosage are a result of bone marrow depression or hepatic toxicity. **Treatment:** Supportive and symptomatic treatment.

In the Adverse Effects section, underline indicates most frequent; CAPS indicates life threatening.

DRUG INTERACTIONS
Aminoglycosides: Increased nephro/audiologic toxicity.

NURSING CONSIDERATIONS
Assessment
General:
Signs/symptoms of anaphylaxis, vital signs.
Physical:
GI tract, infectious disease status, hematopoietic system.
Lab Alterations:
Monitor electrolytes, renal, hematopoietic, and hepatic function prior to and frequently during therapy.

Intervention/Rationale
Anaphylaxis can occur within minutes of administration. ● Bone marrow suppression is dose-related and is increased in patients with impaired renal function. ● Assure that proper antiemetic regimens are prescribed and given regularly to prevent nausea/vomiting.

Patient/Family Education
Perform thorough oral hygiene with a soft toothbrush or sponge brush in the morning and after each meal. Observe closely for signs of infection (fever, sore throat, fatigue), evidence of bleeding (gums, nosebleeds, melena, easy bruising). Avoid crowded environment and persons with known infections. Avoid consumption of fresh fruits and vegetables (during neutropenic periods). Hair loss may affect body image. Use consistent and reliable contraception throughout the duration of therapy due to potential teratogenic and mutagenic effects of drug. Avoid alcohol or over-the-counter products containing aspirin or ibuprofen.

CARDIOPLEGIC SOLUTION
(kar-dee-o-pleege'-ik)
Trade Name(s): Plegisol
Classification(s): Cardioplegic agent
Pregnancy Category: C

PHARMACODYNAMICS/KINETICS
Mechanism of Action: Causes prompt arrest of cardiac electromechanical activity. Combats intracellular ion losses. Buffers ischemic acidosis. Provides a relaxed/bloodless field during operation.

INDICATIONS/DOSAGE

Induces cardiac arrest during open heart surgery, in conjunction with ischemia and hypothermia

Adult/Pediatric/Neonate: Initial infusion rate is 300 mL/m²/min. Solution may be reinfused if electromechanical activity persists or recurs at a rate of 300 mL/m²/min for 2 min. May repeat every 20–30 min, or sooner, if needed.

CONTRAINDICATIONS/PRECAUTIONS
Contraindicated in: Not for IV injection. **Pregnancy/Lactation:** No well-controlled trials to establish safety. Benefits must outweigh risks.

PREPARATION
Availability: Single dose 1000 mL plastic containers. Contains 17.6 mg calcium chloride dihydrate,

In the Adverse Effects section, <u>underline</u> indicates most frequent; CAPS indicates life threatening.

71

325.3 mg magnesium chloride hexahydrate, 119.3 mg potassium chloride and 643 mg sodium chloride per 100 mL. Do not administer without the addition of 8.4% sodium bicarbonate injection.

STABILITY/STORAGE

Infusion: Store at room temperature. Protect from freezing and extreme heat. Use within 24 hr of mixing. Solution contains no preservatives and is intended for single use only. Discard unused portion. Do not use unless solution is clear.

ADMINISTRATION

General: Not intended for IV use. Use only for instillation into cardiac vasculature during cardiopulmonary bypass. Intended for use only by those trained in the procedure of open heart surgery. Infusion is rapidly administered into aortic root after cardiopulmonary bypass and aortic cross-clamp has been initiated. **Continuous Infusion:** Add 10 mL (840 mg) of 8.4% sodium bicarbonate injection to each 1000 mL of cardioplegic solution just prior to administration to adjust pH to approximately 7.8 (measure at room temperature). Cool buffered solution with added sodium bicarbonate to 4°C prior to administration.

ADVERSE EFFECTS

Potential hazards of open heart surgery. **CV:** DYSRHYTHMIAS, ECG abnormalities.

TOXICITY/OVERDOSE

Signs/Symptoms: Unnecessary dilation of myocardial vasculature, leakage into perivascular myocardium, cardiac tissue edema.

NURSING CONSIDERATIONS

Assessment
General:
Continuous ECG monitoring, myocardial temperature monitoring (must maintain hypothermia).

Intervention/Rationale
Induces cardiac standstill. ● Maintenance of hypothermia minimizes oxygen demand/consumption.

CARMUSTINE (BCNU)
(kar-mus'-teen)
Trade Name(s): BiCNU
Classification(s): Antineoplastic
Pregnancy Category: D

PHARMACODYNAMICS/KINETICS

Mechanism of Action: Alkylates DNA and RNA, interferes with synthesis. **Distribution:** Highly lipid-soluble. Crosses blood–brain barrier. **Metabolism/Elimination:** Rapidly converted to active metabolites by the liver. 60%–70% excreted by the kidneys. 10% excreted as respiratory CO_2. **Half-Life:** 15–30 min.

INDICATIONS/DOSAGE

Palliative treatment of brain tumors, multiple myelomas, Hodgkin's disease, and nonHodgkin's lymphomas

For use as a single agent in previously untreated patients.

Adult: 75–100 mg/m^2 for 2 successive days or 150–200 mg/m^2 as a single dose every 6–8 weeks. Base subsequent dose on patient's he-

In the Adverse Effects section, <u>underline</u> indicates most frequent; CAPS indicates life threatening.

matologic response. If platelet count < 75,000/mm^3 and leukocytes count < 3000/mm^3, give 70% of previous dose. If platelet count < 25,000/mm^3 and leukocytes count < 2000/mm^3, give 50% of previous dose.

CONTRAINDICATIONS/ PRECAUTIONS

Contraindicated in: Hypersensitivity. **Pregnancy/Lactation:** No well-controlled trials to establish safety. May cause fetal harm. Documented teratogenicity in rodents. Discontinue nursing or discontinue drug. **Pediatrics:** Safety and efficacy for use in children not established.

PREPARATION

Availability: 100 mg vials with 3 mL sterile diluent. Not intended as a multidose vial. **Reconstitution:** Dissolve powder with provided 3 mL of diluent and add 27 mL sterile water. Yields 3.3 mg/mL carmustine in 10% ethanol. Solution will be clear and colorless or yellowish. **Infusion:** May further dilute with 100–500 mL compatible IV fluid. Use glass containers only.

STABILITY/STORAGE

Vial: Store unopened vials in refrigerator. Unopened vials stable for 7 days at controlled room temperature. Do not use powder vials that have liquified and contain an oily film. Reconstituted solution stable for 8 hr at room temperature or 24 hr refrigerated. **Infusion:** Stable for 8 hr at room temperature and 48 hr refrigerated.

ADMINISTRATION

General: Handle according to institutional guidelines for handling of chemotherapeutic/cytotoxic agents.

Skin contact with the powder or solution may result in hyperpigmentation of area. If contact occurs, thoroughly flush skin or mucosa immediately with water. Avoid extravasation into local tissues. Rapid administration results in skin flushing. **Intermittent Infusion:** Infuse over 1–2 hr to avoid pain/burning at injection and intense skin flushing.

COMPATIBILITY

Solution: Dextrose solutions (only at 0.2 mg/mL final concentration), sodium chloride solutions. **Y-site:** Ondansetron.

ADVERSE EFFECTS

Ophtho: Ocular toxicity, suffusion of the conjunctiva. **Resp:** PULMONARY FIBROSIS/infiltrates (dose related: > 1400 mg/m^2 cumulative dose). **GI:** Reversible hepatotoxicity, <u>nausea</u>, <u>vomiting</u>. **Renal:** Azotemia, diminished kidney size, renal failure. **Heme:** <u>MYELOSUPPRESSION</u> (leukopenia, thrombocytopenia), anemia. *Nadir:* 6–8 weeks. **Other:** Burning at injection site, flushing (within 2 hr, lasting 4 hr).

TOXICITY/OVERDOSE

Signs/Symptoms: Severe myelosuppression. **Treatment:** Symptomatic and supportive.

DRUG INTERACTIONS

Cimetidine: Increased bone marrow suppression. **Digoxin:** Decreased digoxin serum levels. **Phenytoin:** Decreased phenytoin serum levels.

NURSING CONSIDERATIONS

Assessment
General:
Vital signs.

In the Adverse Effects section, <u>underline</u> indicates most frequent; CAPS indicates life threatening.

73

Physical:
Infectious disease status, hematopoietic system.
Lab Alterations:
Monitor electrolytes, renal, hematopoietic, and hepatic function prior to and frequently during therapy.

Intervention/Rationale
Bone marrow suppression is dose-related and is increased in patients with impaired renal function. ● Assure that proper antiemetic regimens are prescribed and given regularly to prevent nausea/vomiting.

Patient/Family Education
Perform thorough oral hygiene with a soft toothbrush or sponge brush in the morning and after each meal. Observe closely for signs of infection (fever, sore throat, fatigue), evidence of bleeding (gums, nosebleeds, melena, easy bruising). Avoid crowded environments and persons with known infections. Avoid consumption of fresh fruits and vegetables (during neutropenic periods). Hair loss may affect body image. Use consistent and reliable contraception throughout the duration of therapy due to potential teratogenic and mutagenic effects of drug. Avoid alcohol or over-the-counter products containing aspirin or ibuprofen.

CEFAMANDOLE
(sef-a-man'-dole)
Trade Name(s): Mandol
Classification(s): Cephalosporin antibiotic, second generation
Pregnancy Category: B

PHARMACODYNAMICS/KINETICS
Mechanism of Action: Bactericidal action, inhibition of bacterial cell wall synthesis. **Distribution:** Widely distributed to most tissues. Does not readily enter CSF except with inflammation. Concentration in bone is usually adequate. Distributed in high concentrations into bile. Protein binding: 70% **Metabolism/Elimination:** Primarily eliminated via kidneys. Removed by hemodialysis. **Half-Life:** 30–60 min. Prolonged in renal impairment.

INDICATIONS/DOSAGE

Treatment or prophylaxis of most gram-positive and many gram-negative organisms

(provides greater gram-negative coverage than first generation cephalosporins, excluding methicillin resistant *S. aureus* and *Pseudomonas* infections) associated with respiratory tract, genitourinary tract, skin/skin structure, bone/joint, and septicemia infections. Dosage interval may need to be adjusted in renal impairment.

Adult:
Uncomplicated UTI: 500 mg every 8 hr.
Complicated UTI: 0.5–1.0 g every 8 hr.
Pneumonia/Skin: 500 mg every 6 hr.
Severe Infections: 1 g every 4–6 hr. Up to 2 g every 4 hr. Not to exceed 12 g/day **Perioperative Prophylaxis: Preoperative:** 1–2 g ½ hr prior to surgery. **Postoperative:** 1–2 g every 6 hr for 24–48 hr after surgery. **C-section:** Administer dose just prior to surgery or just after cord clamping.

Pediatric: 50–100 mg/kg/day in divided doses every 4–8 hr. Not to exceed 150 mg/kg/day in divided

In the Adverse Effects section, underline indicates most frequent; CAPS indicates life threatening.

doses every 4–6 hr in severe infections. Not to exceed adult dosages or 12 g/day. **Perioperative Prophylaxis (> 3 months old):** *Preoperative:* 50–100 mg/kg ½ hr prior to surgery. *Postoperative:* 50–100 mg/kg every 6 hr for 24–48 hr after surgery.

CONTRAINDICATIONS/ PRECAUTIONS

Contraindicated in: Hypersensitivity to cephalosporins/penicillins or related antibiotics. **Use cautiously in:** Impaired renal function. **Pregnancy/ Lactation:** No well-controlled trials to establish safety. Appears to be safe for use in pregnancy when benefits outweigh risk. Crosses placenta. Identified in breast milk in small quantities with infant bowel flora changes and pharmacologic effects. **Pediatrics:** Consider risks and benefits in young children. Safety and efficacy has not been identified in children. Neonates have demonstrated decreased elimination of cephalosporins.

PREPARATION

Availability: 500 mg, 1 g, 2 g vials and 10 g bulk package. Contains 3.3 mEq sodium/g. **Reconstitution:** Dilute each 1 g with at least 10 mL sterile water for injection or compatible diluent for maximum concentration of 50–100 mg/mL. **Intermittent Infusion:** Dilute to a final concentration of 10–30 mg/mL or in 50–100 mL compatible solution.

STABILITY/STORAGE

Vial: Reconstituted vial/solution stable for 24 hr at room temperature and 4 days refrigerated.

ADMINISTRATION

IV Push: Give slowly over at least 3–5 min. **Intermittent Infusion:** Infuse over at least 15–30 min.

COMPATIBILITY

Solution: Amino acids, dextrose solutions, fat emulsion, mannitol, sodium chloride solutions, sterile water for injection. **Syringe:** Heparin. **Y-site:** Acyclovir, cyclophosphamide, hydromorphone, magnesium sulfate, meperidine, morphine, perphenazine.

INCOMPATIBILITY

Solution: Lactated Ringer's, Ringer's injection. **Syringe:** Cimetidine, gentamicin, tobramycin. **Y-site:** Hetastarch.

ADVERSE EFFECTS

CNS: Seizures (especially with high doses in renal impairment), confusion, dizziness, fatigue, headache, lethargy, paresthesia. **CV:** Hypotension. **Resp:** BRONCHOSPASM, interstitial pneumonitis. **GI:** Pseudomembranous colitis, anorexia, cholestasis, cholestatic jaundice, diarrhea, dysguesia, dyspepsia, elevated alkaline phosphatase, bilirubin, LDH, liver enzymes (AST [SGOT], ALT [SGPT], gamma-glutamyl transpeptidase [GGTP]), glossitis, nausea, vomiting. **GU:** Dysuria, genital moniliasis, genitoanal pruritus, hematuria, pyuria, vaginitis. **Renal:** Interstitial nephritis, decreased creatinine clearance, transient elevations in BUN and serum creatinine. **Heme:** Decreased platelet function, hypoprothrombinemia, AGRANULOCYTOSIS, leukopenia, transient neutropenia, thrombocytopenia, anemia, aplastic anemia, bleeding, eosinophilia,

In the Adverse Effects section, underline indicates most frequent; CAPS indicates life threatening.

75

lymphocytosis. **Hypersens:** ANA-PHYLAXIS, angioedema, Stevens Johnson syndrome, chest tightness, edema, eosinophilia, exfoliative dermatitis, joint pain, maculopapular rash, <u>moribilliform eruptions</u>, myalgias, <u>pruritus</u>, rash, <u>urticaria</u>. **Other:** Cellulitis, chills, diaphoresis, fever, flushing, inflammation, local swelling.

TOXICITY/OVERDOSE

Signs/Symptoms: High doses in renal impairment may cause seizures. **Treatment:** Discontinue agent when seizures begin. Administer anticonvulsant therapy and consider hemodialysis.

DRUG INTERACTIONS

Aminoglycosides: Potentiation of aminoglycoside nephrotoxicity. **Bacteriostatic antibiotics (chloramphenicol):** Potential interference with cephalosporin bactericidal action. **Ethanol:** Consumption of alcohol with or up to 72 hr after therapy may result in disulfiram-like reaction beginning within 30 mins of alcohol ingestion and lasting for several hours. **Oral anticoagulants:** Increased hypoprothrombinemic effects of anticoagulants. **Probenecid:** Decreased renal elimination of cephalosporins with potential increase in plasma levels.

NURSING CONSIDERATIONS

Assessment

General:

Allergy history, anaphylaxis.

Physical:

GI tract, signs/symptoms of superinfection (sore throat/stomatitis, vaginal discharge, perianal itching), infectious disease status.

Lab Alterations:

Monitor CBC, coagulation profile, renal, and hepatic function, false-positive direct Coombs', especially in azotemia, false-positive urine glucose with copper sulfate (Clinitest) (use Tes-Tape), false elevation urinary 17-ketosteroid values.

Intervention/Rationale

Patients with history of severe penicillin sensitivity may also have cephalosporin sensitivity (5%–10%). ● May cause pseudomembranous colitis (diarrhea, nausea, vomiting, fluid/electrolyte disturbances—notify physician and obtain culture for *C. difficile* toxin). ● Observe for signs/symptoms of anaphylaxis. ● Obtain cultures for sensitivity, first dose may be given while awaiting preliminary results.

Patient/Family Education

Complete course of therapy. Notify physician if there are any signs/symptoms of worsening infection (persistent fever/diarrhea) or signs of yeast infections (white patches in the mouth or vaginal discharge). Avoid alcohol during or up to 72 hr after stopping therapy (may result in acute alcohol intolerance that begins 30 minutes after alcohol ingestion and subsides 30 minutes to several hours afterwards; the reaction may occur up to 3 days after receiving the last dose).

CEFAZOLIN

(sef-a'-zoe-lin)

Trade Name(s): Ancef, Kefzol

Classification(s): Cephalosporin antibiotic, first generation

Pregnancy Category: B

PHARMACODYNAMICS/KINETICS

Mechanism of Action: Bactericidal action, inhibition of bacterial cell wall synthesis. **Distribution:** Widely distributed to most tissues. Does not readily enter CSF except with inflammation. Concentrations in bone are usually adequate with higher doses in acute inflammation. Protein binding: 80%–86%. **Metabolism/Elimination:** Primarily eliminated by the kidneys. Removed by hemodialysis. **Half-Life:** 90–120 min, prolonged in renal impairment.

INDICATIONS/DOSAGE

Treatment or prophylaxis of most gram-positive and some gram-negative organisms

(excluding methicillin resistant *S. aureus* and *Pseudomonas* infections) associated with respiratory tract, genitourinary tract, skin/skin structure, bone/joint, septicemia infections. Dosage interval may need to be adjusted in renal impairment.

Adult:
Mild Infections: 250–500 mg every 8 hr. **Moderate to Severe Infections:** 0.5–1.0 g every 6–8 hr. Up to 2 g every 4–6 hr. Not to exceed 12 g/day. **Pneumococcal Pneumonia:** 500 mg every 12 hr. **Uncomplicated UTI:** 1 g every 12 hr. **Perioperative Prophylaxis: Preoperative:** 1 g ½ prior to surgery. **Intraoperative (> 2 hr):** 0.5–1.0 g during surgery. **Postoperative:** 0.5–1.0 g every 6–8 hr for 24 hr after surgery.

Pediatric:
Mild to Moderate Infections: 25–50 mg/kg/day in divided doses every 6–8 hr. **Severe Infections:** Up to 100 mg/kg/day in divided doses every 6–8 hr. Not to exceed adult dosages or 6 g/day.

Neonate: Safety in infants < 1 month has not been established. **0–1 week:** 40 mg/kg/day in divided doses every 12 hr. **1–4 weeks:** 60 mg/kg/day in divided doses every 8 hr.

CONTRAINDICATIONS/ PRECAUTIONS

Contraindicated in: Hypersensitivity to cephalosporins/penicillins or related antibiotics. **Use cautiously in:** Impaired renal function. **Pregnancy/ Lactation:** No well-controlled trials to establish safety. Appears to be safe for use in pregnancy when benefits outweigh risk. Crosses placenta. Identified in breast milk in small quantities with potential infant bowel flora changes and pharmacologic effects. **Pediatrics:** Consider risks and benefits in young children. Safety and efficacy has not been identified in children < 1 month. Neonates have demonstrated decreased elimination of cephalosporins.

PREPARATION

Availability: 250 mg, 500 mg, 1 g vials and 5 g, 10 g, 20 g bulk package. Contains 2 mEq sodium/g. **Reconstitution:** Dilute each 500 mg or 1 g with at least 10 mL sterile water for injection or compatible diluent for maximum concentration of 100 mg/mL. **Infusion:** Dilute to a final concentration of 20 mg/mL or 50–100 mL compatible solution.

STABILITY/STORAGE

Vial: Store at room temperature. Reconstituted vial stable for 24 hr at

---

In the Adverse Effects section, underline indicates most frequent;
CAPS indicates life threatening.

room temperature and 4 days refrigerated. **Infusion:** Stable for 24 hr at room temperature and 10 days refrigerated.

ADMINISTRATION

IV Push: Give slowly over at least 3–5 min. **Intermittent Infusion:** Infuse over at least 15–30 min.

COMPATIBILITY

Solution: Amino acids 4.25%/dextrose 25%, dextrose solutions, lactated Ringer's, sodium chloride solutions, sterile water for injection. **Syringe:** Heparin, vitamin B complex. **Y-site:** Acyclovir, atracurium, calcium gluconate, cyclophosphamide, enalaprilat, esmolol, famotidine, foscarnet, hydromorphone, labetalol, lidocaine, magnesium sulfate, meperidine, morphine, multivitamins, ondansetron, pancuronium, perphenazine, vecuronium, vitamin B complex with C.

INCOMPATIBILITY

Syringe: Ascorbic acid, cimetidine, lidocaine, vitamin B with C.

ADVERSE EFFECTS

CNS: Seizures (especially with high doses in renal impairment), confusion, dizziness, fatigue, headache, lethargy, paresthesia. **CV:** Hypotension. **Resp:** BRONCHOSPASM, interstitial pneumonitis. **GI:** <u>Pseudomembranous colitis</u>, anorexia, cholestasis, diarrhea, dysguesia, dyspepsia, elevated alkaline phosphatase, bilirubin, LDH, liver enzymes (AST [SGOT], ALT [SGPT], GGTP), glossitis, <u>nausea</u>, <u>vomiting</u>. **GU:** Dysuria, genital moniliasis, genitoanal pruritus, hematuria, pyuria, vaginitis. **Renal:** Interstitial nephritis, transient elevations in

BUN and serum creatinine. **Heme:** Decreased platelet function, AGRANULOCYTOSIS, leukopenia, transient neutropenia, thrombocytopenia, anemia, aplastic anemia, bleeding, eosinophilia, lymphocytosis. **Hypersens:** ANAPHYLAXIS, angioedema, Stevens Johnson syndrome, chest tightness, edema, eosinophilia, exfoliative dermatitis, joint pain, maculopapular rash, <u>morbilliform eruptions</u>, myalgias, <u>pruritus</u>, rash, <u>urticaria</u>. **Other:** Cellulitis, chills, diaphoresis, fever, flushing, inflammation, local swelling.

TOXICITY/OVERDOSE

Signs/Symptoms: High doses in renal impairment may cause seizures. **Treatment:** Discontinue agent when seizures begin. Administer anticonvulsant therapy and consider hemodialysis.

DRUG INTERACTIONS

Aminoglycosides: Potentiation of aminoglycoside nephrotoxicity. **Bacteriostatic antibiotics (chloramphenicol):** Potential interference with cephalosporin bactericidal action. **Probenecid:** Decreased renal elimination of cephalosporins with potential increase in plasma levels.

NURSING CONSIDERATIONS

Assessment
General:
Allergy history, anaphylaxis.
Physical:
GI tract, signs/symptoms of superinfection (sore throat/stomatitis, vaginal discharge, perianal itching), infectious disease status.
Lab Alterations:
Monitor CBC, coagulation profile, renal and hepatic function, false-

In the Adverse Effects section, <u>underline</u> indicates most frequent; CAPS indicates life threatening.

positive direct Coombs', especially in azotemia, false-positive urine glucose with copper sulfate (Clinitest) (use Tes-Tape), false elevation urinary 17-ketosteroid values.

Intervention/Rationale
Patients with history of severe penicillin sensitivity may also have cephalosporin sensitivity (5%–10%). ● May cause pseudomembranous colitis (diarrhea, nausea, vomiting, fluid/electrolyte disturbances—notify physician and obtain culture for *C. difficile* toxin). ● Observe for signs/symptoms of anaphylaxis. ● Obtain cultures for sensitivity, first dose may be given while awaiting preliminary results.

Patient/Family Education
Complete course of therapy. Notify physician if there are any signs/symptoms of worsening infection (persistent fever/diarrhea) or signs of yeast infections (white patches in the mouth or vaginal discharge).

CEFMETAZOLE
(sef-met′-a-zol)
Trade Name(s): Zefazone
Classification(s): Cephalosporin antibiotic, second generation
Pregnancy Category: B

PHARMACODYNAMICS/KINETICS
Mechanism of Action: Bactericidal action, inhibition of bacterial cell wall synthesis. **Distribution:** Widely distributed to most tissues. Does not readily enter CSF except with inflammation. Concentration in bone is usually adequate. Protein bind-

ing: 65%. **Metabolism/Elimination:** Primarily eliminated via kidneys. Removed by hemodialysis. **Half-Life:** 72 min, prolonged in renal impairment.

INDICATIONS/DOSAGE

Treatment or prophylaxis of most gram-positive and many gram-negative organisms

(provides greater gram-negative coverage than first generation cephalosporins, excluding methicillin resistant *S. aureus* and *Pseudomonas* infections) associated with respiratory tract, genitourinary tract, skin/skin structure, bone/joint, septicemia, and intraabdominal infections. Dosage interval may need to be adjusted in renal impairment.

Adult: 2 g every 6–12 hr for 5–14 days.
Perioperative Prophylaxis: *Vaginal Hysterectomy:* 2 g ½ hr prior to surgery or 1 g ½ prior and repeat 8 and 16 hr later. ***Abdominal Hysterectomy/Cholecystectomy (High Risk):*** 1 g ½ hr prior and repeat 8 and 16 hr later. ***C-section:*** 2 g after cord clamping or 1 g after clamping, then repeat 8 and 16 hr later. ***Colorectal Surgery:*** 2 g ½ prior to surgery or 2 g ½ hr prior and repeat 8 and 16 hr later.

CONTRAINDICATIONS/PRECAUTIONS
Contraindicated in: Hypersensitivity to cephalosporins/penicillins or related antibiotics. **Use cautiously in:** Impaired renal function. **Pregnancy/Lactation:** No well-controlled trials to establish safety. Appears to be safe

In the Adverse Effects section, underline indicates most frequent; CAPS indicates life threatening.

79

for use in pregnancy when benefits outweigh risk. Crosses placenta. Identified in breast milk in small quantities with infant bowel flora changes and pharmacologic effects. **Pediatrics:** Not recommended for use in children. Safety and efficacy has not been established.

PREPARATION
Availability: 1 g, 2 g vials. Contains 2 mEq sodium/g. **Reconstitution:** Dilute each gram with at least 10 mL sterile water for injection or compatible diluent for maximum concentration of 50–100 mg/mL. **Intermittent Infusion:** Dilute to a final concentration of 10–30 mg/mL or in 50–100 mL compatible solution.

STABILITY/STORAGE
Vial: Reconstituted vial/solution stable for 24 hr at room temperature and 7 days refrigerated.

ADMINISTRATION
IV Push: Give slowly over at least 3–5 min. **Intermittent Infusion:** Infuse over at least 15–30 min.

COMPATIBILITY
Solution: Dextrose solutions, lactated Ringer's, sodium chloride solutions, sterile water for injection.

ADVERSE EFFECTS
CNS: Seizures (especially with high doses in renal impairment), confusion, dizziness, fatigue, headache, lethargy, paresthesia. **CV:** Hypotension. **Resp:** BRONCHOSPASM, interstitial pneumonitis. **GI:** <u>Pseudomembranous colitis</u>, anorexia, cholestasis, diarrhea, dysguesia, dyspepsia, elevated alkaline phosphatase, bilirubin, LDH, liver enzymes (AST [SGOT], ALT [SGPT], GGTP), glossitis, <u>nausea</u>, <u>vomiting</u>.

GU: Dysuria, genital moniliasis, genitoanal pruritus, hematuria, pyuria, vaginitis. **Renal:** Interstitial nephritis, transient elevations in BUN and serum creatinine. **Heme:** Leukopenia, thrombocytopenia, transient neutropenia, AGRANULOCYTOSIS, anemia, aplastic anemia, bleeding, eosinophilia, lymphocytosis. **Hypersens:** ANAPHYLAXIS, Stevens Johnson syndrome, angioedema, chest tightness, edema, eosinophilia, exfoliative dermatitis, joint pain, maculopapular rash, <u>moribilliform eruptions</u>, myalgias, <u>pruritus</u>, rash, <u>urticaria</u>. **Other:** Cellulitis, chills, diaphoresis, fever, flushing, inflammation, local swelling.

TOXICITY/OVERDOSE
Signs/Symptoms: High doses in renal impairment may cause seizures. **Treatment:** Discontinue agent when seizures begin. Administer anticonvulsant therapy and consider hemodialysis.

DRUG INTERACTIONS
Aminoglycosides: Potentiation of aminoglycoside nephrotoxicity. **Bacteriostatic antibiotics (chloramphenicol):** Potential interference with cephalosporin bactericidal action. **Probenecid:** Decreased renal elimination of cephalosporins with potential increase in plasma levels.

NURSING CONSIDERATIONS
Assessment
General:
Allergy history, anaphylaxis.
Physical:
GI tract, signs/symptoms of superinfection (sore throat/stomatitis,

In the Adverse Effects section, <u>underline</u> indicates most frequent; CAPS indicates life threatening.

vaginal discharge, perianal itching). Infectious disease status.

Lab Alterations:
Monitor CBC, coagulation profile, renal and hepatic function, false-positive direct Coombs', especially in azotemia, false-positive urine glucose with copper sulfate (Clinitest) (use Tes-Tape). False elevation urinary 17-ketosteroid values.

Intervention/Rationale
Patients with history of severe penicillin sensitivity may also have cephalosporin sensitivity (5%–10%). ● May cause pseudomembranous colitis (diarrhea, nausea, vomiting, fluid/electrolyte disturbances—notify physician and obtain culture for *C. difficile* toxin). ● Observe for signs/symptoms of anaphylaxis. ● Obtain cultures for sensitivity, first dose may be given while awaiting preliminary results.

Patient/Family Education
Complete course of therapy. Notify physician if there are any signs/symptoms of worsening infection (persistent fever/diarrhea) or signs of yeast infections (white patches in the mouth or vaginal discharge).

CEFONICID
(se-fon′-i-sid)
Trade Name(s): Monocid
Classification(s): Cephalosporin antibiotic, second generation
Pregnancy Category: B

PHARMACODYNAMICS/KINETICS
Mechanism of Action: Bactericidal action, inhibition of bacterial cell wall

synthesis. **Distribution:** Widely distributed to most tissues. Does not readily enter CSF except with inflammation. Concentration in bone is usually adequate. Protein binding: 98%. **Metabolism/Elimination:** Primarily eliminated via kidneys. Removed by hemodialysis. **Half-Life:** 270 min, prolonged in renal impairment.

INDICATIONS/DOSAGE

Treatment or prophylaxis of most gram-positive and many gram-negative organisms

(provides greater gram-negative coverage than first generation cephalosporins, excluding methicillin resistant *S. aureus* and *Pseudomonas* infections) associated with respiratory tract, genitourinary tract, skin/skin structure, bone/joint, and septicemia infections. Dosage interval may need to be adjusted in renal impairment.

Adult:
Uncomplicated UTI: 500 mg every 24 hr. **Mild to Moderate Infections:** 1 g every 24 hr. **Severe/life-threatening infections:** 2 g every 24 hr. Not to exceed 2 g/day **Perioperative Prophylaxis:** *Preoperative:* 1 g ½ hr prior to surgery. *C-section:* Administer just after cord clamping.

CONTRAINDICATIONS/ PRECAUTIONS
Contraindicated in: Hypersensitivity to cephalosporins/penicillins or related antibiotics. **Use cautiously in:** Impaired renal function. **Pregnancy/ Lactation:** No well-controlled trials to establish safety. Appears to be safe

In the Adverse Effects section, underline indicates most frequent;
CAPS indicates life threatening.

81

for use in pregnancy when benefits outweigh risk. Crosses placenta. Identified in breast milk in small quantities with infant bowel flora changes and pharmacologic effects. **Pediatrics:** Not recommended for use in children. Safety and efficacy has not been established.

PREPARATION

Availability: 500 mg, 1 g vials and 10 g bulk package. Contains 3.7 mEq sodium/g. **Reconstitution:** Dilute each 1 g with at least 10 mL sterile water for injection or compatible diluent for maximum concentration of 50–100 mg/mL. **Intermittent Infusion:** Dilute to a final concentration of 10–30 mg/mL or in 50–100 mL compatible solution.

STABILITY/STORAGE

Vial: Reconstituted vial/solution stable for 24 hr at room temperature and 3 days refrigerated.

ADMINISTRATION

IV Push: Give slowly over at least 3–5 min. **Intermittent Infusion:** Infuse over at least 15–30 min.

COMPATIBILITY

Solution: Dextrose solutions, lactated Ringer's, Ringer's injection, sodium chloride solutions. **Y-site:** Acyclovir.

ADVERSE EFFECTS

CNS: Seizures (especially with high doses in renal impairment), confusion, dizziness, fatigue, headache, lethargy, paresthesia. **CV:** Hypotension. **Resp:** BRONCHOSPASM, interstitial pneumonitis. **GI:** Pseudomembranous colitis, anorexia, cholestasis, diarrhea, dysguesia, dyspepsia, elevated alkaline phosphatase, bilirubin, LDH, liver en-

zymes (AST [SGOT], ALT [SGPT], GGTP), glossitis, nausea, vomiting. **GU:** Dysuria, genital moniliasis, genitoanal pruritus, hematuria, pyuria, vaginitis. **Renal:** Interstitial nephritis, transient elevations in BUN and serum creatinine. **Heme:** Leukopenia, transient neutropenia, thrombocytopenia, AGRANULO-CYTOSIS, anemia, aplastic anemia, bleeding, eosinophilia, lymphocytosis. **Hypersens:** ANAPHYLAXIS, angioedema, Stevens Johnson syndrome, chest tightness, edema, eosinophilia, exfoliative dermatitis, joint pain, maculopapular rash, moribilliform eruptions, myalgias, pruritus, rash, urticaria. **Other:** Cellulitis, chills, diaphoresis, fever, flushing, inflammation, local swelling.

TOXICITY/OVERDOSE

Signs/Symptoms: High doses in renal impairment may cause seizures. **Treatment:** Discontinue agent when seizures begin. Administer anticonvulsant therapy and consider hemodialysis.

DRUG INTERACTIONS

Aminoglycosides: Potentiation of aminoglycoside nephrotoxicity. **Bacteriostatic antibiotics (chloramphenicol):** Potential interference with cephalosporin bactericidal action. **Probenecid:** Decreased renal elimination of cephalosporins with potential increase in plasma levels.

NURSING CONSIDERATIONS

Assessment

General:

Allergy history, anaphylaxis.

Physical:

GI tract, signs/symptoms of superinfection (sore throat/stomatitis,

vaginal discharge, perianal itching), infectious disease status.
Lab Alterations:
Monitor CBC, coagulation profile, renal and hepatic function, false-positive direct Coombs', especially in azotemia, false-positive urine glucose with copper sulfate (Clinitest) (use Tes-Tape), false elevation urinary 17-ketosteroid values.

Intervention/Rationale
Patients with history of severe penicillin sensitivity may also have cephalosporin sensitivity (5%–10%). ● May cause pseudomembranous colitis (diarrhea, nausea, vomiting, fluid/electrolyte disturbances—notify physician and obtain culture for *C. difficile* toxin). ● Observe for signs/symptoms of anaphylaxis. ● Obtain cultures for sensitivity, first dose may be given while awaiting preliminary results.

Patient/Family Education
Complete course of therapy. Notify physician if there are any signs/symptoms of worsening infection (persistent fever/diarrhea) or signs of yeast infections (white patches in the mouth or vaginal discharge).

CEFOPERAZONE
(sef-oh-per′-a-zone)
Trade Name(s): Cefobid
Classification(s): Cephalosporin antibiotic, third generation
Pregnancy Category: B

PHARMACODYNAMICS/KINETICS
Mechanism of Action: Bactericidal action, inhibition of bacterial cell wall synthesis. **Distribution:** Widely distributed to most tissues, low levels in CSF, concentrations in bone are usually adequate with higher doses. Protein binding: 82%–93%. **Metabolism/Elimination:** Hepatically metabolized and eliminated in bile. **Half-Life:** 102–156 min.

INDICATIONS/DOSAGE

Treatment or prophylaxis of gram-positive and most gram-negative organisms

(provides greater gram-negative coverage than first and second generation cephalosporins) associated with respiratory tract, genitourinary tract, skin/skin structure, bone/joint, septicemia, and intra-abdominal infections. Effective against susceptible *Pseudomonas* infections.

Adult: 1–2 g every 12 hr.
Severe infections: 1.5–4.0 g every 6–12 hr. Not to exceed 16 g/day. Not to exceed 4 g/day in hepatic disease or biliary obstruction.

Pediatric: Safety and efficacy not established. 150 mg/kg/day in divided doses every 8–12 hr. Not to exceed adult dosages or 12 g/day.
Neonate: Safety and efficacy not established. 100 mg/kg/day in divided doses every 12 hr.

CONTRAINDICATIONS/PRECAUTIONS
Contraindicated in: Hypersensitivity to cephalosporins/penicillins or related antibiotics. **Pregnancy/Lactation:** No well-controlled trials to establish safety. Appears to be safe for use in pregnancy when benefits outweigh risk. Crosses placenta.

In the Adverse Effects section, underline indicates most frequent; CAPS indicates life threatening.

83

Identified in breast milk in small quantities demonstrating potential infant bowel flora changes and pharmacologic effects. **Pediatrics:** Consider benefits and risks in young children. Safety and efficacy has not been established. Neonates have demonstrated decreased elimination of cephalosporins.

PREPARATION

Availability: 1 g, 2 g vials. Contains 1.5 mEq sodium/g. **Reconstitution:** Dilute each gram with at least 5 mL sterile water for injection or compatible diluent. **Intermittent Infusion:** Dilute to a final volume of 50–100 mL compatible solution or final concentration of 10–20 mg/mL.

STABILITY/STORAGE

Vial: Store in refrigerator. Reconstituted vial/solution stable for 24 hr at room temperature and 5 days refrigerated.

ADMINISTRATION

IV Push: Give slowly over at least 3–5 min. **Intermittent Infusion:** Infuse over at least 15–30 min.

COMPATIBILITY

Solution: Dextrose solutions, sodium chloride solutions. **Syringe:** Heparin. **Y-site:** Acyclovir, cyclophosphamide, enalaprilat, esmolol, famotidine, foscarnet, hydromorphone, magnesium sulfate, morphine.

INCOMPATIBILITY

Syringe: Doxapram. **Y-site:** Hetastarch, labetalol, meperidine, ondansetron, perphenazine, promethazine.

ADVERSE EFFECTS

CNS: Seizures, confusion, dizziness, fatigue, headache, lethargy, paresthesia. **CV:** Hypotension. **Resp:** BRONCHOSPASM, interstitial pneumonitis. **GI:** <u>Pseudomembranous colitis</u>, anorexia, cholestasis, diarrhea, dysguesia, dyspepsia, elevated alkaline phosphatase, bilirubin, LDH, liver enzymes (AST [SGOT], ALT [SGPT], GGTP), gallbladder sludge, glossitis, <u>nausea</u>, <u>vomiting</u>. **GU:** Dysuria, genital moniliasis, genitoanal pruritus, hematuria, pyuria, vaginitis. **Renal:** Interstitial nephritis, decreased creatinine clearance, transient elevations in BUN and serum creatinine. **Heme:** Decreased platelet function, hypoprothrombinemia, AGRANULOCYTOSIS, leukopenia, transient neutropenia, thrombocytopenia, anemia, aplastic anemia, bleeding, eosinophilia, lymphocytosis. **Hypersens:** ANAPHYLAXIS, angioedema, Stevens Johnson syndrome, chest tightness, edema, eosinophilia, exfoliative dermatitis, joint pain, maculopapular rash, morbilliform eruptions, myalgias, <u>pruritus</u>, rash, <u>urticaria</u>. **Other:** Cellulitis, chills, diaphoresis, fever, flushing, inflammation, local swelling.

TOXICITY/OVERDOSE

Signs/Symptoms: High doses may cause seizures. **Treatment:** Discontinue agent when seizures begin. Administer anticonvulsant therapy and consider hemodialysis.

DRUG INTERACTIONS

Aminoglycosides: Potentiation of aminoglycoside nephrotoxicity. **Bacteriostatic antibiotics (e.g., chloramphenicol):** Potential interference with cephalosporin bactericidal action. **Ethanol:** Consumption of alcohol with or up to 72 hr after therapy

In the Adverse Effects section, <u>underline</u> indicates most frequent; CAPS indicates life threatening.

with these agents may result in disulfiram-like reaction beginning within 30 min of alcohol ingestion and lasting for several hours. **Oral anticoagulants:** Increased hypoprothrombinemic effects of anticoagulants.

NURSING CONSIDERATIONS

Assessment
General:
Allergy history, anaphylaxis.
Physical:
GI tract, signs/symptoms of superinfection (sore throat/stomatitis, vaginal discharge, perianal itching), infectious disease status.
Lab Alterations:
Monitor CBC, coagulation profile, renal and hepatic function, false-positive direct Coombs', especially in azotemia, false-positive urine glucose with copper sulfate (Clinitest) (use Tes-Tape), false elevation urinary 17-ketosteroid values.

Intervention/Rationale
Patients with history of severe penicillin sensitivity may also have cephalosporin sensitivity (5%–10%). ● May cause pseudomembranous colitis (diarrhea, nausea, vomiting, fluid/electrolyte disturbances—notify physician and obtain culture for *C. difficile* toxin). ● Observe for signs/symptoms of anaphylaxis. ● Obtain cultures for sensitivity, first dose may be given while awaiting preliminary results.

Patient/Family Education
Complete course of therapy. Notify physician if there are any signs/symptoms of worsening infection (persistent fever/diarrhea) or signs

of yeast infections (white patches in the mouth or vaginal discharge). Avoid alcohol during or up to 72 hr after stopping therapy (may result in acute alcohol intolerance that begins 30 min after alcohol ingestion and subsides 30 min to several hours afterwards; the reaction may occur up to 3 days after receiving the last dose).

CEFORANIDE
(se-for'-i-nide)
Trade Name(s): Precef
Classification(s): Cephalosporin antibiotic, second generation
Pregnancy Category: B

PHARMACODYNAMICS/KINETICS
Mechanism of Action: Bactericidal action, inhibition of bacterial cell wall synthesis. **Distribution:** Widely distributed to most tissues. Does not readily enter CSF except with inflammation. Concentration in bone is usually adequate. Protein binding: 80%. **Metabolism/Elimination:** Primarily eliminated via kidneys. Removed by hemodialysis. **Half-Life:** 156–180 min, prolonged in renal impairment.

INDICATIONS/DOSAGE

Treatment or prophylaxis of most gram-positive and many gram-negative organisms

(provides greater gram-negative coverage than first generation cephalosporins, excluding methicillin resistant *S. aureus* and *Pseudomonas* infections) associated with respiratory tract, geni-

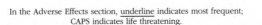
In the Adverse Effects section, <u>underline</u> indicates most frequent; CAPS indicates life threatening.

85

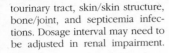

tourinary tract, skin/skin structure, bone/joint, and septicemia infections. Dosage interval may need to be adjusted in renal impairment.

Adult: 0.5–1.0 g every 12 hr.
Perioperative Prophylaxis:
Preoperative: 0.5–1.0 g ½ hr prior to surgery. *Postoperative:* 0.5–1.0 g. May repeat in 12 hr.

Pediatric: 20–40 mg/kg/day in divided doses every 12 hr.

CONTRAINDICATIONS/ PRECAUTIONS
Contraindicated in: Hypersensitivity to cephalosporins/penicillins or related antibiotics. **Use cautiously in:** Impaired renal function. **Pregnancy/ Lactation:** No well-controlled trials to establish safety. Appears to be safe for use in pregnancy when benefits outweigh risk. Crosses placenta. Identified in breast milk in small quantities with infant bowel flora changes and pharmacologic effects. **Pediatrics:** Consider risks and benefits in young children. Safety and efficacy has not been identified in children. Not recommended for neonates < 1 month old. Neonates have demonstrated decreased elimination of cephalosporins.

PREPARATION
Availability: 500 mg, 1 g vials. Contains 0 mEq sodium/g. **Reconstitution:** Dilute each gram with at least 10 mL sterile water for injection or compatible diluent for maximum concentration of 50–100 mg/mL. **Intermittent Infusion:** Dilute to a final concentration of 10–30 mg/mL or in 50–100 mL compatible solution.

STABILITY/STORAGE
Vial: Reconstituted vial/solution stable 48 hr at room temperature and 14 days refrigerated.

ADMINISTRATION
IV Push: Give slowly over at least 3–5 min. **Intermittent Infusion:** Infuse over at least 15–30 min.

COMPATIBILITY
Solution: Dextrose solutions, lactated Ringer's, sodium chloride solutions, sterile water for injection. **Y-site:** Acyclovir, cyclophosphamide, hydromorphone, magnesium sulfate, meperidine, morphine, ondansetron, perphenazine.

ADVERSE EFFECTS
CNS: Seizures (especially with high doses in renal impairment), confusion, dizziness, fatigue, headache, lethargy, paresthesia. **CV:** Hypotension. **Resp:** BRONCHOSPASM, interstitial pneumonitis. **GI:** Pseudomembranous colitis, anorexia, cholestasis, diarrhea, dysguesia, dyspepsia, elevated alkaline phosphatase, bilirubin, LDH, liver enzymes (AST [SGOT], ALT [SGPT], GGTP), glossitis, nausea, vomiting. **GU:** Dysuria, genital moniliasis, genitoanal pruritus, hematuria, pyuria, vaginitis. **Renal:** Interstitial nephritis, transient elevations in BUN and serum creatinine. **Heme:** AGRANULOCYTOSIS, leukopenia, transient neutropenia, thrombocytopenia, anemia, aplastic anemia, bleeding, eosinophilia, lymphocytosis. **Hypersens:** ANAPHYLAXIS, angioedema, Stevens Johnson syndrome, chest tightness, edema, eosinophilia, exfoliative dermatitis, joint pain, maculopapular rash, moribilliform eruptions, myalgias, pruritus, rash

In the Adverse Effects section, underline indicates most frequent; CAPS indicates life threatening.

urticaria. **Other:** Cellulitis, chills, diaphoresis, fever, flushing, inflammation, local swelling.

TOXICITY/OVERDOSE
Signs/Symptoms: High doses in renal impairment may cause seizures. **Treatment:** Discontinue agent when seizures begin. Administer anticonvulsant therapy and consider hemodialysis.

DRUG INTERACTIONS
Aminoglycosides: Potentiation of aminoglycoside nephrotoxicity. **Bacteriostatic antibiotics (chloramphenicol):** Potential interference with cephalosporin bactericidal action. **Probenecid:** Decreased renal elimination of cephalosporins with potential increase in plasma levels.

NURSING CONSIDERATIONS
Assessment
General:
Allergy history, anaphylaxis.
Physical:
GI tract, signs/symptoms of superinfection (sore throat/stomatitis, vaginal discharge, perianal itching), infectious disease status.
Lab Alterations:
Monitor CBC, coagulation profile, renal and hepatic function, false-positive direct Coombs', especially in azotemia, false-positive urine glucose with copper sulfate (Clinitest) (use Tes-Tape), false elevation urinary 17-ketosteroid values.

Intervention/Rationale
Patients with history of severe penicillin sensitivity may also have cephalosporin sensitivity (5%–10%). ● May cause pseudomembranous colitis (diarrhea, nausea, vomiting, fluid/electrolyte disturbances—notify physician and obtain culture for *C. difficile* toxin). ● Observe for signs/symptoms of anaphylaxis. ● Obtain cultures for sensitivity, first dose may be given while awaiting preliminary results.

Patient/Family Education
Complete course of therapy. Notify physician if there are any signs/symptoms of worsening infection (persistent fever/diarrhea) or signs of yeast infections (white patches in the mouth or vaginal discharge).

CEFOTAXIME
(sef-oh-tax′-eem)
Trade Name(s): Claforan
Classification(s): Cephalosporin antibiotic, third generation
Pregnancy Category: B

PHARMACODYNAMICS/KINETICS
Mechanism of Action: Bactericidal action, inhibition of bacterial cell wall synthesis. **Distribution:** Widely distributed to most tissues. Readily crosses into the CSF with inflammation. Concentrations in bone are usually adequate with higher doses. Protein binding: 30%–40%. **Metabolism/Elimination:** Primarily eliminated via kidneys. **Half-Life:** 60 min, prolonged in renal impairment.

INDICATIONS/DOSAGE

Treatment or prophylaxis of gram-positive and most gram-negative organisms
(provides greater gram-negative coverage than first and second gen-

---

In the Adverse Effects section, underline indicates most frequent; CAPS indicates life threatening.

87

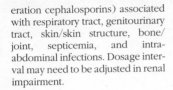

eration cephalosporins) associated with respiratory tract, genitourinary tract, skin/skin structure, bone/joint, septicemia, and intra-abdominal infections. Dosage interval may need to be adjusted in renal impairment.

Adult:
Uncomplicated Infections: 1 g every 12 hr. **Disseminated/Ophthalmia Gonococcal Infections:** 500 mg every 6 hr. **Moderate to Severe Infections:** 1–2 g every 6–8 hr. Up to 2 g every 4 hr. **Perioperative Prophylaxis:** 1 g ½ hr prior to surgery. **C-section:** 1 g after cord clamping then repeat in 6–12 hr.

Pediatric: 50–200 mg/kg/day in divided doses every 4–6 hr. Not to exceed adult dosages or 12 g/day. *Neonate:* 0–1 Week:100 mg/kg/day in divided doses every 12 hr. 1–4 Weeks: 150 mg/kg/day in divided doses every 8 hr.

CONTRAINDICATIONS/PRECAUTIONS
Contraindicated in: Hypersensitivity to cephalosporins/penicillins or related antibiotics. **Use cautiously in:** Impaired renal function. **Pregnancy/Lactation:** No well-controlled trials to establish safety. Appears to be safe for use in pregnancy when benefits outweigh risk. Crosses placenta. Identified in breast milk in small quantities demonstrating potential infant bowel flora changes and pharmacologic effects. **Pediatrics:** Consider benefits and risks in young children. Neonates have demonstrated decreased elimination of cephalosporins.

PREPARATION
Availability: 1 g, 2 g vials and 10 g bulk package. Contains 2.2 mEq sodium/g. **Reconstitution:** Dilute each gram with at least 10 mL sterile water for injection or compatible diluent to a maximum concentration of 50–100 mg/mL. **Intermittent Infusion:** Dilute to a final volume of 50–100 mL compatible solution or final concentration of 10–20 mg/mL.

STABILITY/STORAGE
Vial: Store at room temperature. Reconstituted vial/solution stable for 24 hr at room temperature and 5 days refrigerated.

ADMINISTRATION
IV Push: Give slowly over at least 3–5 min. **Intermittent Infusion:** Infuse over at least 15–30 min.

COMPATIBILITY
Solution: Dextrose solutions, lactated Ringer's, sodium chloride solutions. **Syringe:** Heparin. **Y-site:** Acyclovir, cyclophosphamide, famotidine, gentamicin, hydromorphone, magnesium sulfate, meperidine, morphine, ondansetron, perphenazine, tobramycin, tolazoline.

INCOMPATIBILITY
Syringe: Doxapram. **Y-site:** Hetastarch.

ADVERSE EFFECTS
CNS: Seizures (especially with high doses in renal impairment), confusion, dizziness, fatigue, headache, lethargy, paresthesia. **CV:** Hypotension. **Resp:** BRONCHOSPASM, interstitial pneumonitis. **GI:** Pseudomembranous colitis, anorexia, cholestasis, diarrhea, dysguesia, dyspepsia, elevated alkaline phos-

In the Adverse Effects section, underline indicates most frequent; CAPS indicates life threatening.

phatase, bilirubin, LDH, liver enzymes (AST [SGOT], ALT [SGPT], GGTP), gallbladder sludge, glossitis, <u>nausea</u>, <u>vomiting</u>. **GU:** Dysuria, genital moniliasis, genitoanal pruritus, hematuria, pyuria, vaginitis. **Renal:** Interstitial nephritis, decreased creatinine clearance, transient elevations in BUN and serum creatinine. **Heme:** AGRANULOCYTOSIS, leukopenia, transient neutropenia, thrombocytopenia, anemia, aplastic anemia, bleeding, eosinophilia, lymphocytosis. **Hypersens:** ANAPHYLAXIS, angioedema, Stevens Johnson syndrome, chest tightness, edema, eosinophilia, exfoliative dermatitis, joint pain, maculopapular rash, morbilliform eruptions, myalgias, <u>pruritus</u>, rash, <u>urticaria</u>. **Other:** Cellulitis, chills, diaphoresis, fever, flushing, inflammation, local swelling.

TOXICITY/OVERDOSE
Signs/Symptoms: High doses in renal impairment may cause seizures. **Treatment:** Discontinue agent when seizures begin. Administer anticonvulsant therapy and consider hemodialysis.

DRUG INTERACTIONS
Aminoglycosides: Potentiation of aminoglycoside nephrotoxicity. **Bacteriostatic antibiotics (e.g., chloramphenicol):** Potential interference with cephalosporin bactericidal action.

NURSING CONSIDERATIONS
Assessment
General:
Allergy history, anaphylaxis.
Physical:
GI tract, signs/symptoms of super-

infection (sore throat/stomatitis, vaginal discharge, perianal itching), infectious disease status.
Lab Alterations:
Monitor CBC, coagulation profile, renal and hepatic function, false-positive direct Coombs', especially in azotemia, false-positive urine glucose with copper sulfate (Clinitest) (use Tes-Tape), false elevation urinary 17-ketosteroid values.

Intervention/Rationale
Patients with history of severe penicillin sensitivity may also have cephalosporin sensitivity (5%–10%). ● May cause pseudomembranous colitis (diarrhea, nausea, vomiting, fluid/electrolyte disturbances—notify physician and obtain culture for *C. difficile* toxin). ● Observe for signs/symptoms of anaphylaxis. ● Obtain cultures for sensitivity, first dose may be given while awaiting preliminary results.

Patient/Family Education
Complete course of therapy. Notify physician if there are any signs/symptoms of worsening infection (persistent fever/diarrhea) or signs of yeast infections (white patches in the mouth or vaginal discharge).

CEFOTETAN
(sef´-oh-tee-tan)
Trade Name(s): Cefotan
Classification(s): Cephalosporin antibiotic, second generation
Pregnancy Category: B

PHARMACODYNAMICS/KINETICS
Mechanism of Action: Bactericidal action, inhibition of bacterial cell wall

In the Adverse Effects section, <u>underline</u> indicates most frequent; CAPS indicates life threatening.

89

synthesis. **Distribution:** Widely distributed to most tissues. Does not readily enter CSF except with inflammation. Concentration in bone is usually adequate. Protein binding: 88%–90%. **Metabolism/Elimination:** Primarily eliminated via kidneys. Removed by hemodialysis. **Half-Life:** 180–276 min, prolonged in renal impairment.

INDICATIONS/DOSAGE

Treatment or prophylaxis of most gram-positive and many gram-negative organisms

(provides greater gram-negative coverage than first generation cephalosporins, excluding methicillin resistant *S. aureus* and *Pseudomonas* infections) associated with respiratory tract, genitourinary tract, skin/skin structure, bone/joint, septicemia, and intra-abdominal infections. Dosage interval may need to be adjusted in renal impairment.

Adult:
UTI: 500 mg every 12 hr or 1–2 g every 12–24 hr. **Mild to Moderate Infections:** 1–2 g every 12 hr. **Severe Infections:** 2 g every 12 hr. Up to 3 g every 12 hr. Not to exceed 6 g/day. **Perioperative Prophylaxis:** *Preoperative:* 1–2 g ½ hr prior to surgery. *C-section:* Administer just after cord clamping.

CONTRAINDICATIONS/ PRECAUTIONS

Contraindicated in: Hypersensitivity to cephalosporins/penicillins or related antibiotics. **Use cautiously in:** Impaired renal function. **Pregnancy/ Lactation:** No well-controlled trials to establish safety. Appears to be safe for use in pregnancy when benefits outweigh risk. Crosses placenta. Identified in breast milk in small quantities with infant bowel flora changes and pharmacologic effects. **Pediatrics:** Not recommended for use in children. Safety and efficacy has not been established in children.

PREPARATION

Availability: 1 g, 2 g vials and 10 g bulk package. Contains 3.5 mEq sodium/g. **Reconstitution:** Dilute each gram with at least 10 mL sterile water for injection or compatible diluent for maximum concentration of 50–100 mg/mL. **Intermittent Infusion:** Dilute to a final concentration of 10–30 mg/mL or in 50–100 mL compatible solution.

STABILITY/STORAGE

Vial: Reconstituted vial/solution stable for 24 hr at room temperature and 4 days refrigerated.

ADMINISTRATION

IV Push: Give slowly over at least 3–5 min. **Intermittent Infusion:** Infuse over at least 15–30 min.

COMPATIBILITY

Solution: Dextrose solutions, sodium chloride solutions. **Y-site:** Famotidine, meperidine, morphine.

INCOMPATIBILITY

Syringe: Doxapram.

ADVERSE EFFECTS

CNS: Seizures (especially with high doses in renal impairment), confusion, diaphoresis, dizziness, fatigue, headache, lethargy, paresthesia. **CV:** Hypotension. **Resp:** BRONCHOSPASM, interstitial pneumo-

In the Adverse Effects section, <u>underline</u> indicates most frequent; CAPS indicates life threatening.

90

nitis. **GI:** Pseudomembranous coli-tis, anorexia, cholestasis, diarrhea, dysguesia, dyspepsia, elevated alkaline phosphatase, bilirubin, LDH, liver enzymes (AST [SGOT], ALT [SGPT], GGTP), glossitis, nausea, vomiting. **GU:** Dysuria, genital moniliasis, genitoanal pruritus, hematuria, pyuria, vaginitis. **Renal:** Interstitial nephritis, transient elevations in BUN and serum creatinine. **Heme:** Decreased platelet function, hypoprothrombinemia, AGRANULOCYTOSIS, leukopenia, transient neutropenia, thrombocytopenia, anemia, aplastic anemia, bleeding, eosinophilia, lymphocytosis. **Hypersens:** ANAPHYLAXIS, angioedema, Stevens Johnson syndrome, chest tightness, edema, eosinophilia, exfoliative dermatitis, joint pain, maculopapular rash, moribilliform eruptions, myalgias, pruritus, rash, urticaria. **Other:** Cellulitis, chills, diaphoresis, fever, flushing, inflammation, local swelling.

TOXICITY/OVERDOSE

Signs/Symptoms: High doses in renal impairment may cause seizures. **Treatment:** Discontinue agent when seizures begin. Administer anticonvulsant therapy and consider hemodialysis.

DRUG INTERACTIONS

Aminoglycosides: Potentiation of aminoglycoside nephrotoxicity. **Bacteriostatic antibiotics (chloramphenicol):** Potential interference with cephalosporin bactericidal action. **Ethanol:** Consumption of alcohol with or up to 72 hr after therapy may result in disulfiram-like reaction beginning within 30 min of alcohol ingestion and lasting for sev-eral hours. **Oral anticoagulants:** Increased hypoprothrombinemic effects of anticoagulants. **Probenecid:** Decreased renal elimination of cephalosporins with potential increase in plasma levels.

NURSING CONSIDERATIONS

Assessment
General:
Allergy history, anaphylaxis.
Physical:
GI tract, signs/symptoms of superinfection (sore throat/stomatitis, vaginal discharge, perianal itching), infectious disease status.
Lab Alterations:
Monitor CBC, coagulation profile, renal and hepatic function, false-positive direct Coombs', especially in azotemia, false-positive urine glucose with copper sulfate (Clinitest) (use Tes-Tape), false elevation urinary 17-ketosteroid values, false elevation of serum creatinine with high concentrations (Jaffe measurement method).

Intervention/Rationale
Patients with history of severe penicillin sensitivity may also have cephalosporin sensitivity (5%–10%). ● May cause pseudomembranous colitis (diarrhea, nausea, vomiting, fluid/electrolyte disturbances—notify physician and obtain culture for *C. difficile* toxin). ● Observe for signs/symptoms of anaphylaxis. ● Obtain cultures for sensitivity, first dose may be given while awaiting preliminary results.

Patient/Family Education
Complete course of therapy. Notify physician if there are any signs/

In the Adverse Effects section, underline indicates most frequent; CAPS indicates life threatening.

symptoms of worsening infection (persistent fever/diarrhea) or signs of yeast infections (white patches in the mouth or vaginal discharge). Avoid alcohol during or up to 72 hr after stopping therapy (may result in acute alcohol intolerance that begins 30 min after alcohol ingestion and subsides 30 min to several hours afterwards; the reaction may occur up to 3 days after receiving the last dose).

CEFOXITIN

(se-fox'-i-tin)

Trade Name(s): Mefoxin
Classification(s): Cephalosporin antibiotic, second generation
Pregnancy Category: B

PHARMACODYNAMICS/KINETICS

Mechanism of Action: Bactericidal action, inhibition of bacterial cell wall synthesis. **Distribution:** Widely distributed to most tissues. Does not readily enter CSF except with inflammation. Concentration in bone is usually adequate. *Protein binding:* 73%. **Metabolism/Elimination:** Primarily eliminated via kidneys. Removed by hemodialysis. **Half-Life:** 40–60 min, prolonged in renal impairment.

INDICATIONS/DOSAGE

Treatment or prophylaxis of most gram-positive and many gram-negative organisms

(provides greater gram-negative coverage than first generation cephalosporins, excluding methicillin resistant *S. aureus* and *Pseudomonas* infections) associated with respiratory tract, genitourinary tract, skin/skin structure, bone/joint, septicemia, and intra-abdominal infections. Dosage interval may need to be adjusted in renal impairment.

Adult:
Uncomplicated Infections: 1 g every 6–8 hr. **Disseminated/Ophthalmia Gonococcal Infection:** 1 g every 6 hr for 7 days. **Acute PID:** 2 g every 6 hr. **Moderately/Severe Infections:** 1 g every 4 hr or 2 g every 6–8 hr. Up to 2 g every 4 hr or 3 g every 6 hr. Not to exceed 12 g/day. **Perioperative Prophylaxis:** *Preoperative:* 2 g ½ hr prior to surgery. *Postoperative:* 2 g every 6 hr for 24 hr. *C-section:* Administer 2 g just after cord clamping. If necessary, two additional doses may be given 4 and 8 hr later. *Transurethral prostatectomy:* 1 g prior to surgery then 1 g every 8 hr for 5 days.

Pediatric (> 3 months old): 80–160 mg/kg/day every 4–6 hr. Not to exceed adult dosages or 12 g/day. **Perioperative Prophylaxis (> 3 months old):** *Preoperative:* 30–40 mg/kg ½ hr prior to surgery. *Postoperative:* 120–160 mg/kg in divided doses every 6 hr for 24 hr.

CONTRAINDICATIONS/ PRECAUTIONS

Contraindicated in: Hypersensitivity to cephalosporins/penicillins or related antibiotics. **Use cautiously in:** Impaired renal function. **Pregnancy/ Lactation:** No well-controlled trials to establish safety. Appears to be safe for use in pregnancy when benefits

In the Adverse Effects section, <u>underline</u> indicates most frequent; CAPS indicates life threatening.

outweigh risk. Crosses placenta. Identified in breast milk in small quantities with infant bowel flora changes and pharmacologic effects. **Pediatrics:** Consider risks and benefits in young children. Safety and efficacy has not been identified in children. Not recommended for neonates < 3 months old. Neonates have demonstrated decreased elimination of cephalosporins.

PREPARATION
Availability: 1 g, 2 g vials and 10 g bulk package. Contains 2.3 mEq sodium/g. **Reconstitution:** Dilute each gram with at least 10 mL sterile water for injection or compatible diluent for maximum concentration of 50–100 mg/mL. **Intermittent Infusion:** Dilute to a final concentration of 10–30 mg/mL or in 50–100 mL compatible solution.

STABILITY/STORAGE
Vial: Reconstituted vial/solution stable 24 hr at room temperature and 7 days refrigerated.

ADMINISTRATION
IV Push: Give slowly over at least 3–5 min. **Intermittent Infusion:** Infuse over at least 15–30 min.

COMPATIBILITY
Solution: Dextrose solutions, lactated Ringer's, Ringer's injection, sodium chloride solutions, sterile water for injection. **Syringe:** Heparin. **Y-site:** Acyclovir, aztreonam, cyclophosphamide, famotidine, foscarnet, hydromorphone, magnesium sulfate, meperidine, morphine, ondansetron, perphenazine.

INCOMPATIBILITY
Y-site: Hetastarch.

ADVERSE EFFECTS
CNS: Seizures (especially with high doses in renal impairment), confusion, dizziness, fatigue, headache, lethargy, paresthesia. **CV:** Hypotension. **Resp:** BRONCHOSPASM, interstitial pneumonitis. **GI:** Pseudomembranous colitis, anorexia, cholestasis, diarrhea, dysguesia, dyspepsia, elevated alkaline phosphatase, bilirubin, LDH, liver enzymes (AST [SGOT], ALT [SGPT], GGTP), glossitis, nausea, vomiting. **GU:** Dysuria, genital moniliasis, genitoanal pruritus, hematuria, pyuria, vaginitis. **Renal:** Interstitial nephritis, transient elevations in BUN and serum creatinine. **Heme:** AGRANULOCYTOSIS, leukopenia, transient neutropenia, thrombocytopenia, anemia, aplastic anemia, bleeding, eosinophilia, lymphocytosis. **Hypersens:** ANAPHYLAXIS, angioedema, Stevens Johnson syndrome, chest tightness, edema, eosinophilia, exfoliative dermatitis, joint pain, maculopapular rash, moribilliform eruptions, myalgias, pruritus, rash, urticaria. **Other:** Cellulitis, chills, diaphoresis, fever, flushing, inflammation, local swelling.

TOXICITY/OVERDOSE
Signs/Symptoms: High doses in renal impairment may cause seizures. **Treatment:** Discontinue agent when seizures begin. Administer anticonvulsant therapy and consider hemodialysis.

DRUG INTERACTIONS
Aminoglycosides: Potentiation of aminoglycoside nephrotoxicity. **Bacteriostatic antibiotics (chloramphenicol):** Potential interference with cephalosporin bactericidal action. **Probenecid:** Decreased renal elimi-

In the Adverse Effects section, underline indicates most frequent; CAPS indicates life threatening.

93

nation of cephalosporins with potential increase in plasma levels.

NURSING CONSIDERATIONS

Assessment
General:
Allergy history, anaphylaxis.
Physical:
GI tract, signs/symptoms of superinfection (sore throat/stomatitis, vaginal discharge, perianal itching), infectious disease status.
Lab Alterations:
Monitor CBC, coagulation profile, renal and hepatic function, false-positive direct Coombs', especially in azotemia, false-positive urine glucose with copper sulfate (Clinitest) (use Tes-Tape), false elevation urinary 17-ketosteroid values, false elevations of serum creatinine with high concentrations (Jaffe measurement method).

Intervention/Rationale
Patients with history of severe penicillin sensitivity may also have cephalosporin sensitivity (5%–10%). ● May cause pseudomembranous colitis (diarrhea, nausea, vomiting, fluid/electrolyte disturbances—notify physician and obtain culture for *C. difficile* toxin). ● Observe for signs/symptoms of anaphylaxis. ● Obtain cultures for sensitivity, first dose may be given while awaiting preliminary results.

Patient/Family Education
Complete course of therapy. Notify physician if there are any signs/symptoms of worsening infection (persistent fever/diarrhea) or signs of yeast infections (white patches in the mouth or vaginal discharge).

CEFTAZIDIME
(sef´-tay-zi-deem)
Trade Name(s): Fortaz, Magnacef ♣, Tazicef, Tazidime
Classification(s): Cephalosporin antibiotic, third generation
Pregnancy Category: B

PHARMACODYNAMICS/KINETICS
Mechanism of Action: Bactericidal action, inhibition of bacterial cell wall synthesis. **Distribution:** Widely distributed to most tissues. Readily crosses into the CSF with inflammation. Concentrations in bone are usually adequate with higher doses. Protein binding: 10%–17%. **Metabolism/Elimination:** Primarily eliminated via kidneys. **Half-Life:** 114–120 min, prolonged in renal impairment.

INDICATIONS/DOSAGE

Treatment or prophylaxis of gram-positive and most gram-negative organisms
(provides greater gram-negative coverage than first and second generation cephalosporins) associated with respiratory tract, genitourinary tract, skin/skin structure, bone/joint, septicemia, and intra-abdominal infections. Effective against susceptible *Pseudomonas* infections. Dosage interval may need to be adjusted in renal impairment.

Adult:
Uncomplicated UTI: 250 mg every 12 hr. **Complicated UTI:** 500 mg every 8–12 hr. **Pneumonia/Skin:** 0.5–1.0 g every 8 hr. **Bone/Joint:** 2 g every 12 hr. **Serious Gynecological/Intra-**

In the Adverse Effects section, underline indicates most frequent; CAPS indicates life threatening.

94

abdominal/Meningitis/Life-Threatening Infections: 2 g every 8 hr. **Pseudomonal Lung Infections in Cystic Fibrosis:** 90–150 mg/kg/day in divided doses every 8 hr. Not to exceed 6 g/day.

Pediatric: 90–150 mg/kg/day in divided doses every 8 hr. Not to exceed adult dosages or 6 g/day. *Neonate:* 60 mg/kg/day in divided doses every 12 hr.

CONTRAINDICATIONS/ PRECAUTIONS

Contraindicated in: Hypersensitivity to cephalosporins/penicillins or related antibiotics. **Use cautiously in:** Impaired renal function. **Pregnancy/ Lactation:** No well-controlled trials to establish safety. Appears to be safe for use in pregnancy when benefits outweigh risk. Crosses placenta. Identified in breast milk in small quantities demonstrating potential infant bowel flora changes and pharmacologic effects. **Pediatrics:** Consider benefits and risks in young children. Safety and efficacy has not been established. Neonates have demonstrated decreased elimination of cephalosporins.

PREPARATION

Availability: 500 mg, 1 g, 2 g vials and 6 g bulk package. Contains 2.3 mEq sodium/g. **Reconstitution:** Dilute each gram with at least 10 mL sterile water for injection or compatible diluent to a maximum concentration of 50–100 mg/mL. **Intermittent Infusion:** Dilute to a final volume of 50–100 mL compatible solution or final concentration of 10–20 mg/mL.

STABILITY/STORAGE

Vial: Store at room temperature. Reconstituted vial/solution stable for 24 hr at room temperature and 10 days refrigerated.

ADMINISTRATION

IV Push: Give slowly over at least 3–5 min. **Intermittent Infusion:** Infuse over at least 15–30 min.

COMPATIBILITY

Solution: Dextrose solutions, lactated Ringer's, Ringer's injection, sodium chloride solutions. **Y-site:** Acyclovir, ciprofloxacin, enalaprilat, esmolol, famotidine, foscarnet, labetalol, ondansetron, zidovudine.

ADVERSE EFFECTS

CNS: Seizures (especially with high doses in renal impairment), confusion, dizziness, fatigue, headache, lethargy, paresthesia. **CV:** Hypotension. **Resp:** BRONCHOSPASM, interstitial pneumonitis. **GI:** Pseudomembranous colitis, anorexia, cholestasis, diarrhea, dysguesia, dyspepsia, elevated alkaline phosphatase, bilirubin, LDH, liver enzymes (AST [SGOT], ALT [SGPT], GGTP), gallbladder sludge, glossitis, nausea, vomiting. **GU:** Dysuria, genital moniliasis, genitoanal pruritus, hematuria, pyuria, vaginitis. **Renal:** Interstitial nephritis, decreased creatinine clearance, transient elevations in BUN and serum creatinine. **Heme:** AGRANULOCYTOSIS, leukopenia, transient neutropenia, thrombocytopenia, anemia, aplastic anemia, bleeding, eosinophilia, lymphocytosis. **Hypersens:** ANAPHYLAXIS, angioedema, Stevens Johnson syndrome, chest tightness, edema, eosinophilia, exfoliative dermatitis, joint pain, maculopapu-

In the Adverse Effects section, underline indicates most frequent; CAPS indicates life threatening.

95

lar rash, morbilliform eruptions, myalgias, <u>pruritus</u>, rash, <u>urticaria</u>. **Other:** Cellulitis, chills, diaphoresis, fever, flushing, inflammation, local swelling.

TOXICITY/OVERDOSE
Signs/Symptoms: High doses in renal impairment may cause seizures. **Treatment:** Discontinue agent when seizures begin. Administer anticonvulsant therapy and consider hemodialysis.

DRUG INTERACTIONS
Aminoglycosides: Potentiation of aminoglycoside nephrotoxicity. **Bacteriostatic antibiotics (e.g., chloramphenicol):** Potential interference with cephalosporin bactericidal action.

NURSING CONSIDERATIONS
Assessment
General:
Allergy history, anaphylaxis.
Physical:
GI tract, signs/symptoms of superinfection (sore throat/stomatitis, vaginal discharge, perianal itching), infectious disease status.
Lab Alterations:
Monitor CBC, coagulation profile, renal and hepatic function, false-positive direct Coombs', especially in azotemia, false-positive urine glucose with copper sulfate (Clinitest) (use Tes-Tape), false elevation urinary 17-ketosteroid values.

Intervention/Rationale
Patients with history of severe penicillin sensitivity may also have cephalosporin sensitivity (5%–10%). ● May cause pseudomembranous colitis (diarrhea, nausea,

vomiting, fluid/electrolyte disturbances —notify physician and obtain culture for *C. difficile* toxin). ● Observe for signs/symptoms of anaphylaxis. ● Obtain cultures for sensitivity, first dose may be given while awaiting preliminary results.

Patient/Family Education
Complete course of therapy. Notify physician if there are any signs/symptoms of worsening infection (persistent fever/diarrhea) or signs of yeast infections (white patches in the mouth or vaginal discharge).

CEFTIZOXIME
(sef-ti-zox′-eem)
Trade Name(s): Cefizox
Classification(s): Cephalosporin antibiotic, third generation
Pregnancy Category: B

PHARMACODYNAMICS/KINETICS
Mechanism of Action: Bactericidal action, inhibition of bacterial cell wall synthesis. **Distribution:** Widely distributed to most tissues, readily crosses into the CSF with inflammation, concentrations in bone are usually adequate with higher doses. Protein binding: 30%. **Metabolism/Elimination:** Primarily eliminated via kidneys. **Half-Life:** 84–114 min, prolonged in renal impairment.

INDICATIONS/DOSAGE

Treatment or prophylaxis of gram-positive and most gram-negative organisms

(provides greater gram-negative coverage than first and second generation cephalosporins) associated with respiratory tract, genitourinary tract, skin/skin structure, bone/joint, septicemia, and intra-abdominal infections. Dosage interval may need to be adjusted in renal impairment.

Adult:
Uncomplicated UTI: 500 mg every 12 hr. **Other Sites:** 1 g every 8–12 hr. **Severe Infections:** 1 g every 8 hr or 2 g every 8–12 hr. Up to 3–4 g every 8 hr. Not to exceed 12 g/day.

Pediatric (> 6 months old): 150–200 mg/kg/day in divided doses every 6–8 hr. Not to exceed adult dosages or 12 g/day.

CONTRAINDICATIONS/ PRECAUTIONS

Contraindicated in: Hypersensitivity to cephalosporins/penicillins or related antibiotics. **Use cautiously in:** Impaired renal function. **Pregnancy/ Lactation:** No well-controlled trials to establish safety. Appears to be safe for use in pregnancy when benefits outweigh risk. Crosses placenta. Identified in breast milk in small quantities demonstrating potential infant bowel flora changes and pharmacologic effects. **Pediatrics:** Consider benefits and risks in young children. Safety and efficacy has not been established. Not recommended for use in neonates.

PREPARATION

Availability: 1 g, 2 g vials and 10 g bulk package. Contains 2.6 mEq sodium/g. **Reconstitution:** Dilute each gram with at least 10 mL sterile water for injection or compatible diluent to a maximum concentration of 50–100 mg/mL. **Intermittent Infusion:** Dilute to a final volume of 50–100 mL compatible solution or final concentration of 10–20 mg/mL.

STABILITY/STORAGE

Vial: Store at room temperature. Reconstituted vial/solution stable 24 hr at room temperature and 4 days refrigerated.

ADMINISTRATION

IV Push: Give slowly over at least 3–5 min. **Intermittent Infusion:** Infuse over at least 15–30 min.

COMPATIBILITY

Solution: Dextrose solutions, lactated Ringer's, Ringer's injection, sodium chloride solutions. **Y-site:** Acyclovir, enalaprilat, esmolol, famotidine, foscarnet, hydromorphone, labetalol, meperidine, morphine, ondansetron.

ADVERSE EFFECTS

CNS: Seizures (especially with high doses in renal impairment), confusion, dizziness, fatigue, headache, lethargy, paresthesia. **CV:** Hypotension. **Resp:** BRONCHOSPASM, interstitial pneumonitis. **GI:** <u>Pseudomembranous colitis</u>, anorexia, cholestasis, diarrhea, dysguesia, dyspepsia, elevated alkaline phosphatase, bilirubin, LDH, liver enzymes (AST [SGOT], ALT [SGPT], GGTP), gallbladder sludge, glossitis, <u>nausea</u>, <u>vomiting</u>. **GU:** Dysuria, genital moniliasis, genitoanal pruritus, hematuria, pyuria, vaginitis. **Renal:** Interstitial nephritis, decreased creatinine clearance, transient elevations in BUN and serum creatinine. **Heme:** AGRANULOCYTOSIS, leukopenia, transient neutropenia, thrombocytopenia, anemia, aplastic anemia, bleeding, eosinophilia,

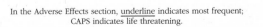
In the Adverse Effects section, <u>underline</u> indicates most frequent; CAPS indicates life threatening.

lymphocytosis. **Hypersens:** ANA-PHYLAXIS, angioedema, Stevens Johnson syndrome, chest tightness, edema, eosinophilia, exfoliative dermatitis, joint pain, maculopapular rash, morbilliform eruptions, myalgias, pruritus, rash, urticaria. **Other:** Cellulitis, chills, diaphoresis, fever, flushing, inflammation, local swelling.

TOXICITY/OVERDOSE

Signs/Symptoms: High doses in renal impairment may cause seizures. **Treatment:** Discontinue agent when seizures begin. Administer anticonvulsant therapy and consider hemodialysis.

DRUG INTERACTIONS

Aminoglycosides: Potentiation of aminoglycoside nephrotoxicity. **Bacateriostatic antibiotics (e.g., chloramphenicol):** Potential interference with cephalosporin bactericidal action.

NURSING CONSIDERATIONS

Assessment

General:
Allergy history, anaphylaxis.
Physical:
GI tract, signs/symptoms of superinfection (sore throat/stomatitis, vaginal discharge, perianal itching), infectious disease status.
Lab Alterations:
Monitor CBC, coagulation profile, renal and hepatic function, false-positive direct Coombs', especially in azotemia, false positive urine glucose with copper sulfate (Clinitest) (use Tes-Tape), false elevation urinary 17-ketosteroid values.

Intervention/Rationale

Patients with history of severe penicillin sensitivity may also have cephalosporin sensitivity (5%–10%). ● May cause pseudomembranous colitis (diarrhea, nausea, vomiting, fluid/electrolyte disturbances—notify physician and obtain culture for *C. difficile* toxin). ● Observe for signs/symptoms of anaphylaxis. ● Obtain cultures for sensitivity, first dose may be given while awaiting preliminary results.

Patient/Family Education

Complete course of therapy. Notify physician if there are any signs/symptoms of worsening infection (persistent fever/diarrhea) or signs of yeast infections (white patches in the mouth or vaginal discharge).

CEFTRIAXONE

(sef-try-ax′-one)
Trade Name(s): Rocephin
Classification(s): Cephalosporin antibiotic, third generation
Pregnancy Category: B

PHARMACODYNAMICS/KINETICS

Mechanism of Action: Bactericidal action, inhibition of bacterial cell wall synthesis. **Distribution:** Widely distributed to most tissues, readily crosses into the CSF with inflammation, concentrations in bone are usually adequate with higher doses. Protein binding: 85%–95%. **Metabolism/Elimination:** Hepatically metabolized and eliminated in bile. **Half-Life:** $5\frac{1}{2}$–$8\frac{1}{2}$ hr.

INDICATIONS/DOSAGE

Treatment or prophylaxis of gram-positive and most gram-negative organisms

(provides greater gram-negative coverage than first and second generation cephalosporins) associated with respiratory tract, genitourinary tract, skin/skin structure, bone/joint, septicemia, and intra-abdominal infections.

Adult: 1–2 g every 24 hr. Up to 2 g every 12 hr. Not to exceed 4 g/day. **Disseminated Gonococcal Infection:** 1 g every 24 hr. **Preoperatiave Prophylaxis:** 1 g ½ prior to surgery.
Pediatric: **Meningitis:** 75–100 mg/kg then 100 mg/kg/day in divided doses every 12 hr or 80 mg/kg every 24 hr. Not to exceed adult dosages or 4 g/day. **Other Infections:** 50–75 mg/kg/day in divided doses every 12–24 hr. Not to exceed adult dosages or 2 g/day.
Neonate: 50 mg/kg/day every 24 hr. **Meningitis:** 100 mg/kg/day in divided doses every 12 hr.

CONTRAINDICATIONS/PRECAUTIONS

Contraindicated in: Hypersensitivity to cephalosporins/penicillins or related antibiotics. **Pregnancy/Lactation:** No well-controlled trials to establish safety. Appears to be safe for use in pregnancy when benefits outweigh risk. Crosses placenta. Identified in breast milk in small quantities demonstrating potential infant bowel flora changes and pharmacologic effects. **Pediatraics:** Consider benefit to risk in young children. Safety and efficacy has not been established. Neonates have demonstrated decreased elimination of cephalosporins.

PREPARATION

Availability: 250 mg, 500 mg, 1 g, 2 g vials and 10 g bulk package. Contains 3.6 mEq sodium/g. **Reconstitution:** Dilute each gram with at least 10 mL sterile water for injection or compatible diluent to a maximum concentration of 50–100 mg/mL. **Intermittent Infusion:** Dilute to a final volume of 50–100 mL compatible solution or final concentration of 10–20 mg/mL

STABILITY/STORAGE

Vial: Store at room temperature. Reconstituted vial/solution stable for 3 days at room temperature and 10 days refrigerated.

ADMINISTRATION

IV Push: Give slowly over at least 3–5 min. **Intermittent Infusion:** Infuse over at least 15–30 min.

COMPATIBILITY

Solution: Amino acid 8.5%, dextrose solutions, lactated Ringer's, mannitol, sodium chloride solutions, sterile water for injection. **Y-site:** Acyclovir, zidovudine.

ADVERSE EFFECTS

CNS: Seizures, confusion, dizziness, fatigue, headache, lethargy, paresthesia. **CV:** Hypotension. **Resp:** BRONCHOSPASM, interstitial pneumonitis. **GI:** Pseudomembranous colitis, anorexia, cholestasis, diarrhea, dysguesia, dyspepsia, elevated alkaline phosphatase, bilirubin, LDH, liver enzymes (AST [SGOT], ALT [SGPT], GGTP), gallbladder sludge, glossitis, nausea,

---

In the Adverse Effects section, <u>underline</u> indicates most frequent; CAPS indicates life threatening.

<u>vomiting</u>. **GU:** Dysiura, genital moniliasis, genitoanal pruritus, hematuria, pyuria, vaginitis. **Renal:** Interstitial nephritis, decreased creatinine clearance, transient elevations in BUN and serum creatinine, urinary casts. **Heme:** AGRANULO-CYTOSIS, leukopenia, transient neutropenia, thrombocytopenia, anemia, aplastic anemia, bleeding, eosinophilia, lymphocytosis. **Hypersens:** ANAPHYLAXIS, angioedema, Stevens Johnson syndrome, chest tightness, edema, eosinophilia, exfoliative dermatitis, joint pain, maculopapular rash, morbilliform eruptions, myalgias, <u>pruritus</u>, rash, <u>urticaria</u>. **Other:** Cellulitis, chills, diaphoresis, fever, flushing, inflammation, local swelling.

TOXICITY/OVERDOSE
Signs/Symptoms: High doses in renal impairment may cause seizures. **Treatment:** Discontinue agent when seizures begin. Administer anticonvulsant therapy and consider hemodialysis.

DRUG INTERACTIONS
Aminoglycosides: Potentiation of aminoglycoside nephrotoxicity. **Bacteriostatic Antibiotics (e.g., chloramphenicol):** Potential interference with cephalosporin bactericidal action.

NURSING CONSIDERATIONS
Assessment
General:
Allergy history, anaphylaxis.
Physical:
GI tract, signs/symptoms of superinfection (sore throat/stomatitis, vaginal discharge, perianal itching), infectious disease status.

Lab Alterations:
Monitor CBC, coagulation profile, renal and hepatic function, false-positive direct Coombs', especially in azotemia, false-positive urine glucose with copper sulfate (Clinitest) (use Tes-Tape), false elevation urinary 17-ketosteroid values.

Intervention/Rationale
Patients with history of severe penicillin sensitivity may also have cephalosporin sensitivity (5%–10%). ● May cause pseudomembranous colitis (diarrhea, nausea, vomiting, fluid/electrolyte disturbances—notify physician and obtain culture for *C. difficile* toxin). ● Observe for signs/symptoms of anaphylaxis. ● Obtain cultures for sensitivity, first dose may be given while awaiting preliminary results.

Patient/Family Education
Complete course of therapy. Notify physician if there are any signs/symptoms of worsening infection (persistent fever/diarrhea) or signs of yeast infections (white patches in the mouth or vaginal discharge).

CEFUROXIME
(sef-ur-ox'-eem)
Trade Name(s): Kefurox, Zinacef
Classification(s): Cephalosporin antibiotic, second generation
Pregnancy Category: B

PHARMACODYNAMICS/KINETICS
Mechanism of Action: Bactericidal action, inhibition of bacterial cell wall synthesis. **Distribution:** Widely distributed to most tissues. Does not readily enter CSF except with in-

In the Adverse Effects section, <u>underline</u> indicates most frequent; CAPS indicates life threatening.

flammation. Concentration in bone is usually adequate. Protein binding: 33%–50%. **Metabolism/Elimination:** Primarily eliminated via kidneys. Removed by hemodialysis. **Half-Life:** 80 min, prolonged in renal impairment.

INDICATIONS/DOSAGE

Treatment or prophylaxis of most gram-positive and many gram-negative organisms

(provides greater gram-negative coverage than first generation cephalosporins, excluding methicillin resistant *S. aureus* and *Pseudomonas* infections) associated with respiratory tract, genitourinary tract, skin/skin structure, bone/joint, and septicemia infections. Dosage interval may need to be adjusted in renal impairment.

Adult: **Uncomplicated UTI/Skin/Disseminated Gonococcal Pneumonia:** 750 mg every 8 hr. **Severe/Complicated/Bone and Joint Infections:** 1.5 g every 8 hr. Up to 1.5 g every 6 hr. Not to exceed 6 g/day. **Bacterial Meningitis:** 1.5–3.0 g every 8 hr. Not to exceed 9 g/day. **Perioperative Prophylaxis:** *Preoperative:* 1.5 g ½ hr prior to surgery. *Intraoperative (if prolonged):* 750 mg every 8 hr. *Open Heart:* 1.5 g with anesthesia induction and 1.5 g every 12 hr for total of 6 g

Pediatric (> 3 months old): 50–100 mg/kg/day in divided doses every 6–8 hr. **Severe Infections:** Up to 100 mg/kg/day in divided doses every 6–8 hr. Not to exceed adult dosages or 6 g/day. **Bone/Joint Infections:** 150 mg/kg/day in divided doses every 8 hr. Not to exceed adult dos-

ages or 6 g/day. **Bacterial Meningitis:** 200–240 mg/kg/day in divided doses every 6–8 hr. Not to exceed adult dosages or 6 g/day. **Acute PID:** 150 mg/kg/day in divided doses every 6 hr.

Neonate: 20–50 mg/kg/day in divided doses every 12 hr. Not to exceed 100 mg/kg/day.

CONTRAINDICATIONS/PRECAUTIONS

Contraindicated in: Hypersensitivity to cephalosporins/penicillins or related antibiotics. **Use cautiously in:** Impaired renal function. **Pregnancy/Lactation:** No well-controlled trials to establish safety. Appears to be safe for use in pregnancy when benefits outweigh risk. Crosses placenta. Identified in breast milk in small quantities with infant bowel flora changes and pharmacologic effects. **Pediatrics:** Consider risks and benefits in young children. Safety and efficacy has not been identified in children. Neonates have demonstrated decreased elimination of cephalosporins.

PREPARATION

Availability: 750 mg, 1.5 g vials. Contains 2.4 mEq sodium/g. **Reconstitution:** Dilute 750 mg with 9 mL and 1.5 g with 14 mL sterile water for injection or compatible diluent. **Intermittent Infusion:** Dilute to a final concentration of 10–30 mg/mL or in 50–100 mL compatible solution.

STABILITY/STORAGE

Vial: Reconstituted vial stable 24 hr at room temperature and 48 hr refrigerated. Infusion stable 24 hr at room temperature and 7 days refrigerated.

In the Adverse Effects section, <u>underline</u> indicates most frequent; CAPS indicates life threatening.

ADMINISTRATION
IV Push: Give slowly over at least 3–5 min. **Intermittent Infusion:** Infuse over at least 15–30 min.

COMPATIBILITY
Solution: Dextrose solutions, lactated Ringer's, Ringer's injection, sodium chloride solutions. **Y-site:** Acyclovir, atracurium, cyclophosphamide, famotidine, foscarnet, hydromorphone, meperidine, morphine, ondansetron, pancuronium, perphenazine, vecuronium.

INCOMPATIBILITY
Syringe: Doxapram.

ADVERSE EFFECTS
CNS: Seizures (especially with high doses in renal impairment), confusion, dizziness, fatigue, headache, lethargy, paresthesia. **CV:** Hypotension. **Resp:** BRONCHOSPASM, interstitial pneumonitis. **GI:** <u>Pseudomembranous colitis</u>, anorexia, cholestasis, diarrhea, dysguesia, dyspepsia, elevated alkaline phosphatase, bilirubin, LDH, liver enzymes (AST [SGOT], ALT [SGPT], GGTP), glossitis, <u>nausea</u>, <u>vomiting</u>. **GU:** Dysuria, genital moniliasis, genitoanal pruritus, hematuria, pyuria, vaginitis. **Renal:** Interstitial nephritis, transient elevations in BUN and serum creatinine. **Heme:** AGRANULOCYTOSIS, leukopenia, transient neutropenia, thrombocytopenia, anemia, aplastic anemia, bleeding, eosinophilia, lymphocytosis. **Hypersens:** ANAPHYLAXIS, angioedema, Stevens Johnson syndrome, chest tightness, edema, eosinophilia, exfoliative dermatitis, joint pain, maculopapular rash, <u>moribilliform eruptions</u>, myalgias, <u>pruritus</u>, rash, <u>urticaria</u>. **Other:** Cellulitis, chills, diaphoresis, fever. flushing, inflammation, local swelling.

TOXICITY/OVERDOSE
Signs/Symptoms: High doses in renal impairment may cause seizures. **Treatment:** Discontinue agent when seizures begin. Administer anticonvulsant therapy and consider hemodialysis.

DRUG INTERACTIONS
Aminoglycosides: Potentiation of aminoglycoside nephrotoxicity. **Bacteriostatic antibiotics (chloramphenicol):** Potential interference with cephalosporin bactericidal action. **Probenecid:** Decreased renal elimination of cephalosporins with potential increase in plasma levels.

NURSING CONSIDERATIONS

Assessment
General:
Allergy history, anaphylaxis.
Physical:
GI tract, signs/symptoms of superinfection (sore throat/stomatits, vaginal discharge, perianal itching), infectious disease status.
Lab Alterations:
Monitor CBC, coagulation profile, renal and hepatic function, false-positive direct Coombs', especially in azotemia, false-positive urine glucose with copper sulfate (Clinitest) (use Tes-Tape), false elevation urinary 17-ketosteroid values.

Intervention/Rationale
Patients with history of severe penicillin sensitivity may also have cephalosporin sensitivity (5%–10%). ● May cause pseudomembranous colitis (diarrhea, nausea,

In the Adverse Effects section, <u>underline</u> indicates most frequent; CAPS indicates life threatening.

vomiting, fluid/electrolyte disturbances—notify physician and obtain culture for *C. difficile* toxin). ● Observe for signs/symptoms of anaphylaxis. ● Obtain cultures for sensitivity, first dose may be given while awaiting preliminary results.

Patient/Family Education

Complete course of therapy. Notify physician if there are any signs/symptoms of worsening infection (persistent fever/diarrhea) or signs of yeast infections (white patches in the mouth or vaginal discharge).

CEPHALOTHIN

(sef-a′-loe-thin)
Trade Name(s): Ceporacin ✿, Keflin
Classification(s): Cephalosporin antibiotic, first generation
Pregnancy Category: B

PHARMACODYNAMICS/KINETICS

Mechanism of Action: Bactericidal action, inhibition of bacterial cell wall synthesis. **Distribution:** Widely distributed to most tissues. Does not readily enter CSF except with inflammation. Protein binding: 70%. **Metabolism/Elimination:** Metabolized to less active compounds by the liver. Metabolites primarily eliminated by the kidneys. Removed by hemodialysis. **Half-Life:** 30–50 min, prolonged in renal impairment.

INDICATIONS/DOSAGE

Treatment or prophylaxis of most gram-positive and some gram-negative organisms

(excluding methicillin resistant *S. aureus* and *Pseudomonas* infections) associated with respiratory tract, genitourinary tract, skin/skin structure, bone/joint, septicemia infections. Dosage interval may need to be adjusted in renal impairment.

Adult:
Mild to Moderate Infections: 500 mg every 6 hr. **Severe Infections:** 500 mg every 4 hr or 1 g every 6 hr. Up to 2 g every 4 hr. Not to exceed 12 g/day.

Pediatric: 100 mg/kg/day in divided doses every 4–6 hr. Not to exceed adult dosages or 10 g/day. **Perioperative Prophylaxis: Preoperative:** 20–30 mg/kg ½ hr prior to surgery. **Intraoperative (> 2 hr):** 20–30 mg/kg during surgery. **Postoperative:** 20–30 mg/kg every 6 hr for 24 hr after surgery.

Neonate:
< 2 kg, < 1 Week: 40 mg/kg/day in divided doses every 12 hr. **< 2 kg, > 1 Week, or > 2 kg, < 1 Week:** 60 mg/kg/day in divided doses every 8 hr. **> 2 kg, > 1 Week:** 80 mg/kg/day in divided doses every 6 hr.

CONTRAINDICATIONS/PRECAUTIONS

Contraindicated in: Hypersensitivity to cephalosporins/penicillins or related antibiotics. **Use cautiously in:** Impaired renal function. **Pregnancy/Lactation:** No well-controlled trials to establish safety. Appears to be safe for use in pregnancy when benefits outweigh risk. Crosses placenta. Identified in breast milk in small quantities with potential infant bowel flora changes and pharmacologic effects. **Pediatrics:** Consider risks and benefits in young chil-

In the Adverse Effects section, underline indicates most frequent; CAPS indicates life threatening.

103

dren. Neonates have demonstrated decreased elimination of cephalosporins.

PREPARATION

Availability: 1 g, 2 g vials and 20 g bulk package. Contains 2.4–2.8 mEq sodium/g. **Reconstitution:** Dilute each 500 mg or 1 g with at least 10 mL sterile water for injection or compatible diluent for maximum concentration of 100 mg/mL. **Infusion:** Dilute to a final concentration of 20 mg/mL or 50–100 mL compatible solution.

STABILITY/STORAGE

Vial: Store at room temperature. Reconstituted vial stable for 24 hr at room temperature and 4 days refrigerated. **Infusion:** Stable for 24 hr at room temperature and 4 days refrigerated.

ADMINISTRATION

IV Push: Give slowly over at least 3–5 min. **Intermittent Infusion:** Infuse over at least 15–30 min.

COMPATIBILITY

Solution: Amino acids 4.25%/dextrose 25%, dextrose solutions, lactated Ringer's, Ringer's injection, sodium chloride solutions, sterile water for injection. **Syringe:** Cimetidine. **Y-site:** Cyclophosphamide, famotidine, heparin, hydrocortisone, hydromorphone, magnesium sulfate, meperidine, morphine, multivitamins, perphenazine, potassium chloride, vitamin B with C.

INCOMPATIBILITY

Syringe: Metoclopramide.

ADVERSE EFFECTS

CNS: Seizures (especially with high doses in renal impairment), confu-

sion, dizziness, fatigue, headache, lethargy, paresthesia. **CV:** Hypotension. **Resp:** BRONCHOSPASM, interstitial pneumonitis. **GI:** <u>Pseudomembranous colitis</u>, anorexia, chol-estasis, diarrhea, dysguesia, dyspepsia, elevated alkaline phosphatase, bilirubin, LDH, liver enzymes (AST [SGOT], ALT [SGPT], GGTP), glossitis, <u>nausea</u>, <u>vomiting</u>. **GU:** Dysuria, genital moniliasis, genitoanal pruritus, hematuria, pyuria, vaginitis. **Renal:** Interstitial nephritis, transient elevations in BUN and serum creatinine. **Heme:** Decreased platelet function, AGRANULOCYTOSIS, leukopenia, transient neutropenia, thrombocytopenia, anemia, aplastic anemia, bleeding, eosinophilia, lymphocytosis. **Hypersens:** ANAPHYLAXIS, angioedema, Stevens Johnson syndrome, chest tightness, edema, eosinophilia, exfoliative dermatitis, joint pain, maculopapular rash, <u>morbilliform eruptions</u>, myalgias, <u>pruritus</u>, rash, <u>urticaria</u>. **Other:** Cellulitis, chills, diaphoresis, fever, flushing, inflammation, local swelling.

TOXICITY/OVERDOSE

Signs/Symptoms: High doses in renal impairment may cause seizures. **Treatment:** Discontinue agent when seizures begin. Administer anticonvulsant therapy and consider hemodialysis.

DRUG INTERACTIONS

Aminoglycosides: Potentiation of aminoglycoside nephrotoxicity. **Bacteriostatic antibiotics (chloramphenicol):** Potential interference with cephalosporin bactericidal action. **Probenecid:** Decreased renal elimination of cephalosporins with potential increase in plasma levels.

In the Adverse Effects section, <u>underline</u> indicates most frequent; CAPS indicates life threatening.

NURSING CONSIDERATIONS

Assessment

General:

Allergy history, anaphylaxis.

Physical:

GI tract, signs/symptoms of super-infection (sore throat/stomatitis, vaginal discharge, perianal itching), infectious disease status.

Lab Alterations:

Monitor CBC, coagulation profile, renal and hepatic function, false-positive direct Coombs', especially in azotemia, false-positive urine glucose with copper sulfate (Clini-test) (use Tes-Tape), false elevation urinary 17-ketosteroid values, false elevations of serum creatinine with high concentrations (Jaffe measurement method).

Intervention/Rationale

Patients with history of severe penicillin sensitivity may also have cephalosporin sensitivity (5%–10%). ● May cause pseudomembranous colitis (diarrhea, nausea, vomiting, fluid/electrolyte disturbances—notify physician and obtain culture for *C. difficile* toxin). ● Observe for signs/symptoms of anaphylaxis. ● Obtain cultures for sensitivity, first dose may be given while awaiting preliminary results.

Patient/Family Education

Complete course of therapy. Notify physician if there are any signs/symptoms of worsening infection (persistent fever/diarrhea) or signs of yeast infections (white patches in the mouth or vaginal discharge).

CEPHAPIRIN

(sef-a-pye'-rin)

Trade Name(s): Cefadyl

Classification(s): Cephalosporin antibiotic, first generation

Pregnancy Category: B

PHARMACODYNAMICS/KINETICS

Mechanism of Action: Bactericidal action, inhibition of bacterial cell wall synthesis. **Distribution:** Widely distributed to most tissues. Does not readily enter CSF except with inflammation. Protein binding: 54%. **Metabolism/Elimination:** Metabolized to less active compounds by the liver. Metabolites primarily eliminated by the kidneys. Removed by hemodialysis. **Half-Life:** 24–36 min, prolonged in renal impairment.

INDICATIONS/DOSAGE

Treatment or prophylaxis of most gram-positive and some gram-negative organisms

(excluding methicillin resistant *S. aureus* and *Pseudomonas* infections) associated with respiratory tract, genitourinary tract, skin/skin structure, bone/joint, septicemia infections. Dosage interval may need to be adjusted in renal impairment.

Adult:

Mild to Moderate Infections: 0.5–1.0 g every 4–6 hr. **Severe/Life-Threatening Infections:** Not to exceed 12 g/day. **Perioperative Prophylaxis:** *Preoperative:* 1–2 g ½ hr prior to surgery. **Intraoperative (> 2 hr):** 1–2 g during surgery. **Postoperative:** 1–2 g every 6 hr for 24 hr after surgery.

In the Adverse Effects section, <u>underline</u> indicates most frequent; CAPS indicates life threatening.

105

Pediatric: 40–80 mg/kg/day in divided doses every 6 hr. Not to exceed adult dosages. Safety in infants < 3 months has not been established.

CONTRAINDICATIONS/ PRECAUTIONS

Contraindicated in: Hypersensitivity to cephalosporins/penicillins or related antibiotics. **Use cautiously in:** Impaired renal function. **Pregnancy/ Lactation:** No well-controlled trials to establish safety. Appears to be safe for use in pregnancy when benefits outweigh risk. Crosses placenta. Identified in breast milk in small quantities with potential infant bowel flora changes and pharmacologic effects. **Pediatrics:** Consider risks and benefits in young children. Neonates have demonstrated decreased elimination of cephalosporins.

PREPARATION

Availability: 500 mg, 1 g, 2 g, 4 g vials and 20 g bulk package. Contains 2.36 mEq sodium/g. **Reconstitution:** Dilute each 500 mg or 1 g with at least 10 mL sterile water for injection or compatible diluent for maximum concentration of 100 mg/mL. **Infusion:** Dilute to a final concentration of 20 mg/mL or 50–100 mL compatible solution.

STABILITY/STORAGE

Vial: Store at room temperature. Reconstituted vial stable at room temperature for 12 hr with sterile water for injection, 24 hr with bacteriostatic water for injection, 24 hr with dextrose and sodium chloride. Stable 10 days refrigerated. **Infusion:** Stable at room temperature for 12 hr with water for injection, 24 hr with bacteriostatic water for injection, 24 hr with dextrose and sodium chloride. Stable 10 days refrigerated.

ADMINISTRATION

IV Push: Give slowly over at least 3–5 min. **Intermittent Infusion:** Infuse over at least 15–30 min.

COMPATIBILITY

Solution: Dextrose solutions, lactated Ringer's, Ringer's injection, sodium chloride solutions, sterile water for injection. **Y-site:** Acyclovir, cyclophosphamide, famotidine, heparin, hydrocortisone, hydromorphone, magnesium sulfate, meperidine, morphine, multivitamins, perphenazine, potassium chloride, vitamin B with C.

INCOMPATIBILITY

Solution: Mannitol.

ADVERSE EFFECTS

CNS: Seizures (especially with high doses in renal impairment), confusion, dizziness, fatigue, headache, lethargy, paresthesia. **CV:** Hypotension. **Resp:** BRONCHOSPASM, interstitial pneumonitis. **GI:** <u>Pseudomembranous colitis</u>, anorexia, cholestasis, diarrhea, dysguesia, dyspepsia, elevated alkaline phosphatase, bilirubin, LDH, liver enzymes (AST [SGOT], ALT [SGPT], GGTP), glossitis, <u>nausea</u>, <u>vomiting</u>. **GU:** Dysuria, genital moniliasis, genitoanal pruritus, hematuria, pyuria, vaginitis. **Renal:** Interstitial nephritis, transient elevations in BUN and serum creatinine. **Heme:** Decreased platelet function, AGRANULOCYTOSIS, leukopenia, transient neutropenia, thrombocytopenia, anemia, aplastic anemia, bleeding,

In the Adverse Effects section, <u>underline</u> indicates most frequent; CAPS indicates life threatening.

eosinophilia, lymphocytosis. **Hypersens:** ANAPHYLAXIS, angioedema, Stevens Johnson syndrome, chest tightness, edema, eosinophilia, exfoliative dermatitis, joint pain, maculopapular rash, <u>morbilliform eruptions</u>, myalgias, <u>pruritus</u>, rash, <u>urticaria</u>. **Other:** Cellulitis, chills, diaphoresis, fever, flushing, inflammation, local swelling.

TOXICITY/OVERDOSE
Signs/Symptoms: High doses in renal impairment may cause seizures. **Treatment:** Discontinue agent when seizures begin. Administer anticonvulsant therapy and consider hemodialysis.

DRUG INTERACTIONS
Aminoglycosides: Potentiation of aminoglycoside nephrotoxicity. **Bacteriostatic antibiotics (chloramphenicol):** Potential interference with cephalosporin bactericidal action. **Probenecid:** Decreased renal elimination of cephalosporins with potential increase in plasma levels.

NURSING CONSIDERATIONS
Assessment
General:
Allergy history, anaphylaxis.
Physical:
GI tract, signs/symptoms of superinfection (sore throat/stomatitis, vaginal discharge, perianal itching), infectious disease status.
Lab Alterations:
Monitor CBC, coagulation profile, renal and hepatic function, false-positive direct Coombs', especially in azotemia, false-positive urine glucose with copper sulfate (Clinitest) (use Tes-Tape), false elevation urinary 17-ketosteroid values.

Intervention/Rationale
Patients with history of severe penicillin sensitivity may also have cephalosporin sensitivity (5%–10%). ● May cause pseudomembranous colitis (diarrhea, nausea, vomiting, fluid/electrolyte disturbances—notify physician and obtain culture for *C. difficile* toxin). ● Observe for signs/symptoms of anaphylaxis. ● Obtain cultures for sensitivity, first dose may be given while awaiting preliminary results.

Patient/Family Education
Complete course of therapy. Notify physician if there are any signs/symptoms of worsening infection (persistent fever/diarrhea) or signs of yeast infection (white patches in the mouth or vaginal discharge).

CEPHRADINE
(sef′-ra-deen)
Trade Name(s): Velosef
Classification(s): Cephalosporin antibiotic, first generation
Pregnancy Category: B

PHARMACODYNAMICS/KINETICS
Mechanism of Action: Bactericidal action, inhibition of bacterial cell wall synthesis. **Distribution:** Widely distributed to most tissues. Does not readily enter CSF except with inflammation. Protein binding: 8%–17%. **Metabolism/Elimination:** Primarily eliminated by the kidneys. Removed by hemodialysis. **Half-Life:** 48–80 min, prolonged in renal impairment.

In the Adverse Effects section, <u>underline</u> indicates most frequent;
CAPS indicates life threatening.

107

INDICATIONS/DOSAGE

Treatment or prophylaxis of most gram-positive and some gram-negative organisms

(excluding methicillin resistant *S. aureus* and *Pseudomonas* infections) associated with respiratory tract, genitourinary tract, skin/skin structure, bone/joint, septicemia infections. Dosage interval may need to be adjusted in renal impairment.

Adult:
Mild to Moderate Infections: 0.5–1.0 g every 6 hr. **Severe Infections:** 1–2 g every 4 hr. Not to exceed 8 g/day. **Perioperative Prophylaxis: Preoperative:** 1 g ½ hr prior to surgery. **Intraoperative (> 2 hr):** 1 g every 4–6 hr for 1–2 doses during surgery. **Postoperative:** 1 g every 4–6 hr for 24 hr after surgery.

Pediatric: 50–100 mg/kg/day in divided doses every 6 hr. Not to exceed adult dosages.

CONTRAINDICATIONS/PRECAUTIONS

Contraindicated in: Hypersensitivity to cephalosporins/penicillins or related antibiotics. **Use cautiously in:** Impaired renal function. **Pregnancy/Lactation:** No well-controlled trials to establish safety. Appears to be safe for use in pregnancy when benefits outweigh risk. Crosses placenta. Identified in breast milk in small quantities with potential infant bowel flora changes and pharmacologic effects. **Pediatrics:** Consider risks and benefits in young children. Safety and efficacy has not been identified in children < 1 month. Neonates have demon-strated decreased elimination of cephalosporins.

PREPARATION

Availability: 250 mg, 500 mg, 1 g, 2 g vials. Contains 6 mEq sodium/g. **Reconstitution:** Dilute each 500 mg or 1 g with at least 10 mL sterile water for injection or compatible diluent for maximum concentration of 100 mg/mL. **Infusion:** Dilute to a final concentration of 30–50 mg/mL.

STABILITY/STORAGE

Vial: Reconstituted vial stable 2 hr at room temperature and 24 hr refrigerated if concentration > 50 mg/mL. Stable 10 hr at room temperature and 48 hr refrigerated at concentrations < 50 mg/mL. **Infusion:** Stable 10 hr at room temperature and 48 hr refrigerated at concentrations < 50 mg/mL.

ADMINISTRATION

IV Push: Give slowly over at least 3–5 min. **Intermittent Infusion:** Infuse over at least 15–30 min.

COMPATIBILITY

Solution: Dextrose and sodium chloride solutions if prepared just prior to administration (stable for < 10 hr), sterile water for injection.

INCOMPATIBILITY

Solution: Dextrose and sodium chloride (incompatible after 10 hr), lactated Ringer's, Ringer's injection.

ADVERSE EFFECTS

CNS: Seizures (especially with high doses in renal impairment), confusion, dizziness, fatigue, headache, lethargy, paresthesia. **CV:** Hypotension. **Resp:** BRONCHOSPASM, interstitial pneumonitis. **GI:** Pseudomembranous colitis, anorexia,

In the Adverse Effects section, underline indicates most frequent; CAPS indicates life threatening.

cholestasis, diarrhea, dysguesia, dyspepsia, elevated alkaline phosphatase, bilirubin, LDH, liver enzymes (AST [SGOT], ALT [SGPT], GGTP), glossitis, <u>nausea</u>, <u>vomiting</u>. **GU:** Dysuria, genital moniliasis, genitoanal pruritus, hematuria, pyuria, vaginitis. **Renal:** Interstitial nephritis, transient elevations in BUN and serum creatinine. **Heme:** Decreased platelet function, AGRANULOCYTOSIS, leukopenia, transient neutropenia, thrombocytopenia, anemia, aplastic anemia, bleeding, eosinophilia, lymphocytosis. **Hypersens:** ANAPHYLAXIS, angioedema, Stevens Johnson syndrome, chest tightness, edema, eosinophilia, exfoliative dermatitis, joint pain, maculopapular rash, <u>morbilliform eruptions</u>, myalgias, <u>pruritus</u>, rash, <u>urticaria</u>. **Other:** Cellulitis, chills, diaphoresis, fever, flushing, inflammation, local swelling.

TOXICITY/OVERDOSE

Signs/Symptoms: High doses in renal impairment may cause seizures. **Treatment:** Discontinue agent when seizures begin. Administer anticonvulsant therapy and consider hemodialysis.

DRUG INTERACTIONS

Aminoglycosides: Potentiation of aminoglycoside nephrotoxicity. **Bacteriostatic antibiotics (chloramphenicol):** Potential interference with cephalosporin bactericidal action. **Probenecid:** Decreased renal elimination of cephalosporins with potential increase in plasma levels.

NURSING CONSIDERATIONS

Assessment
General:
Allergy history, anaphylaxis.
Physical:
GI tract, signs/symptoms of superinfection (sore throat/stomatitis, vaginal discharge, perianal itching), infectious disease status.
Lab Alterations:
Monitor CBC, coagulation profile, renal and hepatic function, false-positive direct Coombs', especially in azotemia, false-positive urine glucose with copper sulfate (Clinitest) (use Tes-Tape), false elevation urinary 17-ketosteroid values, false-positive urinary protein when using sulfosalicylic acid.

Intervention/Rationale
Patients with history of severe penicillin sensitivity may also have cephalosporin sensitivity (5%–10%). ● May cause pseudomembranous colitis (diarrhea, nausea, vomiting, fluid/electrolyte disturbances—notify physician and obtain culture for *C. difficile* toxin). ● Observe for signs/symptoms of anaphylaxis. ● Obtain cultures for sensitivity, first dose may be given while awaiting preliminary results.

Patient/Family Education
Complete course of therapy. Notify physician if there are any signs/symptoms of worsening infection (persistent fever/diarrhea) or signs of yeast infection (white patches in the mouth or vaginal discharge).

In the Adverse Effects section, <u>underline</u> indicates most frequent; CAPS indicates life threatening.

109

CHLORAMPHENICOL

(klor-am-fen'-i-kol)
Trade Name(s): Chloromycetin
Classification(s): Broad
spectrum antibiotic
Pregnancy Category: C

PHARMACODYNAMICS/KINETICS

Mechanism of Action: Bactericidal,
binds to 50S ribosomal units in bacteria and inhibits protein synthesis.
Peak Serum Level: End of infusion.
Therapeutic Serum Levels: Peak 10–20
mcg/mL. Trough 5–10 mcg/mL. **Distribution:** Distribution is rapid but
uneven. Highest concentrations in
liver/kidney. Lowest concentrations in brain/CSF. If no CNS inflammation present, drug enters
CSF at concentrations of 45%–99%
of that of blood. Measurable concentrations have been identified in
pleural/ascitic fluid, saliva, and
aqueous/vitreous humors. In premature neonates, a greater concentration of free drug is present in serum; lower therapeutic serum
levels may be adequate. 60% protein binding. **Metabolism/Elimination:**
Sodium succinate form is hydrolyzed to active form via esterases in
the liver, kidney, and lungs. Most
of the drug is eliminated as inactive
metabolites by the liver through
glucuronidation. 5%–15% free chloramphenicol eliminated via urine.
Half-Life: 4 hr, increased in severe
hepatic/renal impairment.

INDICATIONS/DOSAGE

**Treatment of severe infections asso-
ciated with gram-positive/negative
organisms as well as severe infections**

(associated with *Rickettsia, Lym-
phogranuloma psittacosis, Vibrio
cholerae, Salmonella typhi, Hemophilus influenzae*). Adjust dose
with impaired hepatic/renal function. Monitor serum levels.

Adult: 50 mg/kg/day in divided
doses every 6 hr. Moderately resistant infections may require 100 mg/
kg/day in divided doses every 6 hr.
Decrease high doses as soon as
possible. *Pediatric:* 50–100 mg/
kg/day in divided doses every 6–8
hr. Not to exceed 100 mg/kg/day
or 2 g/day. *Neonates:* Premature
neonates 10–25 mg/kg/day in divided doses every 12–24 hr. Term
neonates (< 2 weeks) 25 mg/kg/
day in divided doses every 12 hr.
Term neonates (> 2 weeks) 25–
50 mg/kg/day in divided doses every 12 hr. Not to exceed 50 mg/kg/
day.

CONTRAINDICATIONS/
PRECAUTIONS

Contraindicated in: History of hyper-
sensitivity/toxicity to chloramphenicol. Infections that are not severe or other than those that are
indicated. **Use cautiously in:** Acute intermittent porphyria or glucose-6-
phosphate deficiency (G6PD),
concurrent use of agents that
have bone marrow suppression
properties, impaired hepatic/renal
function, premature/full-term infants. **Pregnancy/Lactation:** No well-
controlled trials to establish safety.
Crosses placenta. Use particular
caution at term or during labor. Appears in breast milk. **Pediatrics:** Monitor serum levels in newborns to
avoid gray baby syndrome.

In the Adverse Effects section, <u>underline</u> indicates most frequent;
CAPS indicates life threatening.

PREPARATION

Availability: 100 mg/mL, 1 g and 10 g vials. Contains 2.25 mEq sodium/g. **Reconstitution:** Dilute 1 g vial with 10 mL sterile water for injection (do not use bacteriostatic water in neonates) or dextrose 5%. **Syringe:** Administer as 10% (1 g/10 mL) solution. Not to exceed 100 mg/mL. **Infusion:** Dilute in at least 50–100 mL compatible solution.

STABILITY/STORAGE

Vial: Store at room temperature. Reconstituted vial stable for 30 days at room temperature. Slight color change does not indicate potency loss. Solution should be clear. **Infusion:** Stable for 24 hr at room temperature.

ADMINISTRATION

IV Push: Give over at least 1 min. **Intermittent Infusion:** Infuse over 30–60 min.

COMPATIBILITY

Solution: Dextrose solutions, lactated Ringer's, Ringer's injection, sodium chloride solutions. **Syringe:** Ampicillin, heparin, methicillin, penicillin G sodium. **Y-site:** Acyclovir, cyclophosphamide, enalaprilat, esmolol, foscarnet, hydromorphone, labetalol, magnesium sulfate, meperidine, morphine.

INCOMPATIBILITY

Syringe: Glycopyrrolate, metoclopramide.

ADVERSE EFFECTS

CNS: Peripheral neuritis, confusion, delirium, depression, headache. **Ophtho:** Optic neuritis. **GI:** Diarrhea, glossitis, nausea, stomatitis, vomiting. **Heme:** APLASTIC ANEMIA, GRANULOCYTOPENIA, pancy-

topenia, thrombocytopenia. **Hypersens:** ANAPHYLAXIS, angioedema, herxheimer reactions in typhoid fever treatments, rash, urticaria. **Other:** GRAY BABY SYNDROME (associated with high doses in premature infants/newborns presents as abdominal distention), with/without emesis, decreased temperature, loose green stools, progressive cyanosis, refusal to suck, refractory lactic acidosis, vasomotor collapse, fever.

TOXICITY/OVERDOSE

Signs/Symptoms: Gray baby syndrome presentations, severe bone marrow depression. **Treatment:** Discontinue therapy as soon as possible. Begin symptomatic measures. Drug is readily removed by charcoal hemoperfusion.

DRUG INTERACTIONS

Acetaminophen: Elevation of chloramphenicol serum levels requiring dosage alteration. **Chlorpropamide, cyclophosphamide, dicumarol, phenobarbital, phenytoin, tolbutamide:** Chloramphenicol inhibits their metabolism resulting in increased concentrations. **Cyclophosphamide:** Reduced cyclophosphamide activity. **Iron salts, vitamin B$_{12}$:** Decreased hematologic effects of these drugs. **Rifampin:** Decreased chloramphenicol serum levels due to increased metabolism.

NURSING CONSIDERATIONS

Assessment
General:
Allergy history, anaphylaxis.
Physical:
GI tract, signs/symptoms of superinfection (sore throat/stomatitis,

In the Adverse Effects section, <u>underline</u> indicates most frequent; CAPS indicates life threatening.

111

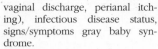

vaginal discharge, perianal itching), infectious disease status, signs/symptoms gray baby syndrome.
Lab Alterations:
Monitor CBC, coagulation profile, renal and hepatic function.

Intervention/Rationale

May cause pseudomembranous colitis (diarrhea, nausea, vomiting, fluid/electrolyte disturbances—notify physician and obtain culture for *C. difficile* toxin). ● Observe for signs/symptoms of anaphylactic reaction. ● Obtain cultures for sensitivity; first dose may be given while awaiting preliminary results. ● Monitor infants and children for signs/symptoms of gray baby syndrome and discontinue drug immediately and call physician.

Patient/Family Education

Follow up examinations to monitor for delayed bone marrow suppression. Avoid excessive acetaminophen. Complete the entire course of therapy. Notify physician/nurse of any signs of gray baby syndrome, excess diarrhea, nausea, vomiting, worsening of the infection, or bleeding.

CHLORDIAZEPOXIDE

(klor-die-az-a-pox'-ide)
Trade Name(s): Librium
Classification(s): Antianxiety agent, anxiolytic, benzodiazepine, sedative/hypnotic
Pregnancy Category: D
Controlled Substance Schedule: IV

PHARMACODYNAMICS/KINETICS

Mechanism of Action: Appears to act at limbic, thalamic, and hypothalamic levels of the CNS. Produces a calming effect on the subcortical levels of the nervous system. **Onset of Action:** 1–5 min. **Duration of Action:** 15–60 min. **Distribution:** Widely distributed into body tissues. 70%–99% protein plasma bound. Crosses the blood–brain barrier. **Metabolism/Elimination:** Metabolized by hepatic biotransformation. Excreted almost entirely in the urine as oxidized and glucuronide-conjugated metabolites. **Half-Life:** 5–30 hr.

INDICATIONS/DOSAGE

Reduce dosage with liver impairment.

Acute alcohol withdrawal

Adult: 50–100 mg initially. May repeat in 2–4 hr if required. Total dose not to exceed 300 mg/24 hr.

Acute/severe anxiety

Adult: 50–100 mg initially. Followed by 25–50 mg 3–4 times per day as required.

Preoperative anxiety/apprehension

Adult: 50–100 mg 1 hr prior to surgery. Preferred route is usually IM.

CONTRAINDICATIONS/ PRECAUTIONS

Contraindicated in: Acute alcohol intoxication with depressed vital signs, childbirth, children < 12 years, coma, hypersensitivity, lactation, psychoses, pregnancy, shock, uncontrolled severe pain, untreated narrow angle glaucoma. **Use cautiously in:** Blood dyscrasias, depressed patients with suicidal ideations, elderly/debilitated, renal/hepatic disease. **Pregnancy/Lactation:** No well-controlled trials to establish safety. Benefits must outweigh risks. Crosses placenta, distributed in breast milk. Known to cause fetal harm when administered to pregnant women. **Pediatrics:** Safety and efficacy not established for children < 12 years.

PREPARATION

Availability: 100 mg per ampule in 5 mL ampules with 2 mL ampule of IM diluent. **Reconstitution:** When reconstituting drug for IV use, do not use IM diluent provided in package. Add 5 mL sodium chloride or sterile water for injection to each 100 mg ampule of drug immediately prior to administration. Agitate gently until completely dissolved.

STABILITY/STORAGE

Vial: Refrigerate. Stable for 14 days at room temperature. Protect from light. Drug is unstable in solution. Use immediately after reconstitution. Discard any unused portions.

ADMINISTRATION

General: Reserve IV route when rapid action is necessary. **IV Push:** Give 100 mg or less slowly over 1 minute via y-site or 3-way stopcock.

COMPATIBILITY

Solution: Dextrose solutions. **Y-site:** Heparin, hydrocortisone, potassium chloride, vitamin B complex with C.

INCOMPATIBILITY

Syringe: Benzquinamide.

ADVERSE EFFECTS

CNS: <u>Dizziness</u>, <u>drowsiness</u>, <u>EEG changes</u>, hiccoughs, <u>lethargy</u>, paradoxical symptoms of acute rage, hallucinations, hyperexcitability. **Ophtho:** Blurred vision. **CV:** Transient hypotension, syncope, tachycardia. **GI:** Abdominal discomfort, constipation, diarrhea, nausea, vomiting. **GU:** Menstrual irregularity, urinary retention. **Derm:** Skin eruptions. **Hypersens:** Rash, urticaria. **Other:** Physical dependence, psychological dependence.

TOXICITY/OVERDOSE

Signs/Symptoms: Overdose: cardiac arrest, respiratory arrest, severe hypotension. **Treatment:** Fluid resuscitation, maintain patent airway, combat hypotension with fluids and pressor agents. With normal kidney function force diuresis with an osmotic diuretic. Dialysis is of limited value. Exchange transfusions may be helpful. Barbiturates are not recommended if hyperexcitability manifestations occur following chlordiazepoxide administration. **Antidote(s):** Flumazenil IV as per physician order (reverses sedation or overdose effects). Physostigmine 0.5–4.0 mg at a rate of 1 mg/min may reverse symptoms resembling central anticholinergic overdose (confusion, delirium, hallucinations, memory disruption, visual disturbances).

DRUG INTERACTIONS

Alcohol, antihistamines, antidepressants, narcotics, sedatives: Additive CNS depression. **Cimetidine:** May increase CNS depressive effects by decreasing metabolism of chlordiazepoxide. **Levodopa:** Antiparkinson efficacy may be decreased.

In the Adverse Effects section, <u>underline</u> indicates most frequent; CAPS indicates life threatening.

Rifampin: Decreases pharmacologic effects of chlordiazepoxide.

NURSING CONSIDERATIONS

Assessment
General:
Vital signs.
Physical:
Neurologic.
Lab Alterations:
Assess liver function tests prior to administration.

Intervention/Rationale
Consider withholding medication if coma or somnolence develops. Assess for CNS effects (dizziness, lethargy, drowsiness, or slurring of speech) and adjust dosage accordingly. ● Protect patient from sustaining injury while receiving drug for acute symptom control. ● Withdraw or taper medication gradually in order to avoid withdrawal symptoms (insomnia, irritability, nervousness, or fine motor tremors).

Patient/Family Education
Drug may cause drowsiness; avoid engaging in tasks requiring mental alertness. Seek assistance with ambulatory activities. Avoid alcohol or other CNS depressants during therapy.

CHLOROTHIAZIDE
(klor-o-thie′-a-zide)
Trade Name(s): Diuril
Classification(s): Thiazide diuretic
Pregnancy Category: D

PHARMACODYNAMICS/KINETICS
Mechanism of Action: Increases urine excretion of sodium and water by inhibiting sodium reabsorption in the cortical dilution site of the nephron. **Onset of Action:** 1–2 hr. **Peak Effect:** 4 hr. **Duration of Action:** 6–12 hr. **Distribution:** Widely distributed into extracellular space. **Metabolism/Elimination:** Excreted unchanged by the kidneys. **Half-Life:** 1–2 hr.

INDICATIONS/DOSAGE

Treatment of edema
Adult: 0.5–2.0 g once or twice daily.

Hypertension
Adult: 0.5–1.0 g daily as a single or divided dose. *Pediatric:* IV use is generally not recommended. **< 2 yr:** 125–375 mg/day in two divided doses. **2–12 yr:** 0.375–1.0 g daily in two divided doses.

CONTRAINDICATIONS/PRECAUTIONS
Contraindicated in: Anuria, hypersensitivity, increasing azotemia/oliguria. **Use cautiously in:** Impaired renal function, lupus erythematosis (may exacerbate symptoms), progressive liver disease. **Pregnancy/Lactation:** No well-controlled trials to establish safety. Benefits must outweigh risks. **Pediatrics:** IV use is generally not recommended.

PREPARATION
Availability: 500 mg powder for injection in 20 mL vials. **Reconstitution:** Each 0.5 g must be diluted with a

In the Adverse Effects section, underline indicates most frequent; CAPS indicates life threatening.

minimum of 18 mL sterile water for injection. **Infusion:** Further dilute in at least 50 mL compatible IV solution.

STABILITY/STORAGE
Vial: Store at room temperature. **Infusion:** Stable for 24 hr at room temperature in concentrations of 1 mg/mL or 25 mg/mL.

ADMINISTRATION
General: IV route should only be used in emergency situations or when patient unable to take oral medication. **IV Push:** Give 0.5 g or less slowly over 5 min. **Intermittent Infusion:** Administer diluted solution over 15–20 minutes via infusion device or in an IV line containing a free flowing compatible solution.

COMPATIBILITY
Solution: Dextrose solutions, lactated Ringer's, Ringer's injection, sodium chloride solutions, sterile water for injection.

ADVERSE EFFECTS
CNS: Anxiety, dizziness, generalized weakness, headache, vertigo. **CV:** Orthostatic hypotension. **Resp:** Respiratory distress, cough. **GI:** Abdominal pain, anorexia, gastric irritation, jaundice, nausea, vomiting. **GU:** Frequent urination, glycosuria, impotence, nocturia. **MS:** Muscle cramps. **Derm:** Dry skin, photosensitivity. **Endo:** Hyperglycemia, <u>hyperuricemia</u>. **Fld/Lytes:** Electrolyte imbalance, <u>hypokalemia</u>, hypovolemia. **Heme:** Leukopenia, neutropenia, thrombocytopenia. **Hypersens:** Anaphylactic reactions, hives, pruritus, rash. **Other:** Venous thrombosis, epistaxis.

TOXICITY/OVERDOSE
Signs/Symptoms: Overdose may produce lethargy progressing to coma within a few hours with minimal decreases of respiratory/cardiovascular function and without evidence of dehydration. **Treatment:** Maintain hydration and electrolyte balance. Support respiratory/cardiovascular/renal function. Resuscitate as necessary.

DRUG INTERACTIONS
Amphotericin B, glucocorticoids, piperacillin, ticarcillin: Increased hypokalemic effects. **Antihypertensives, nitrates:** Additive hypotensive effects. **Diazoxide:** Concomitant administration with thiazide diuretics may result in increased pharmacologic activity. **Digitalis glycoside:** Diuretic induced hypokalemia may increase the potential for digitalis toxicity. **Lithium:** Decreased lithium excretion (results in toxicity). **Nondepolarizing muscle relaxants:** Increased neuromuscular blocking effects with prolonged periods of apnea.

NURSING CONSIDERATIONS

Assessment
General:
Vital signs, intake/output ratio, daily weight.
Physical:
Cardiopulmonary status.
Lab Alterations:
Monitor electrolytes (serum potassium), serum glucose, hepatic/renal function tests, and uric acid concentrations.

In the Adverse Effects section, <u>underline</u> indicates most frequent; CAPS indicates life threatening.

115

Intervention/Rationale

Drug may cause orthostatic hypotension. ● Assess for signs/symptoms of dehydration (skin turgor, mucous membranes, hypotension). Drug may lead to water/electrolyte depletion. Monitor urine output to assess therapeutic response. May cause muscle weakness/cramps. ● Assess patients receiving cardiac glycosides for signs/symptoms of digitalis toxicity (anorexia, confusion, muscle cramps, visual disturbances, nausea, and paresthesias) especially when hypokalemia is present. ● Evaluate diabetic patients for changing insulin needs.

Patient/Family Education

Notify nurse/physician if cramps, muscle weakness, nausea, vomiting occur. Change positions gradually and slowly in order to prevent orthostatic blood pressure changes.

CHLORPROMAZINE
(klor-pro′-ma-zeen)
Trade Name(s): Largactil ♣ , Ormazine, Thorazine
Classification(s): Antiemetic, phenothiazine
Pregnancy Category: C

PHARMACODYNAMICS/KINETICS

Mechanism of Action: Blocks postsynaptic dopamine receptors in the brain. As antiemetic, inhibits the medullary chemoreceptor trigger zone. **Onset of Action:** Rapid. **Peak Serum Level:** Immediately after administration. **Distribution:** Widely distributed throughout tissues and body fluids. Crosses blood–brain barrier.

92%–97% plasma bound. **Metabolism/Elimination:** Extensively metabolized by the liver and kidneys. Excreted by the kidneys. **Half-Life:** 10–20 hr.

INDICATIONS/DOSAGE

Perioperative nausea/vomiting

Adult: 1 mg. May repeat at 2 minute intervals. Not to exceed 0.5 mg/kg. *Pediatric:* 0.275 mg/kg by slow infusion.

Intractable hiccoughs

Adult: 25–50 mg by infusion.

Tetanus

Adult: 0.5 mg/kg every 6–8 hr. *Pediatric:* **< 23 kg:** 0.5 mg/kg. Not to exceed 40 mg/day. **23–45 kg:** 0.5 mg/kg. Not to exceed 75 mg/day except in severe cases.

CONTRAINDICATIONS/PRECAUTIONS

Contraindicated in: Bone marrow depression, cerebral arteriosclerosis, children < 6 months, circulatory collapse, comatose/severely depressed states, coronary disease, hypersensitivity, narrow angle glaucoma. **Use cautiously in:** Acute respiratory disease in children; cardiovascular, liver, or chronic respiratory diseases; children with sleep apnea history; elderly/debilitated; epilepsy; family history of SIDS; hypertension; hypotension; intestinal obstruction; prostatic hypertrophy; Reyes syndrome; subcortical brain damage. **Pregnancy/Lactation:** No well-controlled trials to establish safety. Benefits must outweigh risks. Crosses the placenta. Excreted in breast milk. **Pediatrics:** Not recommended for children < 6 months except where potentially life saving.

PREPARATION

Availability: 25 mg/mL in 1, 2, and 10 mL ampules/vials/cartridges. **Syringe:** Dilute with sodium chloride to 1 mg/mL. **Infusion:** May be further diluted in 500–1000 mL compatible IV fluid.

STABILITY/STORAGE

Vial: Protect from light. Discard if darker than light amber. Store at room temperature. **Infusion:** Stable for 24 hr at room temperature. Prepare immediately prior to infusion.

ADMINISTRATION

General: Individualize dosage based on symptoms. May cause contact dermatitis. Handle drug with care. **IV Push:** Give 1 mg or less over 2 minutes. Do not exceed 1 mg/min in adults or 0.5 mg/min in children. **Intermittent Infusion:** Titrate according to vital signs and symptoms in accordance with physician prescribed rate.

COMPATIBILITY

Solution: Dextrose solutions, lactated Ringer's, Ringer's injection, sodium chloride solutions. **Syringe:** Atropine, butorphanol, diphenhydramine, droperidol, fentanyl, glycopyrrolate, hydromorphone, meperidine, metoclopramide, morphine, pentazocine, perphenazine, prochlorperazine, promethazine, scopolamine. **Y-site:** Heparin, hydrocortisone, potassium chloride, vitamin B complex with C.

INCOMPATIBILITY

Syringe: Cimetidine, dimenhydrinate, pentobarbital, ranitidine, thiopental.

ADVERSE EFFECTS

CNS: Extrapyramidal reactions, EEG changes, dizziness, sedation, tardive dyskinesia, headache, pseudoparkinsonism. **Ophtho:** Blurred vision, ocular changes. **CV:** Orthostatic hypotension, ECG changes, tachycardia. **Resp:** BRONCHOSPASM. **GI:** Hepatitis, abnormal liver function studies, anorexia, cholestatic jaundice, constipation, increased appetite. **GU:** Dark urine, gynecomastia, menstrual irregularities, urine retention. **Derm:** Dermal allergic manifestations, mild photosensitivity, pigment changes. **Heme:** AGRANULOCYTOSIS, transient leukopenia. **Hypersens:** Allergic manifestations, rash. **Other:** Hyperthermia.

TOXICITY/OVERDOSE

Signs/Symptoms: Overdose can cause severe extrapyramidal reactions, CNS depression progressing to coma with areflexia, hypotension, and sedation. Early mild toxicity can cause confusion, excitement, and restlessness. **Treatment:** Symptomatic treatment and supportive care. Epinephrine should not be used for hypotension. CNS stimulants that may cause seizures should be avoided. No specific antidote for overdose. Anticholinergics and antiparkinson drugs may be useful in controlling extrapyramidal symptoms. Hemodialysis is not beneficial. Exchange transfusions may be useful in severe overdosage.

In the Adverse Effects section, underline indicates most frequent;
CAPS indicates life threatening.

DRUG INTERACTIONS

Antihistamines, general anesthetics, narcotics, sedatives/hypnotics: Additive CNS depression. **Antihypertensive agents:** Additive hypotensive effects. **Phenobarbital:** May increase metabolism of drug and decrease effectiveness of phenobarbital drug-lab.

NURSING CONSIDERATIONS

Assessment

General:

Lying/standing blood pressure, ECG, respirations, intake/output ratio.

Physical:

Respiratory status, GI tract, neurologic.

Lab Alterations:

Increased/altered liver function tests, false-positive/negative urine bilirubin, false-positive/negative urine pregnancy test.

Intervention/Rationale

Maintain supine position during therapy. ● Drug may cause depressed cough/gag reflex. ● Drug may cause constipation with prolonged use or mask diagnosis of intestinal obstruction. ● Evaluate patient for development of extrapyramidal symptoms (drooling, rigidity, shuffling gait, tremors) or symptoms of tardive dyskinesia (rhythmical involuntary movements of tongue, face, jaw, or mouth, protrusion of the tongue or chewing-like movements). ● After abrupt withdrawal of long-term therapy, assess for dizziness, feelings of warmth/cold, gastritis, headache, insomnia, nausea, sweating, tachycardia, and/or vomiting.

Patient/Family Education

Dry mouth occurs frequently and may be relieved by sugar free candy/gum or frequent oral care. Notify physician immediately if jaundice, fever, sore throat, cellulitis, or weakness becomes apparent (symptoms of developing blood dyscrasias). Report urinary retention and/or constipation. Wear sunscreen/protective clothing while outside to avoid photosensitivity reactions. Change positions slowly and seek assistance with ambulatory functions to prevent orthostatic hypotension. Avoid alcohol or other CNS depressants. Urine may turn a pink or reddish brown color.

CIMETIDINE

(sye-met′-a-deen)

Trade Name(s): Novocimetine ♣ , Peptol ♣ , Tagamet

Classification(s): Histamine H_2 antagonist

Pregnancy Category: B

PHARMACODYNAMICS/KINETICS

Mechanism of Action: Competitively inhibits action of histamine on H_2 receptors of gastric parietal cells. Reduces gastric output and concentration. Indirectly reduces pepsin secretion by decreasing volume of gastric juice. **Onset of Action:** 0.75–1.5 hr. **Peak Effect:** 35–75 minutes. **Duration of Action:** 4–5 hr. **Distribution:** Widely distributed throughout body. 15%–20% protein bound. **Metabolism/Elimination:** Metabolized by the liver. 75% excreted unchanged in urine, 10% in feces. **Half-Life:** 2 hr.

In the Adverse Effects section, underline indicates most frequent;
CAPS indicates life threatening.

INDICATIONS/DOSAGE

Pathological gastric hypersecretory condition (Zollinger-Ellison syndrome, systemic mastocytosis, multiple endocrine adenomas), upper GI bleeding, stress ulcers

Adult: 300–600 mg every 6 hr. Maximum dose 2400 mg/day.

Treatment of duodenal ulcer, prophylaxis recurrent duodenal ulcer

Adult: Usual dose 300 mg every 6–8 hr. Not to exceed 2400 mg/day. If additional pain relief is needed, increase frequency of dosing. *Pediatric:* 20–40 mg/kg/day in divided doses every 6–8 hr.

Prevention of aspiration pneumonia preanesthesia (*unlabeled use*)

Adult: 300 mg 60–90 min preanesthesia.

CONTRAINDICATIONS/ PRECAUTIONS

Contraindicated in: Hypersensitivity. **Use cautiously in:** Elderly, impaired hepatic/renal function. **Pregnancy/ Lactation:** No well-controlled trials to establish safety. Benefits must outweigh risks. Crosses the placenta. Excreted in breast milk. **Pediatrics:** Not recommended for children < 16 yr unless anticipated benefits outweigh potential risks.

PREPARATION

Availability: 300 mg in 2 mL and 8 mL vials. 2 mL disposable syringes. **Syringe:** Dilute dosage to a total of 20 mL using compatible IV solution. **Intermittent Infusion:** Further dilute in 50–100 mL compatible IV solution. **Continuous Infusion:** Further dilute in 100–1000 mL compatible IV solution.

STABILITY/STORAGE

Vial: Store at room temperature. Protect from light. **Infusion:** Stable for 48 hr at room temperature after dilution.

ADMINISTRATION

General: Rapid parenteral administration has been associated with cardiac dysrhythmias and hypertension. **IV Push:** Inject slowly over at least 2 min. **Intermittent Infusion:** Infuse over 15–20 min. **Continuous Infusion:** Infuse at a rate to administer dose over a 24 hr period via infusion device. Give at no more than 37.5 mg/hr.

COMPATIBILITY

Solution: Amino acids 8.5%, dextrose solutions, lactated Ringer's, Ringer's injection, sodium chloride solutions, sterile water for injection. **Syringe:** Atropine, butorphanol, diazepam, diphenhydramine, doxapram, droperidol, fentanyl, glycopyrrolate, heparin, hydromorphone, lorazepam, meperidine, midazolam, morphine, nafcillin, nalbuphine, penicillin G, pentazocine, perphenazine, prochlorperazine, promethazine, scopolamine, sodium acetate. **Y-site:** Aminophylline, atracurium, enalaprilat, foscarnet, hetastarch, ondansetron, pancuronium, tolazoline, vecuronium.

INCOMPATIBILITY

Syringe: Cefamandole, cefazolin, chlorpromazine, pentobarbital, secobarbital.

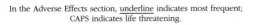

In the Adverse Effects section, <u>underline</u> indicates most frequent; CAPS indicates life threatening.

C ▶

ADVERSE EFFECTS
CNS: <u>Confusion</u>, <u>dizziness</u>, drowsiness, fatigue, hallucinations, headache, somnolence. **CV:** Bradycardia, CARDIAC ARREST, cardiac dysrhythmias, hypotension. **Resp:** BRONCHOSPASM. **GI:** Cholestatic/hepatocellular effects, constipation, diarrhea, hepatitis, nausea. **GU:** Decreased sperm count, gynecomastia, impotence, urinary retention. **Renal:** Reversible interstitial nephritis. **MS:** Arthralgia. **Derm:** Alopecia, erythema multiforme. **Endo:** Pancreatitis. **Heme:** Agranulocytosis, anemia, APLASTIC ANEMIA, granulocytopenia, thrombocytopenia. **Hypersens:** Allergic manifestations, rash, urticaria.

TOXICITY/OVERDOSE
Signs/Symptoms: Toxic doses are manifested by circulatory collapse and cholinergic type effects (diarrhea, emesis, lacrimation, salivation), hypotension, muscle tremors, pallor of mucous membranes, rapid respirations or respiratory failure, redness of mouth/ears, restlessness, tachycardia, vomiting. **Treatment:** Symptomatic and supportive. Physostigmine may arouse obtunded patients with evidence of CNS toxicity.

DRUG INTERACTIONS
Benzodiazepines, caffeine, calcium channel blockers, carbamazepine, chloroquine, labetalol, lidocaine, metroprolol, metronidazole, moricizine, pentoxifylline, phenytoin, propafenone, propranolol, quinidine, quinine, sulfonylureas, theophyllines, triamterene, tricyclic antidepressants, warfarin: Concomitant administration of cimetidine may result in increased pharmacologic effects or toxicity. **Carmustine:** Enhanced bone marrow suppression with concomitant use. **Digoxin:** Decreased serum digoxin concentrations. **Flecainide:** Increased flecainide pharmacologic effects. **Ketoconazole:** Cimetidine decreases pharmacological effects. **Narcotic analgesics:** Increased respiratory depression. **Procainamide:** Increased plasma levels (procainamide, NAPA). **Succinylcholine:** Increased neuromuscular blocking effects with prolonged respiratory depression. **Tocainide:** Decreased pharmacologic effects of tocainide.

NURSING CONSIDERATIONS
Assessment
Physical:
Mental status, GI tract.
Lab Alterations:
Monitor CBC, liver profile, antagonizes effect of histamine and pentagastrin during gastric acid secretion test (avoid administration of cimetidine for at least 24 hr prior to the test). False-negative results in skin tests using allergen extracts (discontinue drug at least 24 hr prior to allergy testing).

Intervention/Rationale
Assess elderly/debilitated for development of CNS findings exhibited by confusion or disorientation. ● Assess gastric pH every 6 hr, and maintain pH > 4 as per physician order. Assess abdominal or epigastric pain in association with medication schedule. Hematest stools/vomitus/nasogastric drainage to assess for presence/absence of occult or frank bleeding.

In the Adverse Effects section, <u>underline</u> indicates most frequent; CAPS indicates life threatening.

Patient/Family Education

Inform physician of concomitant drug therapy including over-the-counter drugs. Clinical effect of reduction of gastric acid is reversed by cigarette smoking. Women taking cimetidine should avoid becoming pregnant or breastfeeding. Drug may cause drowsiness or dizziness; avoid activities that require mental acuity until effects of drug have been determined.

CIPROFLOXACIN

(sip-roe-flox′-a-sin)
Trade Name(s): Cipro IV
Classification(s): Broad spectrum antibiotic
Pregnancy Category: C

PHARMACODYNAMICS/KINETICS

Mechanism of Action: Bactericidal, interferes with bacterial DNA synthesis. **Peak Serum Level:** End of infusion. **Distribution:** Widely distributed throughout the body. Tissue concentrations may exceed serum concentrations, most notably in genital tissue. Diffuses well into CSF. **Metabolism/Elimination:** Metabolized by the liver to active metabolites with less activity than parent drug. Small percent eliminated in feces. Metabolites eliminated by the kidneys. Removed by hemodialysis and peritoneal dialysis. **Half-Life:** 4 hr.

INDICATIONS/DOSAGE

Treatment of infections caused by susceptible organisms

Adult: Adjust dosage with impaired function.

Mild/moderate urinary tract infection:

200 mg every 12 hr.

Severe/complicated urinary tract infection; mild/moderate respiratory tract, bone/joint, and skin/skin structure infections:

400 mg every 12 hr.

CONTRAINDICATIONS/PRECAUTIONS

Contraindicated in: Hypersensitivity to ciprofloxacin or other quinolones. **Use cautiously in:** Patients with predisposition to or seizure history. **Pregnancy/Lactation:** No well-controlled trials to establish safety. Benefits must outweigh risks. Not recommended for use in pregnancy. Distributed in breast milk. Breastfeeding mothers should discontinue either nursing or the drug. **Pediatrics:** Safety and efficacy not established due to bone formation defects in animal studies.

PREPARATION

Availability: 200 mg/20 mL, 20 and 40 mL vials. 200 mg/100 mL, 100 and 200 mL premixed containers. **Infusion:** Further dilute 200 mg in 100 mL and 400 mg in at least 200 mL compatible IV solution.

STABILITY/STORAGE

Vial: Store at room temperature. **Infusion:** Stable 14 days at room temperature or refrigerated.

ADMINISTRATION

General: Consult with physician and if reasonable, temporarily discontinue other drugs/solutions during infusion if common tubing is used. Slow infusions minimize risk of venous irritation/patient discom-

---

In the Adverse Effects section, underline indicates most frequent; CAPS indicates life threatening.

fort. **Intermittent Infusion:** Infuse over at least 60 minutes.

COMPATIBILITY

Solution: Dextrose solutions, sodium chloride solutions. **Y-site:** Aztreonam, ceftazidime, piperacillin, tobramycin.

ADVERSE EFFECTS

CNS: Seizures (with rapid administration), depression, dizziness, drowsiness, hallucinations, <u>headache</u>, insomnia, malaise, paresthesias. **Ophtho:** Eye pain, nystagmus. **CV:** Angina, CARDIAC ARREST, palpitations, postural hypotension. **Resp:** BRONCHOSPASM, dyspnea, pulmonary edema. **GI:** <u>Abdominal discomfort</u>, <u>diarrhea</u>, dry mouth, GI bleeding, increased ALT (SGPT), AST (SGOT), <u>nausea</u>, oral candidiasis, <u>vomiting</u>. **GU:** Polyuria, urethral bleeding, urinary retention, vaginal candidiasis. **Renal:** Increased serum creatinine/BUN, interstitial nephritis, renal tubular acidosis. **MS:** Exacerbation of myasthenia gravis. **Derm:** Hyperpigmentation. **Heme:** Agranulocytosis, eosinophilia, leukopenia. **Hypersens:** ANAPHYLAXIS, <u>rash</u>, urticaria. **Other:** Chills, epistaxis, fever, flushing, venous irritation.

TOXICITY/OVERDOSE

Signs/Symptoms: Extension of adverse effects. **Treatment:** Symptomatic and supportive. Dialysis may be beneficial, especially in impaired renal function.

DRUG INTERACTIONS

Anticoagulants: Increased anticoagulant effect. **Cyclosporine:** Increased nephrotoxicity. **Probenecid:** Increased ciprofloxacin concentration and decreased renal clearance. **Theophylline:** Increased theophylline toxicity and decreased clearance.

NURSING CONSIDERATIONS

Assessment

General:

Allergy history, anaphylaxis.

Physical:

GI tract, signs/symptoms of superinfection (sore throat/stomatitis, vaginal discharge, perianal itching), infectious disease status.

Lab Alterations:

Monitor CBC, coagulation profile, renal/hepatic function.

Intervention/Rationale

Assess neurologic function around scheduled time of infusion (may cause seizures with rapid infusion). ● May cause pseudomembranous colitis (diarrhea, nausea, vomiting, fluid/electrolyte disturbances), notify physician and obtain culture for *C. difficile* toxin). ● Observe for signs/symptoms of anaphylaxis. ● Obtain cultures for sensitivity; first dose may be given while awaiting preliminary results.

Patient/Family Education

Complete course of therapy. Notify physician if any signs/symptoms of worsening infection (persistent fever/diarrhea) or signs of yeast infection (white patches or vaginal discharge). Avoid excess sun exposure during therapy.

In the Adverse Effects section, <u>underline</u> indicates most frequent; CAPS indicates life threatening.

CISPLATIN (CDDP)

(sis-pla′-tin)

Trade Name(s): Platinol, Platinol-AQ

Classification(s): Alkylating agent, antineoplastic

Pregnancy Category: D

PHARMACODYNAMICS/KINETICS

Mechanism of Action: Interferes with DNA and RNA synthesis. **Peak Serum Level:** End of infusion. **Distribution:** Widely distributed throughout body. Concentrates primarily in liver, kidneys, and intestines. 90%–98% protein plasma bound. **Metabolism/Elimination:** Metabolized by the liver. Excreted primarily by the kidneys (only 25%–50% of drug is excreted by the end of 5 days). **Half-Life:** 58–73 hr.

INDICATIONS/DOSAGE

Metastatic testicular tumors

Adult: 20 mg/m²/day IV for 5 days every 3 weeks for 3 courses for remission induction.

Metastatic ovarian tumors

Adult:
Combination Therapy: 50 mg/m²/IV once every 3 weeks. **Single Agent Induction:** 100 mg/m² IV every 4 weeks.

Advanced bladder cancer

Adult: 50–70 mg/m² IV once every 3–4 weeks. Use of radiation therapy or other antineoplastics requires 50 mg/m² every 4 weeks.

Head/neck tumors

Adult:
Combination Therapy: 50–120 mg/m². **Single Agent Induction:** 80–120 mg/m² every 3 weeks or 50 mg/m² on day 1 and day 8 of an every 4 week cycle.

Pediatric: 60 mg/m² daily for 2 days every 3–4 weeks.

Nonsmall cell lung carcinoma

Adult:
Combination Therapy: 40–120 mg/m² every 3–6 weeks. **Single Induction Agent:** 75–120 mg/m² every 3–6 weeks or 50 mg/m² on day 1 and day 8 of an every 4 week cycle.

Osteogenic sarcoma/neuroblastoma

Pediatric: 90 mg/m² every 3 weeks or 30 mg/m² every week.

CONTRAINDICATIONS/PRECAUTIONS

Contraindicated in: Hearing impairment, history of allergic reaction to platinum containing compounds, myelosuppression, preexisting renal failure. **Use cautiously in:** BUN > 25, creatinine > 1.5, electrolyte abnormalities, patients with childbearing capability, platelet count < 100,000 mm³, WBC < 4000 mm³. **Pregnancy/Lactation:** No well-controlled trials to establish safety. Benefits must outweigh risks. Drug is teratogenic in rodents. Mutagenic potential. **Pediatrics:** Increased ototoxicity associated with administration in children.

PREPARATION

Availability: 1 mg/mL in 50, 100 mL vials. Powder for injection in 10 and 50 mg vials. Contains 1.54 mEq so-

In the Adverse Effects section, underline indicates most frequent; CAPS indicates life threatening.

123

dium/10 mg. **Reconstitution:** Dissolve each 10 mg with 10 mL sterile water for injection. Resulting solutions contain 1 mg/mL. **Infusion:** Further dilute in compatible diluent in physician specified volume following adequate hydration.

STABILITY/STORAGE

Vial: Refrigerate dry powder only. Keep reconstituted solutions at room temperature in order to prevent precipitation. **Infusion:** Stable for 20 hr at room temperature.

ADMINISTRATION

General: Handle drug with care and adhere to institutional guidelines for the handling of chemotherapeutic/cytotoxic agents. Aluminum containing IV needles or sets should not be used. **Intermittent Infusion:** Administer each dose over 15–120 min. **Continuous Infusion:** Administer over 24 hr.

COMPATIBILITY

Solution: Dextrose in sodium chloride, sodium chloride solutions. **Syringe:** Bleomycin, cyclophosphamide, doxapram, doxorubicin, droperidol, fluorouracil, furosemide, heparin, leucovorin calcium, methotrexate, metoclopramide, mitomycin, vinblastine, vincristine. **Y-site:** Bleomycin, cyclophosphamide, doxorubicin, droperidol, fluorouracil, furosemide, heparin, leucovorin calcium, methotrexate, metoclopramide, mitomycin, ondansetron, vinblastine, vincristine.

INCOMPATIBILITY

Solution: Sodium bicarbonate.

ADVERSE EFFECTS

CNS: Loss of taste, neurotoxicity, peripheral neuritis, seizures. **Ophtho:** Blurred vision, optic neuritis, papilledema. **CV:** Cardiac abnormalities. **GI:** Diarrhea, hepatotoxicity, <u>nausea</u>, metallic taste beginning 1–4 hr after dose and lasting 24 hr, <u>vomiting</u>. **GU:** Infertility. **Renal:** <u>Nephrotoxicity</u>, renal insufficiency, renal tubular damage. **Fld/Lytes:** Hypocalcemia, hypokalemia, hypomagnesemia. **Heme:** Anemia, LEUKOPENIA, <u>MYELOSUPPRESSION</u>, THROMBOCYTOPENIA, hyperuricemia. *Nadir:* 18–23 days. **Hypersens:** Anaphylactoid reactions. **Other:** Hyperuricemia, ototoxicity, phlebitis at IV site, tinnitus.

DRUG INTERACTIONS

Aminoglycosides, loop diuretics: Additive nephrotoxicity/ototoxicity. **Bone marrow depressants:** Potentiates bone marrow depression. **Phenytoin:** Reduced phenytoin levels.

NURSING CONSIDERATIONS

Assessment
General:
Vital signs, intake/output ratio.
Physical:
Infectious disease status, GI tract, hematopoietic system, signs/symptoms ototoxicity/neurotoxicity (dizziness, hearing loss, loss of coordination, paresthesias of extremities).
Lab Alterations:
Monitor baseline and periodic renal/hepatic function, electrolytes, CBC with differential, and platelet count.

In the Adverse Effects section, <u>underline</u> indicates most frequent; CAPS indicates life threatening.

Intervention/Rationale

Maintain urine output at 100–200 mL/hr for 4 hr before initiating therapy and 24 hr following completion. Encourage patient to drink at least 2000–3000 mL/day to promote adequate urine output and excretion of uric acid. ● Assess for development of fever, chills, or other signs of infection. ● Avoid all IM injections and rectal temperatures when platelet count is < 100,000 mm^3. ● Assess for development of bleeding (bleeding gums, easy bruising, petechiae, hematest positive stools/vomitus/urine). ● Carefully observe for development of hypersensitivity reactions (including wheezing, tachycardia, hypotension). ● Assure that proper antiemetic regimens are prescribed and given regularly to prevent nausea/vomiting.

Patient/Family Education

Review expected outcome and potential adverse effects of drug. Observe for signs of infection (fever, sore throat, fatigue) or bleeding (melena, bleeding gums, nosebleeds, easy bruising). Use a soft toothbrush and electric razor to minimize bleeding tendency. Take and record oral temperature daily and report persistent elevations to physician. Avoid crowded environments and persons with known infections. Report tinnitus or hearing loss immediately. Use consistent and reliable contraception throughout the duration of therapy due to potential teratogenic and mutagenic effects of drug. Seek physician approval prior to receiving live virus vaccinations. Avoid over-the-counter products containing aspirin/ibuprofen throughout course of therapy due to increased potential for bleeding. IV fluids should be administered throughout the course of therapy in an effort to keep the kidneys flushed. Report dizziness, unusual fatigue, or shortness of breath (drug may cause anemia).

CLINDAMYCIN
(klin-da-mye'-sin)

Trade Name(s): Cleocin, Dalacin C ✶

Classification(s): Antibiotic

Pregnancy Category: Unknown

PHARMACODYNAMICS/KINETICS

Mechanism of Action: Inhibits protein synthesis in susceptible organisms by binding to ribosomal units. **Peak Serum Level:** Immediate. **Distribution:** Significant tissue penetration. 60%–95% protein bound. Does not readily penetrate CSF. Not removed by peritoneal/hemodialysis. **Metabolism/Elimination:** 85% metabolized by the liver to active/inactive metabolites. Excreted 10%–15% unchanged by the kidneys. **Half-Life:** 2.4–3.0 hr, increased with significant liver disease.

INDICATIONS/DOSAGE

Treatment of serious infections caused by susceptible aerobic gram-positive cocci or anaerobic bacteria

Adult: 600–1200 mg/day in 2–4 divided doses. Determine dose by severity of infection. *Pediatric (> 1 month):* 15–25 mg/kg/day in 3–4 divided doses.

In the Adverse Effects section, <u>underline</u> indicates most frequent; CAPS indicates life threatening.

Treatment of more severe infections (*B. fragilis, Peptococcus, Clostridium*)

Adult: 1.2–2.7 g/day in 2–4 divided doses. Up to a maximum of 4.8 g/day. Dosage may have to be increased if infection is more serious. *Pediatric (< 1 month):* 25–40 mg/kg/day in 3–4 divided doses. Maximum daily dose 45 mg/kg/day or 4.8 g/day. *Neonate:* 15–20 mg/kg in divided doses every 6–8 hr. Maximum daily dose 300 mg.

Acute pelvic inflammatory disease

Adult: 600 mg every 6–8 hr. Continue for 4 days and at least 48 hr after symptoms improve. Additional aminoglycoside coverage should be given.

CONTRAINDICATIONS/ PRECAUTIONS

Contraindicated in: Hypersensitivity to clindamycin or lincomycin, treatment of minor bacterial/viral infections. **Use cautiously in:** Asthma, colitis, elderly, meningitis, renal/ hepatic disease, significant multiple allergies. **Pregnancy/Lactation:** No well-controlled trials to establish safety. Benefits must outweigh risks. Crosses placenta. No reports of congenital defects are known. Appears in breast milk. Discontinuation of breastfeeding is recommended to avoid potential problems in the infant. **Pediatrics:** Caution when administering to neonates (contains 9.45 mg benzyl alcohol). Organ system functions should be carefully monitored when administered to neonates.

PREPARATION

Availability: 150 mg/mL in 2, 4, and 6 mL vials. **Infusion:** Dilute to a concentration of not more than 12 mg/mL with compatible IV solution.

STABILITY/STORAGE

Vial: Store at room temperature. **Infusion:** Concentrations of 6–12 mg/mLare stable for 16 days at room temperature. Stable for 32 days refrigerated.

ADMINISTRATION

General: Rapid infusion may cause cardiac arrest. Should not be administered undiluted as a bolus injection. **Intermittent Infusion:** Give over at least 10 min. Do not administer more than 1200 mg/hr. **Continuous Infusion:** To maintain serum levels between 4–6 mcg/mL administer a single rapid infusion of the loading dose at 10–20 mg/min for 30 min. Maintenance infusion rate at 0.75–1.25 mg/min for physician prescribed period of time.

COMPATIBILITY

Solution: Amino acid 4.25%/dextrose 25%, dextrose solutions, lactated Ringer's, Ringer's injection, sodium chloride solutions. **Y-site:** Enalaprilat, foscarnet, ondansetron.

ADVERSE EFFECTS

CNS: Dizziness, headache, vertigo. **CV:** CARDIOPULMONARY ARREST (following too rapid administration), dysrhythmias, hypotension. **GI:** Pseudomembranous colitis, abdominal pain, anorexia, diarrhea, esophagitis, jaundice, nausea, vomiting. **Renal:** Azotemia, oliguria, proteinuria. **MS:** Polyarthritis. **Heme:**

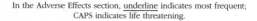
In the Adverse Effects section, underline indicates most frequent; CAPS indicates life threatening.

Agranulocytosis, elevated serum transaminases, eosinophilia, increased AST (SGOT), alkaline phosphatase, and bilirubin, leukopenia, neutropenia, thrombocytopenia. **Hypersens:** ANAPHYLAXIS, erythema multiforme, rash, urticaria. **Other:** Thrombophlebitis of IV site.

DRUG INTERACTIONS
Neuromuscular blocking agents (e.g., tubocurarine, pancuronium): Increased neuromuscular blockade.

NURSING CONSIDERATIONS
Assessment
General:
Allergy history, anaphylaxis, intake/output.
Physical:
GI tract, infectious disease status.
Lab Alterations:
Monitor electrolytes and CBC periodically.

Intervention/Rationale
Obtain specimens for culture and sensitivity prior to initiating therapy (do not withhold initial dose while waiting for results). ● Assess bowel sounds/function for development of diarrhea. Do not treat diarrhea with opiates or diphenoxylate with atropine as condition will worsen. Treat pseudomembranous colitis with fluid, protein, and electrolyte supplementation, IV corticosteroids or corticoid retention enemas. Consider toxicity if bloody stools, abdominal bloating/cramps, or a fever develops. ● Evaluate presence/absence of fever at least every 4 hr. ● Assess skin integrity regularly to note development of rash associated with hypersensitivity reaction. ● Assess for improvement/worsening of infection (temperature, WBC, wound, sputum, chest x-ray, urine, stool).

Patient/Family Education
Notify nurse/physician if diarrhea, bloody stools, abdominal cramping develops. Do not treat diarrhea with standard over-the-counter preparations without consulting physician. Prolonged or repeated use of antibiotics may result in bacterial/fungal overgrowth of nonsusceptible organisms; observe for signs/symptoms of superinfection (furry overgrowth on tongue, vaginal discharge/itching, anal discharge/itching, evidence of new infection sites).

CODEINE
(ko'-deen)
Classification(s): Narcotic analgesic
Pregnancy Category: C (D for prolonged use of high doses at full term)
Controlled Substance Schedule: II

PHARMACODYNAMICS/KINETICS
Mechanism of Action: Binds with opiate receptors at many sites in the brain, brain stem, and spinal cord. Alters perception of and emotional response to pain via an unknown mechanism. **Onset of Action:** 10–30 min. **Peak Effect:** 0.5–1.0 hr. **Duration of Action:** 4–6 hr. **Distribution:** Rapidly distributed to kidneys, liver, and

In the Adverse Effects section, <u>underline</u> indicates most frequent; CAPS indicates life threatening.

127

spleen. Minimally protein bound. **Metabolism/Elimination:** Metabolized by the liver. Excreted primarily by the kidneys. Negligible amounts excreted in feces. **Half-Life:** 3 hr.

INDICATIONS/DOSAGE

Relief of mild–moderate pain

Adult: 15–60 mg every 4–6 hr. Not to exceed 120 mg/24 hr.

CONTRAINDICATIONS/ PRECAUTIONS

Contraindicated in: Delivery of premature infant, hypersensitivity. **Use cautiously in:** Diarrhea of unknown etiology. **Pregnancy/Lactation:** No well-controlled trials to establish safety. Benefits must outweigh risks. Contraindicated during labor and delivery of premature infants. Crosses placenta rapidly. Distributed in breast milk. **Pediatrics:** Safety and efficacy unknown.

PREPARATION

Availability: 30 mg/mL and 60 mg/mL in 1 mL Tubex and vials.

STABILITY/STORAGE

Vial: Store at room temperature.

ADMINISTRATION

General: Do not administer discolored injection solution. **IV Push:** Give slowly (preferably as a 1:1 diluted solution).

COMPATIBILITY

Solution: Sodium chloride solutions, sterile water for injection. **Syringe:** Glycopyrrolate.

ADVERSE EFFECTS

CNS: Clouded sensorium, dizziness, euphoria, sedation, seizures (large doses). **CV:** Bradycardia, hypotension. **Resp:** Respiratory depression. **GI:** Constipation, dry mouth, nausea, paralytic ileus, vomiting. **GU:** Urinary retention. **Other:** Flushing, physical dependence, pruritus.

TOXICITY/OVERDOSE

Signs/Symptoms: Toxic doses may produce circulatory collapse, delirium, excitement, exhilaration, flushed face, hypotension, lassitude, miosis, muscle weakness, narcosis, respiratory paralysis/depression, slow pulse, tachycardia, tinnitus. **Treatment:** Discontinue drug if manifestations develop. Treat symptomatically and supportively. **Antidote(s):** Severe respiratory depression may be reversed by administration of opiate antagonists (naloxone).

DRUG INTERACTIONS

Antihistamines, barbiturates, general anesthetics, phenothiazines, sedative/ hypnotics, tranquilizers, tricyclic antidepressants: Concomitant use may cause coma, hypotension, profound sedation, respiratory depression.

NURSING CONSIDERATIONS

Assessment
General:
Vital signs, pain assessment (if used for analgesia), intake/output ratio.
Physical:
Respiratory, GI tract, neurologic status.

In the Adverse Effects section, underline indicates most frequent; CAPS indicates life threatening.

128

Intervention/Rationale
Evaluate neurological status periodically (note clouding of sensorium, increasing euphoria, or increasing lethargy—all indicative of need for dosage reduction). Use with extreme caution and under close supervision with all head injury patients (may obscure clinical course). ● Administer before intense pain occurs if using for analgesia. Assess pain control/reduction after receiving medication in order to evaluate overall effectiveness of drug. ● Assess bowel sounds/function daily (abdominal discomfort, diarrhea, or constipation). ● Drug may cause urinary retention. ● Discontinue gradually/slowly (physical dependency symptoms may develop if drug has been used for a prolonged period of time).

Patient/Family Education
Avoid all activities requiring mental alertness and seek assistance with ambulatory activities after receiving drug. Avoid alcohol and other CNS depressants. Drug may cause nausea, vomiting, or constipation.

COLCHICINE
(kol'-cha-seen)
Classification(s): Antigout agent
Pregnancy Category: D

PHARMACODYNAMICS/KINETICS
Mechanism of Action: Inhibits leukocyte migration, reduces lactic acid production in leukocytes, resulting in decreased uric acid, interferes with kinin formation, reduces phagocytosis and inflammatory re-

sponse. **Peak Serum Level:** Immediately after administration. **Distribution:** Concentrated in leukocytes. Distributed into kidney, liver, spleen, and GI tract. **Metabolism/Elimination:** Metabolized by the liver. Excreted primarily by biliary and renal routes. **Half-Life:** 20 min (plasma), 60 hr (leukocytes).

INDICATIONS/DOSAGE

Treatment of acute gout
Adult: Initial dose 2 mg followed by 0.5 mg every 6 hr until a satisfactory response is achieved. Do not exceed a total dose of 4 mg/24 hr or a total dose of 4 mg for one course of treatment. If pain recurs administer a daily dose of 1–2 mg for several days.

Prophylaxis/maintenance of recurrent or chronic gouty arthritis
Adult: 0.5–1.0 mg once or twice daily.

CONTRAINDICATIONS/ PRECAUTIONS
Contraindicated in: Hypersensitivity, serious cardiac, GI, or renal disorders. **Use cautiously in:** Geriatric/debilitated patients, hepatic dysfunction. **Pregnancy/Lactation:** No well-controlled trials to establish safety. Benefits must outweigh risks. Use cautiously in breastfeeding. **Pediatrics:** Safety and efficacy has not been established.

PREPARATION
Availability: 1 mg in 2 mL ampule. **Syringe:** May further dilute with sodium chloride or sterile water for injection (no preservative).

In the Adverse Effects section, underline indicates most frequent; CAPS indicates life threatening.

129

STABILITY/STORAGE
Vial: Store at room temperature.

ADMINISTRATION
General: Preferably inject into a tubing of free flowing compatible IV solution. Assess for thrombophlebitis/extravasation. Heat or cold, in conjunction with analgesics, may relieve discomfort from extravasation. Parenteral form of drug is used when rapid response is desired or when GI side effects interfere with oral administration. **IV Push:** Give over 2–5 min.

COMPATIBILITY
Solution: Sodium chloride solutions, sterile water (preservative free).

INCOMPATIBILITY
Solution: Dextrose solutions.

ADVERSE EFFECTS
CNS: Peripheral neuritis. **GI:** Abdominal pain, <u>diarrhea</u>, elevated alkaline phosphatase/AST (SGOT), nausea, vomiting. **GU:** Reversible azoospermia. **Derm:** Alopecia, purpura. **Heme:** Agranulocytosis, aplastic anemia, bone marrow depression, leukopenia, thrombocytopenia (long-term use). **Other:** Phlebitis at IV site.

TOXICITY/OVERDOSE
Signs/Symptoms: Toxic doses may cause generalized vascular damage, oliguria, renal damage with hematuria, severe diarrhea. Overdosage may cause abdominal pain, ascending paralysis, convulsions, diarrhea, delirium, nausea, vascular damage resulting in shock, and vomiting. **Treatment:** Discontinue when symptoms appear irrespective of joint pain relief. No known specific antidote for overdosage.

Use of hemodialysis or peritoneal dialysis may be indicated. Atropine or morphine may be used for abdominal pain relief. Paregoric is useful in controlling diarrhea and abdominal cramps.

DRUG INTERACTIONS
Acidifying agents: Inhibits colchicine effects. **Alkalinizing agents:** Potentiates colchicine. **CNS depressant, sympathomimetic agents:** Colchicine increases sensitivity to drug. **Loop diuretics:** Decreased colchicine efficacy.

NURSING CONSIDERATIONS
Assessment
General:
Pain assessment, intake/output ratio.
Physical:
GI tract.
Lab Alterations:
Monitor baseline and periodic CBC and liver function tests, false-positive urine test for RBC or hemoglobin.

Intervention/Rationale
Assess for pain relief and increased mobility and monitor for improvement every 1–2 hr. ● Encourage fluids to maintain adequate urinary output. ● Evalute GI system including bowel sounds/function; assess for development of nausea, vomiting, or diarrhea.

Patient/Family Education
Notify physician if bruising, fever, numbness, skin rash, sore throat, tingling, tiredness, unusual bleeding, or weakness occur. Discontinue medication as soon as gout

In the Adverse Effects section, <u>underline</u> indicates most frequent; CAPS indicates life threatening.

pain is relieved or at first sign of diarrhea, nausea, stomach pain, or vomiting is noted and notify physician immediately.

CORTICOTROPIN
(kor-ti-ko-troe′-pin)
Trade Name(s): Acthar, ACTH
Classification(s): Adrenal
cortical steroid
Pregnancy Category: C

PHARMACODYNAMICS/KINETICS
Mechanism of Action: Stimulates adrenal cortex to secrete cortisol, corticosterone, weak adrenergic substances, and aldosterone. Does not increase cortisol secretion in primary adrenocortical insufficiency. **Onset of Action:** Rapid. **Peak Serum Level:** 1 hr. **Duration of Action:** 2–4 hr. **Distribution:** Distributed throughout body tissues. **Metabolism/Elimination:** Metabolic reaction is not known. Excreted primarily by the kidneys. **Half-Life:** 15 min.

INDICATIONS/DOSAGE

Diagnosis of adrenocortical functions

Adult: 10–25 units/24 hr. *Pediatric:* 1.6 units/kg or 50 units/m^2 in 3–4 equally divided doses.

Myasthenia gravis (*unlabeled use*)

Adult: 100 units infused daily for 10 days. Repeat dosage after 5–10 days.

CONTRAINDICATIONS/PRECAUTIONS
Contraindicated in: Adrenocortical hyperfunction or primary insufficiency, CHF, Cushing's syndrome, hypertension. IV administration is contraindicated except in the treatment of idiopathic thrombocytopenia or for diagnostic testing of adrenocortical function. Also contraindicated in live vaccinations, ocular herpes simplex, osteoporosis, peptic ulcer, recent surgery, scleroderma, sensitivity to pork and pork products, systemic fungal infections. **Use cautiously in:** Abscess, acute gouty arthritis, cirrhosis, diabetes, diverticulitis, emotional instability or psychotic tendencies, hypothyroidism, latent tuberculosis or tuberculosis reactivity, myasthenia gravis, patients being immunized, pyogenic infections, renal insufficiency. **Pregnancy/Lactation:** No well-controlled trials to establish safety. Benefits must outweigh risks. First trimester pregnancy is a relative contraindication. **Pediatrics:** May retard bone growth. Give intermittently if necessary.

PREPARATION
Availability: 25 and 40 units/vial. **Reconstitution:** Dissolve powder in sterile water for injection or sodium chloride so that individual dose will be contained in 1–2 mL. **Infusion:** Withdraw desired dose from reconstituted vial and dilute with 500 mL compatible IV fluid.

STABILITY/STORAGE
Vial: Store at room temperature. **Infusion:** Reconstituted solution should be refrigerated and used within 24 hr.

In the Adverse Effects section, underline indicates most frequent; CAPS indicates life threatening.

131

ADMINISTRATION
Intermittent Infusion: Infuse over 8 hr.

COMPATIBILITY
Solution: Dextrose solutions, lactated Ringer's, Ringer's injection, sodium chloride solutions.

ADVERSE EFFECTS
CNS: Convulsions, <u>depression</u>, euphoria, headache, vertigo. **Ophtho:** Cataracts, glaucoma, increased intraocular pressure. **CV:** CHF, edema, hypertension, necrotizing angiitis, thromboembolism. **Resp:** Abscess of lung, pneumonia. **GI:** Abdominal distention, pancreatitis, peptic ulcer with possible perforation/hemorrhage, ulcerative esophagitis. **MS:** Aseptic necrosis of bone, muscle weakness, osteoporosis, pathological fracture of the long bones, steroid myopathy. **Derm:** Ecchymoses, impaired wound healing, petechiae. **Endo:** <u>Adrenal suppression</u>, <u>decreased growth in children</u>, hirsutism, hyperglycemia, latent diabetes mellitus, menstrual irregularities. **Fld/Lytes:** Fluid retention, hypocalcemia, hypokalemia, metabolic alkalosis, sodium retention. **Hypersens:** Dizziness, nausea, shock, skin reactions, vomiting. **Other:** Prolonged use may result in antibody production and subsequent loss of stimulation effect of the drug; sepsis.

DRUG INTERACTIONS
Amphotericin B, diuretics, mezlocillin, piperacillin, ticarcillin: Additive hypokalemic effects of corticosteroids. **Aspirin:** Corticotropin may increase renal clearance of salicylates. Increased serum levels of aspirin and salicylate toxicity may occur when steroid therapy is discontinued. **Insulin, oral hypoglycemics:** Increased antidiabetic agent needs.

NURSING CONSIDERATIONS
Assessment
General:
Hypersensitivity, skin testing (with suspected sensitivity to pork/pork products), vital signs, intake/output, daily weight.
Physical:
GI tract.
Lab Alterations:
Monitor serum/urine glucose; baseline and periodic electrolytes, glucose, cholesterol, hematology profile (prolonged use); suppressed reactions to allergy skin testing; decreased I-131 uptake.

Intervention/Rationale
Drug may cause hypertension. ● Hematest stools/vomitus/nasogastric contents for presence of occult blood. ● Assess diabetics for changing insulin and oral hypoglycemic needs. ● Chronic use may result in suppression of the adrenal glands.

Patient/Family Education
Drug may mask infection; record oral temperature daily. Avoid immunization with live vaccine while receiving drug. Diabetics may experience increased requirements for insulin/oral hypoglycemics. Notify physician/nurse with muscle weakness, abdominal pain, seizures, or headache. Weigh daily if on drug for prolonged period of time.

In the Adverse Effects section, <u>underline</u> indicates most frequent; CAPS indicates life threatening.

COSYNTROPIN

(ko-sin-tro'-pin)
Trade Name(s): Cortrosyn, Synacthen ✢
Classification(s): Synthetic pituitary hormone
Pregnancy Category: C

PHARMACODYNAMICS/KINETICS

Mechanism of Action: Stimulates adrenal cortex to secrete cortisol, corticosterone, androgens, aldosterone. Does not increase cortisol secretion in primary adrenocortical insufficiency. **Onset of Action:** 30 min. **Peak Serum Level:** 45–60 min. **Duration of Action:** 2–4 hr. **Distribution:** Distribution and metabolic fate is unknown. **Metabolism/Elimination:** Metabolism unknown. Rapidly removed from plasma by many tissues. **Half-Life:** 15 min.

INDICATIONS/DOSAGE

Rapid screening test of adrenal function, diagnostic drug for adrenocortical insufficiency

Adult: 250 mcg (0.25 mg). Up to 750 mcg (0.75 mg). *Pediatric:* 125 mcg (0.125 mg) for children < 2 yr. May use adult dose for children > 2 yr.

CONTRAINDICATIONS/ PRECAUTIONS

Contraindicated in: Hypersensitivity to drug or its components. **Use cautiously in:** Hypersensitivity to natural corticotropin. **Pregnancy/Lactation:** No well-controlled trial to establish safety. Benefits must outweigh risks. **Pediatrics:** Safety and efficacy not established for children less than 2 yr.

PREPARATION

Availability: 0.25 mg per vial with diluent. **Reconstitution:** Add 1 mL sodium chloride (diluent provided). **Syringe:** May be given direct IV after initial reconstitution. **Infusion:** Further dilute in compatible IV solution.

STABILITY/STORAGE

Vial: Store at room temperature. Stable at room temperature for 24 hr following reconstitution, 21 days if refrigerated. **Infusion:** Stable for 24 hr at room temperature.

ADMINISTRATION

General: Inactivated by enzymes. Not to be added to blood or plasma. **IV Push:** Give over 2 minutes. **Intermittent Infusion:** Infuse diluted solution at 0.04 mg/hr over 4–6 hr.

COMPATIBILITY

Solution: Dextrose solutions, sodium chloride solution.

ADVERSE EFFECTS

CNS: Dizziness, irritability, seizures. **CV:** Bradycardia, fainting. **Resp:** Dyspnea. **Fld/Lytes:** Fluid retention, sodium retention. **Hypersens:** Rash, urticaria. **Other:** Fever, flushing.

DRUG INTERACTIONS

Cortisone, hydrocortisone: Avoid giving on day of test to prevent interference with diagnostic results.

In the Adverse Effects section, underline indicates most frequent; CAPS indicates life threatening.

NURSING CONSIDERATIONS

Assessment

General:

Anaphylaxis, intake/output ratio, daily weight, heart rate.

Lab Alterations:

Falsely elevated plasma cortisol levels.

Intervention/Rationale

Drug may cause bradycardia, fluid/sodium retention. ● Evaluate for hypersensitivity reactions.

Patient/Family Education

Dizziness, faintness, and slow pulse may be noted during administration; notify nurse/physician if any of these effects are experienced.

CYCLOPHOSPHAMIDE

(sye-kloe-foss'-fa-mide)

Trade Name(s): Cytoxan, Neosar, Procytox ✚

Classification(s): Alkylating agent, antineoplastic

Pregnancy Category: D

PHARMACODYNAMICS/KINETICS

Mechanism of Action: Interferes with DNA and RNA synthesis by cross linking of tumor cell DNA. **Peak Serum Level:** 1 hr. **Distribution:** Distributed throughout the body as well as small concentrations in CSF and brain. Protein binding: 0%–10% (a higher percentage for metabolites). **Metabolism/Elimination:** Primarily hepatically metabolized to active metabolites. Active drug (30% unchanged drug) and metabolites excreted within 24 hr. Drug/metabolites may be detected in plasma up to 72 hr. **Half-Life:** 4.0–6.5 hr.

INDICATIONS/DOSAGE

Malignant diseases (including lymphomas, multiple myeloma, leukemias, mycosis fungoides, neuroblastoma, adenocarcinoma of lung, carcinoma of breast, and retinoblastoma.) Reduce dosage with preexisting bone marrow suppression, concurrent immunosuppressants, or chemotherapeutic regimens.

Adult: 40–50 mg/kg (1.5–1.8 g/m^2) in divided doses over 2–5 days. Alternate dosage regimen 10–15 mg/kg every 7–10 days or 3–5 mg/kg twice weekly. *Pediatric:* 2–8 mg/kg/day (60–250 mg/m^2/day) for 6–7 days. Alternate dosage regimen 15–50 mg/kg/week initially, followed by 2–5 mg/kg/dose twice weekly. Additional dosage regimen 10–15 mg/kg/dose weekly or 30 mg/kg/dose every 3–4 weeks.

Amelioration of multiple sclerosis progression, symptoms, and/or frequency (*unlabeled use*)

Adult: Total dose 1–12 g.

Polyarteritis nodosa (*unlabeled use*)

Adult: 4 mg/kg/day initially.

Polymyositis (*unlabeled use*)

Adult: 500 mg over 1 hr every 1–3 weeks.

CONTRAINDICATIONS/PRECAUTIONS

Contraindicated in: Hypersensitivity, severely depressed bone marrow function. **Use cautiously in:** Patients with immunosuppression or receiv-

In the Adverse Effects section, underline indicates most frequent; CAPS indicates life threatening.

ing immunosuppressants. **Pregnancy/Lactation:** No well-controlled trials to establish safety. Teratogenic potential is documented in males and females. Patients should avoid conception/pregnancy. Crosses placenta. Excreted into breast milk. Breastfeeding should be discontinued while receiving this agent.

PREPARATION

Availability: 100 mg, 200 mg, 500 mg, 1 g, 2 g vials. **Reconstitution:** Dilute each 100 mg with 5 mL sterile water for injection or bacteriostatic water for injection. **Infusion:** Further dilute to physician specified volume in compatible IV solution.

STABILITY/STORAGE

Vial: Store at room temperature. Reconstituted solutions stable for 24 hr at room temperature and 6 days refrigerated. If sterile water for injection was used (no preservative), use solution within 6 hr. **Infusion:** Stable for 6 days refrigerated.

ADMINISTRATION

General: Handle drug with care and adhere to institutional guidelines for the handling of chemotherapeutic/cytotoxic agents. **IV Push:** Give slowly direct IV push over 3–5 min. **Intermittent Infusion:** Infuse over physician specified time.

COMPATIBILITY

Solution: Amino acids 4.25%/dextrose 25%, dextrose solutions, lactated Ringer's, sodium chloride solutions. **Syringe:** Bleomycin, cisplatin, doxapram, doxorubicin, droperidol, fluorouracil, furosemide, heparin, leucovorin calcium, methotrexate, metoclopramide, mitomycin, vinblastine, vincristine. **Y-site:** Amikacin, ampicillin, bleomycin, cefazolin, cefoperazone, ceforanide, cefotaxime, cefoxitin, cefuroxime, cephalothin, cephapirin, chloramphenicol, cisplatin, clindamycin, doxorubicin, doxycycline, droperidol, erythromycin, fluorouracil, furosemide, gentamicin, heparin, leucovorin calcium, methotrexate, metoclopramide, mitomycin, vinblastine, vincristine.

ADVERSE EFFECTS

CNS: With high doses: coronary artery vasculitis, hemorrhagic cardiac necrosis, transmural hemorrhages. **Resp:** Interstitial pulmonary fibrosis. **GI:** Abdominal discomfort, anorexia, diarrhea, nausea, stomatitis, vomiting. **GU:** Acute hemorrhagic cystitis. **Renal:** Renal tubular necrosis. **Derm:** Alopecia, pigmentation skin/nails. **Fld/Lytes:** Syndrome of inappropriate antidiuretic hormone (SIADH). **Heme:** LEUKOPENIA, MYELOSUPPRESSION, THROMBOCYTOPENIA. *Nadir:* 8–15 days. **Hypersens:** Rash. **Other:** SECONDARY NEOPLASIA.

TOXICITY/OVERDOSE

Signs/Symptoms: Extension of adverse effects especially cardiotoxicity, myelosuppression, and concurrent infection. **Treatment:** Symptomatic and supportive.

DRUG INTERACTIONS

Anticoagulants: Increased anticoagulant effect. **Chloramphenicol:** Increased cyclophosphamide half-life. **Concomitant chemotherapeutic agents, immunosuppressants:** Increased myelosuppression. **Digoxin:** Decreased digoxin serum levels.

In the Adverse Effects section, underline indicates most frequent; CAPS indicates life threatening.

Doxorubicin: Increased cardiotoxicity. **Succinylcholine:** Increased neuromuscular blockade. **Thiazide diuretics:** Increased cyclosphosphamide levels/toxicity.

NURSING CONSIDERATIONS

Assessment

General:

Vital signs, intake/output ratio.

Physical:

Infectious disease status, GU tract, GI tract, hematopoietic system, cardiopulmonary complications.

Lab Alterations:

Monitor baseline and periodic renal/hepatic function, electrolytes, CBC with differential and platelet count.

Intervention/Rationale

Maintain urine output at 100–200 mL/hr for 4 hr before initiating therapy and 24 hr following completion, encourage patient to drink at least 2–3 L/day (adult) or 1–2 L/day (children) to promote adequate urine output and avoid hemorrhagic cystitis. Avoid administration in the evening to prevent accumulation in the bladder. ● Assess for development of fever, chills, or other signs of infection. ● Avoid all IM injections and rectal temperatures when platelet count is < 100,000 mm³. ● Assess for development of bleeding (bleeding gums, easy bruising, petechiae, hematest positive stools/vomitus/urine). ● Assure that proper antiemetic regimens are prescribed and given regularly to prevent nausea/vomiting. ● Assess for signs/symptoms of pulmonary toxicity with prolonged use (dyspnea, rales, crackles). ● Assess for signs and symptoms of cardiac toxicity that may occur early in therapy (characterized by symptoms of CHF).

Patient/Family Education

Review expected outcome and potential adverse effects of drug, especially expected loss of hair. Observe for signs of infection (fever, sore throat, fatigue) or bleeding (melena, bleeding gums, nosebleeds, easy bruising). Use a soft toothbrush and electric razor to minimize bleeding tendency. Take and record oral temperature daily and report persistent elevations to physician. Avoid crowded environments and persons with known infections. Use consistent and reliable contraception throughout the duration of therapy due to potential teratogenic and mutagenic effects of drug. Seek physician approval prior to receiving live virus vaccinations. Avoid over-the-counter products containing aspirin/ibuprofen throughout course of therapy due to increased potential for bleeding. IV fluids should be administered throughout the course of therapy in an effort to keep the kidneys flushed. Report dizziness, unusual fatigue, or shortness of breath (drug may cause anemia).

CYCLOSPORINE

(sye'-kloe-spor-een)

Trade Name(s): Sandimmune

Classification(s):

Immunosuppressant

Pregnancy Category: C

In the Adverse Effects section, <u>underline</u> indicates most frequent; CAPS indicates life threatening.

PHARMACODYNAMICS/KINETICS

Mechanism of Action: Exact mechanism unknown. Specific and reversible inhibition of immunocompetent lymphocytes, especially T lymphocytes. Inhibition of lymphokine production and release. **Peak Serum Level:** 3.5 hr. **Therapeutic Serum Levels:** 250–800 ng/mL (whole blood, RIA) or 50–300 ng/mL (plasma, RIA). **Distribution:** Distributed outside blood volume (into plasma, erythrocytes, granulocytes, and lymphocytes). 90% bound to plasma proteins, especially lipoproteins. **Metabolism/Elimination:** Extensively hepatically metabolized by cytochrome P-450 hepatic enzymes to active metabolites. Primarily excreted via biliary tract. **Half-Life:** 10–27 hr.

INDICATIONS/DOSAGE

Prophylaxis and treatment of organ rejection in kidney, liver, heart allogeneic transplants in conjunction with immunosuppressants.

Adult/Pediatric: 5–6 mg/kg/day 4–12 hr prior to transplantation. Followed with 5–6 mg/kg/day as a daily dose until oral therapy can be instituted. IV form should be changed to oral as soon as possible. Hepatotoxicity, nephrotoxicity, or bone marrow depression may require dosage to be temporarily decreased.

CONTRAINDICATIONS/ PRECAUTIONS

Contraindicated in: Hypersensitivity to cyclosporine and/or polyoxyethylated castor oil. **Use cautiously in:** Hepatic/renal impairment. **Preg-** nancy/Lactation: No well-controlled trials to establish safety. Benefits must outweigh risks. Breastfeeding should be discontinued while receiving this agent. **Pediatrics:** There are no well-controlled trials in pediatrics. No unusual adverse effects have been noted in children > 6 months.

PREPARATION

Availability: 50 mg/mL, 5 mL ampule. **Infusion:** Dilute each 50 mg (1 mL) in 20–100 mL compatible IV solution. Use glass bottles.

STABILITY/STORAGE

Vial: Store at room temperature. Protect from light. **Infusion:** Prepare just prior to administration. Use glass bottles and nondiethylhexyl phthalate (nonPVC) tubing, if possible, if drug is not prepared just prior to administration (Plasticizer leaching may occur from PVC bags and tubing). Stable for 24 hr (Use within 6 hr in PVC bags, 12 hr in glass).

ADMINISTRATION

General: Must be given by slow IV infusion. **Intermittent Infusion:** Infuse over 2–6 hr.

COMPATIBILITY

Solution: Dextrose solutions (in glass), sodium chloride solutions.

ADVERSE EFFECTS

CNS: Convulsions, headache, paresthesia, tremors **CV:** Hypertension. **Resp:** Sinusitis. **GI:** Hepatotoxicity, abdominal discomfort, anorexia, constipation, diarrhea, gastritis, gum hyperplasia, nausea, vomiting.

In the Adverse Effects section, <u>underline</u> indicates most frequent; CAPS indicates life threatening.

137

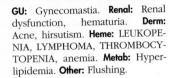

GU: Gynecomastia. **Renal:** Renal dysfunction, hematuria. **Derm:** Acne, hirsutism. **Heme:** LEUKOPENIA, LYMPHOMA, THROMBOCYTOPENIA, anemia. **Metab:** Hyperlipidemia. **Other:** Flushing.

TOXICITY/OVERDOSE

Signs/Symptoms: Transient hepato/nephrotoxicity. **Treatment:** Supportive and symptomatic treatment. Hemodialysis is not beneficial.

DRUG INTERACTIONS

Aminoglycosides, amphotericin B, melphalan, nonsteroidal anti-inflammatory agents, quinolones (ciprofloxacin, norfloxacin, ofloxacin): Increased cyclosporine (CYA) nephrotoxicity. **Azathioprine, corticosteroids, cyclophosphamide, verapamil:** Increased immunosuppression. **Carbamazepine, isoniazid, phenobarbital, phenytoin, rifampin, trimethoprim/sulfamethoxazole:** Decreased CYA serum level. **Danazol, methyltestosterone, oral contraceptives:** Increased CYA serum levels and nephrotoxicity. **Digoxin:** Increased digoxin levels. **Diltiazem, erythromycin, fluconazole, ketoconazole, nicardipine:** Increased CYA serum levels. **Imipenem:** Increased serum levels and CNS toxicity. **Methylprednisolone, prednisolone:** Increased plasma (RIA)/decreased blood (HPLC) levels.

NURSING CONSIDERATIONS

Assessment

General:
Vital signs, intake/output ratio, daily weight.
Physical:
Signs/symptoms of organ rejection.

Lab Alterations:
Monitor CYA serum levels closely. Monitor CBC, platelets, serum creatinine/BUN, and liver profile prior to, and throughout therapy.

Intervention/Rationale

Monitor patient closely for the first 30 minutes following start of the infusion and at frequent intervals thereafter. Observe for signs/symptoms of hypersensitivity reactions (wheezing, dyspnea, flushing). Discontinue the infusion if anaphylaxis occurs.

Patient/Family Education

Review expected outcome and potential adverse effects of drug. Observe for signs of infection (fever, sore throat, fatigue). Patient will require frequent drug serum level assessment.

CYTARABINE (CYTOSINE ARABINOSIDE, ARA-C)

(sye-tare'-a-been)
Trade Name(s): Cytosar-U
Classification(s): Antimetabolite agent, antineoplastic
Pregnancy Category: D

PHARMACODYNAMICS/KINETICS

Mechanism of Action: Inhibition of DNA polymerase resulting in DNA synthesis inhibition. **Peak Effect:** 20–60 minutes. **Distribution:** Rapidly and widely distributed into tissues. Crosses the blood–brain barrier to a limited extent. 13% protein bound. **Metabolism/Elimination:** Rapid and extensive metabolism. Primarily hepatically metabolized; additional

In the Adverse Effects section, underline indicates most frequent; CAPS indicates life threatening.

CYTARABINE (CYTOSINE ARABINOSIDE, ARA-C)

degradation occurs in kidneys, GI mucosa, and granulocytes. Converted intracellularly to active metabolites. Active drug and metabolites excreted in urine (70%–80% in 24 hr, 10% as unchanged drug, and 90% as inactive metabolites). **Half-Life:** Biphasic: Initial phase 10 min, terminal phase 1–3 hr.

INDICATIONS/DOSAGE

Acute lymphocytic leukemia

Adult/Pediatric:
Single Agent: 200 mg/m² daily for 5 days. Repeat every 2 weeks. **Combination Agent:** 2–6 mg/kg/day or 100–200 mg/m² daily for 5–10 days.

Acute nonlymphocytic leukemia combination therapy

Adult/Pediatric: 100 mg/m²/day by continuous infusion days 1 to 7. Alternate dosage regimen 100 mg/m² in divided doses every 12 hr on days 1 to 7.

Meningeal leukemia (intrathecal)

Adult/Pediatric: 5–75 mg/m² once daily for 4 days or once every 4 days. Usual dose is 30 mg/m² every 4 days until CSF findings are normal, followed by one additional treatment.

Refractory acute leukemia

Adult/Pediatric: 3 g/m² every 12 hr for 4–12 doses. Repeat at 2–3 week intervals.

CONTRAINDICATIONS/ PRECAUTIONS

Contraindicated in: Hypersensitivity.
Use cautiously in: Patients with im-

munosuppression. Premature infants due to benzyl alcohol presence in diluent. **Pregnancy/Lactation:** No well-controlled trials to establish safety. Teratogenic potential is documented. Patients should avoid pregnancy during therapy. Breast-feeding should be discontinued while receiving this agent.

PREPARATION

Availability: 100 mg, 500 mg, 1 g, 2 g vials. Provided diluent is bacteriostatic water for injection. **Reconstitution:** Dilute 100 mg with 5 mL, 0.5–1.0 g with 10 mL, and 2 g with 20 mL bacteriostatic water for injection. *High Dose:* Use sterile water for injection (without preservative). **Intrathecal:** Use sodium chloride injection (without preservative). **Syringe:** For intrathecal use, volume should not exceed 5–15 mL. **Infusion:** Further dilute to physician specified volume of compatible IV solution sufficient to run as continuous infusion.

STABILITY/STORAGE

Vial: Store at room temperature. Reconstituted solutions stable 48 hr at room temperature. **Infusion:** Stable for 8 days at room temperature.

ADMINISTRATION

General: Handle drug with care and adhere to institutional guidelines for the handling of chemotherapeutic/cytotoxic agents. **IV Push:** May be given rapidly. **Intermittent Infusion:** Infuse over physician specified time. High dose infusions should be over 1–3 hr.

In the Adverse Effects section, underline indicates most frequent; CAPS indicates life threatening.

COMPATIBILITY
Solution: Amino acid 4.25%/dextrose 25%, dextrose solutions, Elliott's B solution, lactated Ringer's, Ringer's injection, sodium chloride solutions. **Syringe:** Metoclopramide. **Y-site:** Ondansetron.

ADVERSE EFFECTS
CNS: Neurotoxicity, dizziness, headache, neuritis. **Ophtho:** Conjunctivitis. **CV:** Chest pain. **Resp:** Shortness of breath. **GI:** Hepatic dysfunction, abdominal pain, anorexia, diarrhea, esophagitis, nausea, oral/anal inflammation, vomiting. **Renal:** Renal dysfunction. **Derm:** Alopecia, cellulitis, freckling, skin ulceration. **Heme:** ANEMIA, bleeding, LEUKOPENIA, MYELOSUPPRESSION, THROMBOCYTOPENIA, hyperuricemia. *Nadir:* 7–9 days; then a greater decline at 15–24 days. **Hypersens:** Allergic edema, ANAPHYLAXIS, pruritus, rash, urticaria. **Other:** ARA-C SYNDROME occurring 6–12 hr after administration (bone/chest pain, conjunctivitis, fever, maculopapular rash, malaise, myalgia), BACTERIAL, FUNGAL, PARASITIC, VIRAL INFECTIONS, fever, thrombophlebitis.

TOXICITY/OVERDOSE
Signs/Symptoms: Extension of adverse effects especially CNS toxicity and death. **Treatment:** Symptomatic and supportive.

DRUG INTERACTIONS
Aminoglycosides, flucytosine: Decreased activity against Klebsiella pneumoniae and fungi, respectively. **Concomitant chemotherapy agents, immunosuppressants:** Increased myelosuppression. **Digoxin tablets:** Decreased digoxin absorption.

NURSING CONSIDERATIONS
Assessment
General:
Vital signs, intake/output ratio.
Physical:
Infectious disease status, neurologic status, hematopoietic system.
Lab Alterations:
Monitor baseline and periodic renal/hepatic function, electrolytes, CBC with differential, and platelet count.

Intervention/Rationale
Assess for development of fever, chills, or other signs of infection. ● Assess for drug-induced syndromes (bone/chest pain, conjunctivitis, fever, maculopapular rash, malaise, myalgia). ● Avoid all IM injections and rectal temperatures when platelet count is < 100,000 mm³. ● Assess for development of bleeding (bleeding gums, easy bruising, petechiae, hematest positive stools/vomitus/urine). ● Assure that proper antiemetic regimens are prescribed and given regularly to prevent nausea/vomiting.

Patient/Family Education
Review expected outcome and potential adverse effects of drug especially expected loss of hair. Observe for signs of infection (fever, sore throat, fatigue) or bleeding (melena, bleeding gums, nosebleeds, easy bruising). Use a soft toothbrush and electric razor to minimize bleeding tendency. Take and record oral temperature daily and report persistent elevations to

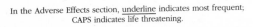

In the Adverse Effects section, underline indicates most frequent; CAPS indicates life threatening.

physician. Avoid crowded environments and persons with known infections. Use consistent and reliable contraception throughout the duration of therapy due to potential teratogenic and mutagenic effects of drug. Seek physician approval prior to receiving live virus vaccinations. Avoid over-the-counter products containing aspirin/ibuprofen throughout course of therapy due to increased potential for bleeding. Report dizziness, unusual fatigue, shortness of breath, or nervous system toxicity (numbness, tingling, loss of sensation).

CYTOMEGALOVIRUS IMMUNE GLOBULIN IV, HUMAN

(sye-toe-meg′-a-loe-vye-rus)
Classification(s): Immune serum globulin
Pregnancy Category: Unknown

PHARMACODYNAMICS/KINETICS
Mechanism of Action: Contains high proportions of antibodies against cytomegalovirus (CMV).

INDICATIONS/DOSAGE

Attenuation of CMV in seronegative CMV transplant recipients of CMV seropositive organs.

Adult/Pediatric: Not to exceed 150 mg/kg/infusion.
Within 72 hr of Transplant: 150 mg/kg.
2–8 Weeks Post-Transplant: 100 mg/kg. **12–16 Weeks Post-Transplant:** 50 mg/kg.

CONTRAINDICATIONS/ PRECAUTIONS
Contraindicated in: Hypersensitivity to drug components or human albumin. **Use cautiously in:** Patients with prior allergic reactions to immunoglobulins. **Pregnancy/Lactation:** Data not available.

PREPARATION
Availability: 2500 mg ± 250 mg/vial. 50 mL sterile water for injection provided as diluent. Contains 5% sucrose and 1% human albumin. **Reconstitution:** Dilute with 50 mL provided diluent via double-ended transfer needle or large syringe. Do not shake. Allow 30 min for complete dissolution. Must be colorless and free of particles. **Infusion:** Slow or temporarily discontinue if minor adverse reactions occur.

STABILITY/STORAGE
Vial: Refrigerate. **Infusion:** Begin infusion within 6 hr and complete within 12 hr of reconstitution.

ADMINISTRATION
General: Complete within 12 hr of reconstitution. Discontinue infusion if anaphylaxis occurs and treat symptomatically. No further dilution necessary. Give via infusion pump through separate IV line containing compatible IV solution. May be piggybacked into preexisting IV line at a dilution of 1 part drug and 2 parts solution. Filtration not needed. **Intermittent Infusion: *Initial dose:*** 15 mg/kg/hr for 30 minutes. Increase to 30 mg/kg/hr if no evidence of reaction. Increase to 60 mg/kg/hr after an additional 30 minutes if no evidence of reaction.

In the Adverse Effects section, underline indicates most frequent; CAPS indicates life threatening.

141

D

Not to exceed 75 mL/hr. *Subsequent Dose:* 15 mg/kg/hr for 15 min. Increase to 30 mg/kg/hr if no evidence of reaction. Increase to 60 mg/kg/hr after an additional 15 minutes if no evidence of reaction. Not to exceed 75 mL/hr.

COMPATIBILITY
Solution: Dextrose solutions, sodium chloride solutions.

ADVERSE EFFECTS
CV: Hypotension. **Resp:** Wheezing. **GI:** Nausea, vomiting. **MS:** Back pain, muscle cramps. **Other:** Chills, fever, flushing.

NURSING CONSIDERATIONS
Assessment
General:
Vital signs.
Physical:
Signs/symptoms of hypersensitivity reactions.

Intervention/Rationale
Reduce flow rate or discontinue and notify physician if vital signs change significantly.

Patient/Family Education
Observe for early signs of allergic reaction (wheezing, chills, fever). Drug is pooled from human serum and risk of transmission of HIV/hepatitis B is present (however, advances in screening techniques reduce risk).

DACARBAZINE (DTIC)
(da-kar'-ba-zeen)
Trade Name(s): DTIC-Dome
Classification(s): Antineoplastic
Pregnancy Category: C

PHARMACODYNAMICS/KINETICS
Mechanism of Action: Exact mechanism unknown. Inhibition of DNA and RNA synthesis. Alkylating effect. **Distribution:** Primarily tissue localization especially in liver. Little penetration into CNS. Minimal protein binding. **Metabolism/Elimination:** Primarily hepatically metabolized to active and inactive metabolites. Eliminated via tubular secretion. 30%–46% active drug recovered in urine after 6 hr (50% as unchanged drug, 50% major active metabolite). **Half-Life:** Biphasic: distributive 19 min, terminal 5 hr. Increased in renal and hepatic impairment.

INDICATIONS/DOSAGE

Metastatic malignant melanoma
Adult: 2.0–4.5 mg/kg/day for 10 days repeated at 4 week intervals. Alternate dosage regimen 250 mg/m^2/day for 5 days and repeated at 3 week intervals.

Combination therapy in Hodgkin's disease
Adult: 150 mg/m^2/day for 5 days repeated at 4 week intervals. Alternate dosage regimen 375 mg/m^2 on day 1 and repeated at 15 day intervals.

CONTRAINDICATIONS/ PRECAUTIONS
Contraindicated in: Hypersensitivity. **Use cautiously in:** Hepatic impairment, patients with immunosuppression. **Pregnancy/Lactation:** No well-controlled trials to establish safety. Benefits must outweigh risks. Breastfeeding should be discontinued while receiving this agent.

In the Adverse Effects section, underline indicates most frequent; CAPS indicates life threatening.

PREPARATION

Availability: 100 mg, 200 mg, 500 mg vials. **Reconstitution:** Dilute 100 mg vial with 9.9 mL, 200 mg with 19.7 mL, 500 mg with 49.5 mL sterile water for injection for a final concentration of 10 mg/mL. **Infusion:** Further dilute up to 250 mL compatible IV solution.

STABILITY/STORAGE

Vial: Store in refrigerator. Reconstituted solution stable for 8 hr at room temperature and 72 hr refrigerated. **Infusion:** Stable for 8 hr at room temperature and 24 hr refrigerated.

ADMINISTRATION

General: Handle drug with care and adhere to institutional guidelines for the handling of chemotherapeutic/cytotoxic agents. Must be administered into vein or by infusion. Avoid subcutaneous extravasation (apply hot packs to minimize local reaction). In the event of a spill, use 10% sulfuric acid for 24 hr to inactivate dacarbazine. **IV Push:** Inject over at least 1 min. **Intermittent Infusion:** Infuse over 15–30 min.

COMPATIBILITY

Solution: Dextrose solutions, sodium chloride solutions. **Y-site:** Heparin (concentration < 10 mg/mL DTIC), ondansetron.

INCOMPATIBILITY

Y-site: Heparin (concentration 25 mg/mL DTIC).

ADVERSE EFFECTS

CNS: Facial paresthesias. **GI:** Abnormal liver function tests, anorexia, diarrhea, hepatoxicity, nausea, vomiting. **Renal:** Serum creatinine abnormalities. **MS:** Myalgia. **Derm:** Alopecia, photosensitivity. **Heme:** LEUKOPENIA, THROMBOCYTOPENIA. **Nadir:** 14–28 days. **Hypersens:** ANAPHYLAXIS, erythematous/urticarial rash. **Other:** Facial flushing, fever, flu-like syndrome, malaise, tissue necrosis.

TOXICITY/OVERDOSE

Signs/Symptoms: Extension of adverse effects. **Treatment:** Symptomatic and supportive.

DRUG INTERACTIONS

Concomitant chemotherapy agents, immunosuppressants: Increased myelosuppression. **Hepatic enzyme inducing agents, phenobarbital, phenytoin:** Increased dacarbazine metabolism resulting in potential decrease in efficacy.

NURSING CONSIDERATIONS

Assessment
General:
Vital signs.
Physical:
Hematopoietic system, signs/symptoms of infection, GI tract.
Lab Alterations:
Evaluate CBC with differential and platelet count throughout course of therapy.

Intervention/Rationale

Assess for development of fever, chills, or other signs of infection and notify physician immediately. ● Assess for development of bleeding (bleeding gums, easy bruising, hematest positive stools/urine/vomitus). ● Avoid intramuscular injections and rectal temperatures. ● Assure that proper antiemetic regimens are prescribed and if needed,

In the Adverse Effects section, underline indicates most frequent; CAPS indicates life threatening.

143

give ½ hr prior to administration of chemotherapy.

Patient/Family Education

Observe for signs of infection (fever, sore throat, fatigue) or bleeding (melena, hematuria, nosebleeds, easy bruising), especially at 2 weeks following administration. Take and record oral temperature daily and report persistent elevation to physician. Use a soft toothbrush and electric razor to minimize bleeding tendency. Avoid crowded environments and persons with known infections. Use reliable contraception throughout the duration of therapy due to potential teratogenic and mutagenic effects of drug. Seek physician approval prior to receiving live virus vaccinations. Avoid over-the-counter drugs containing aspirin or ibuprofen due to increased potential for bleeding. Extended exposure to sunlight may result in photosensitivity reactions.

DACTINOMYCIN (ACTINOMYCIN D)

(dak-ti-noe-mye′-sin)
Trade Name(s): Cosmegen
Classification(s): Antineoplastic antibiotic
Pregnancy Category: C

PHARMACODYNAMICS/KINETICS

Mechanism of Action: Inhibits DNA and RNA synthesis. **Distribution:** Rapidly distributes into tissues. Concentrates in bone marrow cells, granulocytes, and lymphocytes. Little drug is evident in circulation af-

ter 2 minutes. Does not cross blood–brain barrier. **Metabolism/ Elimination:** Primarily eliminated unchanged in urine and feces. **Half-Life:** 36 hr.

INDICATIONS/DOSAGE

Choriocarcinoma, Ewing's sarcoma, nonseminomatous testicular carcinoma, rhabdomyosarcoma, Wilm's tumor

(Calculate based on lean body weight/surface area if obese or edematous). Individualize dosage based on clinical status and laboratory values.

Adult: 0.5 mg daily for a maximum of 5 days. Not to exceed 15 mcg/kg or 400–600 mcg/m² daily for 5 days. A second course may be necessary 3 weeks later if no signs of toxicity present. *Pediatric:* 15 mcg/kg/day (400–600 mcg/m²/day) for a maximum of 5 days. Alternate dosage regimen 2500 mcg/m² in divided doses given over 7 days. A second course may be necessary 3 weeks later if no signs of toxicity present.

CONTRAINDICATIONS/ PRECAUTIONS

Contraindicated in: Hypersensitivity, patients with chickenpox or herpes zoster infections. **Use cautiously in:** Hepatic/renal impairment, immunosuppressed patients, patients who have received radiation therapy. **Pregnancy/Lactation:** No well-controlled trials to establish safety. Benefits must outweigh risks, crosses placenta. Breastfeeding should be discontinued while receiving this agent. **Pediatrics:** Not

In the Adverse Effects section, <u>underline</u> indicates most frequent;
CAPS indicates life threatening.

recommended for children less than 6–12 months old due to increased toxicity potential.

PREPARATION

Availability: 0.5 mg vial. **Reconstitution:** Dilute each vial with 1.1 mL sterile water for injection for a final concentration of 0.5 mg/mL. **Infusion:** Further dilute in volume of compatible IV solution sufficient to run over 15 minutes.

STABILITY/STORAGE

Vial: Store at room temperature. Stable at room temperature for 2–4 hr after reconstitution. **Infusion:** Stable at room temperature for 24 hr.

ADMINISTRATION

General: Handle with care and avoid inhalation and contact to skin, especially the eyes (immediately irrigate eyes or skin with large amounts of water for at least 15 minutes and seek medical attention). Adhere to institutional guidelines for the handling of chemotherapeutic/cytotoxic agents. Must be administered through tubing of running IV solution or by infusion. Avoid extravasation. Notify physician immediately and consider infiltrating area with hydrocortisone (50–100 mg) and/or isotonic sodium thiosulfate injection (4.14% pentahydrate salt, 2.64% anhydrous salt, or a 4% solution prepared by diluting 4 mL of 10% injection with 6 mL sterile water for injection) or ascorbic acid (1 mL of 5% injection); apply cold compresses to minimize local reaction. In the event of a spill, use trisodium phosphate 5% to inactivate dactinomycin. Inline filter not recommended (may partially remove drug). Flush tubing to ensure no residual drug remains. **IV Push:** Inject directly into IV tubing of flowing solution—or—if directly into vein, use two-needle technique using a different sterile needle to inject (do not use same needle used to withdraw from vial). Give slowly over 10–15 min. **Intermittent Infusion:** Infuse over 10–15 min.

COMPATIBILITY

Solution: Dextrose solutions, sodium chloride solutions. **Y-site:** Ondansetron.

ADVERSE EFFECTS

CNS: Fatigue, lethargy, malaise. **GI:** Hepatitis, hepatomegaly, esophagitis, anorexia, dysphagia, GI ulceration, nausea, proctitis, vomiting. **MS:** Myalgia. **Derm:** Mucositis, stomatitis, acne, alopecia, increased erythema/pigmentation of irradiated skin, skin eruptions. **Fld/Lytes:** Hypocalcemia. **Heme:** MYELOSUPPRESSION, AGRANULOCYTOSIS, THROMBOCYTOPENIA, APLASTIC ANEMIA, LEUKOPENIA, PANCYTOPENIA, anemia, reticulopenia. **Nadir:** 14–21 days. **Other:** Fever, tissue necrosis.

TOXICITY/OVERDOSE

Signs/Symptoms: Extension of adverse effects. **Treatment:** Symptomatic and supportive.

DRUG INTERACTIONS

Concomitant chemotherapy agents, immunosuppressants: Increased myelosuppression. **Radiation therapy:** Increased toxicity, especially GI and myelosuppression.

In the Adverse Effects section, <u>underline</u> indicates most frequent;
CAPS indicates life threatening.

145

D

NURSING CONSIDERATIONS

Assessment

General:

Vital signs, hypersensitivity reactions (including wheezing, tachycardia, hypotension).

Physical:

Infectious disease status, hematopoietic system, GI tract.

Lab Alterations:

Monitor CBC with differential and platelet count, BUN, serum creatinine, and liver function prior to and throughout course of therapy. Interferes with bioassay procedures to determine antibacterial drug levels.

Intervention/Rationale

Assess for development of fever, chills, or other signs of infection and notify physician immediately. ● Assess patient for development of bleeding (bleeding gums, easy bruising, hematest positive stools/urine/vomitus). ● Avoid intramuscular injections and rectal temperatures. ● Discontinue if diarrhea, stomatitis, or severe myelosuppression occur. ● Assure that proper antiemetic regimens are prescribed and given regularly to prevent nausea/vomiting.

Patient/Family Education

Hair loss may affect body image. Observe for signs of infection (fever, sore throat, fatigue) or bleeding (melena, hematuria, nosebleeds, easy bruising) especially 1–2 weeks following administration. Take and record oral temperature daily and report persistent elevation to physician. Use a soft toothbrush and electric razor to minimize bleeding tendency. Avoid crowded environments and persons with known infections. Use reliable contraception throughout the duration of therapy due to potential teratogenic and mutagenic effects of drug. Seek physician approval prior to receiving live virus vaccinations. Avoid over-the-counter products containing aspirin or ibuprofen due to increased potential for bleeding. Report dizziness, unusual fatigue, or shortness of breath (drug may cause anemia).

DANTROLENE

(dan'-troe-leen)

Trade Name(s): Dantrium Intravenous

Classification(s): Skeletal muscle relaxant (direct acting)

Pregnancy Category: C

PHARMACODYNAMICS/KINETICS

Mechanism of Action: Direct skeletal muscle relaxation by interfering with calcium ion release in the sarcoplasmic reticulum. In malignant hyperthermia, myoplasm ionized calcium levels are reestablished, which increases bound calcium. **Duration of Action:** Up to 3 hr following infusion discontinuation. **Distribution:** Distributes into erythrocytes to a greater extent than plasma. Substantial, but reversible, plasma protein binding especially to albumin. **Metabolism/Elimination:** Primarily hepatically metabolized. Unchanged drug and metabolites eliminated by kidneys. **Half-Life:** 4–8 hr.

In the Adverse Effects section, underline indicates most frequent;
CAPS indicates life threatening.

INDICATIONS/DOSAGE

Malignant hyperthermia prophylaxis

Adult/Pediatric: 2.5 mg/kg 1.25 hr prior to anesthesia.

Treatment of malignant hyperthermia

Adult/Pediatric: Initially, minimum dose 1 mg/kg. Continue until symptoms subside up to a maximum total dose of 10 mg/kg. Repeat if necessary.

Malignant hyperthermia crisis follow up

Adult/Pediatric: Begin with 1 mg/kg every 6 hr (4–8 mg/kg in 24 hr). Titrate to patient response for 72 hr.

CONTRAINDICATIONS/ PRECAUTIONS

Contraindicated in: History of liver disease, impaired cardiac/pulmonary function. **Pregnancy/Lactation:** No well-controlled trials to establish safety. Benefits must outweigh risks. Crosses placenta. Breastfeeding should be discontinued while receiving this agent. **Pediatrics:** Safety for use in < 5 years old has not been established.

PREPARATION

Availability: 20 mg/vial in 70 mL vials. **Reconstitution:** Dilute with 60 mL sterile water for injection (preservative free) resulting in a final concentration of 0.32 mg/mL. Shake until clear. **Infusion:** Transfer solution to empty sterile plastic bag for infusion. Do not transfer to glass bottles or further dilute.

STABILITY/STORAGE

Vial: Store at room temperature. Reconstituted solution stable at room temperature for only 6 hr. Prepare just prior to use. Protect from light. **Infusion:** Stable for only 6 hr at room temperature. Protect from light.

ADMINISTRATION

General: Avoid extravasation into surrounding tissues. **IV Push:** Give rapidly. **Intermittent Infusion:** Administer over less than 6 hr.

INCOMPATIBILITY

Solution: Dextrose solutions, sodium chloride solutions.

ADVERSE EFFECTS

Resp: Pulmonary edema. **Hypersens:** Erythema, urticaria. **Other:** DEATH, thrombophlebitis.

TOXICITY/OVERDOSE

Signs/Symptoms: Extension of adverse effects. **Treatment:** Symptomatic and supportive, maintain airway, monitor ECG.

DRUG INTERACTIONS

Agents inducing hepatic metabolism: Potential decrease in dantrolene efficacy (diazepam/phenobarbital do not seem to affect metabolism). **Clofibrate, warfarin:** Decreased dantrolene protein binding. **Tolbutamide:** Increased dantrolene protein binding. **Tranquilizers:** Increased sedation/weakness.

NURSING CONSIDERATIONS

Assessment
General:
ECG, vital signs.
Physical:
Neuromuscular, lung sounds.

In the Adverse Effects section, underline indicates most frequent; CAPS indicates life threatening.

147

D

Lab Alterations:
Monitor hepatic function prior to administration, arterial blood gases, electrolytes.

Intervention/Rationale
Assess oxygen needs based on blood gas results. ● Observe for decreased grip strength and increased leg weakness.

Patient/Family Education
Decreased hand grip strength and increased leg weakness may develop during therapy. Avoid alcohol intake and excess sunlight exposure immediately after administration.

DAUNORUBICIN
(daw-noe-roo′-bi-sin)
Trade Name(s): Cerubidine
Classification(s): Anthracycline antineoplastic
Pregnancy Category: D

PHARMACODYNAMICS/KINETICS
Mechanism of Action: Inhibition of DNA/RNA synthesis, antimitotic, cytotoxic, and immunosuppressive effects. **Distribution:** Rapidly taken up by tissues. Concentrated in liver (25%). Extensive plasma and tissue protein binding. Does not cross blood–brain barrier. **Metabolism/Elimination:** Primarily hepatically metabolized to alcohol daunorubicin (daunorubicinol, primary active metabolite). Further metabolized to inactive metabolites. Eliminated as active drug in urine (25%) and in bile (40%) **Half-Life:** Daunorubicin 18.5 hr, daunorubicinol 26.7 hr.

INDICATIONS/DOSAGE
Individualize dosage based on clinical status and laboratory values. Reduce dosage in hepatic or renal impairment.

Remission induction in acute non-lymphocytic leukemia
Adult: 45 mg/m^2/day on days 1–3 of first course and days 1–2 on subsequent courses. If > 60 years old, the dosage may be reduced to 30 mg/m^2/day. Up to three courses may be necessary. Total cumulative dose not to exceed 500–600 mg/m^2.

Remission induction in acute lymphocytic leukemia
Adult: 45 mg/m^2/day on days 1–3. Total cumulative dose not to exceed 500–600 mg/m^2. *Pediatric:* 25 mg/m^2 on day 1 every week for four courses. One or two additional courses may be necessary. If < 2 years old or < 0.5 m^2, base dose on mg/kg. Total cumulative dose not to exceed 300 mg/m^2 if > 2 years or 10 mg/kg if < 2 years or < 0.5 m^2.

CONTRAINDICATIONS/PRECAUTIONS
Contraindicated in: Severe myelosuppression secondary to chemotherapy/radiation. **Use cautiously in:** Impaired hepatic/renal function, patients with bone marrow suppression, preexisting heart disease, previous therapy with anthracycline antineoplastics. **Pregnancy/Lactation:** No well-controlled trials to establish safety. Drug is teratogenic in rodents. Inform patient of potential risk to fetus. Patients should avoid pregnancy. Breastfeeding

---

In the Adverse Effects section, <u>underline</u> indicates most frequent;
CAPS indicates life threatening.

should be discontinued during treatment.

PREPARATION
Availability: 20 mg/vial. **Reconstitution:** Dilute contents of vial with 4 mL sterile water for injection for a final concentration of 5 mg/mL. **Syringe:** Further dilute dose with 10–15 mL sodium chloride. **Infusion:** Further dilute in 50–100 mL compatible IV solution.

STABILITY/STORAGE
Vial: Store at room temperature. Reconstituted solution is stable for 24 hr at room temperature and 48 hr refrigerated. Protect from light. **Infusion:** Prepare just prior to administration.

ADMINISTRATION
General: Handle drug with care and adhere to institutional guidelines for the handling of chemotherapeutic/cytotoxic agents. Administer through rapidly flowing IV infusion. Avoid extravasation. Notify physician immediately and consider infiltrating area with hydrocortisone (50–100 mg) and/or sodium bicarbonate (5 mL of 8.4% injection); apply cold compresses to minimize local reaction. In the event of a spill, use sodium hypochlorite 5% (bleach) to inactivate daunorubicin until a colorless liquid results. **IV Push:** Inject directly into tubing or y-site of rapidly flowing solution of compatible solution over 2–3 minutes. **Intermittent Infusion:** Infuse 50 mL over 10–15 minutes or 100 mL over 30–45 minutes.

COMPATIBILITY
Solution: Dextrose solutions, lactated Ringer's, sodium chloride solutions. **Y-site:** Ondansetron.

ADVERSE EFFECTS
CV: CARDIAC TOXICITY/CARDIOMYOPATHY / CONGESTIVE HEART FAILURE (related to total cumulative dose), ECG abnormalities. **GI:** Acute nausea/vomiting, diarrhea, mucositis. **Renal:** Urine discoloration (red). **Derm:** Alopecia (reversible). **Heme:** MYELOSUPPRESSION. *Nadir:* 10–14 days. **Hypersens:** Rash. **Other:** Chills, fever, tissue necrosis.

TOXICITY/OVERDOSE
Signs/Symptoms: Extension of adverse effects especially cardiac toxicity. **Treatment:** Avoid cumulative doses above those identified with an increased risk. Symptomatic and supportive therapy.

DRUG INTERACTIONS
Concomitant chemotherapy agents, immunosuppressants: Increased myelosuppression. **Radiation therapy:** Increased cardiac toxicity.

NURSING CONSIDERATIONS
Assessment
General:
Vital signs, ECG, intake/output ratio, hypersensitivity reactions.
Physical:
Cardiopulmonary, GU, infectious disease status, hematopoietic system.
Lab Alterations:
Assess CBC with differential and platelet count, BUN, serum creatinine, and liver function prior to and throughout course of therapy, serum uric acid.

Intervention/Rationale
Drug may cause CHF. ● Drug imparts a red color to urine for 1–2

In the Adverse Effects section, <u>underline</u> indicates most frequent; CAPS indicates life threatening.

149

days after administration. ● Assess for development of fever, chills, or other signs of infection and notify physician immediately. ● Maintain adequate hydration during therapy. ● Assess patient for development of bleeding (bleeding gums, easy bruising, hematest positive stools/urine/vomitus). ● Avoid intramuscular injections and rectal temperatures. ● Monitor uric acid levels throughout course of therapy and assure prophylactic allopurinol is prescribed.

Patient/Family Education

Hair loss may affect body image. Secretions (urine/tears/sweat) may be discolored red. Observe for signs of infection (fever, sore throat, fatigue) or bleeding (melena, hematuria, nosebleeds, easy bruising) especially 1 week following administration. Take and record oral temperature daily and report persistent elevation to physician. Use a soft toothbrush and electric razor to minimize bleeding tendency. Avoid crowded environments and persons with known infections. Use reliable contraception throughout the duration of therapy and 4 months following due to potential teratogenic and mutagenic effects of drug. Seek physician approval prior to receiving live virus vaccinations. Avoid over-the-counter products containing aspirin or ibuprofen due to increased potential for bleeding. Report dizziness, unusual fatigue, or shortness of breath (drug may cause anemia).

DEFEROXAMINE
(dee-fer-ox′-a-meen)
Trade Name(s): Desferal
Classification(s): Heavy metal antidote
Pregnancy Category: C

PHARMACODYNAMICS/KINETICS

Mechanism of Action: Chelates iron and other heavy metals (i.e., aluminum) by forming a stable, water-soluble complex that prevents entry into circulation. **Distribution:** Widely distributed into body tissues. **Metabolism/Elimination:** Rapidly metabolized plasma enzymes. Primarily eliminated by kidneys as active drug and reddish complex, ferrioxamine. A small portion is also eliminated via feces as bile. Active drug/metabolite removed by hemodialysis. **Half-Life:** 1 hr.

INDICATIONS/DOSAGE

Acute iron intoxication in patients with cardiovascular collapse

Adult: Initially 1 g, followed by 500 mg every 4 hr for two doses. If needed, 500 mg every 4–12 hr may be administered until urine is no longer salmon pink in color. Not to exceed 15 mg/kg/hr or 6 g/24 hr. *Pediatric (> 3 yrs):* 15 mg/kg/hr. **Alternate Dosage Regimen:** 20 mg/kg initially (600 mg/m²), followed by 10 mg/kg (300 mg/m²) every 4 hr for two doses. If needed, 10 mg/kg (300 mg/m²) every 4–12 hr may be administered until urine is no

In the Adverse Effects section, <u>underline</u> indicates most frequent; CAPS indicates life threatening.

longer pink in color. **Alternate Dosage Regimen:** 50 mg/kg/dose every 6 hr. Not to exceed adult dosages or 15 mg/kg/hr, 2 g/dose or 6 g/24 hr.

Chronic iron overload

Adult: In addition to daily IM dose, 2 g with each unit of blood. Not to exceed 15 mg/kg/hr.

Aluminum-induced dialysis encephalopathy, aluminum bone accumulation in renal failure (*unlabeled use*)

Adult: 40 mg/kg single dose over 2 hr.

CONTRAINDICATIONS/ PRECAUTIONS

Contraindicated in: Hypersensitivity, patients with severe renal disease or anuria, primary hemachromatosis. **Use cautiously in:** Adults without cardiovascular collapse. **Pregnancy/ Lactation:** No well-controlled trials to establish safety. Benefits must outweigh risks. **Pediatrics:** Safety and efficacy has not been established in < 3 years old.

PREPARATION

Availability: 500 mg vial. **Reconstitution:** Dilute each 500 mg vial with 2 mL sterile water for injection resulting in a final concentration of 250 mg/mL. **Infusion:** Further dilute to a sufficient volume of compatible IV solution to infuse at a rate not to exceed 15 mg/kg/hr.

STABILITY/STORAGE

Vial: Store at room temperature. Reconstituted solution stable for 1 week at room temperature. Protect from light. **Infusion:** Must be prepared prior to administration.

ADMINISTRATION

General: Reserve IV route for patients in cardiovascular collapse. **Intermittent Infusion:** Must be infused slowly. Not to exceed 15 mg/kg/hr.

COMPATIBILITY

Solution: Dextrose solutions, lactated Ringer's, sodium chloride solutions.

ADVERSE EFFECTS

Ophtho: Blurred vision (high doses/ long-term use), cataracts, impaired color/night vision. **CV:** Shock, hypotension, tachycardia. **GI:** Abdominal discomfort, diarrhea. **GU:** Dysuria, red urine. **MS:** Leg cramps. **Derm:** Erythema, local irritation/ pain, swelling. **Hypersens:** ANAPHYLAXIS, rash, pruritus, wheal formation, urticaria. **Other:** Fever, high frequency hearing loss.

TOXICITY/OVERDOSE

Signs/Symptoms: GI symptoms, hypotension, tachycardia. **Treatment:** Reduce dosage, consider hemodialysis.

DRUG INTERACTIONS

Other heavy metals: Binding of heavy metal drugs may occur.

NURSING CONSIDERATIONS

Assessment
General:
Vital signs, intake/output ratio, hypersensitivity reactions.
Lab Alterations:
Evaluate liver function studies, serum iron, iron binding capacity, transferrin levels, and urinary iron excretion prior to administration and periodically during therapy.

In the Adverse Effects section, underline indicates most frequent; CAPS indicates life threatening.

151

D

Intervention/Rationale
Maintain adequate hydration. ● Assess patient for development of potential hypersensitivity reactions.

Patient/Family Education
Red color of urine is due to kidney excretion of chelated iron. Reinforce need for follow-up visits to physician and importance of continued lab test monitoring.

DESMOPRESSIN
(des-moe-press'-in)
Trade Name(s): DDAVP
Classification(s): Posterior pituitary hormone
Pregnancy Category: B

PHARMACODYNAMICS/KINETICS
Mechanism of Action: Synthetic arginine vasopressin (antidiuretic hormone). In central diabetes insipidus, antidiuretic hormone replacement. In hemophilia/von Willebrand's, produces a dose-related increase in Factor VIII plasma levels. **Onset of Action:** 30 min. **Peak Effect:** Factor VIII increases in 90 min to 2 hr. **Duration of Action:** Antidiuretic hormone 8–20 hr. **Half-Life:** Biphasic: plasma 7.8 minutes, terminal 75.5 min.

INDICATIONS/DOSAGE

Central diabetes insipidus
Adult: 2–4 mcg (0.5–1.0 mL) daily in two divided doses. Adjust interval based on response and to allow for adequate sleep duration. If controlled on intranasal therapy, administer 1/10 the intranasal dose as injection.

Management of bleeding due to hemophilia A (Type I) with Factor VIII levels > 5% and mild to moderate classic von Willebrand's disease (Type I) with Factor VIII levels > 5%

Administer 30 minutes prior to surgery if needed preoperatively. Repeat dose based on laboratory and clinical response. Tachyphylaxis may occur if administered more frequently than every 48 hr.

Adult: 0.3 mcg/kg/dose. *Pediatric (> 3 months old):* 0.2–0.4 mcg/kg/dose. Alternate dosage 10 mcg/m^2/dose

---

CONTRAINDICATIONS/PRECAUTIONS
Contraindicated in: Hypersensitivity. **Use cautiously in:** Elderly, patients with coronary artery insufficiency and hypertensive cardiovascular disease. **Pregnancy/Lactation:** No well-controlled trials to establish safety. Benefits must outweigh risks. There is no uterotonic activity associated with antidiuretic doses. **Pediatrics:** Use in children requires careful fluid intake restriction. Not recommended for use in < 3 months old for hemophilia/von Willebrand's disease. Not recommended in children < 12 years old for diabetes insipidus.

PREPARATION
Availability: 4 mcg/mL in 1 mL ampules. **Syringe:** Dilute to approximately 0.5 mcg/mL with sodium chloride if necessary. **Infusion:** *Adults/children > 10 kg:* Dilute in 50 mL sodium chloride. *Children < 10 kg:* Dilute in 10 mL sodium chloride.

In the Adverse Effects section, underline indicates most frequent; CAPS indicates life threatening.

STABILITY/STORAGE
Vial: Store in refrigerator. **Infusion:** Prepare just prior to administration.

ADMINISTRATION
IV Push: May be given by direct IV push over 1 min in diabetes insipidus. **Intermittent Infusion:** Administer slowly over 15–30 min in hemophilia.

COMPATIBILITY
Solution: Sodium chloride solutions.

ADVERSE EFFECTS
CNS: Headache. **CV:** Hypotension, slight elevation of blood pressure. **GI:** Mild abdominal cramps, nausea. **GU:** Vulval pain. **Derm:** Burning, local erythema, swelling. **Fld/Lytes:** WATER INTOXICATION, hyponatremia. **Other:** Facial flushing.

TOXICITY/OVERDOSE
Signs/Symptoms: Extension of adverse effect profile, flushing, hypotension, tachycardia, water intoxication. **Treatment:** Symptomatic and supportive.

DRUG INTERACTIONS
Chlorpropamide, clofibrate, fludrocortisone, urea: Increased antidiuretic effect. **Demeclocycline, epinephrine (large doses), ethanol, heparin, lithium:** Decreased antidiuretic effect. **Pressor agents:** Potentiation of hypertension.

NURSING CONSIDERATIONS
Assessment
General:
Blood pressure, heart rate, daily weight, intake/output ratio, endocrine.
Physical:
Hematopoietic system.

Lab Alterations:
Assess urine/serum osmolality and urine specific gravity. Monitor Factor VIII coagulant, antigen, and ristocetin cofactor levels as well as activated partial thromboplastin time. Bleeding time (hemophilia).

Intervention/Rationale
Evaluate need for intravascular fluid replacement. ● Monitor for signs/symptoms of dehydration especially in children.

Patient/Family Education
Contact physician if adverse effects become severe or urine output becomes excessive. Notify physician of signs/symptoms of dehydration. Avoid concurrent alcohol use.

DEXAMETHASONE
(dex-a-meth′-a-sone)
Trade Name(s): Decadron, Dexasone, Hexadrol
Classification(s):
Anti-inflammatory, corticosteroid
Pregnancy Category: C

PHARMACODYNAMICS/KINETICS
Mechanism of Action: Stabilizes leucocyte lysosomal membranes. Suppresses immune response by inhibiting pituitary corticotropin release. Increases protein, fat, and carbohydrate production. **Duration of Action:** 36–54 hr (biologic half-life). **Distribution:** Distributes throughout body especially in intestines, kidneys, liver, muscle, skin. Highly protein bound (unbound drug is pharmacologically active). **Metabolism/Elimination:** Metabolized in tissues and liver to biologically inactive com-

In the Adverse Effects section, underline indicates most frequent;
CAPS indicates life threatening.

153

pounds. Inactive metabolites eliminated by kidneys. **Half-Life:** 110–210 min (plasma).

INDICATIONS/DOSAGE

Dose is variable and dependent on condition. Must be individualized based on need/response. Taper dose gradually.

Acute exacerbation of multiple sclerosis

Adult: 4–8 mg every other day for 1 month.

Airway edema

Pediatric: 1–2 mg/kg/day in divided doses every 6 hr for croup. Begin 24 hr prior to extubation at 1–2 mg/kg/day in divided doses every 4–6 hr for four to six doses.

Cerebral edema, increased intracranial pressure

Adult: Initial IV dose 10 mg, followed by IM maintenance dose. *Pediatric:* Initially 0.5–1.5 mg/kg followed by 0.2–0.5 mg/kg/day in divided doses every 4–6 hr for 5 days. Taper dose.

Immunosuppressant, systemic and local anti-inflammatory agent

Adult: Initial dosage may range from 0.5–9.0 mg daily in divided doses every 12 hr. Use ⅓ to ½ oral dosage if patient stabilized on IV dose. Life-threatening situations may require extremely high doses, up to 24 mg/day. *Pediatric:* 0.03–0.3 mg/kg/day in divided doses every 6–12 hr.

Prevention of chemotherapy induced emesis

Adult: 10–20 mg before chemotherapy. Repeat at a lower dose for 24–72 hr following chemotherapy.

Status asthmaticus

Pediatric: Initially 0.3 mg/kg followed by 0.0125 mg/kg/hr (0.3 mg/kg/day).

Unresponsive shock

Adult: 1–6 mg/kg once. **Alternate Dosage:** 40 mg every 2–6 hr. **Alternate Dosage:** Initially 20 mg followed by 3 mg/kg/day for 48–72 hr.

CONTRAINDICATIONS/PRECAUTIONS

Contraindicated in: Hypersensitivity to any component, patients with immunosuppresant doses receiving live virus vaccines, systemic fungal infections (except as maintenance for adrenocortical insufficiency). **Use cautiously in:** Cirrhosis/hypothyroid patients, diverticulitis, emotionally unstable/psychotic patients, hypertension, myasthenia gravis, nonspecific ulcerative colitis, osteoporosis, peptic ulcer disease, renal insufficiency. **Pregnancy/Lactation:** Animal studies demonstrate cleft palate in first trimester use. Observe neonate for signs/symptoms of hypoadrenalism. Benefits must outweigh risks. Appears in breast milk. May produce growth suppression. Avoid breastfeeding with pharmacologic doses. **Pediatrics:** Prolonged use may produce growth suppression. Avoid products containing benzyl alcohol in premature infants.

In the Adverse Effects section, underline indicates most frequent; CAPS indicates life threatening.

PREPARATION

Availability: 4 mg/mL, 10 mg/mL, 20 mg/mL, 24 mg/mL vials. **Infusion:** Dilute to physician specified volume/concentration in compatible IV solution.

STABILITY/STORAGE

Vial: Store at room temperature. Protect from light. Do not autoclave drug. **Infusion:** Stable at room temperature for 24 hr.

ADMINISTRATION

General: Single daily doses should be administered in the morning prior to 9 AM. **IV Push:** Give doses < 10 mg over 1–5 min. **Intermittent Infusion:** Infuse over 10–20 min. **Continuous Infusion:** Infuse over physician specified time (up to 24 hr).

COMPATIBILITY

Solution: Dextrose solutions, sodium chloride solutions. **Syringe:** Metoclopramide, ranitidine. **Y-site:** Acyclovir, famotidine, foscarnet, heparin, hydrocortisone, ondansetron, potassium chloride, vitamin B complex, zidovudine.

INCOMPATIBILITY

Syringe: Doxapram, glycopyrrolate.

ADVERSE EFFECTS

CNS: Convulsions, headache, hiccups, increased intracranial pressure with papilledema, neuritis, vertigo. **Ophtho:** Exophthalmos, glaucoma, increased intraocular pressure, posterior subcapsular cataracts. **CV:** Cardiac dysrhythmias, hypertension, syncope, thromboembolism. **GI:** Large bowel perforation, peptic ulcer perforation, pancreatitis, ulceratative esophagitis, abdominal distention, increased appetite, nausea, vomiting, weight gain. **MS:** Aseptic necrosis femoral/humeral bones, loss of muscle mass, muscle weakness, osteoporosis, spontaneous fractures, steroid myopathy. **Derm:** Burning, ecchymoses, erythema, hirsutism, hyper/hypopigmentation, impaired wound healing, petechiae, sterile abscess, striae, suppression of skin tests, thin fragile skin, tingling. **Endo:** Cushingoid features, decreased glucose tolerance, growth suppression, menstrual abnormalities, secondary adrenocortical or pituitary unresponsiveness. **Fld/Lytes:** Hypocalcemia, hypokalemia, sodium/water retention. **Hypersens:** Anaphylactoid reaction. **Metab:** Increased cholesterol, metabolic alkalosis, negative nitrogen balance. **Other:** Sweating.

TOXICITY/OVERDOSE

Signs/Symptoms: Symptoms of acute adrenal insufficiency as a result of too rapid withdrawal of drug after long-term use. Cushingoid changes (moonface, central obesity, hypertension, diabetes, fluid/electrolyte imbalance) may result from continuous use of large doses. **Treatment:** Supportive and symptomatic treatment, including fluid resuscitation, vasopressor therapy, and electrolyte replacement.

DRUG INTERACTIONS

Amphotericin, potassium depleting diuretics: Increased hypokalemia. **Attenuated virus vaccines:** Increased viral replication potential. **Cyclophosphamide:** Decreased metabolism cyclophosphamide. **Cyclosporine:** Increased serum levels of both agents. **Digitalis glycoside:** Increased toxicity secondary to hypokalemia.

In the Adverse Effects section, <u>underline</u> indicates most frequent; CAPS indicates life threatening.

155

Insulin: Increased insulin requirements. **Isoniazid:** Decreased antitubercular effect. **Oral contraceptives:** Decreased steroid metabolism. **Phenytoin, rifampin:** Decreased steroid activity. **Salicylates:** Reduced salicylate serum levels. **Somatrem:** Inhibits growth promoting effect. **Theophylline:** Increased theophylline pharmacologic effects. **Warfarin:** Inhibition of warfarin response.

NURSING CONSIDERATIONS

Assessment
General:
Blood pressure, intake/output ratio, daily weight.
Physical:
Infectious disease status.
Lab Alterations:
Serum glucose, electrolytes, altered uptake of Thyroid I-131 and results of brain scan (decreases uptake of radioactive materials).

Intervention/Rationale
Monitor blood pressure. Drug may induce hypertension. ● Notify physician if unusual weight gain is noted or if swelling of lower extremities, muscle weakness, or facial puffiness is observed. ● Drug may increase insulin needs in diabetics. ● Drug may mask signs/symptoms of infection. ● Observe for bruising, petechiae, or other signs of bleeding. ● Monitor signs/symptoms of adrenal insufficiency.

Patient/Family Education
Avoid abrupt withdrawal of therapy. Notify physician/nurse of significant weight gain, extremity swelling, muscle weakness, black tarry stools, facial puffiness, menstrual abnormalities, fever, cold, or infection. Avoid crowds/individuals with known infections and avoid live virus vaccinations without physician approval.

DEXPANTHENOL
(dex-pan′-the-nole)
Trade Name(s): Ilopan, Motilyn ♣ , Panthoderm ♣
Classification(s): GI stimulant, vitamin (water soluble)
Pregnancy Category: C

PHARMACODYNAMICS/KINETICS
Mechanism of Action: Direct mechanism unknown. Coenzyme A precursor that helps to promote synthesis of acetylocholine, thereby increasing smooth muscle contraction and promoting peristalsis. **Distribution:** Widely distributed into body tissues with highest concentration in liver, adrenal glands, heart, and kidneys. **Metabolism/Elimination:** Excreted 70% unchanged in urine and 30% in feces.

INDICATIONS/DOSAGE

Abdominal distention associated with intestinal atony, paralytic ileus, postoperative or postpartum retention of flatus

Adult: 250–500 mg. Repeat dose in 2 hr, then every 6 hr as needed.

CONTRAINDICATIONS/ PRECAUTIONS
Contraindicated in: Hemophilia, hypersensitivity, ileus due to mechanical obstruction. **Pregnancy/Lactation:** No well-controlled trials to establish safety. Benefits must outweigh

In the Adverse Effects section, <u>underline</u> indicates most frequent; CAPS indicates life threatening.

risks. **Pediatrics:** Safety and efficacy not established.

PREPARATION
Availability: 250 mg/mL in 10 and 30 mL vials. **Infusion:** Dilute in 500–1000 mL compatible IV solution.

STABILITY/STORAGE
Vial: Store at room temperature. **Infusion:** Stable for 24 hr after dilution.

ADMINISTRATION
General: Not for direct IV administration. **Intermittent Infusion:** Infuse slowly at physician prescribed rate.

COMPATIBILITY
Solution: Dextrose solutions, lactated Ringer's.

ADVERSE EFFECTS
CNS: Agitation (elderly). **CV:** Slight hypotension. **GI:** Diarrhea, intestinal colic, vomiting. **Derm:** Generalized dermatitis, itching, red patches, tingling. **Heme:** Prolonged bleeding time. **Hypersens:** Urticaria.

DRUG INTERACTIONS
Antibiotics, narcotics: Rare allergic reactions. **Succinylcholine:** Temporary respiratory difficulty (do not give dexpanthenol within 1 hr of succinylcholine).

NURSING CONSIDERATIONS
Assessment
General:
Blood pressure.
Physical:
Abdomen (bowel sounds, abdominal distention, flatus).

Patient/Family Education
Educate about side effects and expected therapeutic effects of drug.

DEXTRAN
(dex'-tran)
Trade Name(s): Dextran 40, Gentran 40, 10% Low molecular weight dextran (LMD), Macrodex ♣, Rheomacrodex
Classification(s): Plasma expander
Pregnancy Category: C

PHARMACODYNAMICS/KINETICS
Mechanism of Action: Causes volume expansion resulting from increase in colloid osmotic pressure (draws fluid from interstitial to intravascular spaces). May also improve microcirculation by decreasing blood viscosity and preventing erythrocyte aggregation. **Onset of Action:** Minutes. **Duration of Action:** 1.5 hr. **Distribution:** Evenly distributed into the vascular system. **Metabolism/Elimination:** 70% of dose excreted unchanged by kidney within 24 hr. Small amounts excreted in feces. **Half-Life:** 44.5 hr.

INDICATIONS/DOSAGE

Shock or impending shock

Adult: Total dosage during the first 24 hr should not exceed 20 mL/kg, with first 10 mL/kg administered rapidly. Dosage beyond 24 hr should not exceed 10 mL/kg, and therapy should not continue for more than 5 days. *Pediatric:* Adjust dose according to body weight. Total dose should not exceed 20 mL/kg.

In the Adverse Effects section, underline indicates most frequent; CAPS indicates life threatening.

157

Priming fluid in pump oxygenators during extracorporeal circulation

Adult: 10–20 mL/kg added to perfusion circuit. *Pediatric:* Adjust dose according to body weight. Total dose should not exceed 20 mL/kg.

Thromboembolism and venous thrombosis prophylaxis

Adult: Initiate therapy during surgical procedure at dosage of 500–1000 mL (approx 10 mL/kg). Continue with 500 mL/day for 2–3 days. Additional doses may be given according to determined risk of complications every second or third day for up to 2 weeks.

CONTRAINDICATIONS/ PRECAUTIONS

Contraindicated in: Hypofibrinogenemia, known hypersensitivity to dextrans or previous anaphylactoid reactions, marked thrombocytopenia, pulmonary edema. **Use cautiously in:** Cardiac decompensation, extreme dehydration, heart failure, pregnancy thrombocytopenia. **Pregnancy/Lactation:** No well-controlled trials to establish safety. Benefits must outweigh risks.

PREPARATION

Availability: 500 mL bottles of 10% dextran in sodium chloride or dextrose.

STABILITY/STORAGE

Vial: Store at room temperature. Protect from freezing.

ADMINISTRATION

General: Discard partially used containers (does not contain preservatives). Dissolve any crystals present before administration by submerging bottle in warm water. Do not administer unless solution is clear.

COMPATIBILITY

Solution: Dextrose solutions, sodium chloride solutions. **Y-site:** Enalaprilat, famotidine.

ADVERSE EFFECTS

CNS: Pulmonary edema (large doses). **Renal:** Nephrotoxicity. **Heme:** Decreased platelet function (large doses), prolonged bleeding (large doses). **Hypersens:** Mild hypersensitivity reactions, SEVERE ANAPHYLACTOID REACTION (rare), urticaria. **Other:** Extravasation, venous thrombosis/phlebitis at injection site.

NURSING CONSIDERATIONS

Assessment

General:

Vital signs, urine output, central venous pressure (if available), intake/output ratio, state of hydration, signs/symptoms of hypersensitivity reactions.

Lab Alterations:

Monitor hematocrit (avoid depressing hematocrit below 30% volume). May interfere with blood glucose, blood typing, crossmatching, or total protein determination (false high or inaccurate results).

Intervention/Rationale

Administer additional IV fluid if signs of deyhdration are present. ● Monitor for signs of CHF and circulatory overload (increase in heart rate or BP, crackles/rales, coughing, dyspnea, jugular venous distention, hepatosplenomegaly). Discontinue infusion if central venous pressure precipitously rises or if signs of circulatory overload are present. ● Hypersensitivity reactions are most-

---

In the Adverse Effects section, <u>underline</u> indicates most frequent; CAPS indicates life threatening.

likely to occur at beginning of infusion.

Patient/Family Education
Educate regarding adverse effects and therapeutic outcome of therapy.

DEXTROSE
(dex'-trose)
Classification(s): Caloric agent
Pregnancy Category: C

PHARMACODYNAMICS/KINETICS
Mechanism of Action: Caloric and fluid source, 5% solution is isotonic.
Onset of Action: Rapid. **Distribution:** Widely distributed. **Metabolism/Elimination:** Rapidly metabolized to carbon dioxide and water.

INDICATIONS/DOSAGE

Provides hydration and calories (lower concentrations, 2.5%–11.5%), provides calories for parenteral nutrition in combination with amino acids

Adult/Pediatric: 0.5–0.8 g/kg/hr.

Treatment of hypoglycemia (higher concentrations up to 70%)

Adult: 20–50 mL of 50% solution at rate of 3 mL/min. *Pediatric/Neonate:* 2 mL/kg of 10%–15% solution infused slowly.

CONTRAINDICATIONS/PRECAUTIONS
Contraindicated in: Delirium tremens in dehydrated patients, diabetic coma while blood glucose is excessively high, glucose-galactose malabsorption syndrome, intracranial or intraspinal hemorrhage (concentrated solutions). **Use cautiously in:** Carbohydrate intolerance, CHF, diabetes mellitus; inappropriate insulin secretion may result from long-term use of hypertonic solutions for parenteral nutrition, overhydration, pulmonary edema. **Pregnancy/Lactation:** No well-controlled trials to establish safety. Benefits must outweigh risks. **Pediatrics:** Caution with use in neonates of diabetic mothers, except in hypoglycemic neonates.

PREPARATION
Availability: 2.5%, 5%, 7.7%, 10%, 11.5%, 20%, 25%, 30%, 38%, 40%, 50%, 60% and 70% solutions in volumes ranging from 10–1000 mL. Contains 3.4 kcal/g (D_5W contains 170 calories/L, $D_{10}W$ contains 340 calories/L). Not all percentages available in all volumes.

STABILITY/STORAGE
Infusion: Do not use unless solution is clear. Discard unused portions. Protect from freezing and extreme heat.

ADMINISTRATION
General: May be mixed with amino acids or other compatible IV solutions to provide calories for parenteral nutrition. 2.5%–11.5% solutions may be administered via peripheral vein. Hypertonic solutions (greater than 11.5%) should be administered through a central vein. Concentrated (hypertonic) solutions should be gradually withdrawn and followed with 5% or 10% dextrose to prevent rebound

---

In the Adverse Effects section, underline indicates most frequent; CAPS indicates life threatening.

hypoglycemia. Do not use dextrose containing solutions as a diluent or priming solution when administering blood or blood products. **IV Push:** Hypertonic solutions used for the emergency treatment of hypoglycemia may be administered slowly via a large peripheral vein.

ADVERSE EFFECTS

CNS: Mental confusion. **Endo:** Hyperglycemia, hyperosmolar syndrome (hypertonic solutions). **Fld/Lytes:** Dehydration, hypervolemia, hypokalemia, hypomagnesemia, hyponatremia, hypophosphatemia, hypovolemia. **Other:** Infection at injection site, pain and irritation at injection site (more frequent with hypertonic solutions), tissue necrosis with extravasation (hypertonic solutions).

TOXICITY/OVERDOSE

Signs/Symptoms: Fluid volume overload, hyperosmolar syndrome. **Treatment:** Discontinue infusion and notify physician. Treat symptomatically.

DRUG INTERACTIONS

Insulin, oral hypoglycemic agents: Altered insulin requirements.

NURSING CONSIDERATIONS

Assessment
General:
Intake/output ratio, hydration status.
Physical:
Nutritional status.
Lab Alterations:
Monitor serum glucose, electrolytes, and acid-base balance.

Intervention/Rationale

Electrolytes should be added to solutions of patients requiring long-term IV fluid therapy. ● Dextrose solutions alone do not provide sufficient calories to meet nutritional needs.

Patient/Family Education

Educate regarding possible side effects and therapeutic outcome of therapy.

DEZOCINE
(dez'-oh-seen)
Trade Name(s): Dalgan
Classification(s): Narcotic agonist–antagonist analgesic
Pregnancy Category: C

PHARMACODYNAMICS/KINETICS

Mechanism of Action: Binds to CNS opiate receptors. **Onset of Action:** 15 minutes. **Peak Effect:** 1.0–1.5 hr. **Duration of Action:** 2–4 hr. **Distribution:** Distributed throughout the body. **Metabolism/Elimination:** Metabolized primarily by the liver. Metabolites excreted by the kidneys. **Half-Life:** 2.4 hr.

INDICATIONS/DOSAGE

Management of pain

Adult: 2.5–10.0 mg. May repeat every 2–4 hr. Usual initial dose 5 mg. Reduce dosage in hepatic/renal impairment.

CONTRAINDICATIONS/PRECAUTIONS

Contraindicated in: Hypersensitivity, sulfite sensitivity. **Use cautiously in:**

In the Adverse Effects section, <u>underline</u> indicates most frequent; CAPS indicates life threatening.

Bronchial asthma, head injury/increased intracranial pressure, obstructive respiratory disease, renal/hepatic impairment, respiratory depression, those prone to drug abuse/emotionally unstable. **Pregnancy:** No well-controlled trials to establish safety. Benefits must outweigh risks. **Pediatrics:** Safety and efficacy not established in children < 18 years.

PREPARATION
Availability: 5 mg/mL in 2 mL vials. 10 mg/mL in 2 and 10 mL vials. 15 mg/mL in 2 mL vials.

STABILITY/STORAGE
Vial: Store at room temperature.

ADMINISTRATION
IV Push: Give slowly over 1 min.

COMPATIBILITY/INCOMPATIBILITY
Data not available.

ADVERSE EFFECTS
CNS: <u>Sedation</u>, confusion, <u>dizziness</u>, anxiety, headache. **Ophtho:** Blurred vision, diplopia. **CV:** Chest pain, edema, hypertension, hypotension, irregular heartbeat/rate, pallor. **Resp:** RESPIRATORY DEPRESSION, atelectasis, hiccoughs. **GI:** Abdominal pain, constipation, diarrhea, dry mouth, increased alkaline phosphatase/AST, <u>nausea</u>, <u>vomiting</u>. **GU:** Urinary frequency/retention. **MS:** Cramping. **Derm:** Erythema. **Heme:** Low hemoglobin. **Other:** Chills, flushing, sweating, slurred speech, pruritus, rash, thrombophlebitis, tinnitus.

TOXICITY/OVERDOSE
Signs/Symptoms: Respiratory depression, cardiovascular compromise, delirium. **Treatment:** Symptomatic and supportive (IV fluids, supplemental oxygen, vasopressors, ventilatory support). **Antidote(s):** Naloxone.

DRUG INTERACTIONS
CNS depressants, general anesthetics, narcotic analgesics, tranquilizers: Additive pharmacologic effects.

NURSING CONSIDERATIONS
Assessment
General:
Vital signs, pain assessment (alleviating/aggravating factors).

Intervention/Rationale
Narcotic dependent patients may experience withdrawal symptoms after discontinuation.

Patient/Family Education
Have patient request pain medication before pain becomes too severe. Inform nurse if pain medication does not relieve pain. Medication may cause drowsiness or dizziness. Avoid activities requiring mental alertness. Call for assistance with ambulation activities. Avoid alcohol use. Cough, turn, and deep breathe to avoid atelectasis.

DIAZEPAM
(dye-az′-e-pam)
Trade Name(s): Valium
Classification(s): Anticonvulsant, anxiolytic, benzodiazepine, sedative/hypnotic, skeletal muscle relaxant
Pregnancy Category: D
Controlled Substance Schedule: IV

In the Adverse Effects section, <u>underline</u> indicates most frequent; CAPS indicates life threatening.

161

PHARMACODYNAMICS/KINETICS

Mechanism of Action: Depresses subcortical levels of the CNS. Calming effect may be a result of actions on limbic system and reticular formation. Potentiates effects of inhibitory transmitters by binding to benzodiazepine receptor sites. Anticonvulsant properties are a result of CNS depression. **Onset of Action:** Rapid. **Distribution:** Highly lipid soluble, Highly protein bound (may be greatly reduced in renal insufficiency), Widely distributed to body tissues (reduced lipid binding may occur in chronic alcoholics, cirrhosis, newborns). **Metabolism/Elimination:** Metabolized by the liver. Excreted by the kidney. Not removed by hemodialysis. **Half-Life:** 20–50 hr.

INDICATIONS/DOSAGE

Reduce dose in elderly or debilitated and when other sedatives are given.

Moderate to severe anxiety

Adult: 2–10 mg. May repeat dose every 3–4 hr as needed.

Acute alcohol withdrawal

Adult: 10 mg initially followed by 5–10 mg every 3–4 hr if needed.

Status epilepticus/recurrent convulsive seizures

Adult: 5–10 mg initially. Repeat if necessary at 10–15 min intervals up to a maximum dose of 30 mg. Dose may be repeated in 2–4 hr if needed.

Pediatric:
Infants (over 30 Days of Age)/Children under 5 Years: 0.2–0.5 mg slowly every 2–5 minutes up to a maximum of 5 mg. Repeat in 2–4 hr, if needed.

Children over 5 Years: 1 mg every 2–5 min up to a maximum of 10 mg. May repeat in 2–4 hr if needed.

Sedation for endoscopic procedures

Adult: Titrate dose to desired sedative response (usually 10 mg or less is required). Administer slowly just prior to procedure. May use up to 20 mg, especially when *not* combined with narcotics.

Sedation for cardioversion

Adult: 5–15 mg 5–10 min prior to procedure.

Skeletal muscle relaxation

Adult: 5–10 mg followed by 5–10 mg in 3–4 hr, if necessary.

Tetanic muscle spasms

Pediatric:
Infants (over 30 Days of Age): 1–2 mg slowly. Repeat every 3–4 hr as needed.
Children (5 Years or Older): 5–10 mg. Repeat every 3–4 hr as needed.

CONTRAINDICATIONS/PRECAUTIONS

Contraindicated in: Hypersensitivity, untreated acute narrow angle glaucoma, children < 6 months.
Use cautiously in: Depressed patients with suicidal ideation, elderly/debilitated, significant renal/hepatic disease.
Pregnancy/Lactation: No well-controlled trials to establish safety. Benefits must outweigh risks. Distributed in breast milk. Known to cause fetal harm when administered to pregnant women.

In the Adverse Effects section, underline indicates most frequent; CAPS indicates life threatening.

Pediatrics: Safety and efficacy not established for children < 12 years.

PREPARATION
Availability: 5 mg/mL in 2 and 10 mL ampules/vials.

STABILITY/STORAGE
Vial: Store at room temperature. Protect from light and freezing.

ADMINISTRATION
General: Do not mix or dilute with other solutions or drugs (may precipitate). Administer slowly through infusion tubing as close to the vein insertion site as possible. Do not use small veins (dorsum of hands, or wrist).
IV Push: Too rapid administration may cause apnea, hypotension, bradycardia, or cardiopulmonary arrest. **Adults:** Give 5 mg (1 mL) slowly per minute. **Children:** Give slowly over 3–5 min.

COMPATIBILITY
Syringe: Cimetidine, ranitidine.
Y-site: Dobutamine, nafcillin, quinidine gluconate.

INCOMPATIBILITY
Syringe: Atropine, benzquinamide, doxapram, glycopyrrolate, heparin, nalbuphine, scopolamine.
Y-site: Atracurium, foscarnet, heparin, hydrocortisone, pancuronium, potassium chloride, vecuronium, vitamin B complex with C.

ADVERSE EFFECTS
CNS: <u>Dizziness</u>, <u>drowsiness</u>, disorientation, depression. **Ophtho:** Blurred vision, diplopia. **CV:** Bradycardia, hypotension. **Resp:** Respiratory depression. **GI:** Abdominal cramps, constipation, diarrhea, dry mouth, increased salivation, vomiting. **GU:** Dysuria, incontinence, urinary retention. **Heme:** Blood dyscrasias (long-term use). **Hypersens:** Rash. **Other:** Thrombosis/thrombophlebitis at injection sites.

TOXICITY/OVERDOSE
Signs/Symptoms: Ataxia, confusion, coma, drowsiness, hypotension, hypnosis, lethargy.
Treatment: Monitor respiration, pulse, blood pressure, maintain patent airway, combat hypotension with IV fluids and vasopressors, force diuresis with IV fluids, osmotic diuretics (if normal renal function is present).
Antidote(s): Flumazenil IV as per physician order (reverses sedation or overdose). Physostigmine 0.5–4.0 mg at a rate of 1 mg/min may reverse symptoms resembling central anticholinergic overdose (confusion, delirium, hallucinations, memory disruption, visual disturbances).

DRUG INTERACTIONS
Alcohol, CNS depressants: Increased effects of both drugs. **Cimetidine, disulfiram, erythromycin, isoniazid, ketoconazole, metroprolol, oral contraceptives, propoxyphene, propranolol, valproic acid:** Decreased elimination of diazepam resulting in excessive sedation/impaired psychomotor function. **Cigarette smoking:** Increased sedation. **Digoxin:** Increased effect/toxicity. **Levodopa:** Decreased antiparkinson effect. **Rifampin:** Decreased benzodiazepine effect. **Scopolamine:** Increased sedation, hallucinations, irrational behavior.

In the Adverse Effects section, <u>underline</u> indicates most frequent; CAPS indicates life threatening.

163

D

NURSING CONSIDERATIONS

Assessment
General:
Vital signs.
Physical:
Neurologic status.
Lab Alterations:
Monitor CBC and hepatorenal function periodically throughout therapy (long-term use).

Intervention/Rationale
Document degree of patient anxiety prior to and after administration. ● Consider withholding medication if coma or somnolence develops. Adjust dosage accordingly if CNS effects develop (dizziness, lethargy, drowsiness, or slurring of speech). ● Protect seizure and alcohol withdrawal patients from injury. Observe and document duration, location, and intensity of seizure activity. Notify physician for repeated doses of medication if seizure activity is not obliterated.

Patient/Family Education
Drug may cause drowsiness; avoid engaging in tasks requiring mental alertness. Seek assistance with ambulatory activities. Avoid alcohol or other CNS depressants during therapy.

DIAZOXIDE
(dye-as-oxd'-ide)
Trade Name(s): Hyperstat
Classifications: Antihypertensive
Pregnancy Category: C

PHARMACODYNAMICS/KINETICS
Mechanism of Action: Exact mechanism unknown. Causes vasodilation of arterioles and decreased peripheral resistance. **Onset of Action:** 1 min. **Peak Effect:** 2–5 min. **Duration of Action:** 2–12 hr. **Distribution:** Highly bound to albumin (reduced in uremia). **Metabolism/Elimination:** Metabolized by the liver. Metabolites excreted by the kidneys. **Half-Life:** 21–36 hr (normal renal function). Anuria 20–53 hr (plasma half-life is much longer than the hypotensive effect and accumulation occurs with repeated doses).

INDICATIONS/DOSAGE

Emergency reduction of blood pressure
(for short-term use in hospitalized patients only).

Adult: 1–3 mg/kg up to a maximum of 150 mg in a single injection. Dose may be repeated in 5–15 min intervals until satisfactory reduction of blood pressure is obtained. May repeat dose at intervals of 4–24 hr if needed. Maximum daily dose 1.2 g. Do not use for longer than 10 days. Administer with loop diuretic 30–60 min prior to diazoxide to obtain maximum antihypertensive effect and prevent CHF due to sodium and water retention.

Pediatric: 1–3 mg/kg. Repeat in 5–15 min if necessary. Dose may be repeated at intervals of 4–24 hr if needed.

In the Adverse Effects section, <u>underline</u> indicates most frequent; CAPS indicates life threatening.

CONTRAINDICATIONS/ PRECAUTIONS

Contraindicated in: Aortic coarctation, arteriovenous shunt, hypersensitivity to diazoxide, thiazide diuretics, or sulfa drugs, pheochromocytoma.

Use cautiously in: Cardiovascular disease, diabetes mellitus, impaired cerebral or cardiac circulation, liver disease, renal disease, uremia.

Pregnancy/Lactation: No well-controlled trials to establish safety. Benefits must outweigh risks. Crosses placenta. Animal studies show decreased parturition and tetratogenic effects.

PREPARATION

Availability: 15 mg/mL in 20 mL vials.

STABILITY/STORAGE

Vial: Store at room temperature. Protect from freezing. Protect from light. Do not use darkened solutions.

ADMINISTRATION

General: Patient should be in a supine position during and for 1 hr after administration.

IV Push: Give undiluted drug rapidly over 30 seconds or less (slower administration may reduce or shorten response because of extensive protein binding).

COMPATIBILITY

Syringe: Heparin.

INCOMPATIBILITY

Y-site: Hydralazine, propranolol.

ADVERSE EFFECTS

CNS: Confusion, drowsiness, headache. **CV:** dysrhythmias, <u>hypotension</u>, <u>tachycardia</u>, CHF angina, peripheral edema. **GI:** Abdominal discomfort, constipation, diarrhea, elevated alkaline phosphatase, elevated AST (SGOT), nausea, vomiting. **Derm:** Hirsutism. **Endo:** <u>Hyperglycemia</u>. **Fld/Lytes:** <u>Sodium and water retention</u>. **Heme:** Decreased hemoglobin/hematocrit, leukopenia, hyperuricemia. **Hypersens:** Rash. **Renal:** Decreased creatinine clearance, elevated BUN. **Other:** Fever, flushing, pain at injection site, phlebitis.

TOXICITY/OVERDOSE

Signs/Symptoms: Severe hypotension, marked hyperglycemia.

Treatment: *Severe Hypotension:* Trendelenburg position, dopamine, norepinephrine. *Marked Hyperglycemia:* Conventional glucose lowering methods, close observation.

DRUG INTERACTIONS

Hydantoins (phenytoin): Increased hepatic metabolism. **Phenytoin, corticosteroids, estrogen/progesterone:** Increased hyperglycemic effect. **Peripheral vasodilators (hydralazine, nitroprusside):** Increased diazoxide effect. **Sulfonylureas:** Decreased pharmacologic effect of both drugs. **Thiazide diuretics:** Potentiation of hyperuricemic and antihypertensive effects.

NURSING CONSIDERATIONS

Assessment

General:
Blood pressure (every 5 minutes until stable, then hourly), intake/output ratio, daily weight.
Physical:
Cardiovascular status.

In the Adverse Effects section, <u>underline</u> indicates most frequent; CAPS indicates life threatening.

Lab Alterations:
Monitor serum glucose during and after therapy.

Intervention/Rationale
Assess for signs/symptoms of CHF. ● Place in Trendelenburg position if severe hypotension develops. Patient should remain supine for 1 hr following administration. ● Assess for orthostatic hypotension before allowing to ambulate.

Patient/Family Education
Change positions slowly to avoid orthostatic hypotension.

DIETHYLSTILBESTROL (DES)
(dye-eth-il-stil-bess'-trole)
Trade Name(s): Stilphostrol
Classification(s): Estrogen hormone
Pregnancy Category: X

PHARMACODYNAMICS/KINETICS
Mechanism of Action: Estrogen competes with androgens for tumor receptor sites.
Distribution: Widely distributed. 50%–80% bound to plasma proteins.
Metabolism/Elimination: Metabolized and excreted by the liver.

INDICATIONS/DOSAGE

Palliative treatment for inoperable prostatic carcinoma

Adult: Initially, 500 mg followed by 1 g daily for 5 days. Adjust dose depending on patient response. Subsequent dose 250–500 mg 1–2 times weekly if needed.

CONTRAINDICATIONS/PRECAUTIONS
Contraindicated in: Estrogen-dependent neoplasia, hypersensitivity, thromboembolic disorders (current or history of).
Use cautiously in: Cardiovascular disease, severe hepatic or renal dysfunction.
Pregnancy/Lactation: Not safe for use during pregnancy. Crosses placenta and causes serious fetal toxicity. Probably distributed into breast milk. Not safe for use in breastfeeding mothers.
Pediatrics: Safety and efficacy not established.

PREPARATION
Availability: 0.25 g in 5 mL ampules.
Infusion: Dilute 500 mg–1 g with at least 250 mL compatible IV solution.

STABILITY/STORAGE
Vial: Store at room temperature.
Infusion: Stable for 24 hr at room temperature.

ADMINISTRATION
Intermittent Infusion: Infuse over 1 hr. Begin infusion slowly (20–30 drops per minute for the first 10–15 min).

COMPATIBILITY
Solution: Dextrose solutions, sodium chloride solutions.

ADVERSE EFFECTS
CNS: Depression, dizziness, headache, dizziness, stroke, subarachnoid hemorrhage. **Ophtho:** Intolerance to contact lenses. **CV:** <u>Edema</u>, <u>hypertension</u>, MI, thromboembolism. **GI:** Abdominal cramps, changes in appetite, diarrhea, nausea, vomiting, weight changes. **GU:** <u>Breast tender-</u>

In the Adverse Effects section, <u>underline</u> indicates most frequent; CAPS indicates life threatening.

ness, changes in libido, gyneco-mastia, testicular atrophy. **MS:** Leg cramps. **Derm:** Acne, increased pigmentation, oily skin, photosensitivity. **Endo:** Decreased free T_3 resin uptake, hyperglycemia, increased thyroid binding globulin. **Fld/Lytes:** Hypercalcemia, hypernatremia, sodium and water retention. **Heme:** Decreased antithrombin III, increased prothrombin, Factor VII, VIII, IX, and X. **Hypersens:** Urticaria. **Metab:** Increased serum triglycerides, decreased serum folate.

DRUG INTERACTIONS

Anticoagulants: Decreased hypoprothrombinemic effect. **Barbiturates, carbamazepine, phenylbutazone, phenytoin, primidone, rifampin:** Increased metabolism of estrogen. **Corticosteroids:** Decreased steroid metabolism resulting in increased steroid effects.

NURSING CONSIDERATIONS

Assessment
General:
Blood pressure, intake/output ratio, daily weight.
Lab Alterations:
Monitor serum calcium in patients with metastatic bone lesions.

Patient/Family Education
Report signs of fluid retention (swelling of hands and feet, shortness of breath, weight gain) and thromboembolic disorders (tenderness/pain in extremities, shortness of breath, chest pain, blurred vision, headache) to physician. ● Wear sunscreen and protective clothing to avoid photosensitivity reactions. ● Eat solid foods in small amounts if nausea is present. ● Cigarette smoking during estrogen therapy increases the incidence of serious side effects. ● Remind of the importance of follow-up physical examinations with physician.

DIGOXIN

(di-jox-in)
Trade Name(s): Lanoxin
Classification(s): Cardiac glycoside
Pregnancy Category: C

PHARMACODYNAMICS/KINETICS

Mechanism of Action: Direct action on cardiac muscle to increase force of contraction. Prolongs conduction through the SA and AV nodes. Increases refractory period through AV node. Increases total peripheral resistance. **Onset of Action:** 5–30 min. **Peak Effect:** 1–5 hr. **Therapeutic Serum Levels:** 0.5–2.0 ng/mL. **Distribution:** Widely distributed in tissues, especially in myocardium, liver, kidneys, and skeletal muscle. 20%–25% protein bound. **Metabolism/Elimination:** Primarily eliminated by the kidneys (50%–70% unchanged). Not removed by hemodialysis. **Half-Life:** 30–40 hr. Anuria 100+ hr.

INDICATIONS/DOSAGE

Base dosage on lean body weight. Reduce dosage in renal impairment.

Atrial fibrillation, atrial flutter, cardiogenic shock, CHF, paroxysmal atrial tachycardia (PAT)

Adult/Pediatric (> 10 yrs): Initial digitalization dose 0.5–1.0 mg in

In the Adverse Effects section, underline indicates most frequent; CAPS indicates life threatening.

167

divided doses. Maintenance dose 0.125–0.5 mg daily. May give additional fractions of total dose at 4–8 hr intervals if needed.

Pediatric:

5–10 Years: 15–30 mcg/kg initially in several divided doses every 6–8 hr. Maintenance dose 25%–35% of daily loading dose. **2–5 Years:** 25–35 mcg/kg initially in several divided doses every 6–8 hr. Maintenance dose 25%–35% of daily loading dose. **1–24 months:** 30–50 mcg/kg initially in several divided doses every 6–8 hr. Maintenance dose 25%–35% of daily loading dose.

Neonate:

Full Term: 20–30 mcg/kg initially in several divided doses every 6–8 hr. Maintenance dose 25%–35% of daily loading dose. **Premature:** 15–25 mcg/kg initially in several divided doses every 6–8 hr. Maintenance dose 25%–35% of daily loading dose.

CONTRAINDICATIONS/ PRECAUTIONS

Contraindicated in: Beriberi heart disease, digitalis toxicity, hypersensitivity, uncontrolled ventricular dysrhythmias. **Use cautiously in:** Elderly, electrolyte abnormalities (hypokalemia, hypercalcemia, and hypomagnesemia may predispose to digitalis toxicity), idiopathic hypertrophic subaortic stenosis, incomplete AV block, renal impairment, sick sinus syndrome, Wolf-Parkinson-White syndrome (WPW). **Pregnancy/Lactation:** Drug has been safely used in some pregnant women. Crosses the placenta. Benefits must outweigh risks. Animal studies have not demonstrated teratogenic effects. Distributed into breast milk. Safe use in breastfeeding mothers not established. **Pediatrics:** Premature and immature infants are particularly sensitive to the drug. Reduce dose and individualize digitalization dose based on infant's degree of maturity.

PREPARATION

Availability: 2 mL amps 0.25 mg/mL (adult). 1 mL amps 0.1 mg/mL (pediatric).

STABILITY/STORAGE

Vial: Store at room temperature. Protect from light.

ADMINISTRATION

General: Divide loading dose and give 50% initially. Give remaining loading dose in two separate doses at 2–6 hr intervals. **IV Push:** Give undiluted over 5 min. May also dilute with at least four times volume of compatible IV solution.

COMPATIBILITY

Solution: Dextrose solutions, dextrose 5% in sodium chloride 0.45% with potassium chloride 20 mEq, lactated Ringer's, sodium chloride solutions. **Syringe:** Heparin, milrinone. **Y-site:** Famotidine, heparin, hydrocortisone, milrinone, potassium chloride, vitamin B complex with C.

INCOMPATIBILITY

Syringe: Doxapram. **Y-site:** Foscarnet.

ADVERSE EFFECTS

CNS: Confusion, drowsiness, fatigue, headache, weakness,. **Optho:** Visual disturbances (blurred vision, halo effect, yellow or green

In the Adverse Effects section, <u>underline</u> indicates most frequent; CAPS indicates life threatening.

vision). **CV:** Bradycardia, dysrhythmias, ECG changes. **GI:** Anorexia, diarrhea, nausea, vomiting. **GU:** Gynecomastia. **Heme:** Thrombocytopenia. **Hypersens:** Rash.

TOXICITY/OVERDOSE

Signs/Symptoms: Early symptoms are anorexia, vomiting, and diarrhea; also headache, visual disturbances (see adverse effects), drowsiness, confusion, restlessness, disorientation, ECG changes/dysrhythmias. **Treatment:** Discontinue drug until all signs of toxicity are abolished. Monitor therapeutic serum levels. Monitor electrolytes (hypokalemia, hypercalcemia, and hypomagnesemia may precipitate digitalis toxicity). Do not administer potassium salts if hyperkalemia or heart block are present. Cardiac dysrhythmias are one of the first signs of toxicity in infants and small children. Digitalis-induced dysrhythmias may be treated with phenytoin, lidocaine, atropine, countershock, and digoxin immune FAB. **Antidote:** Digoxin immune FAB (binds digoxin molecule in the blood and is then excreted by the kidneys).

DRUG INTERACTIONS

Amiodarone, benzodiazepines, captopril, diltiazem, esmolol, flecainide, nifedipine, quinidine, verapamil: Increased serum digoxin levels. **Loop and thiazide diuretics:** Increased urinary loss of potassium and hypokalemia. **Penicillamine, thyroid hormones:** Decreased therapeutic effect of digoxin.

NURSING CONSIDERATIONS

Assessment
General:
Apical heart rate, ECG monitoring (recommended).
Lab Alterations:
Monitor serum digoxin levels (at least 6–8 hr after the last dose to allow time for equilibration). Monitor serum electrolytes (especially potassium), calcium, and phosphate levels.

Intervention/Rationale
Check apical heart rate for 1 full minute prior to administration and check with physician before giving if rate is < 60 beats per minute (bpm) in adults, < 70 bpm in children or < 90 bpm in infants. ● Notify physician if bradycardia, dysrhythmias, or AV block develop or increase. ● Monitor for signs/symptoms of toxicity.

Patient/Family Education
Call physician/nurse if heart rate is much slower, faster, or more irregular than usual. Teach signs of toxicity and notify physician/nurse if present. Emphasize importance of follow-up appointments with physician.

DIGOXIN IMMUNE FAB
(di-jox'-in im-myoon'-fab)
Trade Name(s): Digibind
Classification(s): Antidote for digoxin
Pregnancy Category: C

In the Adverse Effects section, underline indicates most frequent;
CAPS´indicates life threatening.

169

PHARMACODYNAMICS/KINETICS

Mechanism of Action: Binds digoxin molecule and renders it inactive. **Onset of Action:** 30 min,. **Distribution:** Distributes rapidly into extracellular space, plasma, and interstitial fluid. **Metabolism/Elimination:** FAB-digoxin complex eliminated by the kidneys. FAB fragments not removed by hemodialysis. **Half-Life:** 15–20 hr.

INDICATIONS/DOSAGE

Treatment of potentially life-threatening digoxin-digitoxin intoxication/overdosage

Adult/Pediatric: Give when manifestations of life-threatening toxicity are present (include ventricular tachycardia, ventricular fibrillation, progressive bradydysrhythmias not responsive to atropine). Serum digoxin concentrations of > 10 ng/ml or serum potassium concentrations of > 5 mEq/L are indications for digoxin FAB therapy. Dosage varies according to the amount of digoxin to be neutralized.

1. First, calculate total body load to determine number of vials needed
a. If exact dose is known:
total body load (mg) = mg ingested (multiplied by 0.8 if tablets)
b. If serum concentration available:
total body load (mg) =

$$\frac{\text{serum conc in ng/mL} \times \begin{matrix} 5.6 \text{ (digoxin)} \\ \text{or} \\ 0.56 \text{ (digitoxin)} \end{matrix} \times \text{wt (kg)}}{1000}$$

2. Then calculate number of vials needed

$$\frac{\text{total body load (mg)}}{0.6 \text{ (mg/vial)}}$$

If calculated dose significantly differs from serum concentration, use higher calculated dose.

CONTRAINDICATIONS/PRECAUTIONS

Contraindicated in: None known. **Use cautiously in:** History of allergic reactions to ovine protein or previous exposure to antibodies of FAB fragments derived from ovine serum. **Pregnancy/Lactation:** No well-controlled trials to establish safety. Benefits must outweigh risks. **Pediatrics:** Drug has been successfully used in infants with no apparent adverse reactions. Use only if benefits clearly outweigh risks.

PREPARATION

Availability: 40 mg per vial with 75 mg sorbitol. Each vial will bind approximately 0.6 mg digoxin or digitoxin. **Reconstitution:** Dissolve the contents of each vial with 4 mL sterile water and mix gently. Use reconstituted product promptly. If not used immediately, refrigerate for up to 4 hr. **Syringe:** May dilute reconstituted product with sterile saline to a physician specified volume.

STABILITY/STORAGE

Vial: Store vial at room temperature. Reconstituted drug stable for 4 hr if refrigerated.

ADMINISTRATION

General: Postpone redigitalization until all FAB fragments have been eliminated (normal renal function: several days, impaired renal function: 1 week or longer). **IV Push:** Give as a bolus injection only if cardiac arrest is imminent. **Intermittent Infusion:** Give over 30 minutes through a 0.22 micron membrane filter.

In the Adverse Effects section, <u>underline</u> indicates most frequent; CAPS indicates life threatening.

COMPATIBILITY
Solution: Sodium chloride solutions.

ADVERSE EFFECTS
CV: CHF. **Fld/Lytes:** Hypokalemia. **Hypersens:** Facial swelling, urticarial rash.

NURSING CONSIDERATIONS
Assessment
General: Blood pressure, ECG, body temperature, hypersensitivity reactions.
Lab Alterations:
Monitor serum potassium concentrations closely (hypokalemia may develop rapidly, especially during the first several hours after therapy). Serum digoxin levels are unreliable for 5–7 days following administration.

Intervention/Rationale
Patients with preexisting atrial fibrillation may develop a rapid ventricular rate during therapy due to the effects of decreasing digoxin level. ● Skin testing should be performed whenever possible because of the limited experience with this agent, if the time delay for testing will not jeopardize patient safety.

Patient/Family Education
Educate regarding potential adverse effects and outcome of therapy.

DIHYDROERGOTAMINE
(dye-hye′-droe-err-got-a-meen)
Trade Name(s): DHE 45
Classification(s): Agent for migraine
Pregnancy Category: X

PHARMACODYNAMICS/KINETICS
Mechanism of Action: Peripheral vasoconstrictor. **Onset of Action:** Within minutes. **Peak Effect:** 30–45 min. **Duration of Action:** 3–4 hr. **Distribution:** 90% protein bound. **Metabolism/Elimination:** Metabolized by the liver. 10% of drug eliminated by the kidneys, 90% eliminated in feces. **Half-Life:** 21–32 hr.

INDICATIONS/DOSAGE

Vascular headaches (migraine, cluster)

Adult: 1 mg, followed by 1 mg in 1 hr if needed. Maximum dose 2 mg. Total weekly dosage not to exceed 6 mg.

CONTRAINDICATIONS/PRECAUTIONS
Contraindicated in: Coronary artery disease, impaired hepatic or renal function, lactation, peripheral vascular disease, pregnancy, sensitivity to ergot alkaloids, sepsis, uncontrolled hypertension. **Pediatrics:** Safety and efficacy not established.

PREPARATION
Availability: 1 mg/mL in 1 mL ampules.

STABILITY/STORAGE
Vial: Store at room temperature.

ADMINISTRATION:
General: IV use reserved for when rapid effect desired/required. **IV Push:** Give slowly over 1–2 min.

In the Adverse Effects section, <u>underline</u> indicates most frequent; CAPS indicates life threatening.

ADVERSE EFFECTS

CNS: Confusion, dizziness, syncope. **CV:** Bradycardia, edema, tachycardia, vasospasm. **GI:** Nausea, vomiting. **Hypersens:** Itching. **MS:** Leg weakness.

TOXICITY/OVERDOSE

Signs/Symptoms: Severe vasospasm (cold extremities, muscle pain in extremities, numbness and tingling in fingers and toes, chest pain). **Treatment:** Discontinue the drug. Keep extremities warm. Supportive care to prevent tissue damage. Vasodilators if necessary (sodium nitroprusside).

DRUG INTERACTIONS

Beta blockers: Increased peripheral ischemia. **Ergot alkaloids:** Concomitant use results in severe vasospasm. **Nitrates:** Decreased antianginal effect. **Vasodilators:** Increased hypertension.

NURSING CONSIDERATIONS

Assessment
General:
Vital signs.
Physical:
Neurologic/neurovascular status.

Intervention/Rationale
Assess patient for signs/symptoms of vascular headache prior to and after administration. Initiate therapy at first sign of headache for best effect. Allow patient to rest quietly in darkened room after administration. ● Assess for signs of cerebral and peripheral vasospasm (changes in mentation/level of consciouness, tingling/paresthesias of extremities).

Patient/Family Education
Avoid alcohol, tobacco, and increased exposure to cold (may cause increased vasospasm).

DILTIAZEM

(dill-tie'-a-zem)
Trade Name(s): Cardizem
Classification(s): Calcium channel blocker
Pregnancy Category: C

PHARMACODYNAMICS/KINETICS

Mechanism of Action: Inhibits movement of calcium ions across the cell membrane resulting in depression of mechanical contraction (myocardial and smooth muscle), automaticity, and conduction velocity. **Onset of Action:** Immediate. **Peak Effect:** 2–5 min. **Distribution:** Distributed throughout the body. **Metabolism/Elimination:** Metabolized by the liver to desacetyldiltiazem, a less active metabolite. Eliminated by the kidneys as metabolite and 2%–4% unchanged drug. **Half-Life:** 3.5–6.0 hr (parent), 5–7 hr (metabolite).

INDICATIONS/DOSAGE

Treatment of atrial fibrillation/flutter

(not associated with accessory bypass tracts, i.e., WPW syndrome, paroxysmal supraventricular tachycardia)

Adult: Initially 0.25 mg/kg as a single bolus. Average dose 20 mg. If inadequate response in 15 minutes, 0.35 mg/kg (actual body weight). Subsequent doses should be based on patient response. Continuous infusion 10 mg/hr (some patients

In the Adverse Effects section, underline indicates most frequent;
CAPS indicates life threatening.

may need 5 mg/hr), increased in 5 mg/hr increments, up to 15 mg/hr as needed for up to 24 hr.

CONTRAINDICATIONS/ PRECAUTIONS

Contraindicated in: Sick sinus syndrome/second or third degree AV block (except with functioning ventricular pacemaker), severe hypotension or cardiogenic shock, hypersensitivity, patients with accessory bypass tract (i.e., WPW) associated with atrial fibrillation/flutter, concomitant use (within a few hours) of IV beta blockers, ventricular tachycardia. **Use cautiously in:** CHF, hypotension, hepatic impairment. **Pregnancy/Lactation:** No well-controlled trials to establish safety. Benefits must outweigh risks. **Pediatrics:** Safety and efficacy not established.

PREPARATION

Availability: 5 mg/mL, 5 and 10 mL vials. **Infusion:** Dilute each 125 mg (25 mL) in at least 100 mL of compatible IV solution.

STABILITY/STORAGE

Vial: Store in refrigerator. May be stored at room temperature for 1 month only after removal from refrigerator. **Infusion:** Store in refrigerator. Stable for 24 hr after preparation.

ADMINISTRATION

IV Push: Administer over 2 min. **Continuous Infusion:** 10–15 mg/hr.

COMPATIBILITY

Solution: Dextrose solutions, sodium chloride solutions.

ADVERSE EFFECTS

CNS: Paresthesia, dizziness. **Ophtho:** Amblyopia. **CV:** VENTRICULAR FIBRILLATION, hypotension, dysrhythmias, ventricular tachycardia. **Resp:** Dyspnea. **GI:** Constipation, nausea, vomiting, elevated AST (SGOT) and alkaline phosphatase, dry mouth. **Fld/Lytes:** Edema. **Heme:** Hyperuricemia. **Hypersens:** Pruritus. **Other:** Injection site irritation, flushing, sweating.

TOXICITY/OVERDOSE

Signs/Symptoms: Bradycardia, high degree AV block, cardiac failure, hypotension. **Treatment:** Symptomatic and supportive treatment. Treat bradycardia and AV block with cardiac pacing. Cardiac failure requires inotropic support. Hypotension treated with vasopressor agents.

DRUG INTERACTIONS

Anesthetics, beta blockers, digoxin: Additive effect on contractility and/or SA/AV node conduction.

NURSING CONSIDERATIONS

Assessment
General:
Blood pressure, continuous ECG monitoring.
Physical:
Cardiovascular status.

Intervention/Rationale
Continuous ECG monitoring required during administration. Rapid treatment of extrasystoles and AV block may be required. Emergency equipment and defibrillator must be readily available.

In the Adverse Effects section, underline indicates most frequent; CAPS indicates life threatening.

173

Patient/Family Education

Educate regarding side effects and expected therapeutic effects of drug. Seek assistance with ambulatory activities.

DIPHENHYDRAMINE

(dye-fen-hye'-dra-meen)

Trade Name(s): Bena-D, Benadryl, Benahist, Benoject-10, Dihydrex, Diphenacen, Hyrexin, Nordryl, Wehdryl

Classification(s): Antihistamine

Pregnancy Category: B

PHARMACODYNAMICS/KINETICS

Mechanism of Action: Antagonizes histamine at receptor sites thereby blocking the effects of histamine. Has anticholinergic, antipruritic, and sedative effects.

Distribution: 80%–85% protein bound. **Metabolism/Elimination:** Metabolized by the liver. Metabolites and small amounts of unchanged drug excreted by the kidneys.

INDICATIONS/DOSAGE

Reduce dosage in elderly.

Treatment of allergic reaction to blood or plasma, of anaphylaxis as an adjunct to epinephrine, and of motion sickness and nausea associated with chemotherapy.

Adult: 10–50 mg. Maximum limit per dose is 100 mg. Maximum daily dose 400 mg.

Pediatric: 5 mg/kg/day. Maximum daily dose is 300 mg in divided doses.

Treatment of Parkinson's disease

(for elderly unable to tolerate more potent agents, used in combination with centrally-acting anticholinergics).

Adult: 10–50 mg. Maximum limit per dose is 100 mg. Maximum daily dose 400 mg.

CONTRAINDICATIONS/PRECAUTIONS

Contraindicated in: Asthmatic attack, bladder neck obstruction, hypersensitivity, narrow-angle glaucoma, peptic ulcer, symptomatic prostatic hypertrophy, pyloroduodenal obstruction, patients on monoamine oxidase (MAO) inhibitors. **Use cautiously in:** Elderly (more likely to cause dizziness, excessive sedation, confusion, hypotension), hypertension, liver disease. **Pregnancy/Lactation:** No well-controlled trials to establish safety. Crosses placenta. Benefits must outweigh risks. Distributed in breast milk. Not for use in breastfeeding women. **Pediatrics:** Give to children under age 6 only under the direction of a physician. Not for use in neonates and premature infants.

PREPARATION

Availability: 10 mg/mL and 50 mg/mL in 1, 10, and 30 mL vials/amps.

STABILITY/STORAGE

Vial: Store at room temperature. Protect from light.

ADMINISTRATION

IV Push: Give slowly over 5 min.

COMPATIBILITY
Solution: Dextrose solutions, lactated Ringer's, Ringer's injection, sodium chloride solutions. **Syringe:** Atropine, butorphanol, chlorpromazine, cimetidine, dimenhydrinate, droperidol, fentanyl, glycopyrrolate, hydromorphone, meperidine, metclopramide, midazolam, morphine, nalbuphine, pentazocine, periphenazine, promethazine, ranitidine, scopolamine. **Y-site:** Acyclovir, heparin, hydrocortisone, ondansetron, potassium chloride, vitamin B complex with C.

INCOMPATIBILITY
Syringe: Pentobarbital, thiopental. **Y-site:** Foscarnet.

ADVERSE EFFECTS
CNS: Disturbed coordination, dizziness, <u>drowsiness</u>, faintness, paradoxical excitation (children), <u>sedation</u>. **CV:** Bradycardia, hypotension, tachycardia. **Resp:** Nasal stuffiness, thickening of bronchial secretions. **GI:** Anorexia, diarrhea, dry mouth, epigastric distress, vomiting. **GU:** Dysuria, urinary retention/frequency.

DRUG INTERACTIONS
Alcohol/CNS depressants: Additive depressant effects. **MAO inhibitors:** Intensified drying effects, hypotension, extrapyramidal reactions.

NURSING CONSIDERATIONS
Assessment
Physical:
Neurologic status, GI tract, GU tract.

Intervention/Rationale
Drug has many different uses. Determine why drug was ordered and individualize assessment to specific patient.

Patient/Family Education
Drug may cause drowsiness/sedation; avoid performing activities that require mental alertness. Dry mouth may be alleviated with gum, sugar-free hard candy, and good oral hygiene. Avoid alcohol or other CNS depressants while taking drug.

DIPYRIDAMOLE
(die-pa-rid′-a-mole)
Trade Name(s): Persantine IV
Classification(s): Vasodilator
Pregnancy Category: B

PHARMACODYNAMICS/KINETICS
Mechanism of Action: Adenosine uptake inhibition resulting in coronary vasodilation. **Peak Effect:** 6.5 min. **Duration of Action:** 30 min. **Distribution:** Distributed throughout the body. Protein binding to alpha-acid glycoprotein (99%). **Metabolism/Elimination:** Metabolized to glucuronide conjugates by the liver. Excreted via bile. **Half-Life:** Triphasic: 3–12 min, 33–62 min, 11.6–15.0 hr.

INDICATIONS/DOSAGE

Alternative to exercise in thallium myocardial perfusion imaging in coronary artery disease
Adult: Adjust dose based on weight. 0.142 mg/kg/min (0.57 mg/kg total). Single dose should not exceed 60 mg.

In the Adverse Effects section, <u>underline</u> indicates most frequent; CAPS indicates life threatening.

175

CONTRAINDICATIONS/ PRECAUTIONS

Contraindicated in: Hypersensitivity. **Use cautiously in:** Asthma, unstable angina. **Pregnancy/Lactation:** No well-controlled trials to establish safety. Benefits must outweigh risks. **Pediatrics:** Safety and efficacy not established.

PREPARATION

Availability: 10 mg/2 mL amp. **Syringe:** Dilute in at least a 1:2 ratio (i.e., dilute each 10 mg [2 mL] with 4 mL) with compatible solution for a total volume of 20–50 mL. Must be diluted to avoid local irritation.

STABILITY/STORAGE

Vial: Store at room temperature. Avoid freezing. Protect from light.

ADMINISTRATION

General: Inject thallium-201 within 5 min of dipyridamole administration. **IV Push/Intermittent Infusion:** Administer as a single dose over 4 min.

COMPATIBILITY

Solution: Dextrose solutions, sodium chloride solutions.

ADVERSE EFFECTS

CNS: Paresthesia, hypothesia, hypertonia, nervousness/anxiety, tremor, somnolence, <u>headache</u>, migraine, <u>vertigo</u>, syncope. **Ophtho:** Vision abnormalities, eye pain. **CV:** <u>ECG abnormalities</u> (ST-T changes/ extrasystoles), dysrhythmias, palpitations, bradycardia, <u>ventricular tachycardia</u>, <u>MI</u>, AV block, <u>chest pain/angina</u>, <u>orthostatic hypotension</u>, atrial fibrillation, cardiomyopathy, edema, hypertension. **Resp:** BRONCHOSPASM, pharyngitis, hyperventilation, cough. **GI:** Dyspepsia, dry mouth, abdominal pain, flatulence, vomiting, dysphagia, increased appetite, <u>nausea</u>. **GU:** Kidney pain. **MS:** Arthralgia, myalgia, back pain, intermittent claudication. **Other:** Diaphoresis, tinnitus, earache, <u>flushing</u>.

DRUG INTERACTIONS

Theophylline: False-negative thallium imaging by decreasing vasodilatory effect.

NURSING CONSIDERATIONS

Assessment
General:
Vital signs, continuous ECG monitoring.
Physical:
Cardiopulmonary status, neurologic status.

Intervention/Rational
Continuous ECG monitoring required during infusion. Rapid treatment of extrasystoles and AV block needed. ● Observe for neurologic deficits during or following administration.

Patient/Family Education
Educate regarding side effects and expected therapeutic effects of drug. Seek assistance with ambulatory activities especially immediately following procedure.

DOBUTAMINE HYDROCHLORIDE
(doe-byoo'-ta-meen)
Trade Name(s): Dobutrex
Classification(s): Inotropic agent
Pregnancy Category: C

In the Adverse Effects section, <u>underline</u> indicates most frequent; CAPS indicates life threatening.

D

PHARMACODYNAMICS/KINETICS

Mechanism of Action: Stimulates beta-1 receptors of the heart while producing chronotropic, hypertensive, arrhythmogenic, and vasodilatative effects. Increases cardiac output. **Onset of Action:** 1–2 min. **Peak Effect:** 10 min. **Duration of Action:** Brief (minutes). **Metabolism/Elimination:** Metabolized by the liver and other tissues. Excreted via the kidneys. **Half-Life:** 2 min.

INDICATIONS/DOSAGE

Short-term inotropic support in cardiac decompensation from decreased myocardial contractility resulting from organic heart disease or as a result of cardiac surgical procedures

Adult: 2.5–10 mcg/kg/min. Rate adjusted according to desired response. Maximum dose up to 40 mcg/kg/min.

Cardiac catheterization of children with congenital heart disease (*unlabeled use*)

Pediatric: 2.0–7.75 mcg/kg/min infused for 10 min.

CONTRAINDICATIONS/ PRECAUTIONS

Contraindicated in: Hypersensitivity, idiopathic hypertrophic subaortic stenosis. **Use cautiously in:** MI, uncorrected hypovolemia. **Pregnancy/ Lactation:** No well-controlled trials to establish safety. Benefits must outweigh risks. **Pediatrics:** Safety and efficacy has not been established.

PREPARATION

Availability: 250 mg in 20 mL vials. Each vial contains 250 mg mannitol.

Reconstitution: If available in powder form, add 10 mL sterile water for injection or 5% destrose in water to vial. Add an additional 10 mL if not completely dissolved.

Infusion: Must be further diluted to final volume of at least 50 mL in compatible IV solution.

STABILITY/STORAGE

Vial: Store at room temperature. Following reconstitution, stable for 48 hr when refrigerated or 6 hr at room temperature.

Infusion: Use within 24 hr. Solution may be pink in color due to slight oxidation without loss of potency. Freezing is not recommended due to possible crystallization.

ADMINISTRATION

General: Administer via infusion device. Hypovolemia should be corrected before initiation of dobutamine administration.

Continuous Infusion: Begin with recommended dose for weight and overall condition. Gradually increase to obtain desired response as indicated by improvement of vital signs, heart rate, presence/absence of ectopics, urine flow, and hemodynamic parameters.

COMPATIBILITY

Solution: Dextrose solution, lactated Ringer's, sodium chloride solutions. **Syringe:** Heparin, ranitidine. **Y-site:** Amiodarone, amrinone, atracu-

---

In the Adverse Effects section, <u>underline</u> indicates most frequent; CAPS indicates life threatening.

rium, bretylium, calcium chloride, calcium gluconate, diazepam, dopamine, enalaprilat, famotidine, insulin, lidocaine, magnesium sulfate, nitroglycerin, pancuronium, potassium chloride, ranitidine, sodium nitroprusside, streptokinase, tolazoline, vecuronium, verapamil, zidovudine.

INCOMPATIBILITY

Solution: 5% sodium bicarbonate. **Syringe:** Doxapram. **Y-site:** Acyclovir, alteplase, aminophylline, foscarnet, phytonadione.

ADVERSE EFFECTS

CNS: Headache. **CV:** Angina, <u>hypertension</u>, nonspecific chest pain, <u>palpitation</u>, <u>premature ventricular contractions</u>, <u>tachycardia</u>. **Resp:** Shortness of breath. **GI:** Nausea, vomiting. **Other:** Local phlebitis.

TOXICITY/OVERDOSE

Signs/Symptoms: Excessive alteration of blood pressure or tachycardia are the usual manifestations of overdosage. **Treatment:** Notify physician of all side effects. Decrease infusion rate if extrasystoles, heart rate, or blood pressure increase. Due to short half-life no other treatment is usually required.

DRUG INTERACTIONS

Bretylium: Potentiates vasopressor action resulting in dysrhythmias. **Halogenated hydrocarbon anesthetic agents:** Sensitizes myocardium to catecholamine response; may produce serious dysrhythmias. **Oxytocic drugs (obstetrics):** May cause severe, persistent hypertension.

NURSING CONSIDERATIONS

Assessment

General:
Vital signs, baseline/daily weight, hydration status, continuous ECG (recommended), intake/output ratio.

Physical:
Cardiovascular status, hemodynamic parameters (recommended).

Lab Alterations:
Acidosis decreases effectiveness of vasopressor activity. Monitor serum glucose in diabetics.

Intervention/Rationale

Obtain baseline weight for accurate drug calculation. ● Correct hypovolemia with IV fluids prior to initiation of therapy. ● May cause rebound tachycardia or supraventricular tachydysrhythmias. Continuously monitor heart rate, ectopic activity, blood pressure, and urinary output. ● Hourly measurement of central venous pressure, pulmonary wedge pressure, and cardiac output assists in determining drug's effectiveness. ● When discontinuing infusion it is necessary to gradually decrease dose. ● Drug may increase insulin/oral hypoglycemic agent requirements.

Patient/Family Education

Notify physician immediately if chest pain or shortness of breath occur. Review rationale for instituting drug therapy and the need for frequent vital sign assessment and continuous monitoring. Notify physician/nurse immediately if pain/discomfort occurs at site of infusion.

In the Adverse Effects section, <u>underline</u> indicates most frequent; CAPS indicates life threatening.

DOPAMINE
(dope'-a-meen)
Trade Name(s): Intropin, Revimine ♣
Classification(s): Inotropic agent, vasopressor
Pregnancy Category: C

PHARMACODYNAMICS/KINETICS
Mechanism of Action: Endogenous catecholamine. Dose related stimulation of dopaminergic, beta-adrenergic, and alpha-adrenergic receptors of sympathetic nervous system. Dilates renal and mesenteric blood vessels. **Onset of Action:** 5 min. **Duration of Action:** 10 min or less. **Distribution:** Widely distributed throughout the body. Does not cross blood–brain barrier. **Metabolism/Elimination:** Metabolized in liver, kidneys, and plasma by MAO and catechol-O-methyltransferase to inactive compounds. 80% of drug is excreted in the urine within 24 hr. **Half-Life:** 2 min.

INDICATIONS/DOSAGE

Treatment of shock and correction of hemodynamics. Improve perfusion of vital organs, increase cardiac output, and blood pressure

Adult: 2–5 mcg/kg/min. 0.5–2.0 mcg/kg/min stimulates dopaminergic receptors producing renal vasodilation. 2–10 mcg/kg/min stimulates dopaminergic and beta-1 adrenergic receptors causing cardiac stimulation. Doses greater than 10 mcg/kg/min stimulate alpha adrenergic receptors causing vasoconstriction.

CONTRAINDICATIONS/PRECAUTIONS
Contraindicated in: Pheochromocytoma, uncorrected tachydysrhythmias, ventricular fibrillation. **Use cautiously in:** Arterial embolism, cold related injuries, diabetic endarteritis, hypovolemia, MAO inhibitors, occlusive vascular damage. **Pregnancy/Lactation:** No well-controlled trials to establish safety. Benefits must outweigh risks. **Pediatrics:** Safety and efficacy has not been established.

PREPARATION
Availability: 40, 80, 160 mg/mL in 5 mL amps, 5, 10, 20 mL vials and 5, 10 mL syringes. **Infusion:** Dilute each 200 or 400 mg in 250–500 mL of compatible IV solution. Concentrations used range from 400–1500 mcg/mL.

STABILITY/STORAGE
Vial: Store at room temperature. **Infusion:** Stable for 24 hr at room temperature.

ADMINISTRATION
General: Administer via an infusion device. Assess IV site regularly for evidence of infiltration or irritation. If extravasation occurs 10–15 mL 0.9% sodium chloride containing 5–10 mg phentolamine should be infiltrated throughout affected area under physician's direction. **Continuous Infusion:** Usually begin at rate of 1–5 mcg/kg/min and increase by 1–4 mcg/kg/min at 15–30 minute intervals until optimal response is obtained.

COMPATIBILITY
Solution: Dextrose solutions, lactated Ringer's, sodium chloride so-

In the Adverse Effects section, underline indicates most frequent; CAPS indicates life threatening.

179

lutions. **Syringe:** Doxapram, heparin, ranitidine. **Y-site:** Amiodarone, amrinone, atracurium, dobutamine, enalaprilat, esmolol, famotidine, foscarnet, heparin, hydrocortisone, labetalol, lidocaine, nitroglycerin, pancuronium, potassium chloride, ranitidine, sodium nitroprusside, streptokinase, tolazoline, vecuronium, verapamil, vitamin B complex with C, zidovudine.

INCOMPATIBILITY
Solution: 5% sodium bicarbonate. **Y-site:** Acyclovir, alteplase.

ADVERSE EFFECTS
CNS: Headache. **CV:** <u>Hypotension</u>, angina, <u>dysrhythmias</u>, ECG changes, palpitations, tachycardia, <u>vasoconstriction</u>, widened QRS complex. **Resp:** Dyspnea. **GI:** Nausea, vomiting. **Renal:** Azotemia. **Derm:** Piloerection. **Other:** Tissue necrosis (extravasation).

TOXICITY/OVERDOSE
Signs/Symptoms: Accidental overdose is manifested by excessive blood pressure. **Treatment:** Decrease rate of administration or temporarily discontinue until condition is stabilized. If blood pressure does not return to normal consider the use of a short acting alpha-adrenergic blocking agent (ex: phentolamine).

DRUG INTERACTIONS
Guanethidine: Partial or total reversal of antihypertensive effect. **Halogenated hydrocarbon anesthetic agents:** Serious dysrhythmias (results from myocardial sensitization). **MAO inhibitors:** Increased vasopressor response. **Oxytocic drugs:** Severe persistent hypertension in obstetrics.

Phenytoin: Concomitant infusion may lead to seizures, severe hypotension, and bradycardia. **Tricyclic antidepressants:** Vasopressor response of dopamine may be decreased.

NURSING CONSIDERATIONS
Assessment
General:
Vital signs, baseline/daily weight, hydration status, intake/output ratio.
Physical:
Cardiovascular status.
Lab Alterations:
Acidosis decreases effectiveness of vasopressor activity.

Intervention/Rationale
Obtain baseline weight for accurate drug calculation. ● Drug has dose-dependent effect; low doses lead to cardiac stimulation and renal vascular dilation; large doses cause vasoconstriction. ● Monitor blood pressure every 5 min until stabilization occurs. Arterial catheter may be inserted to monitor blood pressure continuously throughout therapy. ● Assess peripheral pulses regularly, carefully noting color, temperature, motion, and sensation of extremities, or if mottling is noted. ● If hypotension continues or worsens, dosage of drug should be titrated within specified parameters. Need for continuous monitoring of ECG throughout administration of drug is probable during hypotensive manifestations. ● When discontinuing infusion it is necessary to gradually decrease dose and expand blood volume with IV fluid to prevent recurrence of hypoten-

In the Adverse Effects section, <u>underline</u> indicates most frequent; CAPS indicates life threatening.

sion. Renal perfusion rates of drug may also require gradual weaning of continuous infusion in order to prevent rebound hypotension.

Patient/Family Education
Routinely monitor blood pressure. Notify physician/nurse immediately if chest pain, numbness, tingling, or burning of extremities occurs. Change positions slowly in order to minimize orthostatic effects.

DOXACURIUM

(dox-a-cure′-e-um)
Trade Name(s): Nuromax
Classification(s): Nondepolarizing neuromuscular blocking agent
Pregnancy Category: C

PHARMACODYNAMICS/KINETICS
Mechanism of Action: Causes partial paralysis by interfering with neural transmission at myoneural junction, prevents acetylcholine from binding to receptors at muscle end plate. **Onset of Action:** 4 min. **Peak Effect:** 5 min. **Duration of Action:** 100 min. **Distribution:** Distributes rapidly throughout the body. **Metabolism/ Elimination:** Not metabolized. Eliminated unchanged in urine and bile. **Half-Life:** 60–100 min.

INDICATIONS/DOSAGE

Intubation and maintenance of neuromuscular blockade

Adult: Individualize dose according to patient needs. Reduce dosage in elderly or severe renal impairment.

Initial dose: 0.025 mg/kg. **Maintenance dose:** 0.005–0.01 mg/kg every hour. Adjust doses for shorter or longer durations.

Maintenance of neuromuscular blockade during prolonged operative procedures

Adult: Individualize dose according to patient needs. Reduce dosage in elderly or severe renal impairment.
Initial Dose: 0.05 mg/kg. 0.08 mg/kg for prolonged blockade. **Maintenance Dose:** 0.005–0.01 mg/kg every hour. Adjust dose for shorter or longer durations.

Pediatric: Individualize dose according to patient needs. Reduce dosage in severe renal impairment. 0.03–0.05 mg/kg. Adjust doses for shorter or longer durations. Higher doses and more frequent administration may be necessary.

CONTRAINDICATIONS/ PRECAUTIONS
Contraindicated in: Hypersensitivity. **Use cautiously in:** Bronchial asthma, myasthenia gravis, severe electrolyte disturbances, cardiovascular disease, bronchogenic cancer, neuromuscular diseases. **Pregnancy/ Lactation:** No well-controlled trials to establish safety. Benefits must outweigh risks. **Pediatrics:** Safety and efficacy has not been established for children < 2 years old.

PREPARATION
Availability: 1 mg/mL in 5 mL vials. **Infusion:** May be diluted as a 1:10 ratio (1 mL drug/10 mL compatible IV solution). Dilute just prior to administration.

In the Adverse Effects section, underline indicates most frequent; CAPS indicates life threatening.

D

STABILITY/STORAGE

Vial: Store at room temperature. **Infusion:** Stable for 8 hr after dilution. Use within 24 hr.

ADMINISTRATION

General: Unconsciousness must be established prior to administration to prevent patient distress. **IV Push:** Give initial bolus over 30–60 sec. **Continuous Infusion:** Give at physician specified rate.

COMPATIBILITY

Solution: Dextrose solutions, lactated Ringer's, sodium chloride solutions. **Y-site:** Alfentanil, fentanyl, sufentanil.

INCOMPATIBILITY

Y-site: Barbiturates.

ADVERSE EFFECTS

Ophtho: Diplopia. **CV:** Hypotension, myocardial infarction, VENTRICULAR FIBRILLATION. **Resp:** BRONCHOSPASM, prolonged dose-related apnea, wheezing. **MS:** Inadequate blockade, prolonged neuromuscular blockade. **Hypersens:** Urticaria. **Other:** Fever, flushing.

TOXICITY/OVERDOSE

Signs/Symptoms: Apnea, airway closure, hypersensitivity, including anaphylaxis, respiratory insufficiency. **Treatment:** Provide cardiovascular support, assure patent airway and ventilation, resuscitate as necessary. **Antidote(s):** Reverse blockade symptoms with anticholinesterase reversing agents (edrophonium, neostigmine, pyridostigmine) and anticholinergic agents (atropine, glycopyrrolate).

DRUG INTERACTIONS

Aminoglycosides, carbamazepine, clindamycin, diuretics, general anesthetics (enflurane, isoflurane, halothane), lincomycin, lithium, magnesium sulfate, muscle relaxants, polypeptide antibiotics (bacitracin, polymyxin B), verapamil: Increased neuromuscular blockade. **Phenytoin, theophylline:** Resistance to or reversal of neuromuscular blockade. **Succinylcholine:** Increased onset and depth of neuromuscular blockade.

NURSING CONSIDERATIONS

Assessment

General:

Vital signs.

Physical:

Respiratory status, neurologic/neuromuscular status.

Lab Alterations:

Assess electrolyte status, correct deficiencies prior to surgery.

Intervention/Rationale

Produces apnea; maintain patent airway and have emergency respiratory support available (endotracheal equipment, ventilator, oxygen, ambu bag, and suction). ● Monitor response to drug during intraoperative period by use of a peripheral nerve stimulator. ● Assess postoperatively for presence of any residual muscle weakness. Evaluate hand grip, head lift, and ability to cough in order to ascertain full recovery from residual effects of drug.

Patient/Family Education

Discuss the rationale for hand grip, head lift, and cough demonstration in the immediate postoperative

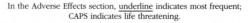

In the Adverse Effects section, underline indicates most frequent; CAPS indicates life threatening.

phase in order to assure patient co-operation.

DOXAPRAM

(dox'-a-pram)
Trade Name(s): Dopram
Classification(s): Analeptic CNS stimulant, respiratory and cerebral stimulant
Pregnancy Category: B

PHARMACODYNAMICS/KINETICS

Mechanism of Action: Produces respiratory stimulation by activating peripheral carotid chemoreceptors. Increased dosage stimulates medullary respiratory centers. **Onset of Action:** 20–40 sec. **Peak Effect:** 1–2 min. **Duration of Action:** 5–12 min. **Metabolism/Elimination:** Metabolized rapidly by liver. Eliminated by the kidneys. **Half-Life:** 2.4–4.1 hr.

INDICATIONS/DOSAGE

Treatment of drug-induced postanesthesia respiratory depression or apnea

Adult:
Single IV Injection: 0.5–1.0 mg/kg. Total dose not to exceed 1.5 mg/kg. **Alternate Dose Infusion:** 5 mg/min until satisfactory response. Maintenance infusion 1–3 mg/min. Maximum recommended dose 4 mg/kg.

Drug induced CNS depression

Adult: 2 mg/kg, repeat in 5 min. May repeat every 1–2 hr. Total maximum dose 3 g. If no response, begin infusion at 1–3 mg/min. Discontinue after 2 hr or if patient awakens. Not to exceed 3 g/24 hr.

Pulmonary disease (chronic) in conjunction with increased P_{CO_2}

Adult: Infusion: 1–2 mg/min. May increase to maximum 3 mg/min. Administration time should not exceed 2 hr.

CONTRAINDICATIONS/ PRECAUTIONS

Contraindicated in: Contains benzyl alcohol, do not use in newborns, acute bronchial asthma, cardiovascular impairment, cerebrovascular accident, epilepsy and convulsive states, pneumothorax, pulmonary fibrosis, pulmonary restrictive disease, severe hypertension. **Use cautiously in:** Hyperthyroidism, increased intracranial pressure, lactating women, pheochromocytoma. **Pregnancy/Lactation:** No well-controlled trials to establish safety. Benefits must outweigh risks. **Pediatrics:** Safety and efficacy for children less than 12 years has not been established.

PREPARATION

Availability: 20 mg/mL in 20 mL vials. **Syringe:** May be given undiluted or diluted with equal parts of sterile water for injection. **Infusion:** Dilute 250 mg in 230 mL of compatible IV solution to deliver a 1 mg/mL solution.

STABILITY/STORAGE

Vial: Store at room temperature. Avoid freezing. **Infusion:** Stable for 24 hr at room temperature.

ADMINISTRATION

General: Not effective for muscle relaxation or narcotic induced respiratory depression. Rapid infusion may cause hemolysis. **IV Push:** Administer slowly over 5 min. **Intermit-**

In the Adverse Effects section, underline indicates most frequent; CAPS indicates life threatening.

183

tent Infusion: Give loading dose of 2 mg/kg followed by an infusion at 1–3 mg/min according to patient size and depth of coma. Discontinue at the end of 2 hr or if patient awakens. **Continuous Infusion:** Begin at 5 mg/min, decrease to 1–3 mg/min with close observation of respiratory response. To be discontinued after 2 hr. Temporarily discontinue infusion for 1–2 hr, if still needed, repeat procedure.

COMPATIBILITY
Solution: Dextrose solutions, sodium chloride solutions. **Syringe:** Amikacin, bumetanide, chlorpromazine, cimetidine, cisplatin, cyclophosphamide, deslanoside, dopamine, doxycycline, epinephrine, methotrexate, netilmicin, phytonadione, pyridoxine, terbutaline, thiamine, tobramycin.

INCOMPATIBILITY
Syringe: Aminophylline, ascorbic acid, cefoperazone, cefotaxime, cefuroxime, dexamethasone, diazepam, digoxin, dobutamine, folic acid, furosemide, hydrocortisone, methylprednisolone, thiopental, ticarcillin.

ADVERSE EFFECTS
CNS: Seizures, apprehension, disorientation, dizziness, headache, hyperpyrexia, paresthesia, pupil dilation. **CV:** Chest pain, chest tightness, dysrhythmias, hypertension, hypotension, T-wave inversion. **Resp:** LARYNGOSPASM, BRONCHOSPASM, coughing, hiccough, sneezing. **GI:** Diarrhea, nausea, vomiting. **GU:** Perineal or genital burning sensation, spontaneous voiding, urinary retention. **MS:** Involuntary movements, muscle spasticity. **Hypersens:** Pruritus. **Other:** Sweating, flushing, irritation at IV site.

TOXICITY/OVERDOSE
Signs/Symptoms: Drug is known to have a narrow margin of safety. May cause excessive increase in blood pressure, tachycardia, and other dysrhythmias. Skeletal muscle hyperactivity including increased deep tendon reflexes, muscle spasticity, involuntary movements, and dyspnea may be considered early signs of overdose. More serious symptoms include clonus and generalized seizures. **Treatment:** Seizures may be treated with IV injection of anticonvulsant. Oxygen and resuscitative equipment should be available. No evidence to support that drug is dialyzable.

DRUG INTERACTIONS
Inhalant anesthetic agents (halothane, cyclopropane, enflurane): Initiation of therapy should be delayed for at least 10 min following discontinuance of anesthetic agents known to sensitize the myocardial cells (due to catecholamine release). **Muscle relaxants:** May temporarily mask symptoms of muscle relaxation. **MAO inhibitors, sympathomimetics:** Additive pressor effects.

NURSING CONSIDERATIONS
Assessment
General:
Vital signs, hemodynamic alterations, continuous ECG (recommended).
Physical:
Neurologic status (level of consciousness, deep tendon reflexes,

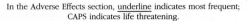
In the Adverse Effects section, underline indicates most frequent; CAPS indicates life threatening.

pupillary response), cardiopulmonary status.

Lab Alterations:
Evaluate ABGs for effectiveness of oxygenation.

Intervention/Rationale
Increases blood pressure, heart rate, cardiac output, and pulmonary artery pressure. ● Assess regularly for deepening/lightening of coma. Close observation is required until fully alert for a minimum of 1 hr. Regularly assess respiratory status, including rate, depth, and regularity of respirations. ● Drug may cause dysrhythmias, rate changes, or T-wave inversions.

Patient/Family Education
Review expected outcome of drug therapy and potential adverse effects.

DOXORUBICIN
(dox-oh-roo'-bi-sin)
Trade Name(s): Adriamycin
Classification(s): Antineoplastic antibiotic
Pregnancy Category: D

PHARMACODYNAMICS/KINETICS
Mechanism of Action: Forms a complex with DNA causing inhibition of DNA synthesis. Immunosuppressive action. **Distribution:** Widely distributed in plasma and tissues. Does not cross blood–brain barrier (ineffective in brain tumors/CNS metastasis). **Metabolism/Elimination:** Metabolized rapidly by liver to active and inactive metabolites. Excreted primarily via bile. **Half-Life:** Plasma disappearance follows a triphasic pattern with mean half-lives 12 min, 3.3 hr, 29.6 hr.

INDICATIONS/DOSAGE

Treatment of acute lymphoblastic leukemia, acute myeloblastic leukemia, neuroblastoma, solid tumor treatment including breast/ovarian cancer and Wilm's tumor

Adult: 60–75 mg/m² administered as a single dose at 21 day intervals. Alternate dose 20 mg/m² once weekly. Total dose should not exceed 550 mg/m² (risk of cumulative cardiotoxicity). Reduce dose 50% if serum bilirubin is 1.2–3 mg/dL. Reduce by 25% if serum bilirubin > 3 mg/dL.

Pediatric: 30 mg/m² as single injection each day for 3 days. Repeat every 4 weeks.

CONTRAINDICATIONS/PRECAUTIONS
Contraindicated in: Colon cancer, malignant melanoma, myelosuppression from previous therapy, renal cancer. **Use cautiously in:** Dysrhythmias, infections, patients with childbearing potential, previous CHF history. **Pregnancy/Lactation:** No well-controlled trials to establish safety. Benefits must outweigh risks.

PREPARATION
Availability: Lyophilized powder for injection in 10, 20, 50, or 100 mg/vial, rapid dissolution formula in 150 mg multidose vial, preserative free injection in 5, 10, and 25 mL vials. **Reconstitution:** Dilute with 5–25 mL 0.9% sodium chloride or sterile water for injection to provide

In the Adverse Effects section, underline indicates most frequent; CAPS indicates life threatening.

185

D

a final concentration of 2 mg/mL. Bacteriostatic diluents are not recommended.

STABILITY/STORAGE

Vial: Store at room temperature. Protect from light. **Infusion:** Unstable in solution with pH less than 3 or greater than 7. In pH range of 3–7, stable for 48 hr under refrigeration and 24 hr at room temperature.

ADMINISTRATION

General: Handle drug with care and adhere to institutional guidelines for the handling of chemotherapeutic/cytotoxic agents. Administer through rapidly flowing IV infusion. Extremely irritating to tissues. Avoid extravasation. Notify physician immediately and consider infiltrating area with hydrocortisone (50–100 mg) and/or sodium bicarbonate (5 mL of 8.4% injection). Apply cold compresses to minimize local reaction. In the event of a spill, use sodium hypochlorite 5% (bleach) to inactivate doxorubicin until a colorless liquid results. If powder/solution comes in direct contact with skin or mucosa wash thoroughly and immediately flush with soap and water. **Intermittent Infusion:** Administer slowly into the tubing of a free flowing IV over at least 3–5 min. Rate dependent on the vein size and total dosage.

COMPATIBILITY

Solution: Dextrose solutions, lactated Ringer's, sodium chloride solutions. **Syringe:** Bleomycin, cisplatin, cyclophosphamide, droperidol, fluorouracil, leucovorin calcium, methotrexate, metoclopramide, mitomycin, vinblastine, vincristine. **Y-site:** Bleomycin, cisplatin, cyclophosphamide, droperidol, fluorouracil, leucovorin calcium, methotrexate, metoclopramide, mitomycin, ondansetron, vinblastine, vincristine.

INCOMPATIBILITY

Syringe: Furosemide, heparin. **Y-site:** Furosemide, heparin.

ADVERSE EFFECTS

CV: Abnormal ECG findings, CARDIOMYOPATHY, dysrhythmias. **GI:** <u>Diarrhea</u>, <u>esophagitis</u>, <u>nausea</u>, <u>stomatitis</u>, <u>vomiting</u>, anorexia. **GU:** Red urine. **Derm:** <u>Alopecia</u>, hyperpigmentation of nail beds, tissue necrosis with extravasation. **Heme:** LEUKOPENIA, THROMBOCYTOPENIA, <u>ANEMIA</u>, hyperuricemia. **Hypersens:** ANAPHYLAXIS. **Other:** Chills, fever, flushing.

TOXICITY/OVERDOSE

Signs/Symptoms: Acute overdose enhances toxic effects of mucositis, leukopenia, and thrombocytopenia. Chronic overdose increases risk of cardiomyopathy with resultant CHF. **Treatment:** Treat severe myelosuppression by hospitalization, antibiotics, platelets, WBC transfusions, and symptomatic treatment of mucositis. Treatment of chronic overdose consists of vigorous management of CHF with digitalis preparations and diuretics. Peripheral vasodilator therapy is also recommended.

DRUG INTERACTIONS

Digoxin: Decreased digoxin plasma levels and renal excretion. **Other antineoplastic agents:** Potentiation of antineoplastic agent toxicity. **Radiation:** Increased toxicity to the myocardium, mucosa, skin, and liver.

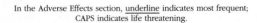

In the Adverse Effects section, <u>underline</u> indicates most frequent; CAPS indicates life threatening.

NURSING CONSIDERATIONS

Assessment

General:
Vital signs, ECG, intake/output ratio, hypersensitivity reactions.

Physical:
Cardiopulmonary status, GU tract, infectious disease status, hematopoietic system.

Lab Alterations:
Assess CBC with differential and platelet count, BUN, serum creatinine, and liver function prior to and throughout course of therapy. Serum uric acid evaluation.

Intervention/Rationale

Drug may cause CHF and imparts a red color to urine for 1–2 days after administration. ● Assess for development of fever, chills, or other signs of infection and notify physician immediately. ● Maintain adequate hydration during therapy. ● Assess patient for development of bleeding (bleeding gums, easy bruising, hematest positive stools/urine/vomitus). ● Avoid intramuscular injections and rectal temperatures. ● Monitor uric acid levels throughout course of therapy and assure prophylactic allopurinol is prescribed.

Patient/Family Education

Hair loss may affect body image. Secretions (urine/tears/sweat) may be discolored red. Observe for signs of infection (fever, sore throat, fatigue) or bleeding (melena, hematuria, nosebleeds, easy bruising) especially 1 week following administration. Take and record oral temperature daily and report persistent elevation to physician. Use a soft toothbrush and electric razor to minimize bleeding tendency. Avoid crowded environments and persons with known infections. Use reliable contraception throughout the duration of therapy and 4 months following due to potential teratogenic and mutagenic effects of drug. Seek physician approval prior to receiving live virus vaccinations or chloroquine. Avoid over-the-counter products containing aspirin or ibuprofen due to increased potential for bleeding. Report dizziness, unusual fatigue, shortness of breath (drug may cause anemia), or irregular heart beat.

DOXYCYCLINE

(dox-i-sye'-kleen)
Trade Name(s): Vibramycin
Classification(s): Broad spectrum antibiotic, semisynthetic tetracycline
Pregnancy Category: D

PHARMACODYNAMICS/KINETICS

Mechanism of Action: Bacteriostatic, inhibits microorganism protein synthesis by binding to ribosomes. **Onset of Action:** Rapid. **Peak Serum Level:** End of infusion. **Distribution:** 60%–90% protein bound. Highly lipid soluble. Readily penetrates cerebrospinal fluid, the eye, and the prostate. **Metabolism/Elimination:** Partially inactivated in the intestine. Undergoes enterohepatic circulation with some excretion via the bile and feces. 20%–40% excreted unchanged in the urine. **Half-Life:** 14–25 hr.

In the Adverse Effects section, underline indicates most frequent; CAPS indicates life threatening.

187

INDICATIONS/DOSAGE

Treatment of acute pelvic inflammatory disease, chlamydia trachomatis, gonococcal infections, and mycoplasma infections

Adult: Usual dose is 200 mg IV on first day of treatment. Subsequent daily dose of 100–200 mg dependent on severity of infection. 200 mg administered in one to two infusions.

Treatment of primary and secondary syphilis

Adult: 300 mg daily in divided doses for at least 10 days.

Pediatric: > 8 years and 45 kg: 4.4 mg/kg divided into two doses on day 1, followed by 2.2 mg/kg given as single dose or divided into two doses on subsequent days.
> 45 kg: Usual adult dosage.

CONTRAINDICATIONS/ PRECAUTIONS

Contraindicated in: Known hypersensitivity to tetracyclines. Not recommended for children < 8 years. **Use cautiously in:** Impaired liver function, lactation, postpartum, pregnancy. **Pregnancy/Lactation:** No well-controlled trials to establish safety. Benefits must outweigh risks. Crosses placenta. Secreted in breast milk. **Pediatrics:** May cause skeletal retardation in infants and in the fetus. Can cause permanent tooth discoloration in children < 8 years, including in utero or via lactation process.

PREPARATION

Availability: 100 and 200 mg powder for injection in vials. **Reconstitution:** Add 10 mL sterile water or compatible IV solution to each 100 mg. **Infusion:** Dilute each 100 mg in 100–1000 mL compatible IV solution. Resulting recommended concentration of 0.1 mg/mL.

STABILITY/STORAGE

Vial: Store at room temperature. Must be stored away from heat and light. **Infusion:** If diluted with 0.9% sodium chloride, 5% dextrose in water or Ringer's injection, stable for 72 hr prior to infusion if refrigerated. If diluted with D5/LR or lactated Ringer's solution, stable for 6 hr. Protect from direct sunlight during infusion.

ADMINISTRATION

General: Avoid rapid administration. Determine absolute patency of vein to avoid tissue extravasation. Assess for irritation, phlebitis, or infiltration of injection site. **Intermittent Infusion:** Duration of infusion varies with dose, but is usually 1–4 hr. Recommended *minimum* infusion time for 100 mg of 0.5 mg/mL solution is 1 hr.

COMPATIBILITY

Solution: Dextrose solutions, Ringer's injection, sodium chloride solutions. **Syringe:** Doxapram. **Y-site:** Acyclovir, cyclophosphamide, hydromorphone, magnesium sulfate, meperidine, morphine, ondansetron, perphenazine.

ADVERSE EFFECTS

GI: Anogenital lesions, anorexia, bulky loose stools, <u>diarrhea</u>, epigastric distress, <u>nausea</u>, steatorrhea, stomatitis, <u>vomiting</u>. **Derm:** Photosensitivity. **Heme:** HEMOLYTIC ANEMIA, neutropenia, thrombocy-

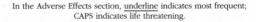
In the Adverse Effects section, <u>underline</u> indicates most frequent; CAPS indicates life threatening.

topenia, anemia. **Hypersens:** ANA-
PHYLAXIS, urticaria, maculopapu-
lar/erythematous rash. **Other:**
Phlebitis, superinfection.

TOXICITY/OVERDOSE
Signs/Symptoms: Hypersensitivity
reactions including but not limited
to anaphylaxis, liver damage, photosensitivity, systemic moniliasis.
Treatment: Notify physician, discontinue drug, treat allergic reaction
according to manifestations, resuscitate as necessary.

DRUG INTERACTIONS
Anticoagulants: Depresses plasma
prothrombin activity. Concomitant
administration may require a decrease in anticoagulant dosage. **Barbiturates, carbamazepine, phenytoin:**
Decreased doxycycline half-life.
Digoxin: Increased digoxin bioavailability resulting in toxicity. **Methoxyflurane:** Avoid concomitant use;
may enhance nephrotoxicity. **Oral
contraceptives:** Decreased pharmacologic action of oral contraceptives causing breakthrough bleeding or pregnancy.

NURSING CONSIDERATIONS
Assessment
General:
Allergy history, anaphylaxis.
Physical:
Hematopoietic system, dermatologic system, GI tract, infectious
disease status, signs/symptoms superinfection (sore throat/stomatitis,
vaginal discharge, perianal itching).
Lab Alterations:
Monitor liver enzymes, CBC with
differential, BUN, creatinine prior
to and throughout course of ther-

apy. False-positive or false-negative
readings with Clinitest.

Intervention/Rationale
Obtain specimens for culture and
sensitivity prior to initiating therapy. Do not withhold first dose
prior to obtaining culture results. ●
Assess skin regularly throughout
course of therapy to identify development of maculopapular rash.

Patient/Family Education
Review expected outcome and potential adverse effects of drug.
Complete course of therapy. Be
alert for photosensitivity skin reactions. Use sunscreen when outdoors for extended periods of time.
Be alert for new sources of infection. Report pruritus, urticaria, or
skin rash to nurse/physician.

DROPERIDOL
(droe-per'-i-dole)
Trade Name(s): Inapsine
Classification(s): Antiemetic,
general anesthetic, tranquilizer
Pregnancy Category: C

PHARMACODYNAMICS/KINETICS
Mechanism of Action: Acts at subcortical level to produce tran-
quilization, peripheral vascular
vasodilatation, sedation, mild
alpha-adrenergic blockade, and an-
tiemesis. **Onset of Action:** 3–10 min.
Peak Effect: 30 min. **Duration of Action:**
2–4 hr. **Metabolism/Elimination:** Metabolized in the liver. Excreted in
feces. 1% is excreted unchanged in
the urine. **Half-Life:** 2.2 hr.

In the Adverse Effects section, <u>underline</u> indicates most frequent;
CAPS indicates life threatening.

189

D

INDICATIONS/DOSAGE

Individualize dosage.

Treatment of postoperative nausea/vomiting

Adult: 0.5 mg every 4 hr.

Adjunct to general/regional anesthesia used to produce tranquilization

Adult: Premedication: 2.5–10 mg administered 30–60 min before induction of general anesthesia. Repeat 1.25–2.5 mg if indicated. **Anesthesia Induction:** 0.22–0.275 mg/kg administered concomitantly with an analgesic and general anesthesia. Anesthesia maintenance: 1.25–2.5 mg; individualized according to age, weight, physical status, and underlying pathologic condition. **Diagnostic Procedure without Anesthesia:** 1.25–5.0 mg. Additional doses may be required. Usually preceded by a 2.5–10.0 mg IM dose 30–60 min prior to procedure.

Pediatric (2–12 years): **Premedication:** 0.88–0.165 mg/kg. **Anesthesia Induction:** 0.088–0.165 mg/kg.

CONTRAINDICATIONS/PRECAUTIONS

Contraindicated in: Bone marrow depression, CNS depression, hypersensitivity, known intolerance, narrow angle glaucoma, severe liver or cardiac disease. **Use cautiously in:** Bone marrow depression, cardiac/liver disease, CNS depression, CNS tumors, diabetics, elderly or debilitated patients, intestinal obstruction, narrow angle glaucoma, prostatic hypertrophy, respiratory insufficiency, severely ill/compromised patients, seizures. **Pregnancy/Lactation:** No well-controlled trials to establish safety. Benefits must outweigh risks. Has been used during cesarean section without respiratory depression to the newborn. Exercise caution when administering to a nursing mother. **Pediatrics:** Not recommended for children less than 2 years.

PREPARATION

Availability: 2.5 mg/mL in 2, 5, 10 mL amps/vials. **Infusion:** Dilute in compatible IV solution.

STABILITY/STORAGE

Vial: Store at room temperature. Protect from light. **Infusion:** Stable for 7–10 days at concentrations of 1 mg/50 mL.

ADMINISTRATION

General: Used primarily under direct observation of anesthesiologist/nurse anesthetist. **IV Push:** 10 mg or less over 1 min period. Give through Y-site of an infusing IV or via 3-way stopcock. **Continuous Infusion:** Administer as per physician directions. Titrate to desired patient response.

COMPATIBILITY

Solution: Dextrose solutions, lactated Ringer's, Ringer's injection, sodium chloride solutions. **Syringe:** Atropine, buprenorphine, butorphanol, chlorpromazine, dimenhydrinate, diphenhydramine, fentanyl, glycopyrrolate, meperidine, metoclopramide, morphine, nalbuphine, pentazocine, perphenazine, prochlorperazine, promethazine, scopolamine. **Y-site:** Ondansetron.

In the Adverse Effects section, <u>underline</u> indicates most frequent; CAPS indicates life threatening.

INCOMPATIBILITY
Syringe: Pentobarbital. **Y-site:** Foscarnet.

ADVERSE EFFECTS
CNS: Anxiety, decreased seizure threshold, dizziness, drowsiness, <u>extrapyramidal symptoms</u> (dystonia, akathisia, oculogyric crisis), hallucinatory episodes, hyperactivity, restlessness. **Ophtho:** Blurred vision, dry eyes. **CV:** Hypertension, <u>hypotension</u>, <u>tachycardia</u>. **Resp:** Apnea, BRONCHOSPASM, LARYNGOSPASM, muscle rigidity, respiratory depression. **GI:** Constipation, dry mouth. **Other:** Chills, facial sweating, shivering.

TOXICITY/OVERDOSE
Signs/Symptoms: Apnea, extrapyramidal symptoms, severe hypotension, respiratory depression, respiratory arrest. **Treatment:** Discontinue drug. Treat symptomatically with supportive therapy. Reverse hypotension with fluid resuscitation and vasopressors. Epinephrine is contraindicated; further hypotension will occur due to alpha-adrenergic blocking action of drug. **Antidote(s):** Use benztropine or diphenhydramine for extrapyramidal symptom control.

DRUG INTERACTIONS
CNS depressant drugs, conduction anesthetic agents (spinal and peridural): May cause peripheral vasodilation and hypotension due to sympathetic blockade. **Narcotics:** Respiratory depressant effect lasts longer than analgesic effect.

NURSING CONSIDERATIONS
Assessment
General:
Continuous monitoring of vital signs.
Physical:
Respiratory status, mentation, GI tract, sedation level, neurologic status.

Intervention/Rationale
Prevent rapid changes in moving and positioning patient because of increased potential for hypotension. ● Fluids and other countermeasures to manage hypotension must be available. ● Monitor blood pressure, heart rate, and respiratory rate and pattern throughout administration period. ● Evaluate level of sedation and analgesia following administration. ● Carefully assess patient for the potential development of extrapyramidal effects of drug. ● Reduced dose of narcotics for pain control will be required postoperatively for at least 24 hr due to potential for CNS depression and respiratory depression.

Patient/Family Education
Change positions slowly in order to minimize orthostatic hypotension. Report immediately extrapyramidal reactions (unusual twitching, jerky movements). Medication causes drowsiness. Call for assistance during ambulatory activities.

In the Adverse Effects section, <u>underline</u> indicates most frequent; CAPS indicates life threatening.

191

EDETATE CALCIUM DISODIUM (CALCIUM EDTA)

(ee'-de-tate kal'-see-yum dye-sode'-ee-yum)

Trade Name(s): Calcium Disodium Versenate

Classification(s): Antidote, heavy metal antagonist, lead chelator

Pregnancy Category: C

PHARMACODYNAMICS/KINETICS

Mechanism of Action: Forms stable soluble complexes with heavy metals particularly lead. Removes toxic levels of lead or other heavy metals by displacing calcium. **Onset of Action:** 1 hr. **Peak Effect:** 24–48 hr. **Distribution:** Distributed primarily throughout extracellular fluid. Does not penetrate erythrocytes or CSF. **Metabolism/Elimination:** Not metabolized. Readily displaced by heavy metals. 50% excreted in the urine in 1 hr, 95% within 24 hr. **Half-Life:** 20–60 min.

INDICATIONS/DOSAGE

Management of acute/chronic lead poisoning, heavy metal poisoning, removal of radioactive/nuclear fission products

Total dose of drug depends on severity of lead intoxication and patient's response. Dosage reduction required if serum creatinine > 2 mg/dL.

Diagnosis of lead poisoning

Adult/Pediatric: 500 mg/m^2. Not to exceed 1 g.

Lead poisoning without encephalopathy

Adult/Pediatric: 1.0–1.5 g/m^2/24 hr in two divided doses for 3–5 days (not to exceed two courses). Wait at least 2–4 days but preferably 2–3 weeks between courses.

Lead poinsoning with encephalopathy

Adult/Pediatric: Continuous infusion of 1.5 g/m^2/24 hr for 5 days beginning 4 hr after dimercaprol.

CONTRAINDICATIONS/PRECAUTIONS

Contraindicated in: Anuria, increased intracranial pressure. **Use cautiously in:** Cardiac dysrhythmias, underlying renal disease (potentially nephrotoxic). **Pregnancy/Lactation:** No well-controlled trials to establish safety. Benefits must outweigh risks.

PREPARATION

Availability: 200 mg/mL in 5 mL vials. **Infusion:** Dilute each dose in 250–500 mL of compatible IV solution.

STABILITY/STORAGE

Vial: Store at room temperature. **Infusion:** Stable for 24 hr at room temperature.

ADMINISTRATION

General: In patients with incipient or overt lead encephalopathy, the drug must be infused slowly (rapid administration may increase intracranial pressure to lethal levels). Administer via IV infusion device. When administering continuously, interrupt infusion for 1 hr before a blood lead concentration is measured in order to prevent false val-

In the Adverse Effects section, <u>underline</u> indicates most frequent; CAPS indicates life threatening.

ues. **Intermittent Infusion:** Administer 50% daily dose over at least 1 hr, at least 2 hr if patient is symptomatic. **Continuous Infusion:** When given as a single infusion daily doses are usually infused over 8–24 hr.

COMPATIBILITY
Solution: Dextrose 5%, sodium chloride 0.9%.

INCOMPATIBILITY
Solution: Dextrose 10%, lactated Ringer's, Ringer's injection.

ADVERSE EFFECTS
CNS: Paresthesia, fatigue, headache, malaise, numbness. **CV:** Cardiac dysrhythmias, hypotension, inverted T-waves. **GI:** Nausea, vomiting. **GU:** <u>Hematuria</u>, <u>proteinuria</u>, urinary frequency, urinary urgency, glycosuria. **Renal:** <u>Nephrotoxicity with renal tubular necrosis leading to fatal NEPHROSIS</u>. **MS:** Arthralgia, leg cramps, myalgia. **Fld/Lytes:** Depletion of trace metals, hypercalcemia. **Heme:** Transient bone marrow depression with prolonged administration. **Hypersens:** Histamine-like reaction. **Other:** Thrombophlebitis, sudden fever, chills, fatigue, excessive thirst, sneezing, nasal congestion (4–8 hr after infusion).

TOXICITY/OVERDOSE
Signs/Symptoms: Prolonged administration of drug in high doses may produce bone marrow depression and skin/mucous membrane lesions, including cheilosis. Severe depletion of trace metals is also possible. **Treatment:** To avoid toxicity, use with dimercaprol. Discontinue drug if above signs or symptoms occur.

NURSING CONSIDERATIONS

Assessment
General:
Strict intake/output ratio, vital signs, ECG monitoring (recommended), daily weight.
Physical:
Neurologic status, cardiovascular status, renal status.
Lab Alterations:
Monitor urine/blood lead levels and BUN/creatinine regularly. Discontinue infusion for 1 hr before measuring blood lead concentration.

Intervention/Rationale
Force fluids to facilitate lead excretion in all patients except those with signs/symptoms of lead encephalopathy. ● If patient is anuric drug should be held, physician notified, and urine flow reestablished by means of IV fluid resuscitation. ● Assess neurologic status frequently throughout administration of drug, note development of encephalopathy. ● If increased intracranial pressure signs/symptoms are noted, notify physician and restrict fluids as per order. ● Monitor cardiac status and evaluate development of dysrhythmias, peaked T-waves.

Patient/Family Education
Critical need for outpatient follow-up to regularly monitor lead levels and the need to evaluate other family members for lead poisoning. Contact public health department regarding sources or potential sources of lead poisoning in the home, school, recreation area, or work place.

In the Adverse Effects section, <u>underline</u> indicates most frequent; CAPS indicates life threatening.

EDETATE DISODIUM (EDTA)

(ee'-de-tate dye-sode'-ee-yum)
Trade Name(s): Chealamide, Disotate, Endrate
Classification(s): Chelating agent
Pregnancy Category: C

PHARMACODYNAMICS/KINETICS

Mechanism of Action: Forms chelates with divalent/trivalent metals. Because of affinity for calcium, will lower serum calcium levels. Severely depletes calcium stores of body. Negative inotropic effect on heart. **Distribution:** Widely distributed in extracellular fluid. Does not enter CSF. **Metabolism/Elimination:** Not metabolized. Excreted rapidly via urine. 95% eliminated within 24 hr. **Half-Life:** 20–60 min.

INDICATIONS/DOSAGE

Emergency treatment of hypercalcemia, treatment of cardiac dysrhythmias associated with digitalis toxicity

Adult: 50 mg/kg/24 hr. Total dose not to exceed 3 g/24 hr. Administer for 5 days, hold for 2 days. May repeat to total of 15 doses. *Pediatric:* 40 mg/kg/24 hr. Not to exceed 70 mg/kg/24 hr or adult dosage.

CONTRAINDICATIONS/PRECAUTIONS

Contraindicated in: Anuria, hypersensitivity to any component. **Use cautiously in:** Incipient CHF, intracranial lesions, patients with limited cardiac reserve, renal disease, sei-

zures. **Pregnancy/Lactation:** No well-controlled trials to establish safety. Benefits must outweigh risks.

PREPARATION

Availability: 150 mg/mL in 20 mL vials. **Infusion:** Must be diluted prior to administration in 500 mL compatible IV solution. Use less diluent in children if necessary. Final concentrations must not exceed 3% (3 g/100 mL).

STABILITY/STORAGE

Vial: Store at room temperature. **Infusion:** Mix immediately prior to use. Stable for 24 hr at room temperature.

ADMINISTRATION

General: Confirm vein patency prior to initiation of administration. Avoid extravasation, tissue necrosis can result. If pain occurs reduce infusion rate and further dilute. **Continuous Infusion:** Total dose usually administered over 3–4 hr period. Not to exceed more than 15 mg/min. Do not exceed patient's cardiac reserve.

COMPATIBILITY

Solution: Dextrose solution, sodium chloride solutions.

INCOMPATIBILITY

Solution: 5% dextrose in alcohol.

ADVERSE EFFECTS

CNS: <u>Headache</u>, <u>numbness</u>, <u>transient circumoral paresthesia</u>. **CV:** Hypotension. **GI:** Abdominal cramps, anorexia, diarrhea, nausea, vomiting. **GU:** Glycosuria, nocturia, oliguria, polyuria, proteinuria, urinary urgency. **Renal:** Acute tubular necrosis, nephrotoxicity. **Derm:** Erythematous skin eruptions, exfo-

---

In the Adverse Effects section, <u>underline</u> indicates most frequent; CAPS indicates life threatening.

liative dermatitis. **Fld/Lytes:** Hypocalcemia. **Heme:** Anemia, hyperuricemia. **Other:** Fever, chills.

TOXICITY/OVERDOSE

Signs/Symptoms: Rapid infusion or high serum concentration of drug may cause a sudden decrease in serum calcium concentrations resulting in hypocalcemic tetany, seizures, severe cardiac dysrhythmias, and death from respiratory arrest. **Treatment:** Symptomatic/supportive, IV calcium salt (calcium gluconate) may be required as replacement therapy.

DRUG INTERACTIONS

Insulin: Concomitant use may result in lower requirements in insulin dependent diabetics.

NURSING CONSIDERATIONS

Assessment

General:

Vital signs, intake/output ratio, ECG monitoring (recommended), baseline/daily weight.

Physical:

Cardiopulmonary status, neurologic status, GI tract.

Lab Alterations:

Assess baseline electrolytes and trace metals prior to initiation of drug therapy, evaluate periodically throughout course of treatment. Serum calcium concentrations must be determined by atomic absorption spectrometry. Evaluate renal function (BUN/creatinine) periodically throughout therapy.

Intervention/Rationale

Monitor vital signs and ECG frequently before, during, and after therapy to observe for transient drop in systolic/diastolic blood pressure and changes in ECG. Keep patient in supine position after administration of drug for 15–30 minutes in order to avoid postural hypotensive effects of drug. ● Evaluate patient for development of CHF signs/symptoms (edema, weight gain, jugular venous distention, adventitious sounds, dyspnea). ● Assess for presence of numbness, tingling, and circumoral paresthesias.

Patient/Family Education

Insulin needs may be altered while receiving drug. Generalized systemic reaction may occur 4–8 hr after drug administration; symptoms include fever, chills, back pain, emesis, muscle cramps, and urinary urgency. Notify physician of symptom development. Symptoms usually disappear within 12 hr.

EDROPHONIUM

(ed-roe-fone′-ee-yum)

Trade Name(s): Enlon, Reversol, Tensilon, Enlon Plus (contains atropine)

Classification(s): Anticholinesterase, cholinergic muscle stimulant

Pregnancy Category: C

PHARMACODYNAMICS/KINETICS

Mechanism of Action: Inhibits destruction of acetylcholine released from both somatic efferent nerves and parasympathetic nerves. Acetylcholine accumulates and increases stimulation of myoneural receptors. Inhibits enzyme cholinesterase. **Onset of Action:** 30–60 sec. **Duration of Action:** 5–10 min. **Metabolism/Elimination:** Unknown.

In the Adverse Effects section, underline indicates most frequent; CAPS indicates life threatening.

195

INDICATIONS/DOSAGE

Curare antagonist, reversal of non-depolarizing neuromuscular blocker

Adult: 10 mg. Not to exceed 40 mg.

Diagnostic aid in myasthenia gravis

Adult: 1–2 mg within 15–30 sec. Followed by 8 mg if no response.

Pediatric: Initially 1 mg (< 34 kg) or 2 mg (> 34 kg). If no response may administer 1 mg every 30–45 sec to a total dose of 10 mg. Cholinergic response is treated with atropine.

Differentiation between myasthenic/cholinergic crisis

Adult: 1 mg. If no response in 1 min may repeat dosage. Increased muscle strength confirms myasthenic crisis. No increase in strength or exaggerated weakness confirms a cholinergic crisis.

Treatment of supraventricular tachycardia (*unlabeled use*)

Adult: 5–10 mg IV over 1 min. *Pediatric:* 2 mg over 1 min.

CONTRAINDICATIONS/PRECAUTIONS

Contraindicated in: Hypersensitivity, mechanical obstruction of the GI or GU tract. **Use cautiously in:** Cardiac dysrhythmias, epilepsy, history of asthma, hyperthyroidism, myasthenia gravis treated with anticholinesterase drugs, ulcer disease. **Pregnancy/Lactation:** No well-controlled trials to establish safety. Benefits must outweigh risks. May cause uterine irritability when ad

ministered near term.
Pediatrics: Newborns may display muscle weakness.

PREPARATION

Availability: 10 mg/mL, 1 mL amps and 10 mL, 15 mL vials. Enlon Plus 10 mg edrophonium and 0.14 mg atropine per mL, 5 mL and 15 mL vials. **IV Push:** May be given undiluted. **Infusion:** For myasthenic crisis, may be given as continuous IV infusion in physician specified volume of compatible IV solution.

STABILITY/STORAGE

Vial: Store at room temperature. **Infusion:** Stable for 24 hr at room temperature.

ADMINISTRATION

General: Assure patent airway prior to administration and before subsequent doses; carefully observe the effect of each dosage on the respiratory and cardiac state. **IV Push:** 2 mg or less over 15–30 sec. *Curare Antagonist:* Administer single dose over 30–45 sec. **Infusion:** Infuse as per physician specified rate.

COMPATIBILITY

Solution: Dextrose solutions, sodium chloride solutions. **Y-site:** Heparin, hydrocortisone, potassium chloride, vitamin B complex with C.

ADVERSE EFFECTS

CNS: Seizures. **Ophtho:** Diplopia, increased lacrimation, miosis. **CV:** Bradycardia, hypotension. **Resp:** Respiratory muscle paralysis, BRONCHOSPASM, excess secretions. **GI:** Abdominal cramps, diarrhea, dysphagia, excess salivation,

In the Adverse Effects section, underline indicates most frequent; CAPS indicates life threatening.

nausea, vomiting. **GU:** Urinary frequency. **MS:** Muscle cramps, muscle fasiculations. **Hypersens:** Rash. **Other:** Weakness, sweating.

TOXICITY/OVERDOSE

Signs/Symptoms: Overdose may cause cholinergic crisis characterized by nausea, vomiting, diarrhea, increased salivation, sweating, increased bronchial secretions, lacrimation, bradycardia or tachycardia, bronchospasm, hypotension. Death may result from cardiac arrest, respiratory paralysis, or pulmonary edema. **Treatment:** Discontinue drug immediately. Initiate supportive and resuscitative therapies. **Antidote(s):** 0.4–0.5 mg atropine sulfate IV every 3–10 min as needed. More than 2 mg is rarely needed. Pralidoxime chloride 50–100 mg/min up to a maximum of 1 g may be used as a cholinesterase reactivator.

DRUG INTERACTIONS

Anticholinergic drugs (including antihistamines, antidepressants, atropine, phenothiazines, and disopyramide): Antagonizes the effects of edrophonium. **Depolarizing muscle relaxants:** Prolongs muscle relaxant effects. **Digitalis:** Increases sensitivity to drug.

NURSING CONSIDERATIONS

Assessment

General:

Vital signs, continuous ECG monitoring (recommended), respiratory parameters.
Physical:

Pulmonary status, neurologic/neuromuscular status.

Intervention/Rationale

Monitor blood pressure, heart rate, and ECG prior to and throughout administration of drug to assess the development of supraventricular dysrhythmias and/or hypotension. Bradycardia may be noted if receiving digitalis preparations. ● Vital capacity should be measured during testing for myasthenia gravis. Assure patent airway prior to and during administration. Adequate facilities for CPR, cardiac monitoring, and endotracheal intubation should be available. ● All other cholinergic drugs should be stopped before receiving this drug if at all possible. ● Evaluate neurological/neuromuscular findings, particularly noting cranial nerve deficits, diplopia, dysphagia, and overall muscle strength/weakness of the extremities. Evaluate Glasgow coma score prior to and following drug therapy.

Patient/Family Education

Explain therapeutic/diagnostic effects of drug and reassure that physician/nurse will be present during administration. Effects of drug may last up to 30 min. Stress importance of the need for cooperation with vital capacity measurements.

EFLORNITHINE

(e-flor′-na-theen)
Trade Name(s): Ornidyl
Classification(s): Antiprotozoal agent
Pregnancy Category: C

In the Adverse Effects section, underline indicates most frequent;
CAPS indicates life threatening.

PHARMACODYNAMICS/KINETICS

Mechanism of Action: Inhibition of ornithine decarboxylase, an enzyme required for growth in protozoal organisms. **Distribution:** Distributed throughout the body tissues. Crosses the blood-brain barrier. **Metabolism/Elimination:** Primarily eliminated unchanged by the kidneys. **Half-Life:** 3 hr.

INDICATIONS/DOSAGE

Treatment of meningoencephalitic stage of *Trypanosoma brucei gambiense* infection (sleeping sickness).

Adult: 100 mg/kg every 6 hr for 14 days. Reduce dosage in renal impairment.

CONTRAINDICATIONS/ PRECAUTIONS

Use cautiously in: Bone marrow depression, history of seizures, renal impairment. **Pregnancy/Lactation:** No well-controlled trials to establish safety. Benefits must outweigh risks. **Pediatrics:** Safety and efficacy not established.

PREPARATION

Availability: 200 mg/mL, 100 mL vials. **Infusion:** Dilute each 25 mL of drug in 100 mL sterile water for injection.

STABILITY/STORAGE

Vial: Store at room temperature. Protect from light. **Infusion:** Stable for 24 hr at room temperature.

ADMINISTRATION

General: Hypertonic solution must be diluted prior to administration. Do not administer other drugs concomitantly. **Intermittent Infusion:** Infuse over at least 45 min (without interruption).

COMPATIBILITY

Solution: Sterile water for injection.

ADVERSE EFFECTS

CNS: <u>Seizures</u>, headache, asthenia, dizziness. **GI:** <u>diarrhea</u>, vomiting, anorexia, abdominal pain. **Derm:** Alopecia. **Heme:** <u>Anemia</u>, <u>leukopenia</u>, thrombocytopenia, eosinophilia. **Other:** <u>Hearing impairment</u>, facial edema.

TOXICITY/OVERDOSE

Signs/Symptoms: Seizures. **Treatment:** Symptomatic treatment.

NURSING CONSIDERATIONS

Assessment
Physical:
Hematopoietic system, neurologic status, GI tract.
Lab Alterations:
Monitor CBC with differential and platelets (evaluate throughout course of therapy).

Intervention/Rationale
Assess for development of infection and/or bleeding (bleeding gums, easy bruising, hematest positive stools/urine/vomitus). ● Avoid intramuscular injections or rectal temperatures.

Patient/Family Education
Educate regarding side effects and expected therapeutic effects of drug. Observe for signs of infection (fever, sore throat, fatigue) or bleeding (melena, hematuria, nosebleeds, easy bruising). Avoid over-the-counter products containing aspirin or ibuprofen due to increased

In the Adverse Effects section, <u>underline</u> indicates most frequent; CAPS indicates life threatening.

potential for bleeding. Report dizziness, unusual fatigue, or shortness of breath (drug may cause anemia). Notify physician/nurse if severe diarrhea occurs.

ENALAPRILAT
(e-nal'-a-pril-at)
Trade Name(s): Vasotec IV
Classification(s): Angiotensin converting enzyme (ACE) inhibitor, antihypertensive
Pregnancy Category: D

PHARMACODYNAMICS/KINETICS
Mechanism of Action: Angiotensin converting enzyme inhibitor that prevents conversion of angiotensin I to angiotensin II resulting in systemic vasodilation. **Onset of Action:** 15 min. **Peak Effect:** 1–4 hr. Peak effects of subsequent doses may be greater than that of the initial dose. **Duration of Action:** 6 hr. **Metabolism/ Elimination:** Eliminated via bile and urine. Removed by hemodialysis. **Half-Life:** 11 hr. Increased in renal impairment.

INDICATIONS/DOSAGE

Used alone or in combination with other drugs for the control/treatment of hypertension

Adult: Loading dose of 1.25 mg every 6 hr. IV and PO daily dose is the same. Clinical studies have not shown need for doses > 1.25 mg. Reduce loading dose to 0.625 mg for patients on diuretics with serum creatinine > 3 mg/dL or creatinine clearance < 30 mL/min. If dose is ineffective may be repeated in 1 hr.

Maintenance dose of 1.25 mg may be given every 6 hr. Decrease dose to 0.625 mg every 6 hr for hemodialysis patients.

CONTRAINDICATIONS/ PRECAUTIONS
Contraindicated in: Hypersensitivity to ACE inhibitors. **Use cautiously in:** Aortic stenosis, cerebrovascular disease, coronary insufficiency, elderly, patients receiving diuretics, renal impairment, surgical patients undergoing anesthesia or with agents that produce hypotension. **Pregnancy/Lactation:** Crosses placenta. Causes fetal/neonatal morbidity and mortality. First trimester effects unknown; oligohydramnios may occur in second/third trimester. Alternate therapy recommended. **Pediatrics:** Safety and efficacy not established.

PREPARATION
Availability: 1.25 mg/mL in 1 and 2 mL vials. **Infusion:** Dilute in up to 50 mL of compatible IV solution.

STABILITY/STORAGE
Vial: Store at room temperature. **Infusion:** Stable at room temperature for up to 24 hr.

ADMINISTRATION
General: Reduced dosage required for patients on diuretics, impaired renal function, or hemodialysis. **IV Push:** Give over at least 5 minutes. May be given through Y-site or three-way stopcock through an infusing IV solution. **Intermittent Infusion:** Administer at physician prescribed rate.

E

In the Adverse Effects section, underline indicates most frequent;
CAPS indicates life threatening.

E

COMPATIBILITY

Solution: Dextrose solutions, lactated Ringer's, sodium chloride solutions. **Y-site:** Amikacin, aminophylline, ampicillin, ampicillin-sulbactam, aztreonam, butorphanol, calcium gluconate, cefazolin, cefoperazone, ceftazidime, ceftizoxime, chloramphenicol, cimetidine, clindamycin, dobutamine, dopamine, erythromycin lactobionate, esmolol, famotidine, fentanyl, gentamicin, heparin, hydrocortisone, labetalol, lidocaine, magnesium sulfate, methylprednisolone, metronidazole, morphine, nafcillin, nicardipine, penicillin G potassium, piperacillin, potassium chloride, potassium phosphate, ranitidine, sodium acetate, sodium nitroprusside, tobramycin, trimethoprim-sulfamethoxazole, vancomycin.

ADVERSE EFFECTS

CNS: <u>Dizziness</u>, <u>fatigue</u>, <u>headache</u>, insomnia, paresthesias. **CV:** ANGIOEDEMA, <u>hypotension</u>, angina, palpitations, tachycardia. **Resp:** Cough, dyspnea. **GI:** Anorexia, diarrhea, nausea. **GU:** Impotence. **MS:** Muscle cramps. **Fld/Lytes:** Hyperkalemia. **Heme:** <u>AGRANULOCYTOSIS</u>, neutropenia. **Hypersens:** Pruritus, rash.

TOXICITY/OVERDOSE

Signs/Symptoms: Angioedema (laryngeal edema, swelling of the face, eyes, lips, tongue). **Treatment:** Discontinue drug, and notify physician immediately. Use epinephrine immediately for angioedema. Support patient as required.

DRUG INTERACTIONS

Allopurinol: Increased frequency of various hypersensitivity reactions. **Antihypertensive agents:** Cause renin release; augment the effect of enalaprilat. **Diuretics:** Cause a precipitous fall in blood pressure within the first hour after administering initial dose. **Probenecid, potassium sparing diuretics, potassium supplements:** Increased serum potassium.

NURSING CONSIDERATIONS

Assessment

General:

Vital signs, hemodynamic monitoring (recommended), intake/output ratio, baseline/daily weight.

Physical:

Cardiopulmonary status.

Lab Alterations:

Assess electrolytes prior to and periodically throughout therapy.

Intervention/Rationale

Monitor blood pressure and heart rate frequently during initial dosage adjustment (may cause significant decrease in blood pressure following initial dose). ● Peripheral arterial resistance decreases in patients with hypertension. ● CHF patients may become hypotensive at any point in time; monitor hemodynamics carefully and at least hourly during initial and subsequent doses. ● Diuretics given concomitantly may cause significant decrease in blood pressure within the first hour of the initial dose; monitor closely. ● Anaphylactoid reactions may occur with polyacrylonitrile (PAN) dialyzers (discontinue dialysis immediately).

In the Adverse Effects section, <u>underline</u> indicates most frequent; CAPS indicates life threatening.

Patient/Family Education

Review hypertensive disease state and present therapy. Review potential adverse reactions. May cause drowsiness, especially during first days of therapy or when dose is increased. Seek assistance with ambulatory activities. Avoid salt substitutes or foods containing high levels of sodium or potassium unless specifically instructed by physician/nurse.

EPHEDRINE

(e-fed'-drin)

Classification(s): Alpha/beta adrenergic agonist, bronchodilator, vasopressor

Pregnancy Category: C

PHARMACODYNAMICS/KINETICS

Mechanism of Action: Stimulates both alpha- and beta-adrenergic receptors causing smooth muscle relaxation of bronchial tree. If norepinephrine stores are not depleted causes cardiac stimulation and increased systolic and usually diastolic blood pressure. **Duration of Action:** 1 hr. **Distribution:** Widely distributed throughout body fluids. Crosses blood–brain barrier. **Metabolism/Elimination:** Metabolized slowly by liver. Excreted by the kidneys. **Half-Life:** 3–6 hr depending on urine pH (3 hr if pH acidic).

INDICATIONS/DOSAGE

Management of acute hypotension and bradycardia associated with overdosage of antihypertensive agents

Adults: 10–25 mg. Additional doses may be given in 5–10 min, not to exceed 150 mg/24 hr.

Pediatric: 3 mg/kg/24 hr or 25–100 mg/m^2/24 hr in four to six divided doses.

CONTRAINDICATIONS/PRECAUTIONS

Contraindicated in: Cyclopropane or halothane anesthesia, diabetes, hypersensitivity, hypertension, narrow angle-closure glaucoma, severe cardiovascular disease, thyrotoxicosis. **Use cautiously in:** Cardiovascular disease including coronary insufficiency, angina, cardiac dysrhythmias, and organic heart disease; elderly males (with enlarged prostates); hyperthyroidism. **Pregnancy/Lactation:** No well-controlled trials to establish safety. Benefits must outweigh risks. If given during spinal anesthesia can cause acceleration of fetal heart rate and should not be used in patients when maternal systolic/diastolic blood pressure > 130/80.

PREPARATION

Availability: 25 mg/mL and 50 mg/mL in 1 mL ampules and 10 mL bristojects. **Syringe:** May be given undiluted.

STABILITY/STORAGE

Vial: Store at room temperature. Gradually decomposes and darkens on exposure to light. Should be stored in light resistant containers and not be exposed to excessive heat.

ADMINISTRATION

General: IV route should be used only if immediate effect is required. **IV Push:** Administer 10 mg over at

In the Adverse Effects section, underline indicates most frequent; CAPS indicates life threatening.

201

least 1 min. May be injected via Y-site or three-way stopcock of infusing IV solution.

COMPATIBILITY
Solution: Dextrose solutions, lactated Ringer's, sodium chloride solutions.

INCOMPATIBILITY
Syringe: Thiopental.

ADVERSE EFFECTS
CNS: <u>Insomnia</u>, <u>nervousness</u>, dizziness, headache, paranoid state (long-term use), vertigo. **Ophtho:** Dilated pupils. **CV:** Dysrhythmias, tachycardia, angina, hypertension, palpitations. **Resp:** Dyspnea, shortness of breath. **GI:** Anorexia, dryness of nose and throat, mild epigastric distress, nausea, vomiting. **GU:** Painful urination due to sphincter spasm, urinary retention. **Renal:** Constriction of renal blood vessels, decreased urine formation. **MS:** Muscle weakness. **Other:** Rapid development of tolerance (tachyphylaxis), sweating.

TOXICITY/OVERDOSE
Signs/Symptoms: Confusion, delirium, euphoria, hallucinations (high doses); convulsions, pulmonary edema, respiratory failure, or arrest may occur with overdose. **Treatment:** Notify physician and discontinue drug. Treat hypotension with fluid resuscitation. Vasopressors are contraindicated. Treat hypertension with phentolamine. Convulsions may be treated with diazepam. Treat dysrhythmias with beta blockers.

DRUG INTERACTIONS
Halogenated anesthetics: Sensitize the myocardium to the effects of catecholamines and precipitate dysrhythmic effects. **MAO inhibitors:** Increase pressor response and pontentiate hypertensive crises and intracranial hemorrhage. **Oxytocic drug (obstetrics):** Concomitant use may cause severe hypertensive state. **Tricyclic antidepressants:** Decrease pressor response resulting in higher dose requirement.

NURSING CONSIDERATIONS
Assessment
General:
Vital signs, ECG monitoring (recommended), hemodynamic monitoring (recommended), intake/output ratio, hydration status.
Physical:
Cardiopulmonary status, neurologic status.
Lab Alterations:
Electrolytes, ABG analysis for hypoxia, hypercapnia, acidosis determination.

Intervention/Rationale
Monitor blood pressure, heart rate, ECG, and respiratory rate and pattern during administration. ● Prolonged use may cause an anxiety state response. To prevent insomnia, avoid administration, if possible, within 2 hr of bedtime. ● Hypoxia, hypercapnia, acidosis may decrease the effectiveness of the drug or increase the incidence of adverse effects and must be assessed and treated prior to or during administration. ● Not a substitute for blood or fluid volume deficit. Preload should be increased before vasopressor therapy is initiated.

In the Adverse Effects section, <u>underline</u> indicates most frequent; CAPS indicates life threatening.

Patient/Family Education
Contact physician/nurse immediately if shortness of breath is not relieved by medication or is accompanied by diaphoresis, palpitations, or angina. Drug may produce nervous, excitable state. Seek assistance when engaging in ambulatory activities as drug can cause dizziness or lightheadedness.

EPINEPHRINE
(ep-i-nef′-rin)
Trade Name(s): Adrenalin
Classification(s):
Bronchodilator, cardiac stimulant, sympathomimetic
Pregnancy Category: C

PHARMACODYNAMICS/KINETICS
Mechanism of Action: Acts directly on alpha and beta adrenergic receptors of tissues innervated by sympathetic nervous system (in usual doses). Acts primarily on beta receptors of heart, vascular, and smooth muscle. Exhibits predominantly alpha effects in higher doses. Main therapeutic effects are bronchial smooth muscle relaxation, cardiac stimulation, and skeletal vasculature dilation. **Onset of Action:** Rapid. **Duration of Action:** Short. **Distribution:** Does not cross blood–brain barrier. Drug becomes fixed in tissues. **Metabolism/Elimination:** Rapidly inactivated by hepatic enzymes to metanephrine or normetanephrine. Conjugated/glucuronidated in the liver. Metabolites are eliminated by the kidneys.

INDICATIONS/DOSAGE

Advanced life support during cardiopulmonary resuscitation
Adult: 0.1–1.0 mg IV push, usually as 1–10 mL of a 1:10,000 injection. Repeat every 5 minutes as needed. Alternate dose 1–4 mcg/min. 1 mg (10 mL of a 1:10,000 solution) may be given tracheobronchially if no IV access is available. 0.1–1.0 mg (1–10 mL of a 1:10,000 injection) may be given by intracardiac injection only if other administration routes are persistently unavailable.
Pediatric: 0.01 mg/kg IV push (0.1 mL/kg of a 1:10,000 injection). Repeat every 5 min as needed. Alternate dose 0.1 mcg/min. May be increased in 0.1 mcg/min increments to a maximum of 1 mcg/min. Tracheobronchial dose is the same as IV dose. Intracardiac dose 0.005–0.01 mg/kg (0.05–0.1 mL/kg of a 1:10,000 injection).
Neonate: 0.01–0.03 mg/kg IV push (0.1–0.3 mL/kg of a 1:10,000 injection).

Vasopressor
Adult: 1–4 mcg/min. *Pediatric:* 0.1 mcg/min. May be increased by 0.1 mcg/min increments to a maximum of 1 mcg/min.

Severe anaphylaxis or asthma
Adult: 0.1–0.25 mg (1.0–2.5 mL of 1:10,000 injection) slowly over 5–10 min. Repeat every 5–15 minutes as necessary. May be followed by an infusion at 1–4 mcg/min. *Pediatric:* 0.1 mg over 5–10 min (10 mL of 1:1000 injection). May be followed by an infusion at initial

In the Adverse Effects section, <u>underline</u> indicates most frequent;
CAPS indicates life threatening.

203

rate of 0.1 mcg/kg/min. Increase to maximum of 1.5 mcg/kg/min.

CONTRAINDICATIONS/ PRECAUTIONS

Contraindicated in: Angle-closure glaucoma, cerebral arteriosclerosis, general anesthesia with chloroform, trichloroethylene, or cyclopropane, hypersensitivity to sympathomimetic amines or drug components, local anesthesia of fingers or toes, organic brain damage. **Use cautiously in:** Cardiovascular disease, diabetes mellitus, elderly, halogenated hydrocarbon anesthetics, long-standing bronchial asthma/emphysema with concurrent degenerative heart disease, psychoneurotic disorders. **Pregnancy/Lactation:** No well-controlled trials to establish safety. Crosses the placenta. May cause anoxia to fetus. Benefits must outweigh risks. Distributed into breast milk; potential for serious neonatal side effects. **Pediatrics:** Use cautiously in infants and children. Use special caution in asthmatic children to avoid snycope.

PREPARATION

Availability: 1 mg/mL (1:1000 solution) in 1 and 30 mL amps/vials and 1 and 2 mL syringes. 0.1 mg/mL (1:10,000 solution) in 3, 5, and 10 mL syringes/bristojects. **Infusion:** Dilute 1–2 mg (1:1000) in compatible IV solution.

STABILITY/STORAGE

Vial: Store at room temperature. Protect from light, extreme heat, and freezing. Do not use if solution is brown or contains a precipitate. **Infusion:** Stable for 24 hr at room temperature.

ADMINISTRATION

IV Push: Give rapidly. **Continuous Infusion:** Give via infusion device. **Tracheobronchial Instillation:** This route may be used in an emergency situation when IV access has not been established. Dose may be diluted in 10 mL normal saline to aid delivery. **Intracardiac:** Well-trained personnel may use this route only when other routes are unavailable. Dose must be followed by external cardiac massage to ensure entry of drug into coronary circulation.

COMPATIBILITY

Solution: Dextrose solutions, lactated Ringer's, Ringer's injection, sodium chloride solutions. **Syringe:** Doxapram, heparin. **Y-site:** Amrinone, atracurium, calcium chloride, calcium gluconate, famotidine, heparin, hydrocortisone, pancuronium, phytonadione, potassium chloride, vecuronium, vitamin B complex with C.

INCOMPATIBILITY

Solution: Sodium bicarbonate 5%. **Y-site:** Ampicillin.

ADVERSE EFFECTS

CNS: CEREBRAL HEMORRHAGE, SUBARACHNOID HEMORRHAGE, dizziness, anxiety, headache, restlessness, hemiplegia, fear, syncope (children). **CV:** Dysrhythmias, hypertension, palpitations, angina. **GI:** Nausea, vomiting. **Endo:** Transient blood glucose elevation. **Hypersens:** Urticaria, wheal. **Metab:** Elevated serum lactate levels with SEVERE METABOLIC ACIDOSIS (prolonged use or overdose).

TOXICITY/OVERDOSE

Signs/Symptoms: Unusually elevated blood pressure (may result in cere-

In the Adverse Effects section, underline indicates most frequent; CAPS indicates life threatening.

brovascular hemorrhage, especially in elderly), precordial distress, vomiting, headache, dyspnea, pallor, cold skin, metabolic acidosis, kidney failure, severe peripheral vasoconstriction, cardiac stimulation resulting in pulmonary arterial hypertension or fatal pulmonary edema, ventricular hyperirritability, cardiac dysrhythmias (especially ventricular premature contractions/ventricular tachycardia), ventricular fibrillation, transient bradycardia followed by tachycardia. **Treatment:** Counteract toxic effect with injection of alpha- and beta-adrenergic blockers. Counter marked pressor effects with rapid acting vasodilators (nitrates) or alpha-adrenergic blockers. Treatment may result in prolonged hypotension—treat with another pressor drug, such as norepinephrine. Treat pulmonary edema interfering with respiration with rapid acting alpha-adrenergic agent (i.e., phentolamine) or positive pressure ventilation. Treat cardiac dysrhythmias with beta-adrenergic blockers (i.e., propranolol).

DRUG INTERACTIONS
Beta-adrenergic blockers: Hypertension with concomitant use. **Bretylium:** Possible enhanced action on adrenergic receptors leading to dysrhythmias. **Guanethidine:** Increased pressor effect and severe hypertension. **Halogenated hydrocarbon anesthetics:** Dysrhythmias resulting from catecholamine sensitization of myocardium. **Oxytocic drugs:** Severe persistent hypertension. **Tricyclic antidepressants:** Potentiated pressor response.

NURSING CONSIDERATIONS
Assessmen
General:
Blood pressure (continuous during first 5 minutes, then every 3–5 min until stabilized), continuous ECG, respiratory rate, signs/symptoms of hypersensitivity.
Physical:
Cardiopulmonary status.
Lab Alterations:
Monitor serum glucose/lactate levels.

Intervention/Rationale
Assess lung sounds before, during, and after treatment when drug given as bronchodilator. ● Transient elevations of serum glucose/lactate may occur due to sympathomimetic action.

Patient/Family Education
Notify physician/nurse of increased heart rate, irregular pulse, or chest pain.

EPOETIN ALFA (ERYTHROPOIETIN)
(e-poe′-i-tin al′-fa)
Trade Name(s): Epogen, Procrit
Classification(s): Hormone-recombinant human erythropoietin
Pregnancy Category: C

PHARMACODYNAMICS/KINETICS
Mechanism of Action: A glycoprotein that stimulates red blood cell production. Has the same biological effects as endogenous erythropoi-

In the Adverse Effects section, underline indicates most frequent; CAPS indicates life threatening.

205

etin. **Onset of Action:** 10 days (increased reticulocytes). **Peak Effect:** 2–6 weeks (RBC, hemoglobin/hematocrit increase). **Metabolism/Elimination:** Unknown. **Half-Life:** Chronic renal failure 4–13 hr.

INDICATIONS/DOSAGE

Treatment of anemia associated with chronic renal failure

Adult: Initial dose 50–100 units/kg three times weekly. Maintenance dose for dialysis patients 75 units/kg three times weekly. Nondialysis patients 75–150 units/kg per week. Dose is adjusted based on hematocrit. Individualize maintenance dose once hematocrit is within target range (target hematocrit range 30%–33%). Decrease dosage by approximately 25 units/kg three times weekly to avoid exceeding target range. Allow 2–6 weeks for stabilization of response (first evidence of response to drug is increased reticulocyte count within 10 days, followed by increases in red cell count, hemoglobin/hematocrit).

Treatment of anemia in AZT-treated HIV-infected patients

Adult: Initial dose 100 units/kg three times weekly. May increase by 50–100 units/kg three times weekly after 8 weeks. Maintenance dose based on desired patient response/hematocrit.

CONTRAINDICATIONS/ PRECAUTIONS

Contraindicated in: Uncontrolled hypertension, sensitivity to human albumin or mammalian cell-derived products. **Use cautiously in:** Known porphyria (rare exacerbation has been observed but drug has not caused urinary excretion of porphyrin metabolites in normal volunteers). **Pregnancy/Lactation:** No well-controlled trials to establish safety. Benefits must outweigh risks. **Pediatrics:** Safety and efficacy not established in children.

PREPARATION

Availability: 2000, 3000, 4000, and 10,000 units/1 mL single dose vials.

STABILITY/STORAGE

Vial: Refrigerate.

ADMINISTRATION

General: Do not shake vial (may render drug inactive). Do not administer in conjunction with other drug solutions. May be given into the venous line at the end of dialysis. **IV Push:** May be given by direct IV push (SC route preferred for patients not receiving dialysis).

ADVERSE EFFECTS

CNS: Seizures (too rapid hematocrit rise, > 4 percent increase in a 2 week period), headache. **CV:** Clotted vascular access, hypertension, tachycardia. **Resp:** Shortness of breath. **GI:** Diarrhea, nausea, vomiting. **Endo:** Resumption of menses. **Fld/Lytes:** Hyperkalemia. **Hypersens:** Skin rash, urticaria.

TOXICITY/OVERDOSE

Signs/Symptoms: Polycythemia develops if hematocrit is not closely monitored. Maximum amount for safe administration not established. Doses of up to 1500 units/kg three times weekly for 3–4 weeks have been given without any direct toxic effects. **Treatment:** Temporarily with-

In the Adverse Effects section, <u>underline</u> indicates most frequent; CAPS indicates life threatening.

hold drug until hematocrit returns to target range. Phlebotomy may be necessary if polycythemia problematic.

NURSING CONSIDERATIONS
Assessment
General:
Blood pressure, intake/output ratio, daily weight.
Physical:
Neurologic status.
Lab Alterations:
Monitor reticulocyte count, CBC with differential, and platelet count regularly. Closely monitor renal function (BUN, creatinine, uric acid, phosphorus). Iron stores (transferrin, serum ferritin) should be evaluated prior to and during therapy.

Intervention/Rationale
Carefully monitor and aggressively control blood pressure throughout course of treatment. ● Too rapid increase in hematocrit (> 4 points in any 2 week period) may exacerbate hypertension or cause seizures. Monitor closely for presence of neurologic symptoms. ● Hemodialysis patients may require increased anticoagulation to prevent clotting of access graft/shunt or artificial kidney. ● Patient may require supplemental iron.

Patient/Family Education
Encourage compliance with dietary restrictions (erythropoietin therapy may result in an increased sense of well-being, however, underlying disease is still present). Avoid driving or other potentially hazardous activities such as operating heavy machinery during treatment period until tolerance is ascertained (increased seizure risk). Report signs/symptoms of hypertension to physician (headache, dizziness, fatigue). Discuss need for compliance with possible antihypertensive therapy. Patients receiving supplemental iron may normally have black stools. Inform patients with return of menses to discuss contraception option with physician.

ERGONOVINE
(er-goe-noe'-veen)
Trade Name(s): Ergotrate
Classification(s): Oxytocic
Pregnancy Category: Unknown

PHARMACODYNAMICS/KINETICS
Mechanism of Action: Directly stimulates contraction of uterine and smooth muscle. Increases amplitude and frequency of uterine contractions and tone, which impedes uterine blood flow. **Onset of Action:** 40 sec. **Duration of Action:** 45 min. **Distribution:** Distributes rapidly into plasma, extracellular fluid, and tissues. **Metabolism/Elimination:** Primarily metabolized in liver. Excreted in feces. Small amount excreted in urine. Elimination may be prolonged in neonates. **Half-Life:** 0.5–2.0 hr.

INDICATIONS/DOSAGE

Prevention and treatment of postpartum and postabortal hemorrhage due to uterine atony or subinvolution

---

In the Adverse Effects section, <u>underline</u> indicates most frequent; CAPS indicates life threatening.

207

Adult: Initial dose 0.2 mg. May repeat every 2–4 hr for a maximum of five doses.

Diagnostic use to identify variant angina (Prinzmetal's angina) (*unlabeled use*)

Adult: 0.05–0.2 mg IV during coronary angiography.

CONTRAINDICATIONS/ PRECAUTIONS

Contraindicated in: Known hypersensitivity or idiosyncratic reactions, induction of labor, threatened spontaneous abortion, obstetrical patient prior to placental delivery. **Use cautiously in:** Coronary artery disease, essential hypertension, heart disease, hypocalcemia, mitral valve stenosis, occlusive peripheral vascular disease, pregnancy-induced hypertension, renal or hepatic impairment, sepsis, toxemia of pregnancy, venoatrial shunts. **Pregnancy/Lactation:** No well-controlled trials to establish safety. Benefits must outweigh risks. Should not be administered prior to delivery of placenta (captivation of placenta may occur). High doses given prior to delivery may cause problems in infant (hypoxia, intracranial hemorrhage). Distributed into breast milk. May cause ergotism in infant.

PREPARATION
Availability: 1 mL ampules.

STABILITY/STORAGE
Vial: Refrigerate. Intact ampules stable for 60–90 days at room temperature. Protect from light and freezing.

ADMINISTRATION
General: Not for long-term or chronic use. IV use limited to patients with severe uterine bleeding or other emergent conditions. Use recommended in pregnancy only when surgical and intensive care facilities are immediately available. **Diagnostic Use:** Provokes spontaneous coronary artery spasms that result in Prinzmetal's angina. Effects reversible with nitroglycerine. May precipitate dysrhythmias, ventricular tachycardia, or MI. **IV Push:** Give slowly over 1 minute. May be diluted to a 5 mL volume with normal saline before injection.

COMPATIBILITY
Solution: Sodium chloride solutions.

ADVERSE EFFECTS
CNS: Headache. **CV:** Extreme blood pressure elevation, myocardial infarction (rare). **GI:** Nausea, vomiting (rare, with overdose).

DRUG INTERACTIONS

Vasoconstrictors, vasopressors, other ergot alkaloids, heavy tobacco smoking:

Enhanced vasoconstriction.

TOXICITY/OVERDOSE
Signs/Symptoms: *Acute Ergotism:* Convulsions, nausea, vomiting, diarrhea, hyper/hypotension, dyspnea, weak pulse, numb/cold extremities, tingling, chest pain, gangrene of fingers and toes, hypercoagulability, loss of consciousness, confusion, excitement, delirium, hallucinations, coma. **Chronic Ergotism:** Gangrene. **Treatment:** Support airway and hemodynamic status with conventional methods. Treat sei-

In the Adverse Effects section, <u>underline</u> indicates most frequent; CAPS indicates life threatening.

zures with conventional methods. Control hypercoagulability with heparin and maintain blood clotting times three times normal. Nitroglycerin is helpful in treating chest pain secondary to coronary vasospasm. Gangrene may require surgical intervention. **Antidote:** Vasodilators.

NURSING CONSIDERATIONS

Assessment
General:
Vital signs, uterine response, ECG (when used for variant angina diagnosis).
Physical:
Uterine findings.

Intervention/Rationale
Report sudden vital sign changes, observe and record character of vaginal bleeding, report frequent periods of uterine relaxation.

Patient/Family Education
Strong uterine cramping may be experienced.

ERYTHROMYCIN
(eh-rith-roe-mye'-sin)
Trade Name(s): Erythrocin
Classification(s): Antibacterial
Pregnancy Category: B

PHARMACODYNAMICS/KINETICS
Mechanism of Action: Bactericidal or bacteriostatic agent that binds to ribosomal subunit of susceptible bacteria. Suppresses bacterial protein synthesis. **Onset of Action:** Rapid. **Peak Serum Level:** Immedi-

ately after infusion. **Distribution:** 70% protein bound. Widely distributed into most body tissues. Low concentrations (2%–13% of serum concentration) found in spinal fluid. Crosses blood–brain barrier. **Metabolism/Elimination:** Concentrated in the liver and bile with normal hepatic function. Mainly excreted unchanged in bile. 12%–15% excreted in active form in the urine. Not removed by peritoneal or hemodialysis. **Half-Life:** 1.5–2.0 hr. Anuria: 6 hr.

INDICATIONS/DOSAGE

Treatment of various infections due to susceptible organisms
(including: upper/lower respiratory infections, pneumonia, Legionnaires' disease, gonorrhea, chlamydia, genitourinary infections, skin and soft tissue infections). Diphtheria (as adjunct to diphtheria antitoxin).

Adult: 250–500 mg every 6 hr up to a maximum dose of 4–6 g daily.

Pediatric: 3.75–5.0 mg/kg of body weight every 6 hr.

CONTRAINDICATIONS/ PRECAUTIONS
Contraindicated in: Hypersensitivity. **Use cautiously in:** Impaired hepatic function. **Pregnancy/Lactation:** No well-controlled trials to establish safety. No evidence of fetal harm in animal studies. Benefits must outweigh risks. Excreted in breast milk with no infant adverse effects reported. May modify infant's bowel flora or interfere with fever work-up.

In the Adverse Effects section, <u>underline</u> indicates most frequent; CAPS indicates life threatening.

PREPARATION

Availability: 500, and 1000 mg vials.
Reconstitution: *Syringe:* Add at least 10 mL diluent to each 500 mg vial. Use only sterile water for injection without preservative. Do not use sodium chloride in the initial reconstitution. **Intermittent Infusion:** Dilute 500 mg in 100 mL or 1 g in 250 mL compatible. **Continuous Infusion:** May be further diluted to a final concentation of 1 g/L in compatible IV solution.

STABILITY/STORAGE

Vial: Store at room temperature. Stable after reconstitution for 7 days refrigerated. **Infusion:** Stable for 8 hr at room temperature or 24 hr refrigerated.

ADMINISTRATION

General: Not to be given IV push. **Intermittent Infusion:** Infuse over 20–60 minutes. **Continuous Infusion:** Infuse over physician specified time.

COMPATIBILITY:

Solution: Sodium chloride solutions. **Syringe:** Methicillin. **Y-site:** Acylovir, cyclophosphamide, enalaprilat, esmolol, famotidine, foscarnet, hydromorphone, labetalol, magnesium sulfate, meperidine, morphine, multivitamin, perphenazine, vitamin B complex with C, zidovudine.

INCOMPATIBILITY:

Solution: Dextrose solutions, Ringer's injection. **Syringe:** Ampicillin, heparin.

ADVERSE EFFECTS

GI: Nausea, vomiting, altered liver function (high doses or prolonged therapy), diarrhea, pseudomembranous colitis. **Hypersens:** ANAPHYLAXIS, mild allergic reactions (rash, urticaria, bullous fixed eruption, eczema). **Other:** Local venous irritation, reversible ototoxicity (renal impairment, high doses > 4 g/day), superinfection.

DRUG INTERACTIONS

Carbamazepine: Increased carbamazepine toxic effect. **Cyclosporine:** Increased cyclosporine toxic effects (inhibited cyclosporine clearance). **Digoxin:** Increased digoxin therapeutic and toxic effects (increased bioavailability of digoxin). **Methylprednisolone:** Increased methylprednisolone effects. **Penicillin:** Increased antimicrobial effectiveness with coadministration. **Sulfonamide:** Synergy against *Hemophilus influenzae*. **Theophylline:** Increased pharmacologic or toxic effects. **Warfarin:** Increased warfarin effects (reduce anticoagulant dose).

NURSING CONSIDERATIONS

Assessment
General:
Infectious disease status.
Physical:
GI tract.
Lab Alterations:
False elevations of urinary catecholamines.

Intervention/Rationale
Obtain specimens for culture and organism susceptibility prior to administration (first dose may be given while awaiting results). ● Drug may cause diarrhea, nausea, vomiting, or pseudomembranous colitis. Report frequent, loose, foul-smelling stools to physician.

In the Adverse Effects section, underline indicates most frequent; CAPS indicates life threatening.

Patient/Family Education

Complete entire course of therapy. Drug may cause nausea, vomiting, and diarrhea. Notify physician if severe abdominal pain, yellow discoloration of the skin or eyes, darkened urine, pale stools, or unusual tiredness occurs. Educate about signs/symptoms of superinfection.

ESMOLOL

(ez'-moe-lole)
Trade Name(s): Brevibloc
Classification(s): Beta-adrenergic blocker (beta$_1$ selective)
Pregnancy Category: C

PHARMACODYNAMICS/KINETICS

Mechanism of Action: Short-acting beta$_1$-selective adrenergic agent blocks cardiac beta$_1$-adrenergic receptors. Has little effect on beta$_2$-adrenergic receptors of bronchial muscle and vascular smooth muscle. Selectivity for beta$_1$ receptors decreases at high doses (> 300 mcg/kg/min). Clinical effects include slowing of sinus rate, decreased AV conduction, decreased cardiac output, and systolic and diastolic BP reduction. **Onset of Action:** Rapid. **Peak Effect:** 10–30 min. **Duration of Action:** Rapid decline following discontinuation. **Distribution:** Rapidly and widely distributed. Approximately 55% bound to plasma proteins. Minimal distribution into the CNS. **Metabolism/Elimination:** Rapidly and extensively metabolized via esterases in the cytosol of erythrocytes. Deesterified metabolite excreted principally by the kidneys. **Half-Life:** 9 min.

INDICATIONS/DOSAGE

Short-term treatment of supraventricular tachycardia and control of rapid ventricular rate in patients with atrial fibrillation or atrial flutter

Adult: Loading dose 500 mcg/kg/min over 1 min followed by a maintenance infusion of 50 mcg/kg/min for 4 min. If adequate therapeutic response is not observed within 5 minutes, repeat loading dose over 1 min (500 mcg/kg/min) and increase maintenance infusion to 100 mcg/kg/min until maximum of 200 mcg/kg/min is reached. When desired heart rate or safety endpoint is reached (lowered BP), omit the loading infusion and reduce maintenance infusion in increments of 25 mcg/kg/min. Adjust dose according to patient tolerance and response (indicated by heart rate and BP).

Controlled hypotension during anesthesia to reduce bleeding from surgical procedures (*unlabeled use*)

Adult: Titrate to level necessary to maintain required BP reduction or to a maximum of 300 mcg/kg/min.

CONTRAINDICATIONS/PRECAUTIONS

Contraindicated in: Known hypersensitivity, sinus bradycardia, greater than first degree heart block, cardiogenic shock, CHF (unless secondary to a tachydysrhythmia treatable with beta-blockers), overt cardiac failure. **Use cautiously in:** Hypertensive patients with CHF controlled with digitalis and beta-blockers, peripheral vascular disease, bronchospastic disease, dia-

In the Adverse Effects section, <u>underline</u> indicates most frequent; CAPS indicates life threatening.

211

betes mellitus, hypoglycemia, renal impairment. **Pregnancy/Lactation:** No well-controlled trials to establish safety. Benefits must outweigh risks. **Pediatrics:** Safety and efficacy in children not established.

PREPARATION

Availability: 10 mg/mL and 250 mg/mL in 10 mL amps/vials.

STABILITY/STORAGE

Vial: Store at room temperature. **Infusion:** Diluted solution stable for 24 hr at room temperature.

ADMINISTRATION

General: Must be diluted prior to administration. Administer via infusion device. Do not use butterfly needle to administer. Concentrations > 10 mg/mL may cause burning, swelling, and skin discoloration at injection site. **Intermittent Infusion:** Dilute to final concentration of 10 mg/mL by removing 20 mL from a 500 mL bag of compatible IV solution and adding 5 g (20 mL).

COMPATIBILITY

Solution: Dextrose solutions, lactated Ringer's, sodium chloride solutions. **Y-site:** Amikacin, aminophylline, ampicillin, atracurium, butorphanol, calcium chloride, cefazolin, cefoperazone, ceftazidime, ceftizoxime, chloramphenicol, cimetidine, clindamycin, dopamine, enalaprilat, erythromycin, famotidine, fentanyl, gentamicin, heparin, hydrocortisone, magnesium sulfate, methyldopa, metronidazole, morphine, nafcillin, pancuronium, penicillin G potassium, phenytoin, piperacillin, polymyxin, potassium chloride, potassium phosphate, ranitidine, sodium acetate, streptomycin, tobramycin, trimethoprim, vancomycin, vecuronium.

INCOMPATIBILITY

Y-site: Furosemide.

ADVERSE EFFECTS

CNS: Agitation, confusion, dizziness, somnolence, syncope, headache. **Ophtho:** Visual disturbances. **CV:** Bradycardia, chest pain, heart block, <u>hypotension</u> (reversed in 30 minutes after drug discontinued or dose reduced), increased pulmonary pressures, peripheral ischemia, premature ventricular contractions, pulmonary edema, transient ST segment changes on ECG. **Resp:** Bronochoconstriction, wheezing. **GI:** <u>Nausea</u>, vomiting. **GU:** Urinary retention. **Hypersens:** Rash. **Other:** Diaphoresis, flushing, local skin necrosis (extravasation), inflammation/induration of injection site, thrombophlebitis.

TOXICITY/OVERDOSE

Signs/Symptoms: Limited information available on acute toxicity. Toxic effects are extensions of pharmacologic effects (hypotension, symptomatic bradycardia, advanced AV block, intraventricular conduction defects, acute cardiac failure, seizures, bronchospasm, hypoglycemia). **Treatment:** Discontinue infusion. Treat symptomatic bradycardia with atropine and/or isoproterenol. Treat cardiac failure with diuretics and/or cardiac glycoside. Manage symptomatic hypotension with fluids or pressor agents. Treat bronchospasm with beta-adrenergic agonist and/or theophylline derivative. Myocardial depression and hypotension may also be managed with IV glucagon.

DRUG INTERACTIONS

Digoxin: Increased serum digoxin levels. **Catecholamine-depleting drugs (i.e., reserpine):** Additive catecholamine effects. **Morphine:** Increased blood esmolol concentrations. **Neuromuscular blocking agents:** Prolonged neuromuscular blockade.

NURSING CONSIDERATIONS

Assessment
General:
Continuous ECG, BP, and heart rate.
Physical:
Cardiopulmonary status.
Lab Alterations:
Monitor blood glucose (especially in diabetics).

Intervention/Rationale
Incidence of hypotension is greatest in first 30 minutes of infusion. Reduce or discontinue drug at first sign of impending cardiac failure. Infusion can be restarted if needed at lower rate after successful treatment of cardiac failure. ● May mask signs/symptoms of hypoglycemia and may potentiate insulin-induced hypoglycemia. Monitor blood sugars closely in diabetic patients. ● Exacerbation of angina or precipitation of MI may occur if drug is abruptly withdrawn in patients with coronary artery disease. After achieving adequate control of heart rate and stabilizing patient, con-

sider transition to alternative antiarrhythmic therapy (longer acting beta-adrenergic blockers, digoxin, verapamil). Reduce esmolol dose by one-half 30 min following first dose of alternative agent, discontinue esmolol if adequate response is maintained for 1 hr following the second dose of the alternative agent.

Patient/Family Education
Educate about adverse effects and expected therapeutic outcome.

ESTROGENS (CONJUGATED)

(ess'-troe-jenz)
Trade Name(s): Premarin
Classification(s): Hormone-estrogen
Pregnancy Category: X

PHARMACODYNAMICS/KINETICS

Mechanism of Action: Promotes the growth, development, and maintenance of female reproductive system and secondary sex characteristics. **Distribution:** Widely distributed. **Metabolism/Elimination:** Degraded in liver to less active estrogenic compounds conjugated with sulfuric and glucuronic acids. Excreted mainly in urine. Small amount present in feces.

INDICATIONS/DOSAGE

Abnormal uterine bleeding causing hormonal imbalance

Adult: 25 mg. May repeat in 6–12 hr if needed.

In the Adverse Effects section, <u>underline</u> indicates most frequent;
CAPS indicates life threatening.

CONTRAINDICATIONS/ PRECAUTIONS

Contraindicated in: Pregnancy, breast cancer (except for patients being treated for metastic disease), estrogen-dependent neoplasia, undiagnosed abnormal genital bleeding, history/active thrombophlebitis/ thromboembolic disorders, hypersensitivity. **Use cautiously in:** Severe hepatic or renal impairment. **Pregnancy/Lactation:** Do not use during pregnancy—serious fetal damage may occur. Crosses placenta. Distributed into breast milk.

PREPARATION

Availability: 25 mg vial with 5 mL sterile diluent. **Reconstitution:** *Syringe:* Reconstitute with 5 mL of provided diluent (sterile water for injection containing benzyl alcohol). Diluent will be easier to add if 5 mL of air is withdrawn from vial containing powder before adding. Using sterile technique, slowly add diluent to vial, directing the flow against inner wall. Gently agitate container to dissolve contents. Avoid vigorous shaking.

STABILITY/STORAGE

Vial: Refrigerate unreconstituted vials. Reconstituted drug stable for 60 days refrigerated.

ADMINISTRATION

IV Push: Give drug slowly to avoid flushing.

COMPATIBILITY

Solution: Dextrose solutions, sodium chloride solutions. **Y-site:** Heparin, hydrocortisone, potassium chloride, vitamin B complex with C.

ADVERSE EFFECTS

CNS: Dizziness, chorea, convulsions, <u>headache</u>, migraine. **Ophtho:** Steepening of corneal curvature, intolerance to contact lenses. **CV:** Edema/fluid retention, <u>hypertension</u>, <u>thromboembolism</u>. **GI:** Acute pancreatitis, abnormal cramps, bloating, cholestatic jaundice, <u>nausea</u>, vomiting. **GU:** Amenorrhea, breakthrough bleeding, <u>breast tenderness</u>, cervical erosions, changes in libido, dysmenorhea, gynecomastia (males), vaginal candidiasis. **Derm:** Acne, oily skin. **Endo:** Hyplerglycemia. **Hypersens:** Urticaria. **Metab:** Reduced carbohydrate tolerance. **Other:** Aggravation of porphyria, pain at injection site, <u>weight changes</u>.

DRUG INTERACTIONS

Tricyclic antidepressants: Increased antidepressant toxicity. **Insulin:** Increased insulin requirements. **Oral anticoagulants:** Reduced anticoagulant effect. **Anticonvulsants:** Decreased estrogen effect.

NURSING CONSIDERATIONS

Assessment
General:
Monitor BP prior to and during therapy.
Physical:
GU tract.
Lab Alterations:
Increased prothrombin and factors VII, VIII, IX, and X. Decreased antithrombin III. Increased thyroid binding globulin. Decreased from T_3 resin uptake.

Intervention/Rationale
Assess for breakthrough bleeding, amenorrhea, breast tenderness,

and gynecomastia (males). ● Evaluate blood pressure for untoward changes.

Patient/Family Education
Emphasize need for gynecological follow-up every 6–12 months. Cigarette smoking during estrogen therapy may increase incidence of side effects (especially in women over 35).

ETHACRYNIC ACID
(eth-a-krin′-ic)
Trade Name(s): Edecrin
Classification(s): Loop diuretic
Pregnancy Category: B

PHARMACODYNAMICS/KINETICS
Mechanism of Action: Inhibits reabsorption of sodium/chloride primarily in the Loop of Henle and to a lesser extent in the proximal/distal renal tubules. Results in enhanced excretion of sodium, chloride, potassium, hydrogen, calcium, and magnesium. Has little or no effect on glomerular filtration rate or renal blood flow. **Onset of Action:** 5 min. **Peak Effect:** 15–30 min. **Duration of Action:** 2 hr. **Distribution:** Does not enter the CNS. **Metabolism/Elimination:** Metabolized to a cysteine conjugate and an unidentified compound (animal studies). 30%–65% of dose is secreted by proximal tubules and excreted in urine. 35%–40% excreted in bile as cysteine conjugate. **Half-Life:** 1 hr.

INDICATIONS/DOSAGE

Management of edema associated with CHF (may be effective in pa-tients with substantial renal impairment and those refractory to other diuretics). Short-term management of ascites caused by malignancy, idiopathic edema of lymphedema

Adult: 0.5–1.0 mg/kg or 50 mg for adult of average size. Single IV dose not to exceed 100 mg. May repeat in 2–4 hr if necessary.

Use in hypercalcemia to increase renal excretion of calcium. Concomi-tant use with mannitol in manage-ment of ethylene glycol poisoning. Management of bromide intoxica-tion to increase bromide excretion. Treatment of nephrogenic diabetes insipidus not responsive to vaso-pressin or chlorpropamide (unla-beled uses)

Adult: 50 mg. Maximum 100 mg/dose. May repeat in 2–4 hr if nec-essary.

Short-term management of hospital-ized children with congenital heart disease or nephrotic syndrome (un-labeled use)

Pediatric: 0.5–1.0 mg/kg/dose. Not to exceed 2 mg/kg/dose or > 3 mg/kg in 30 minutes. Repeat doses are not recommended al-though doses every 8–12 hr have been used.

CONTRAINDICATIONS/ PRECAUTIONS
Contraindicated in: Hypersensitivity, anuria, hypotension, dehydration with low serum sodium. **Use cau-tiously in:** Acute MI with cardiogenic shock and pulmonary edema, fluid and electrolyte depletion, elderly, patients with chronic cardiac dis-ease with prolonged sodium re-striction, advanced hepatic cirrho-

---

In the Adverse Effects section, underline indicates most frequent;
CAPS indicates life threatening.

sis. **Pregnancy/Lactation:** No well-controlled trials to establish safety. Benefits must outweigh risks. Poly-hydramnios, neonatal diuresis, and nephrolithiasis have occurred with chronic oral use of ethacrynic acid. **Pediatrics:** Drug should not be administered to infants.

PREPARATION

Availability: 50 mg vials for reconstitution. **Reconstitution:** Add 50 mL dextrose injection or sodium chloride injection to 50 mg vial of ethacrynic acid for a final concentration of 1 mg/mL. Do not use dextrose solutions with pH below 5 (hazy or opalescent solution will result).

STABILITY/STORAGE

Vial: Store vial at room temperature. Reconstituted solution stable for 24 hr at room temperature. **Infusion:** 24 hr at room temperature.

ADMINISTRATION

General: Choose new injection site if second dose is required to prevent possible thrombophlebitis. **IV Push:** Give **slowly** over 5–10 min (too rapid administration may result in temporary/permanent hearing loss). **Intermittent Infusion:** Infuse **slowly** over 20–30 min.

COMPATIBILITY

Solution: Dextrose solutions, lactated Ringer's, Ringer's injection, sodium chloride solutions, sterile water for injection. **Y-site:** Heparin, hydrocortisone, potassium chloride, vitamin B complex with C.

ADVERSE EFFECTS

CNS: Dizziness, hearing loss (rate related; temporary/permanent), Acute hypotension, CIRCULATORY COLLAPSE (too vigorous diuresis), orthostatic hypotension. **GI:** Acute GI bleeding (especially with concomitant heparin therapy), acute necrotizing pancreatitis, anorexia, abdominal discomfort/pain, diarrhea, dysphagia, HEPATIC COMA (patients with hepatic cirrhosis), nausea, vomiting. **Fld/Lytes:** Dehydration, hypokalemia, hypochloremia, hypomagnesemia, hyponatremia, hypovolemia, reversible hyperuricemia. **Heme:** Agranulocytosis, hemoconcentration, SEVERE NEUTROPENIA, thrombocytopenia. **Hypersens:** Rash. **Metab:** Acid-base disturbances, metabolic alkalosis. **Other:** Local pain, irritation, or thrombophlebitis at injection site.

TOXICITY/OVERDOSE

Signs/Symptoms: Acute profound water loss, volume and electrolyte depletion, dehydration, circulatory collapse, possible vascular thrombosis and embolism due to hemoconcentration. **Treatment:** Replace fluid/electrolyte losses. Supportive measures.

DRUG INTERACTIONS

Aminoglycosides/other ototoxic agents: Enhanced ototoxic potential. **Antihypertensive agents:** Enhanced antihypertensive effects. **Cardiac glycosides:** Glycoside toxicity (if electrolyte depletion present). **Diuretics:** Enhanced diuretic effects. **Insulin/oral antidiabetic agents:** Increased blood sugar. **Lithium:** Enhanced lithium therapeutic and toxic effects. **Nephrotoxic agents:** Enhanced nephrotoxic potential.

216   In the Adverse Effects section, underline indicates most frequent; CAPS indicates life threatening.

Probenecid: Decreased effectiveness of ethacrynic acid. **Tubocurarine:** Prolonged neuromuscular blockade. **Warfarin:** Enhanced coagulation.

NURSING CONSIDERATIONS

Assessment
General:
Blood pressure, intake/output ratio, daily weight.
Physical:
Cardiopulmonary status, hearing, GI tract, hematopoietic system.
Lab Alterations:
Monitor electrolytes, BUN, and creatinine at least daily. Monitor calcium, magnesium, CBC with differential, and platelet count periodically.

Intervention/Rationale
Assess for signs of electrolyte depletion/dehydration. Administer electrolyte replacement therapy as ordered. ● Monitor hypokalemic patients concomitantly receiving cardiac glycosides for signs of digitalis toxicity (hypokalemia may potentiate digoxin toxicity). ● Assess patient for hearing loss. ● Drug may cause muscle weakness and cramps. ● Monitor for signs/symptoms of GI bleeding (especially in patients receiving concomitant heparin therapy).

Patient/Family Education
Change positions slowly in bed to minimize orthostatic hypotension. Notify nurse/physician if muscle cramps/weakness occur.

ETIDRONATE DISODIUM (EHDP)

(eh-tih-droe′-nate di-soe′-dee-um)
Trade Name(s): Didronel IV
Classification(s): Antihypercalcemic
Pregnancy Category: C

E

PHARMACODYNAMICS/KINETICS
Mechanism of Action: Acts on bone to reduce normal/abnormal bone resorption. Osteoclastic activity is reduced. **Duration of Action:** 6 hr. **Distribution:** Approximately 50% of drug is distributed almost exclusively into bone. Almost no uptake into soft tissues. **Metabolism/Elimination:** Not metabolized. 40%–60% of dose excreted unchanged in urine within 24 hr. Nonrenal clearance is a result of uptake by bone. Drug is eliminated slowly by bone turnover. **Half-Life:** 6 hr. Bone half-life 3–6 months.

INDICATIONS/DOSAGE

Treatment of hypercalcemia associated with malignant neoplasms not adequately controlled by dietary modifications and/or fluid therapy and malignancy-associated hypercalcemia that persists after adequate hydration

Adult: 7.5 mg/kg daily for 3 consecutive days. May require treatment up to 7 days. May repeat dose after 7 days for recurrent hypercalcemia (begin oral dose on last day of IV dose to maintain therapeutic calcium levels). Treatment not recommended for longer than 90 days.

In the Adverse Effects section, <u>underline</u> indicates most frequent; CAPS indicates life threatening.

217

Reduce dosage in renal impairment.

CONTRAINDICATIONS/ PRECAUTIONS
Contraindicated in: Known hypersensitivity. **Use cautiously in:** Serum creatinine 2.5–4.9 mg/dL. **Pregnancy/ Lactation:** No well-controlled trials to establish safety. Benefits must outweigh risks. **Pediatrics:** Safety and efficacy not established.

PREPARATION
Availability: 50 mg/mL in 6 mL amps.
Infusion: Dilute in at least 250 mL sodium chloride.

STABILITY/STORAGE
Vial: Store vial at room temperature.
Infusion: Stable for 48 hr at room temperature.

ADMINISTRATION
Intermittent Infusion: May be diluted in larger volumes and given over an extended infusion time if desired. Administer by slow IV infusion over 2 hr regardless of diluted volume.

COMPATIBILITY
Solution: Sodium chloride solutions.

ADVERSE EFFECTS
GI: Diarrhea, nausea, metallic, altered, or loss of taste (reversible).
Renal: Nephrotoxicity. **Fld/Lytes:** Hypocalcemia.

TOXICITY/OVERDOSE
Signs/Symptoms: Significant hypocalcemia (evidenced by tetany, seizures, paresthesias, muscle twitching, cardiac dysrhythmias, Chvostek's or Trousseau's sign), renal insufficiency, proximal renal tubule damage, ECG changes. **Treatment:** Symptomatic/supportive therapy, IV calcium gluconate.

DRUG INTERACTIONS
Nephrotoxic agents: Increased nephrotoxicity.

NURSING CONSIDERATIONS
Assessment
General:
Intake/output ratio, daily weight.
Physical:
Signs of hypo/hypercalcemia.
Lab Alterations:
Monitor total serum calcium and renal function (BUN, creatinine).

Intervention/Rationale
Pretreatment or simultaneous treatment with IV saline and loop diuretics will enhance calcium excretion. Rate of renal excretion is directly related to renal sodium excretion. ● Avoid overhydration in elderly or patients with cardiac failure. ● Maintain adequte nutrition.

Patient/Family Education
Metallic taste after administration is associated with drug and will disappear. Instruct in dietary modifications, including eating adequate amounts of vitamin D and calcium. Inform nurse/physician of signs of hypercalcemia (bone pain, nausea, thirst, lethargy, vomiting) or hypocalcemia. Nurse/physician follow-up after discharge important to detect or prevent relapse.

In the Adverse Effects section, underline indicates most frequent; CAPS indicates life threatening.

ETOMIDATE

(e-tome'-i-date)
Trade Name(s): Amidate
Classification(s): General anesthetic
Pregnancy Category: C

PHARMACODYNAMICS/KINETICS

Mechanism of Action: Nonbarbiturate hypnotic without analgesic activity. **Onset of Action:** 1 min. **Duration of Action:** 3–5 min. **Metabolism/Elimination:** Rapidly metabolized in the liver. 75% excreted as inactive metabolite in urine, 10% in bile, 13% in feces. **Half-Life:** 75 minutes.

INDICATIONS/DOSAGE

Induction of general anesthesia

Adult/Pediatric (children > 10 years): 0.2–0.6 mg/kg (usual dose 0.3 mg/kg over 30–60 sec). Dose should be individualized for patient.

Concomitant anesthesia for short operative procedures

Adult: Small increments may be given during short procedures to supplement subpotent anesthetic agents.

CONTRAINDICATIONS/PRECAUTIONS

Contraindicated in: Hypersensitivity. **Use cautiously in:** Consider exogenous corticosteroid replacement in patients undergoing severe stress. **Pregnancy/Lactation:** No well-controlled trials to establish safety.

Benefits must outweigh risks. Fetal effects unknown. **Pediatrics:** Safety and efficacy not established in children under the age of 10.

PREPARATION

Availability: 2 mg/mL in 10 and 20 mL amps.

STABILITY/STORAGE

Vial: Store at room temperature. Protect from freezing and extreme heat.

ADMINISTRATION

General: To be given only by personnel trained in intubation and mechanical ventilation. **IV Push:** Give dose over 30–60 sec.

ADVERSE EFFECTS

CV: Bradycardia, dysrhythmias, hypertension, hypotension. **Resp:** LARYNGOSPASM, hyperventilation, hypoventilation, hiccoughs, snoring. **GI:** Postoperative nausea/vomiting. **MS:** Transient skeletal muscle movements. **Other:** Transient pain at injection site.

NURSING CONSIDERATION

Assessment
General:
Continuous blood pressure and ECG monitoring.
Physical:
Pulmonary status.

Intervention/Rationale
Maintain adequate airway and ventilation. ● Evaluate blood pressure and ECG continuously to prevent hypotension and dysrhythmias.

In the Adverse Effects section, underline indicates most frequent; CAPS indicates life threatening.

Patient/Family Education
Educate about adverse effects and therapeutic outcome.

ETOPOSIDE (VP-16)
(e-toe'-poe-side)
Trade Name(s): VePesid
Classification(s): Antineoplastic, antimitotic
Pregnancy Category: D

PHARMACODYNAMICS/KINETICS
Mechanism of Action: Inhibits DNA synthesis prior to mitosis. **Peak Serum Levels:** 1.0–1.5 hr. **Distribution:** 97% bound to plasma proteins. Animal studies indicate concentrations in small intestine, kidneys, and liver. **Metabolism/Elimination:** Metabolized primarily to inactive metabolites. Primarily eliminated in urine. Fecal excretion is variable. **Half-Life:** Biphasic-initial 0.6–2.0 hr, terminal 5.3–10.8 hr.

INDICATIONS/DOSAGE

Refractory testicular tumors
Adult: 50–100 mg/m^2/day on days 1–5. 100 mg/m^2/day on days 1, 3, and 5. Repeat course at 3–4 week intervals after recovery from toxicity.

Small cell lung cancer
Adult: 35 mg/m^2/day for 4 days. 50 mg/m^2/day for 5 days. Repeat course at 3–4 week intervals after recovery from toxicity.

CONTRAINDICATIONS/PRECAUTIONS
Contraindicated in: Hypersensitivity. **Use cautiously in:** Severe myelosuppression, chronic debilitating illnesses. **Pregnancy/Lactation:** Causes fetal harm. Benefits must outweigh risks. Women of childbearing age should be instructed to use contraceptives. Patients becoming pregnant during therapy should be apprised of the risks to fetus. **Pediatrics:** Safety and efficacy in children not established.

PREPARATION
Availability: 20 mg/mL in 5 mL amps. **Infusion:** Dilute with dextrose injection or sodium chloride injection to give a final concentration of 0.2 or 0.4 mg/mL.

STABILITY/STORAGE
Vial: Store at room temperature. **Infusion:** Diluted concentrations (0.2 or 0.4 mg/mL) stable for 96 and 48 hr, respectively, in both glass and plastic containers.

ADMINISTRATION
General: Prepare and handle solution according to institutional guidelines for the handling of chemotherapeutic/cytotoxic agents. Immediately wash skin with soap and water if contact occurs. In the event of a spill, add 5% sodium hypochlorite (household bleach) or 1% potassium permanente to spill to inactivate. **IV Push:** Do not give by rapid IV injection (may cause hypotension). **Intermittent Infusion:** Administer over 30–60 min.

In the Adverse Effects section, underline indicates most frequent; CAPS indicates life threatening.

COMPATIBILITY
Solution: Dextrose solutions, sodium chloride solutions. **Y-site:** Ondansetron.

ADVERSE EFFECTS
CV: Hypotension (too rapid infusion), hypertension. **GI:** Anorexia, constipation, diarrhea, dysphagia, nausea, stomatitis, vomiting. **Derm:** Pigmentation, reversible alopecia. **Heme:** SEVERE LEUKOPENIA, SEVERE THROMBOCYTOPENIA, anemia. **Nadir:** Granulocyte 7–14 days. Platelet 9–16 days. **Hypersens:** Anaphylactic-like reactions (chills, fever, tachycardia, bronchospasm, dyspnea, hypotension), pruritus, rash. **Other:** Peripheral neurotoxicity.

DRUG INTERACTIONS
Other antineoplastics/radiation therapy: Additive bone marrow suppression.

NURSING CONSIDERATIONS
Assessment
General:
Monitor BP prior to and every 15 min during infusion, hypersensitivity reactions, intake/output ratio.
Physical:
Infectious disease status, hematpoietic system, GI tract.
Lab Alterations:
Monitor platelet count, hemoglobin, WBC count, and differential at start of therapy and prior to each subsequent dose. Monitor liver and renal function studies periodically.

Intervention/Rationale
Stop infusion if hypotension occurs. May resume infusion at lower rate after successful treatment of hypotension with IV fluids and other supportive measures. ● Withhold subsequent therapy for a platelet count < 50,000/mm^3 or a neutrophil count < 500/mm^3 (treatment may be resumed when counts have sufficiently recovered). ● Avoid IM injections and rectal temperatures. ● Assess for bleeding (bruising, petechiae, bleeding gums). ● Administer antiemetics if nausea and vomiting become problematic. ● Assess for signs/symptoms of infection and notify physician immediately if present.

Patient/Family Education
Maintain good oral hygiene using soft toothbrush and alcohol-free mouthwash. Use an electric razor for shaving. Avoid persons with known infections and crowded environments. Assess for signs/symptoms of infection/bleeding and notify physician immediately if present. Inspect mouth for presence of oral sores; use sponge toothbrushes and warm water rinses after eating. Oral viscous lidocaine may relieve oral pain associated with eating. Follow-up lab tests and physician visits important to monitor for toxicity. Hair loss may affect body image. Use consistent and reliable contraception throughout the duration of therapy due to potential teratogenic and mutagenic effects of drug. Avoid over-the-counter products containing aspirin or ibuprofen.

In the Adverse Effects section, underline indicates most frequent; CAPS indicates life threatening.

FACTOR IX COMPLEX

(fak'-tor nine)
Trade Name(s): Konyne-HT, Profilnine Heat-Treated, Proplex T, Proplex SX-T
Classification(s): Antihemophilic factor (AHF)
Pregnancy Category: C

PHARMACODYNAMICS/KINETICS
Mechanism of Action: Increases plasma levels and restores hemostasis, increases Factor II, VII, IX, X. **Onset of Action:** Instantaneous rise in coagulant level. **Duration of Action:** 24–48 hr. **Metabolism/Elimination:** Rapidly cleared from plasma. **Half-Life:** Factor IX: 24–32 hr. Factor VII: 3–6 hr.

INDICATIONS/DOSAGE

Adult/Pediatric: Dose is individualized depending on patient's weight, severity of deficiency, severity of hemorrhage, presence of inhibitors, and Factor IX level desired. One unit of Factor IX activity equals 1 mL average normal fresh plasma. Dose required to achieve a % increase in plasma F-IX level:

Units required = weight (kg) × 0.8–1.0 × desired F-IX increase (% normal)

Prevention/Control of Bleeding in Factor IX Deficiency (Hemophilia B): Minimum dosage for hemostasis after trauma or prior to/after surgery is 25% normal. Maintain these levels for at least 1 week. Loading dose 40–60 units/kg. Maintenance 10–20 units/kg/day. **Prophylaxis of Factor IX Spontaneous Bleeding:** 10–20 units/kg once or twice weekly.

Bleeding with Factor VIII (Hemophilia A) Inhibitors: 75 units/kg. Second dose may be administered after 8–12 hr if necessary. **Reversal of Coumarin-Induced Anticoagulant Effects:** 15 units/kg. **Factor VII Deficiency (Proplex T Only):** Calculate a dose to raise level 40%–60% normal. Administer every 4–6 hr as needed:

Units required =
weight (kg) × 0.5 units/kg
× desired F-VII increase (% normal)

CONTRAINDICATIONS/PRECAUTIONS
Contraindicated in: Factor VII deficiencies (except for Proplex T), liver disease with signs of intravascular coagulation/fibrinolysis. **Use cautiously in:** Liver disease, postoperative patients, patients predisposed to thrombosis. **Pregnancy/Lactation:** No well-controlled trials to establish safety. Benefits must outweigh risks.

PREPARATION
Availability: Actual number of AHF units indicated on vials with diluent. **Reconstitution:** Warm vial and diluent (sterile water for injection) to room temperature (not to exceed 37°C). Use diluent provided. Add diluent to vial and gently agitate until the powder is completely dissolved. Drug must be completely dissolved to avoid removal of active components through filter needle. **Infusion:** Add contents of reconstituted vial to empty sterile IV bag or buretrol device using a filter needle to transfer.

STABILITY/STORAGE
Vial: Refrigerate lyophilized powder; do not freeze. Reconstituted

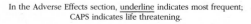

In the Adverse Effects section, <u>underline</u> indicates most frequent; CAPS indicates life threatening.

solution stable for 12 hr. Administer within 3 hr after reconstitution. Do not refrigerate reconstituted solution (to avoid precipitation of active ingredients). **Infusion:** Use within 3 hr of reconstitution. Store at room temperature.

ADMINISTRATION

General: Administer slowly via infusion device. Must be filtered prior to administration. **IV Push/Intermittent Infusion:** Infuse slowly. **Konyne-HT:** Not to exceed 100 units/min. **Profilnine:** Not to exceed 10 mL/min. **Proplex T:** 2–3 mL/min; not to exceed 3 mL/min.

COMPATIBILITY

Syringe: Heparin. **Y-site:** Heparin.

ADVERSE EFFECTS

CNS: Headache (rapid infusion). **CV:** Changes in heart rate/blood pressure (rapid infusion), myocardial infarction (high doses). **Resp:** Pulmonary embolism (high doses). **GI:** Nausea, vomiting (rapid infusion). **Heme:** Disseminated intravascular coagulation, venous thrombosis. **Hypersens:** Urticaria (rapid infusion). **Other:** Chills, fever (high doses), flushing (rapid infusion).

DRUG INTERACTIONS

Aminocaproic acid: Increased risk of thrombosis.

NURSING CONSIDERATIONS

Assessment
General:
Vital signs.
Physical:
Signs/symptoms of hypersensitivity reactions, hematologic profile.

Lab Alterations:
Monitor Factor IX (or VII) levels daily. If treatment is prolonged, monitor Factor II, IX, and X levels.

Intervention/Rationale
Evaluate vital signs prior to and periodically during infusion. If infusion related effects or pulse rate increases, reduce flow rate or discontinue and notify physician. ● Assess Factor II, IX, and X levels to assure adequate levels are reached and maintained. If levels fail to reach expected range or bleeding is uncontrolled, inhibitors may be present.

Patient/Family Education
Observe for early signs of allergic reactions. Risk of transmission of HIV/hepatitis B is present (however, advances in screening techniques reduce risk). Avoid situations likely to increase bleeding potential. Notify nurse/physician if bleeding occurs from gums, stools, skin, or urine. Patient should carry identification of disease status.

FAMOTIDINE

(fa-moe′-ti-deen)
Trade Name(s): Pepcid
Classification(s): Histamine (H_2) receptor antagonist
Pregnancy Category: B

PHARMACODYNAMICS/KINETICS

Mechanism of Action: Competitively inhibits action of histamine on H_2 receptors of gastric parietal cells. Reduces gastric output and concentration. Indirectly reduces pepsin secretion by decreasing volume of

In the Adverse Effects section, <u>underline</u> indicates most frequent; CAPS indicates life threatening.

223

gastric juice. **Peak Effect:** 0.5–3.0 hr. **Duration of Action:** 10–12 hr. **Distribution:** Widely distributed throughout body especially in kidneys, liver, pancreas, and submandibular gland. 15%–20% protein bound. **Metabolism/Elimination:** Metabolized by the liver to S-oxide metabolite (no antisecretory activity). Primarily eliminated via glomerular/tubular secretion. 65%–80% excreted unchanged in urine. **Half-Life:** 2.5–4.0 hr. Increased in renal impairment; 12–24 hr.

INDICATIONS/DOSAGE

Short-term treatment/maintenance of duodenal ulcer or benign gastric ulcer

Adult: 20 mg every 12 hr. Adjust dose in renal impairment. (Creatinine clearance < 10 mL/min: 10–20 mg every 24–48 hr.)

Pathological hypersecretory conditions (Zollinger-Ellison syndrome)

Adult: 20 mg every 6–12 hr. May require up to 160 mg every 6 hr. Adjust dose in renal impairment.

CONTRAINDICATIONS/ PRECAUTIONS

Contraindicated in: Hypersensitivity. **Use cautiously in:** Elderly, impaired hepatic/renal function. **Pregnancy/ Lactation:** No well-controlled trials to establish safety. Benefits must outweigh risks. Crosses placenta. Excreted in breast milk. **Pediatrics:** Safety and efficacy not established.

PREPARATION

Availability: 10 mg/mL, 2- and 4-mL vials. **Syringe:** Dilute dosage to a total of 5–10 mL using compatible IV solution. **Infusion:** Further dilute in 50–100 mL compatible IV solution.

STABILITY/STORAGE

Vial: Store in refrigerator. May be stored at room temperature for 26 weeks. **Infusion:** Stable for 48 hr at room temperature. 14 days refrigerated.

ADMINISTRATION

General: Rapid administration may cause hypotension. **IV Push:** Inject slowly over at least 2 min. Not to exceed 10 mg/min. **Intermittent Infusion:** Infuse over 15–30 min. **Continuous Infusion:** Infuse at a rate to administer dose over a 24 hr period via infusion device. Not to exceed usual total daily intermittent dose.

COMPATIBILITY

Solution: Dextrose solutions, fat emulsion, lactated Ringer's, sodium bicarbonate, sodium chloride solutions, sterile water for injection. **Y-site:** Aminophylline, ampicillin, ampicillin-sulbactam, amrinone, atropine, bretylium, calcium gluconate, cefazolin, cefoperazone, cefotaxime, cefotetan, cefoxitin, ceftazidime, ceftizoxime, cefuroxime, cephalothin, cephapirin, dexamethasone, dextran, digoxin, dobutamine, dopamine, enalaprilat, epinephrine, erythromycin, esmolol, folic acid, furosemide, gentamicin, heparin, hydrocortisone, imipenem, insulin, isoproterenol, labetalol, lidocaine, magnesium sulfate, methylprednisolone, metoclopramide, mezlocillin, midazolam, morphine, nafcillin, nitroglycerin, norepinephrine, ondansetron, oxacillin, perphenazine, phenylephrine, phenytoin, phytonadione, piperacillin, potassium chloride,

In the Adverse Effects section, underline indicates most frequent; CAPS indicates life threatening.

potassium phosphate, procainamide, sodium bicarbonate, sodium nitroprusside, theophylline, thiamine, ticarcillin, ticarcillin-clauvulanate, verapamil.

ADVERSE EFFECTS
CNS: Seizures, dizziness, headache, paresthesia, tinnitus. **Ophtho:** Conjunctival injection, orbital edema. **CV:** Hypotension, palpitations. **GI:** Anorexia, constipation, diarrhea, dry mouth, taste disorders. **MS:** Musculoskeletal pain. **Derm:** Acne, alopecia, dry skin. **Other:** Fever, flushing.

TOXICITY/OVERDOSE
Signs/Symptoms: No reports of toxicity. Animal studies demonstrate rapid respiration, respiratory failure, tachycardia, muscle tremors, vomiting, restlessness, hypotension, lacrimation, salivation, miosis, diarrhea. **Treatment:** Symptomatic treatment. Hemodialysis is not effective.

DRUG INTERACTIONS
Ketoconazole: Inhibits ketoconazole absorption.

NURSING CONSIDERATIONS
Assessment
General:
GI tract, neurologic status.
Lab Alterations:
Monitor CBC with differential, false-negative results in skin tests using allergen extracts (discontinue drug at least 24 hr prior to allergy testing).

Intervention/Rationale
Assess elderly/debilitated for development of CNS findings. ● Assess gastric pH every 6 hr and maintain pH > 4 as per physician order. Assess abdominal or epigastric pain in association with medication schedule. Hematest stools/vomitus/nasogastric drainage to assess for presence/absence of occult or note frank bleeding.

Patient/Family Education
Clinical effect of reduction of gastric acid is reversed by cigarette smoking. Avoid becoming pregnant or breastfeeding while taking drug. Avoid drugs/food that will aggravate ulcer condition (aspirin, alcohol, etc.). Drug may cause drowsiness or dizziness; avoid activities that require mental acuity until effects of drug have been determined.

FAT EMULSION, INTRAVENOUS
(fat ee-mul'-shun)
Trade Name(s): Intralipid, Liposyn II, Liposyn III, Nutrilipid, Soyacal
Classification(s): Intravenous nutritional therapy
Pregnancy Category:
B—Nutrilipid 10%, Soyacal 10%.
C—Intralipid, Liposyn II, Liposyn III, Nutrilipid

PHARMACODYNAMICS/KINETICS
Mechanism of Action: Provide a caloric source of fatty acids for energy from heat production, oxygen consumption, and decreased respiratory quotient. Fatty acids include linoleic, oleic, palmitic, linolenic, and stearic acids. Contains soybean

In the Adverse Effects section, underline indicates most frequent; CAPS indicates life threatening.

225

oil and/or safflower oil. **Distribution:** Distributed throughout intravascular space. **Metabolism/Elimination:** Converted to triglycerides that are hydrolyzed to free fatty acids and glycerol. The free fatty acids enter tissues for oxidation or triglyceride synthesis for storage. May circulate bound to albumin. May reenter systemic circulation via hepatic oxidation or VLDL conversion. Glycerin is metabolized to carbon dioxide and glycogen or is used in fat synthesis.

INDICATIONS/DOSAGE

Dosage is dependent on nutritional/metabolic needs of patient.

Total parenteral nutrition needs for extended period of time (usually for more than 5 days):

Fat emulsion should comprise no more than 60% of total caloric need.

Adult:
10%: 1 mL/min for the first 15–30 minutes. Infuse no more than 500 mL the first day. Increase dose the following day. Should not exceed 3 g/kg/day. **20%:** 0.5 mL/min for the first 15–30 min. Infuse no more than 250 mL (Soyacal) or 500 mL (Intralipid) the first day. Increase dose the following day. Should not exceed 3 g/kg/day.

Pediatric:
10%: 0.1 mL/min for the first 10–15 min. **20%:** 0.05 mL/min for the first 10–15 min. If no untoward reaction, increase 1 g/kg in 4 hr. Not to exceed a rate of 50 mL/hr (20%) or 100 mL/hr (10%). Should not exceed 4 g/kg/day.

Neonates: Not to exceed 1 g/kg in 4 hr (due to poor fat clearance).

Fatty acid deficiency

Adult/Pediatrics: Supply 8%–10% caloric intake by fat emulsion to provide an adequate amount of linoleic acid.

CONTRAINDICATIONS/ PRECAUTIONS

Contraindicated in: Disturbances of normal fat metabolism, severe egg allergy (contains egg yolk phospholipids). **Use cautiously in:** Anemia, blood coagulation disorders, pulmonary disease, severe liver damage. **Pregnancy/Lactation:** No well-controlled trials to establish safety. Benefits must outweigh risks. **Pediatrics:** Use with caution in premature or jaundiced infants because bilirubin bound to albumin may be displaced.

PREPARATION

Availability: 50 mL, 100 mL, 250 mL, 500 mL glass bottles with non-phthalate infusion sets (provided with product). 10% contains 1.1 calories/mL. 20% contains 2.0 calories/mL.

STABILITY/STORAGE

Vial: Store at room temperature in intact containers. **Infusion:** Store at room temperature. Infusion and total nutrient admixtures may hang for 24 hr.

ADMINISTRATION

General: Do not use filters (although data suggests a 1.2 micron filter is acceptable for particulate matter extraction). Use nonphthalate infusion sets (provided with product) to avoid extraction into PVC tubing. If other tubing is used, do not prime the set until just prior to administration. Change tubing every 24 hr or per institutional policy. Administer via peripheral or central venous catheter (may be infused through a separate peripheral site). May be simultaneously infused with amino acid–dextrose mixtures with a Y-connector using separate flow controls. Keep the lipid infusion higher than the amino acid-dextrose line so that it will not be taken up into the other line because of the lower specific gravity of fat. Monitor peripheral sites to avoid phlebitis. **IV Push/Infusion:** Administer as per dosage guideline rates. Rapid infusion may cause fluid or fat overload. Heparin, 1–2 units/mL, may be added to activate lipoprotein lipase that enhances the hydrolysis of triglycerides to free fatty acids and glycerol.

COMPATIBILITY
Solution: Amino acids 8.5%, dextrose 5%, dextrose 50%, lactated Ringer's, sodium chloride solutions. **Y-site:** Ampicillin, cefamandole, cefazolin, cefoxitin, cephapirin, clindamycin, digoxin, dopamine, erythromycin, furosemide, gentamicin, isoproterenol, lidocaine, norepinephrine, oxacillin, penicillin G, potassium chloride, ticarcillin, tobramycin. **Additive:** It is recommended that no other drugs or solution be added to fat emulsion because of potential disturbance to stability.

INCOMPATIBILITY
Solution: Amino acids 10%, dextrose 10%, dextrose 25%. **Y-site:** Amikacin.

ADVERSE EFFECTS
CNS: Dizziness, headache. **Ophtho:** Eye pressure. **CV:** Chest pain. **Resp:** Cyanosis, dyspnea. **GI:** Hepatomegaly (long-term), hyperlipemia, jaundice (long-term), transient liver enzyme increases, nausea, splenomegaly, vomiting. **MS:** Back pain. **Heme:** Hypercoagulability, leukopenia (long-term), thrombocytopenia (long-term). **Hypersens:** Urticaria. **Other:** Increased temperature, flushing, sweating, overloading syndrome (with long-term use); fever, leukocytosis, seizures, splenomegaly, shock, sepsis, thrombophlebitis.

TOXICITY/OVERDOSE
Signs/Symptoms: Extension of immediate adverse effects. **Treatment:** Discontinue infusion, symptomatic treatment.

NURSING CONSIDERATIONS
Assessment
General:
Intake/output ratio, nutritional status.
Physical:
Hematopoietic system, GI tract.
Lab Alterations:
Monitor plasma lipid profile, liver function, PT/PTT, platelet count periodically during therapy.

Intervention/Rationale
Monitor fat clearance from circulation by assessment of above lab values. Lipemia must clear between daily infusions. Draw serum triglyceride level just prior to next administration to allow complete metabolism (note time of blood drawn for lipid profile with respect to infusion

---

In the Adverse Effects section, underline indicates most frequent; CAPS indicates life threatening.

time). ● Monitor patient for unto-ward adverse effects with initial administration.

Patient/Family Education

Advise patient of necessity of the use of fat emulsions for improvement of nutritional status.

F

FENTANYL

(fen'-ta-nil)
Trade Name(s): Sublimaze, Innovar (with droperidol)
Classification(s): Narcotic analgesic
Pregnancy Category: C
Controlled Substance Schedule: II

PHARMACODYNAMICS/KINETICS

Mechanism of Action: Binds to opiate receptors in the CNS. **Onset of Action:** Rapid. **Peak Effect:** Within several minutes. **Duration of Action:** 0.5–1.0 hr. **Metabolism:** Hepatic metabolism to active metabolites. **Elimination:** Metabolites and unchanged (10%–25%) drug eliminated in the urine. **Half-Life:** 1.5–6.0 hr.

INDICATIONS/DOSAGE

Consider the total dose of all narcotic analgesics; use ¼–⅓ less narcotic doses than recommended when used in conjunction with fentanyl. Respiratory depressant effects persist longer than analgesic effects. Reduce dosage in elderly, debilitated, patients with concur-rent CNS depressants, or high risk patients.

Adjunct to general anesthesia

Adult:
Total Low Dosage: 2 mcg/kg for minor, painful surgical procedures and postoperative pain relief. **Total Moderate Dosage:** 2–20 mcg/kg. Artificial ventilation and observation postoperatively is necessary. **Maintenance Moderate Dosage:** 25–100 mcg when movement or vital sign changes indicate anesthesia lightening or surgical stress. **Total High Dosage:** 20–50 mcg/kg for "stress free" anesthesia when surgery is prolonged or complicated. Inject with nitrous oxide/oxygen. Postoperative ventilation and observation are required. **Maintenance High Dosage:** 25 mcg to 50% loading dose. Individualize dose. Administer when vital sign changes indicate anesthesia lightening or surgical stress.

Pediatric:
1–3 Years Old: 2–3 mcg/kg/dose; may repeat after 30–60 min as needed. **3–12 Years Old:** 1–2 mcg/kg/dose; may repeat after 30–60 min as needed. **> 12 Years Old:** 0.5–1.0 mcg/kg/dose; may repeat after 30–60 min as needed.

Adjunct to regional anesthesia

Adult: 50–100 mcg.

General anesthetic

Adult: 50–100 mcg/kg with oxygen and skeletal muscle relaxant. Up to 150 mcg/kg may be needed.
Pediatric: 1.7–3.3 mcg/kg/dose.

In the Adverse Effects section, underline indicates most frequent; CAPS indicates life threatening.

228

CONTRAINDICATIONS/ PRECAUTIONS

Contraindicated in: Acute bronchial asthma, narcotic hypersensitivity, upper airway obstruction. **Use cautiously in:** Asthma/other respiratory conditions, patients prone to hypotension. **Pregnancy/Lactation:** No well-controlled trials to establish safety. Benefits must outweigh risks. Use is not recommended since it crosses the placenta. **Pediatrics:** Safety and efficacy has not been established in children < 2 years old.

PREPARATION

Availability: 50 mcg/mL in 2, 5, 10, 20 and 50 mL amp/vials.

STABILITY/STORAGE

Vial: Store at room temperature. Protect from light.

ADMINISTRATION

General: Rapid injection may result in respiratory paralysis or apnea. To be given only by individuals trained in anesthesia administration/emergency airway management. **IV Push:** Give undiluted slowly over 1–2 min. **Pediatric:** Give over 3–5 min.

COMPATIBILITY

Solution: Dextrose solutions, sodium chloride solutions. **Syringe:** Atropine, butorphanol, chlorpromazine, cimetidine, dimenhydrinate, diphenhydramine, droperidol, heparin, hydromorphone, meperidine, metoclopramide, midazolam, morphine, pentazocine, perphenazine, prochlorperazine, promethazine, ranitidine, scopolamine. **Y-site:** Atracurium, enalaprilat, esmolol, heparin, hydrocortisone, labetalol, nafcillin, pancuronium, potassium chloride, vecuronium, vitamin B complex with C.

INCOMPATIBILITY

Syringe: Methohexital, pentobarbital, thiopental.

ADVERSE EFFECTS

CNS: Seizures, <u>dizziness</u>, dysphoria, <u>lightheadedness</u>, <u>sedation</u>. **CV:** CARDIAC ARREST, CIRCULATORY DEPRESSION, bradycardia, hypotension, shock. **Resp:** Apnea, RESPIRATORY ARREST/DEPRESSION. **GI:** Constipation, nausea, vomiting. **GU:** Ureteral spasm. **Hypersens:** Pruritus, urticaria. **MS:** Skeletal/thoracic muscle rigidity. **Other:** Diaphoresis, flushing.

TOXICITY/OVERDOSE

Signs/Symptoms: CNS depression, miosis, respiratory depression, hypotension, hypothermia, pulmonary edema, pneumonia, shock, apnea, bradycardia, cardiac arrest, circulatory collapse, seizures, death. **Treatment:** Supportive measures, maintain ventilation. **Antidote(s):** In significant respiratory or circulatory depression, administer naloxone as per physician order.

DRUG INTERACTIONS

Cimetidine: Increased CNS toxicity. **CNS depressants:** Increased respiratory/CNS depression. **Diazepam:** Cardiovascular depression. **Droperidol:** Increased hypotension. **Monoamine oxidase inhibitors:** Fatal reaction if used within 14 days of MAO-inhibitor use. **Nitrous oxide:** Cardiovascular depression.

In the Adverse Effects section, <u>underline</u> indicates most frequent; CAPS indicates life threatening.

NURSING CONSIDERATIONS

Assessment

General:
Vital signs, pain assessment/evaluation.
Physical:
Respiratory status.
Lab Alterations:
Increased amylase/lipase levels for 24 hr following administration.

Intervention/Rationale
Ascertain time of last fentanyl administration prior to administering narcotic analgesics in immediate postanesthesia period. ● Evaluate vital signs for development of adverse effects.

Patient/Family Education
Change positions slowly following administration. Avoid alcohol and CNS depressants for 24 hr after administration. Inform physician of monoamine oxidase inhibitor use (avoid within 14 days of fentanyl).

FILGRASTIM
(fill-gra′-stim)
Trade Name(s): Neupogen
Classification(s): Colony stimulating factor
Pregnancy Category: C

PHARMACODYNAMICS/KINETICS
Mechanism of Action: Binds to specific cell surface receptors resulting in proliferation and differentiation of neutrophil lineage. **Onset of Action:** 2–4 hr. **Peak Serum Level:** 2–6 hr. **Duration of Action:** 4 days. **Distribution:** Distributed throughout body specifically into bone marrow. **Metabolism/Elimination:** Eliminated by kidneys. **Half-Life:** 3.5 hr.

INDICATIONS/DOSAGE

Decrease infection incidence (severe neutropenia with fever) associated with myelosuppressive anticancer regimens

Adult/Pediatric: 5 mcg/kg/day as a single injection. If necessary, increase dose by 5 mcg/kg for each cycle. Begin at least 24 hr after the last dose of chemotherapy and continue beyond nadir until absolute neutrophil count > 10,000 mm³. Discontinue at least 24 hr prior to next dose of chemotherapy.

CONTRAINDICATIONS/ PRECAUTIONS
Contraindicated in: Hypersensitivity to *E. coli* derived proteins. **Use cautiously in:** Preexisting cardiac conditions. **Pregnancy/Lactation:** No well-controlled trials to establish safety. Benefits must outweigh risks. **Pediatrics:** No difference in toxicity profile in comparison to adults.

PREPARATION
Availability 300 mcg/mL, 1 and 1.6 mL vials (single dose). **Infusion:** May dilute in compatible IV solution to a volume sufficient to infuse over 24 hr or physician specified time. If concentration < 15 mcg/mL, albumin must be added to prevent adsorption to plastic at a final concentration of 2 mg/mL albumin.

STABILITY/STORAGE
Vial: Store in refrigerator. Stable at room temperature for 6 hr. Discard after single dose removed. **Infusion:** Prepare just prior to administration.

In the Adverse Effects section, underline indicates most frequent; CAPS indicates life threatening.

ADMINISTRATION
Intermittent/Continuous Infusion (Unlabeled route): Infuse over 24 hr or at physician specified rate.

COMPATIBILITY
Solution: Dextrose solutions.

INCOMPATIBILITY
Solution: Sodium chloride solutions.

ADVERSE EFFECTS
CV: Dysrhythmias, myocardial infarction, transient hypotension. **Resp:** Adult respiratory distress syndrome. **GI:** Elevated lactic dehydrogenase/alkaline phosphatase. **MS:** Medullary bone pain. **Heme:** Increased uric acid, leukocytosis. **Other:** Fever.

TOXICITY/OVERDOSE
Signs/Symptoms: No toxic effects reported.

DRUG INTERACTIONS
Cytotoxic chemotherapeutic drugs: Decreased neutropenia incidence.

NURSING CONSIDERATIONS
Assessment
General:
Vital signs, infectious disease status.
Physical:
Hematopoietic status, pulmonary status.
Lab Alterations:
Obtain baseline CBC, differential, and platelets at least twice a week throughout course of treatment.

Intervention/Rationale
Evaluate blood pressure for development of transient hypotension. Assess apical pulse for 1 full minute regularly, and consider continuous ECG monitoring if irregular heart rate is noted. ● Discontinue therapy when absolute neutrophil count reaches 10,000 mm³ after the expected nadir.

Patient/Family Education
Notify physician of signs of infection, fever/bone pain (correlating to actual drug administration). Review expected outcome and potential adverse effects.

FLUCONAZOLE
(flu-con′-a-zoll)
Trade Name(s): Diflucan
Classification(s): Antifungal agent
Pregnancy Category: C

PHARMACODYNAMICS/KINETICS
Mechanism of Action: Inhibition of fungal growth by selective inhibition of fungal cytochrome P-450 and sterol alpha-demethylation. **Distribution:** Distributes throughout body. Concentrates in skin, urine, blistered skin, sputum, saliva, CSF (independent of inflammation). 11%–12% protein bound. **Metabolism/Elimination:** Minimal hepatic metabolism. Primarily eliminated as unchanged drug (80%) and metabolites (11%) in urine. Removed 50% by hemodialysis. **Half-Life:** 30 hr. Increased in renal impairment.

INDICATIONS/DOSAGE
Dosage reduction in renal impairment based on creatinine clearance (Clcr):
- Initial dose: 50–400 mg
- Clcr > mL/min: 100% recommended dose.

In the Adverse Effects section, underline indicates most frequent; CAPS indicates life threatening.

231

- Clcr 21–50 mL/min: 50% recommended dose.
- Clcr 11–20 mL/min: 25% recommended dose.
- Hemodialysis: administer 100% recommended dose after each dialysis.

Treatment of cryptococcal meningitis

Adult: 400 mg on first day, followed by 200 mg daily for 10–12 weeks after CSF negative. 400 mg daily may be used based on patient response.

Pediatric (3–13 Years) (unlabeled use): 3–6 mg/kg/day as a single daily dose.

Treatment of oropharyngeal/esophageal candidiasis

Adult: 200 mg on first day, followed by 100 mg daily. Doses up to 400 mg daily may be used for refractory esophageal infections based on patient response. Continue therapy for at least 2 weeks following symptomatic response.

Pediatric (3–13 Years) (unlabeled use): 3–6 mg/kg/day as a single daily dose.

Treatment of systemic candidiasis

Adult: 400 mg on first day, followed by 200 mg daily for 4 weeks. Continue therapy for at least 2 weeks following symptomatic response.

Pediatric (3–13 Years) (unlabeled use): 3–6 mg/kg/day as a single daily dose.

CONTRAINDICATIONS/ PRECAUTIONS

Contraindicated in: Hypersensitivity to fluconazole/related products or components. **Use cautiously in:** Patients sensitive to other related agents (e.g., ketoconazole, miconazole). **Pregnancy/Lactation:** No well-controlled trials to establish safety. Benefits must outweigh risks. **Pediatrics:** Efficacy has not been established.

PREPARATION

Availability: 200 mg/100 mL and 400 mg/200 mL ready-to-use vials/viaflex containers. **Infusion:** Ready-to-use containers.

STABILITY/STORAGE

Vial/Infusion: Store at room temperature. If viaflex packaging is used, do not remove overwrap until ready to use since overwrap protects sterility.

ADMINISTRATION

General: Do not use plastic containers in series connections to avoid air embolism possibility. **Intermittent Infusion:** Not to exceed 200 mg/hr.

COMPATIBILITY

Solution: Sodium chloride solutions.

ADVERSE EFFECTS

CNS: Dizziness, <u>headache</u>. **GI:** HEPATOTOXICITY, abdominal pain, diarrhea, increased serum transaminase levels, <u>nausea</u>, vomiting. **Hypersens:** STEVENS JOHNSON SYNDROME, rash.

TOXICITY/OVERDOSE

Signs/Symptoms: Animal studies show decreased motility and respiration, ptosis, lacrimation, salivation, urinary incontinence, cyanosis, convulsions, death. **Treatment:** Symptomatic/supportive treatment. Hemodialysis may be beneficial.

In the Adverse Effects section, <u>underline</u> indicates most frequent; CAPS indicates life threatening.

DRUG INTERACTIONS

Cimetidine: Decreased fluconazole serum concentration. **Cyclosporine (CYA):** Slight increase in CYA levels. **Glipizide, glyburide, tolbutamide:** Increased hypoglycemia. **Oral contraceptives:** Decreased ethinyl estradiol levels. **Phenytoin:** Increased phenytoin levels. **Rifampin:** Decreased fluconazole levels. **Warfarin:** Increased prothrombin time.

NURSING CONSIDERATIONS

Assessment
General:
Hypersensitivity.
Physical:
GI tract.
Lab Alterations:
Monitor BUN/creatinine and liver enzymes to assess for hepatorenal toxicity and consider drug discontinuation.

Intervention/Rationale
Obtain specimens for fungal culture, serology, and histopathology prior to therapy to identify causative organism. ● Monitor renal function to adjust dosage. ● Evaluate or treat nausea, vomiting, or abdominal discomfort.

Patient/Family Education
Explain purpose of drug and potential therapeutic outcome. Report excess fatigue, malaise, abdominal pain to physician/nurse.

FLUDARABINE
(floo-dare'-a-been)
Trade Name(s): Fludara
Classification(s): Antimetabolite antineoplastic agent
Pregnancy Category: D

PHARMACODYNAMICS/KINETICS

Mechanism of Action: Inhibits DNA synthesis. **Distribution:** Distributed throughout the body. **Metabolism/ Elimination:** Rapidly converted to an active metabolite. Excreted by the kidneys. **Half-Life:** 10 hr (metabolite).

INDICATIONS/DOSAGE

Treatment of unresponsive chronic lymphocytic leukemia
Adult: 25 mg/m² daily for 5 days. Repeat every 28 days. Reduce dosage based on hematologic profile.

CONTRAINDICATIONS/ PRECAUTIONS

Contraindicated in: Hypersensitivity to the drug or its components. **Use cautiously in:** Renal impairment, severe bone marrow depression. **Pregnancy/Lactation:** No well-controlled trials to establish safety. Teratogenic/mutagenic potential is documented. Benefits must outweigh risks. Patient should avoid conception/pregnancy. **Pediatrics:** Safety and efficacy has not been established.

PREPARATION

Availability: 50 mg vials. **Reconstitution:** Dilute with 2 mL sterile water for injection. Final concentration 25 mg/mL. **Infusion:** Further dilute in 100–125 mL compatible IV solution.

STABILITY/STORAGE

Vial: Refrigerate vial. Stable for 8 hr after reconstitution. **Infusion:** Stable for 24 hr at room temperature.

In the Adverse Effects section, underline indicates most frequent; CAPS indicates life threatening.

ADMINISTRATION

General: Handle drug with care and adhere to institutional guidelines for the handling of chemotherapeutic/cytotoxic agents. Avoid exposure to skin and/or inhalation. **Intermittent Infusion:** Infuse over 30 min.

COMPATIBILITY

Solution: Dextrose solutions, sodium chloride solutions.

ADVERSE EFFECTS

CNS: Coma, agitation, confusion. **Ophtho:** Visual disturbances. **CV:** Pericardial effusion, edema. **Resp:** Cough, dyspnea, interstitial pulmonary infiltrates, pneumonia. **GI:** Anorexia, diarrhea, GI bleeding, stomatitis, <u>nausea/vomiting</u>. **Derm:** Skin rash. **Heme:** <u>MYELOSUPPRESSION</u>, anemia, thrombocytopenia, neutropenia. **Nadir:** 13 days. **Other:** <u>Fever</u>, <u>chills</u>, <u>infection</u>, fatigue, tumor lysis syndrome (hyperuricemia, hyperphosphatemia, hyperkalemia, hypocalcemia, metabolic acidosis, renal failure).

TOXICITY/OVERDOSE

Signs/Symptoms: Irreversible CNS toxicity, severe bone marrow depression. **Treatment:** Symptomatic and supportive.

DRUG INTERACTIONS

Immunosuppressants: Increased myelosuppression.

NURSING CONSIDERATIONS

Assessment

General:
Vital signs.
Physical:
Infectious disease status, GI tract, hematopoietic system, neurologic status, cardiopulmonary system.

Lab Alterations:
Monitor baseline and periodic electrolytes, BUN/creatinine, uric acid, CBC with differential, and platelet count.

Intervention/Rationale

Assess for development of fever, chills, or other signs of infection. ● Avoid all IM injections and rectal temperatures when platelet count < 100,000 mm³. ● Assess for development of bleeding (bleeding gums, easy bruising, petechiae, hematest positive stools/vomitus/urine). ● Assure that proper antiemetic regimens are prescribed and given regularly to prevent nausea/vomiting. ● Discontinue therapy with signs of toxicity (stomatitis, rapidly falling WBC count, leukopenia, intractable vomiting, diarrhea, GI ulcers/bleeding, thrombocytopenia/hemorrhage). ● Evaluate mental status for confusion or agitation.

Patient/Family Education

Review expected outcome and potential adverse effects of drug especially expected loss of hair. Drink plenty of fluids. Observe for signs of infection (fever, sore throat, fatigue) or bleeding (melena, bleeding gums, nosebleeds, easy bruising). Use a soft toothbrush and electric razor to minimize bleeding tendency. Take and record oral temperature daily and report persistent elevations to physician. Avoid crowded environments and persons with known infections especially 13 days after treatment. Use consistent and reliable contra-

In the Adverse Effects section, <u>underline</u> indicates most frequent; CAPS indicates life threatening.

ception throughout the duration of therapy and 4 months after due to potential teratogenic and mutagenic effects of drug. Seek physician approval prior to receiving live virus vaccinations. Avoid over-the-counter products containing aspirin/ibuprofen throughout course of therapy due to increased potential for bleeding. Report dizziness, unusual fatigue, or shortness of breath (drug may cause anemia) or unusual GI symptoms.

FLUMAZENIL
(flu-maz′-a-nil)
Trade Name(s): Mazicon
Classification(s): Benzodiazepine antagonist
Pregnancy Category: C

PHARMACODYNAMICS/KINETICS
Mechanism of Action: Competitive antagonist at benzodiazepine receptor sites. **Onset of Action:** 1–2 min. **Peak Effect:** 6–10 min. **Distribution:** Distributed throughout body especially in CNS. 50% protein binding. **Metabolism/Elimination:** Primarily hepatically metabolized. Metabolites excreted in urine (complete within 72 hr). **Half-Life:** 41–79 min.

INDICATIONS/DOSAGE

Complete or partial reversal of sedative effects of benzodiazepine.

Reversal of conscious sedation, reversal in general anesthesia
Adult: 0.2 mg. If response is not adequate after 45 sec, dose may be repeated. Additional doses may be

given every 60 sec, up to a maximum of four additional times.

Suspected benzodiazepine overdose management
Adult: 0.2 mg. If response is not adequate after 30 sec, 0.3 mg may be given. Additional 0.5 mg doses may be given every 60 seconds, up to a cumulative dose of 3 mg. If resedation occurs, repeated doses may be given every 20 minutes; not to exceed 3 mg in 1 hr.

CONTRAINDICATIONS/PRECAUTIONS
Contraindicated in: Hypersensitivity, severe cyclic antidepressant overdose, patients given benzodiazepine for control of potentially, life-threatening condition (e.g., status epilepticus, increased intracranial pressure). **Use cautiously in:** Cardiovascular disease, concomitant neuromuscular blocking agents, drug/alcohol dependent patients, head injury, liver disease, psychiatric patients, respiratory disease. **Pregnancy/Lactation:** No well-controlled trials to establish safety. Benefits must outweigh risks. **Pediatrics:** Safety and efficacy has not been established.

PREPARATION
Availability: 0.1 mg/mL, 5 and 10 mL multidose vials.

STABILITY/STORAGE
Vial: Store at room temperature. **Syringe:** Stable for 24 hr in syringe. Recommended to prepare just prior to administration.

ADMINISTRATION
General: Administer through freely running IV solution into a large

In the Adverse Effects section, underline indicates most frequent; CAPS indicates life threatening.

235

vein. Provide for secure airway prior to administration. Initiate therapy slowly. **IV Push:** *Reversal of Conscious Sedation or in General Anesthesia:* Give over 15 seconds. **Reversal of Overdose:** Give over 30 sec.

COMPATIBILITY
Solution: Dextrose solutions, lactated Ringer's, sodium chloride solutions.

ADVERSE EFFECTS
CNS: Anxiety, dizziness, emotional lability, insomnia, nervousness, paresthesia, tremor. **Ophtho:** Abnormal vision, diplopia. **CV:** Bradycardia, chest pain, dysrhythmia, tachycardia. **GI:** Dry mouth, nausea, vomiting. **Other:** Fatigue, flushing, hot flashes, pain at injection site, rigors, shivering, sweating, tinnitus.

TOXICITY/OVERDOSE
Signs/Symptoms: Extension of pharmacologic effects. Excessive doses may produce anxiety, agitation, increased muscle tone, hyperesthesia, and seizures. **Treatment:** Symptomatic and supportive therapy.

NURSING CONSIDERATIONS
Assessment
General:
Vital signs.
Physical:
Mental status, cardiopulmonary status, patent airway.

Intervention/Rationale
Monitor for resedation, respiratory depression, or other persistent/recurrent benzodiazepine effects for an adequate period of time after administration. Secure airway/ventilation and venous access since patient may become confused and agitated on arousal and attempt to remove endotracheal tube and/or IV lines. ● Evaluate vital signs for dysrhythmia development.

Patient/Family Education
Amnesic effects of benzodiazepines are not reversed; reinforce postprocedural instructions in writing or with responsible family members. Avoid activities requiring mental alertness for up to 18–24 hr after administration and effects of benzodiazepines are no longer evident. Avoid alcohol or over-the-counter medications for 18–24 hr after administration.

FLUOROURACIL (5-FU)
(floor-oh-yoor′-a-sill)
Trade Name(s): Adrucil
Classification(s): Antimetabolite antineoplastic agent
Pregnancy Category: D

PHARMACODYNAMICS/KINETICS
Mechanism of Action: Interferes with DNA and RNA synthesis. **Distribution:** Distributes into tumors, intestinal mucosa, bone marrow, liver, and body tissues. Diffuses readily into CSF and brain tissue. **Metabolism/Elimination:** Major portion degraded in liver to inactive metabolites with a small portion converted to an active metabolite. Unchanged drug is eliminated in urine (7%–20%). Inactive metabolites are excreted through respiration as carbon dioxide and as urea in the urine. **Half-Life:** 8–20 min (dose dependent).

In the Adverse Effects section, <u>underline</u> indicates most frequent; CAPS indicates life threatening.

INDICATIONS/DOSAGE

Palliative management of carcinoma of colon, rectum, breast, stomach, and pancreas

Adult: Individualize dosage and base on actual body weight. (Use ideal body weight in obese patients).

Initial dose: 12 mg/kg once daily for 4 days (not to exceed 800 mg/day). If no toxic symptoms, 6 mg/kg on days 6, 8, 10, 12. Discontinue after day 12. If poor risk or nutritional status, 6 mg/kg once daily for 3 days (not to exceed 400 mg/day). If no toxic symptoms, 3 mg/kg on days 5, 7, 9. Discontinue a course of therapy with any signs of toxicity.

Maintenance Dose: Repeat dosage of first course every 30 days after last day of previous treatment—OR, if toxic signs have subsided, 10–15 mg/kg/week as a single dose (not to exceed 1 g/week). Use reduced doses for poor risk patients. Some patients have received 9–45 courses over 12–60 months.

CONTRAINDICATIONS/ PRECAUTIONS

Contraindicated in: Depressed bone marrow function, hypersensitivity, poor nutritional status, potentially serious infections. **Use cautiously in:** Patients with preexisting coronary artery disease. **Pregnancy/Lactation:** No well-controlled trials to establish safety. Teratogenic/mutagenic potential is documented. Crosses the placenta. Benefits must outweigh risks. Patients should avoid conception/pregnancy. Excreted in breast milk. Breastfeeding should

be discontinued while receiving this agent. **Pediatrics:** Safety and efficacy has not been established.

PREPARATION

Availability: 50 mg/mL in 10, 20, 50, 100 mL vials/amps. **Syringe:** No further dilution required. **Infusion:** Dilute in physician specified volume of compatible IV solution sufficient to infuse over specified time.

STABILITY/STORAGE

Vial: Store at room temperature. Protect from light. Solution may discolor during storage (potency/safety not adversely affected). If crystals form, heat to 140° F (60° C) and shake vigorously. Cool to body temperature prior to using. **Infusion:** Stable for 7 days at room temperature.

ADMINISTRATION

General: Handle drug with care and adhere to institutional guidelines for the handling of chemotherapeutic/cytotoxic agents. Avoid extravasation. In the event of a spill, use a 5% sodium hypochlorite solution (household bleach) to inactivate fluorouracil. **IV Push:** May be given by direct IV push over 1–2 min. **Continuous Infusion:** Administer over physician specified time.

COMPATIBILITY

Solution: Amino acids 4.25%/dextrose 25%, dextrose solutions, sodium chloride solutions. **Syringe:** Bleomycin, cisplatin, cyclophosphamide, doxorubicin, furosemide, heparin, leucovorin calcium, methotrexate, metoclopramide, mitomycin, vinblastine, vincristine. **Y-site:** Bleomycin, cisplatin, cyclophosphamide, doxorubicin, furosemide,

In the Adverse Effects section, <u>underline</u> indicates most frequent; CAPS indicates life threatening.

237

heparin, hydrocortisone, leucovorin calcium, methotrexate, metoclopramide, mitomycin, potassium chloride, vinblastine, vincristine, vitamin B complex.

INCOMPATIBILITY
Syringe: Droperidol. **Y-site:** Droperidol.

ADVERSE EFFECTS
CNS: Acute cerebellar syndrome, confusion, disorientation, euphoria, headache, lethargy, malaise, weakness. **Ophtho:** Decreased vision, diplopia, lacrimation, nystagmus, photophobia, visual changes. **CV:** Myocardial ischemia, angina. **GI:** Anorexia, bleeding, cramps, <u>diarrhea</u>, <u>enteritis</u>, esophagopharyngitis, gastritis, GI ulceration, glossitis, increased alkaline phosphatase, serum transaminase, bilirubin, lactic dehydrogenase, <u>nausea</u>, pharyngitis, <u>stomatitis</u>, <u>vomiting</u>. **Derm:** <u>Alopecia</u>, dermatitis, dry skin, fissuring, nail changes/losses, photosensitivity, vein pigmentation. **Heme:** AGRANULOCYTOSIS, <u>ANEMIA</u>, <u>LEUKOPENIA</u>, PANCYTOPENIA, <u>THROMBOCYTOPENIA</u>. **Nadir:** 9–14 days. **Hypersens:** ANAPHYLAXIS. **Other:** Epistaxis, fever.

TOXICITY/OVERDOSE
Signs/Symptoms: Extension of adverse effects especially bone marrow depression and GI effects. **Treatment:** Symptomatic and supportive. Monitor hematologic profile closely for 4 weeks.

DRUG INTERACTIONS
Immunosuppressants: Increased myelosuppression. **Leucovorin calcium:** Increased response rate and reduced time to progression. May increase 5-FU adverse effects.

NURSING CONSIDERATIONS
Assessment
General:
Vital signs.
Physical:
Infectious disease status, GI tract, hematopoietic system.
Lab Alterations:
Monitor baseline and periodic hepatic function, BUN/creatinine, uric acid, CBC with differential, and platelet count.

Intervention/Rationale
Assess for development of fever, chills, or other signs of infection. ● Avoid all IM injections and rectal temperatures when platelet count < 100,000 mm³. ● Assess for development of bleeding (bleeding gums, easy bruising, petechiae, hematest positive stools/vomitus/urine). ● Assure that proper antiemetic regimen are prescribed and given regularly to prevent nausea/vomiting. ● Discontinue therapy with signs of toxicity (stomatitis/esophagopharyngitis, rapidly falling WBC count, leukopenia, intractable vomiting, diarrhea, GI ulcers/bleeding, thrombocytopenia/hemorrhage). ● Monitor all vital signs for development of adverse effects.

Patient/Family Education
Review expected outcome and potential adverse effects of drug especially expected loss of hair. Drink plenty of fluids. Observe for signs of infection (fever, sore throat, fatigue) or bleeding (melena, bleeding gums, nosebleeds, easy bruising). Use a soft toothbrush and electric razor to minimize bleeding

In the Adverse Effects section, <u>underline</u> indicates most frequent; CAPS indicates life threatening.

tendency. Take and record oral temperature daily and report persistent elevations to physician. Avoid crowded environments and persons with known infections especially days 9–14 after treatment. Use consistent and reliable contraception throughout the duration of therapy and 4 months after due to potential teratogenic and mutagenic effects of drug. Seek physician approval prior to receiving live virus vaccinations. Avoid over-the-counter products containing aspirin/ibuprofen throughout course of therapy due to increased potential for bleeding. Report dizziness, unusual fatigue, or shortness of breath (drug may cause anemia). Observe for GI symptoms (mouth ulcerations, yellowing of skin/eyes, abdominal pain, significant diarrhea) and notify physician/nurse.

FOLIC ACID

(foe'-lik-a'-sid)
Trade Name(s): Folvite
Classification(s): Water soluble vitamin
Pregnancy Category: A

PHARMACODYNAMICS/KINETICS
Mechanism of Action: Incorporated in nucleic acid synthesis and RBC development/function. **Distribution:** Distributed in all body tissues and into liver (50%). Concentrated in CSF. **Metabolism/Elimination:** Transported and stored in the body as methyltetrahydrofolic acid (tetrahydrofolic acid is a cofactor in protein synthesis). Excess folate is eliminated in the urine. Removed by hemodialysis.

INDICATIONS/DOSAGE
Patients with alcoholism, hemolytic anemia, and those receiving anticonvulsants may require higher doses.

Treatment of megaloblastic anemias
Adult/Pediatrics: 0.25–1.0 mg daily.

Supplement in pregnancy for fetal development
Adult: 0.8–1.0 mg daily.

Maintenance therapy in folic acid deficiency and prophylaxis
Adult: 0.4–1.0 mg daily.

Pediatric: > 4 years old: 0.4 mg daily. < 4 years old: 0.3 mg daily. *Neonate:* 0.1 mg daily. Premature infants 0.05 mg (15 mcg/kg/day) daily.

CONTRAINDICATIONS/ PRECAUTIONS
Contraindicated in: Aplastic, normocytic, and pernicious anemias (ineffective). **Use cautiously in:** Pernicous anemia to avoid masking diagnosis. **Pregnancy/Lactation:** Folate administration during pregnancy is necessary for normal fetal development.

PREPARATION
Availability: 5 mg/mL and 10 mg/mL in 10 mL vials. **Infusion:** Dilute 5 mg (1 mL) with at least 49 mL compatible IV solution for a final concentation 100 mcg/mL.

STABILITY/STORAGE
Vial: Store at controlled room temperature. Protect from light. **Infusion:** Stable under fluorescent lighting for 48 hr.

F

In the Adverse Effects section, <u>underline</u> indicates most frequent; CAPS indicates life threatening.

ADMINISTRATION
IV Push: Give by direct IV push at a rate of 5 mg/min. **Intermittent Infusion:** Administer at physician specified rate.

COMPATIBILITY
Solution: Amino acids 4.25%/dextrose 25%, dextrose 5%, dextrose 20%. **Y-site:** Famotidine.

INCOMPATIBILITY
Syringe: Doxapram.

ADVERSE EFFECTS
Resp: BRONCHOSPASM. **Hypersens:** ANAPHYLAXIS, erythema, itching, rash. **Other:** Malaise.

TOXICITY/OVERDOSE
Signs/Symptoms: Relatively nontoxic.

DRUG INTERACTIONS
Chloramphenicol: Antagonizes hematopoietic response to folic acid. **Oral contraceptives:** May produce folate depletion. **Phenytoin:** Increased phenytoin metabolism/decreased serum levels. **Pyrimethamine:** Inhibits antimicrobial effects against toxoplasmosis. Interferes with folic acid use. **Trimethoprim, triamterene:** Interferes with folic acid use.

NURSING CONSIDERATIONS
Assessment
General:
Overall nutritional status.
Physical:
Observe for improvement of presenting symptoms, GI tract, hematologic profile.
Lab Alterations:
Falsely low serum/erythrocyte folate levels with *L. casei* assay with concurrent anti-infective agent use.

Monitor hematologic profile including folate levels, hemoglobin/hematocrit, and reticulocyte count (response indicated by increases in 2–5 days).

Intervention/Rationale
Prior to instituting therapy, diagnosis should exclude pernicious anemia. ● Dietary history, baseline weight, and daily nutritional needs should be evaluated.

Patient/Family Education
Increased folic acid requirements may be associated with pregnancy, lactation, alcoholism, hemolytic anemia, and patients receiving anticonvulsant therapy. Continue therapy as per physician instructions. Supplement medication with a diet high in folic acid (fresh vegetables, fruit, organ meats) to enhance therapy. Urine may become intensely dark yellow during therapy.

FOSCARNET
(foss'-car-net)
Trade Name(s): Foscavir
Classification(s): Antiviral
Pregnancy Category: C

PHARMACODYNAMICS/KINETICS
Mechanism of Action: Inhibits viral replication of CMV as well as herpes simplex (HSV-1 and HSV-2), Epstein Barr, and varicella zoster. **Peak Serum Level:** 1 hr. **Distribution:** Preferential distribution into viral infected cells. Accumulates in bone. Variable penetration into CSF. 14%–17% plasma protein binding. **Metabolism/Elimination:** Primarily eliminated unchanged by the kidneys (80–90%) via tubular

In the Adverse Effects section, underline indicates most frequent; CAPS indicates life threatening.

secretion and glomerular filtration. **Half-Life:** 2–8 hr. Increased in renal impairment.

INDICATIONS/DOSAGE

Treatment of cytomegalovirus retinitis in patients with acquired immune deficiency syndrome (AIDS).

Adult:
Induction: 60 mg/kg every 8 hr for 2–3 weeks based on patient response. **Maintenance:** 90–120 mg/kg/day. Reduce dosage in renal impairment based on creatinine clearance

CONTRAINDICATIONS/ PRECAUTIONS

Contraindicated in: Hypersensitivity. **Use cautiously in:** Concurrent nephrotoxins and hypocalcemic agents, elderly, electrolyte imbalance, neurotoxicity, renal impairment, seizure history. **Pregnancy/Lactation:** No well-controlled trials to establish safety. Benefits must outweigh risks. **Pediatrics:** Safety and efficacy not established.

PREPARATION

Availability: 24 mg/mL in 250 and 500 mL infusion bottles. **Infusion:** Must be infused into a central vein if undiluted. Dilute to 12 mg/mL with compatible IV solution if given through a peripheral vein.

STABILITY/STORAGE

Vial: Store at room temperature. **Infusion:** Stable for 24 hr after first entry of sterile IV bottle.

ADMINISTRATION

General: Handle drug with care and adhere to institutional guidelines for the handling of chemotherapeutic/cytotoxic agents. Avoid rapid or bolus IV injection. Carefully control rate of infusion via use of infusion pump. Hydration is required prior to and during treatment to minimize renal toxicity. **Intermittent Infusion:** Infuse over at least 1 hr for induction or over 2 hr for maintenance.

COMPATIBILITY
Solution: Dextrose 5%, sodium chloride 0.9%.

INCOMPATIBILITY
Solution: Dextrose 30%, Ringer's injection.

ADVERSE EFFECTS
CNS: Seizures, aphasia, ataxia, dementia, dizziness, headache, involuntary muscle contractions, paresthesias, stupor, tremors. **Ophtho:** Conjunctivitis, diplopia, eye/vision abnormalities, photophobia. **CV:** Cardiomyopathy, ECG abnormalities (sinus tachycardia, first degree AV block), hypertension, hypotension. **Resp:** Respiratory insufficiency/failure, coughing, dyspnea, pneumonia, pharyngitis, rhinitis, sinustitis. **GI:** Abdominal pain, anorexia, constipation, diarrhea, nausea, vomiting. **GU:** Gynecomastia, hematuria, nocturia, penile inflammation, perineal pain (women), polyuria, urinary incontinence/retention. **Renal:** Acute renal failure, altered renal function. **MS:** Arthralgia, myalgia, synovitis, torticollis. **Derm:** Skin ulceration. **Endo:** Antidiuretic hormone disorders, diabetes mellitus. **Fld/Lytes:** Mineral/electrolyte imbalance (hypokalemia, hypocalcemia, hypomagnesemia, hy-

In the Adverse Effects section, underline indicates most frequent; CAPS indicates life threatening.

241

po/hyperphosphatemia). **Heme:** Anemia, granulocytopenia, leukopenia. **Hypersens:** Pruritus, rash. **Other:** Flushing, increased sweating, pain at injection site.

TOXICITY/OVERDOSE

Signs/Symptoms: Bone marrow depression, extension of adverse effects especially paresthesia, seizures, electrolyte disturbance (magnesium/phosphate), and impaired renal function. **Treatment:** Supportive, hemodialysis and hydration may be beneficial.

DRUG INTERACTIONS

Aminoglycosides, amphotericin B, nephrotoxic agents: Increased nephrotoxicity potential. **Pentamidine IV:** Increased nephrotoxic hypocalcemia risk. **Zidovudine:** Additive anemia effects.

NURSING CONSIDERATIONS

Assessment
General:
Maintain adequte hydration, intake/output ratio.
Physical:
Neurologic/mental status, cardiopulmonary status, skin and mucosal lesions (assess for improvement/change), ophthalmologic findings.
Lab Alterations:
Monitor BUN, creatinine, CBC/differential, platelet count, and electrolytes especially calcium/magnesium.

Intervention/Rationale
Adequate hydration should be given concurrently to enhance renal elimination. ● Neutrophil and platelet counts should be monitored every 2 days initially and weekly once maintenance therapy has begun. If prior history of foscarnet-bone marrow suppression, monitor counts daily. Severe neutropenia (ANC < 500) or thrombocytopenia (< 25,000) require interruption of therapy until recovery is observed (ANC ≥ 750). ● If renal impairment is identified, dosage adjustment should be done. ● Evaluate patient for neurologic changes (grand mal seizures).

Patient/Family Education
Treatment is not a cure for CMV; use is reserved for immunocompromised patients only. Regular opthalmic examinations are necessary to minimize progression of the disease. Maintain good oral fluid intake/hydration. Avoid persons with known infections and crowds. Notify physician/nurse of signs of decreased WBC counts, and/or infection (fever, sore throat, fatigue), and bleeding (increased bruising, nosebleeds, bleeding gums, melena). Instruct patient to use a soft toothbrush and electric razor to minimize bleeding tendency. Check oral temperatures daily. Caution male and female patients of teratogenic potential effects and to use contraceptive measures during therapy and for up to 4 months following treatment.

FUROSEMIDE
(fur-oh′-se-mide)
Trade Name(s): Lasix
Classification(s): Loop diuretic
Pregnancy Category: C

In the Adverse Effects section, underline indicates most frequent; CAPS indicates life threatening.

PHARMACODYNAMICS/KINETICS

Mechanism of Action: Inhibits sodium and chloride reabsorption in the ascending loop of Henle and to a lesser extent in the proximal and distal tubules. Increases excretion of sodium, chloride, potassium, hydrogen, calcium, magnesium, ammonium, phosphate, and bicarbonate. Dilates renal vasculature and increases renal blood flow. **Onset of Action:** Within 5 min. **Peak Effect:** 30 min. **Duration of Action:** 2 hr. **Distribution:** Highly protein bound (> 90%). **Metabolism/Elimination:** Metabolized by the liver (30%–40%). Excreted primarily unchanged by the kidneys (60%–70%). **Half-Life:** 120 min. Increased in renal failure, CHF, and in neonates.

INDICATIONS/DOSAGE

Individualize dosage. Higher dosages may be necessary especially in renal impairment. Not to exceed 600 mg/day.

Treatment of acute pulmonary edema

Adult: Initially 40 mg. If no response, give 80 mg after 1 hr.

Pediatric: 1 mg/kg/dose. If no diuretic response, increase dosage by 1 mg/kg at intervals of 6–12 hr. Not to exceed 6 mg/kg/dose.

Neonates (Premature): 1–2 mg/kg/dose every 12–24 hr.

Treatment of edema

Adult: Initially 20–40 mg. Increase dose by 20 mg and repeat dose in 2 hr if necessary until response is achieved.

Pediatric: 1 mg/kg/dose. If no diuretic response, increase dosage by 1 mg/kg at intervals of 6–12 hr. Not to exceed 6 mg/kg/dose.

Neonates (Premature): 1–2 mg/kg/dose every 12–24 hr.

CONTRAINDICATIONS/PRECAUTIONS

Contraindicated in: Anuria, hypersensitivity to furosemide or related agents. **Use cautiously in:** Allergy to sulfa drugs/bumetanide, hepatic coma, hyperuricemia, hypokalemia, increasing BUN and creatinine, ototoxicity, severe electrolyte imbalance. **Pregnancy/Lactation:** No well-controlled trials to establish safety. Animal studies demonstrate fetal hydronephrosis. Benefits must outweigh risks. Appears in breast milk. Breastfeeding should be discontinued. **Pediatrics:** Increased incidence of patent ductus arteriosus and renal calcifications (concomitant chlorothiazide is required to prevent) in premature infants.

PREPARATION

Availability: 10 mg/mL in 2, 4, and 10 mL ampules/vials. **Infusion:** Dilute in compatible IV solution to physician specified volume.

STABILITY/STORAGE

Vial: Store at room temperature. Protect from light. **Infusion:** Prepare just prior to administration and use within 24 hr.

ADMINISTRATION

General: Administer maintenance dose once or twice daily. Tinnitus, reversible or permanent hearing impairment have occurred follow-

In the Adverse Effects section, underline indicates most frequent; CAPS indicates life threatening.

243

ing rapid IV administration. **IV Push:** Give undiluted slowly over 1–2 min. Not to exceed 40 mg/min. **Intermittent/Continuous Infusion:** Administer at physician specified rate. High doses (greater than 120–200 mg) should not exceed 4 mg/min (adult) or 0.5 mg/kg/min (pediatric) to avoid ototoxicity.

COMPATIBILITY
Solution: Amino acid 4.25%/dextrose 25%, dextrose solutions, lactated Ringer's, Ringer's injection, sodium chloride solutions. **Syringe:** Bleomycin, cisplatin, cyclophosphamide, fluorouracil, heparin, leucovorin calcium, methotrexate, mitomycin, vinblastine, vincristine. **Y-site:** Amikacin, cisplatin, cyclophosphamide, famotidine, fluorouracil, foscarnet, heparin, hydrocortisone, leucovorin calcium, methotrexate, mitomycin, potassium chloride, tobramycin, tolazoline, vitamin B complex with C.

INCOMPATIBILITY
Solution: Acidic solutions with pH < 5.5. **Syringe:** Doxapram, doxorubicin, droperidol, metoclopramide, milrinone. **Y-site:** Doxorubicin, droperidol, esmolol, gentamicin, hydralazine, metoclopramide, milrinone, netilmicin, ondansetron, quinidine gluconate, vinblastine, vincristine.

ADVERSE EFFECTS
CNS: Blurred vision, dizziness, headache, paresthesias. **CV:** <u>Orthostatic hypotension</u>, irregular heartbeat. **GI:** Encephalopathy (especially with preexisting liver disease), diarrhea, dry mouth, nausea, vomiting. **GU:** Glycosuria, urinary bladder spasm. **Renal:** Increased serum creatinine. **MS:** <u>Muscle cramps</u>, <u>muscle weakness</u>. **Derm:** Photosensitivity. **Endo:** Hyperglycemia. **Fld/Lytes:** Dehydration, <u>electrolyte disturbances</u> (hypomagnesemia, hypocalcemia, hyponatremia), <u>hypokalemia</u>. **Heme:** Anemia, asymptomatic hyperuricemia, leukopenia. **Hypersens:** Rash. **Metab:** Acid-base disturbances, metabolic alkalosis. **Other:** Ototoxicity (hearing loss), thrombophlebitis.

TOXICITY/OVERDOSE
Signs/Symptoms: Acute profound water loss/dehydration, circulatory collapse. **Treatment:** Fluid/electrolye replacement, supportive therapy.

DRUG INTERACTIONS
Aminoglycosides, amphotericin B, nephrotoxic agents: Increased risk of oto/nephrotoxicity. **Antihypertensives:** Additive hypotensive effect. **Digitalis glycosides:** Increased potential for digitalis toxicity and hypokalemic-induced dysrhythmia. **Diuretics:** Concurrent use enhances volume depletion. **Lithium:** Decreased excretion, possible lithium toxicity. **Neuromuscular blocking agents:** Enhanced neuromuscular blockade.

NURSING CONSIDERATIONS
Assessment
General:
Blood pressure, intake/output ratio, baseline and daily weight.
Physical:
Hearing function, musculoskeletal system.
Lab Alterations:
Monitor electrolytes (serum potassium daily), hepatic and renal function tests, serum glucose, and uric acid concentrations prior to and during therapy.

In the Adverse Effects section, <u>underline</u> indicates most frequent; CAPS indicates life threatening.

Intervention/Rationale

Assess for signs/symptoms of dehydration (skin turgor, mucous membranes, hypotension). Drug may lead to profound water/electrolyte depletion. Monitor urine output to assess therapeutic response. Drug may cause muscle weakness and cramps due to hypokalemia. ● Assess patients receiving digitalis glycosides for signs/symptoms of toxicity (nausea, vomiting, anorexia, visual disturbances, confusion, cardiac rhythm disturbances), especially when hypokalemia is present.

Patient/Family Education

Change positions slowly to avoid orthostatic hypotension. Notify nurse/physician if muscle cramps/weakness occur. Note any signs of dehydration (decreased urination, loss of skin turgor, excessive thirst, and leg cramps). Avoid excessive exposure to sunlight. Encourage diet high in potassium containing foods.

GALLIUM NITRATE
(gal-ee′-um nye′-trate)
Trade Name(s): Ganite
Classification(s): Hypocalcemic agent
Pregnancy Category: C

PHARMACODYNAMICS/KINETICS
Mechanism of Action: Inhibits bone calcium resorption by reducing increased bone turnover, resulting in a hypocalcemic effect. **Onset of Action:** 24–48 hr. **Duration of Action:** 7.5 days. **Distribution:** Distributed throughout body. **Metabolism/Elimination:** Primarily excreted unchanged by the kidneys. **Half-Life:** 25–111 hr.

INDICATIONS/DOSAGE

Treatment of symptomatic cancer-related hypercalcemia unresponsive to hydration
Adult: 200 mg/m^2 daily for 5 consecutive days. Mild symptomatic patients may use 100 mg/m^2 daily. Treatment may be discontinued if serum levels normalize prior to day 5. Discontinue therapy if serum creatinine > 2.5 mg/dL.

CONTRAINDICATIONS/PRECAUTIONS
Contraindicated in: Severe renal impairment (serum creatinine > 2.5 mg/dL). **Use cautiously in:** Compromised cardiovascular states, mild renal impairment. **Pregnancy/Lactation:** No well-controlled trials to establish safety. Benefits must outweigh risks. **Pediatrics:** Safety and efficacy not established.

PREPARATION
Availability: 25 mg/mL in 20 mL vials. **Infusion:** Dilute dose in 1000 mL compatible IV solution, discard unused portion (no preservative).

STABILITY/STORAGE
Vial: Store at room temperature. **Infusion:** Stable for 48 hr at room temperature and 7 days refrigerated.

ADMINISTRATION
General: Adequate oral/IV hydration must be established with good urine output (2 L/day) prior to initiation of therapy. **Continuous Infusion:** Infuse over 24 hr.

In the Adverse Effects section, <u>underline</u> indicates most frequent; CAPS indicates life threatening.

COMPATIBILITY
Solution: Dextrose solutions, sodium chloride solutions.

ADVERSE EFFECTS
CNS: Confusion, lethargy, paresthesia. **Ophtho:** Acute optic neuritis, impaired vision. **CV:** Tachycardia, lower extremity edema, hypotension. **Resp:** Dyspnea, rales/rhonchi, pleural effusion. **GI:** Constipation, diarrhea, nausea, vomiting. **Renal:** Acute renal failure, increased BUN/creatinine. **Fld/Lytes:** Hypocalcemia, decreased sodium bicarbonate (asymptomatic), transient hypophosphatemia. **Heme:** Anemia, neutropenia. **Hypersens:** Rash. **Metab:** Hypothermia. **Other:** Decreased hearing, fever.

TOXICITY/OVERDOSE
Signs/Symptoms: Nausea, vomiting, renal insufficiency. **Treatment:** Discontinue infusion, monitor calcium, symptomatic/supportive especially hydration.

DRUG INTERACTIONS
Aminoglycosides, amphotericin B, nephrotoxic agents: Increased potential of renal insufficiency.

NURSING CONSIDERATIONS
Assessment
General:
Intake/output ratio, vital signs, daily weight.
Physical:
Cardiopulmonary status, hydration status.
Lab Alterations:
Monitor renal function (serum creatinine/BUN), calcium, phosphorus at baseline and during therapy.

Intervention/Rationalenur
Assess lung fields for development of adventitious sounds. ● Maintain adequate hydration prior to and during therapy. ● Evaluate blood pressure and heart rate/rhythm for development of hypotensive resultant dysrhythmias.

Patient/Family Education
Review therapeutic outcome and expected adverse effects.

GANCICLOVIR (DHPG)
(gan-sye'-kloe-vir)
Trade Name(s): Cytovene
Classification(s): Antiviral
Pregnancy Category: C

PHARMACODYNAMICS/KINETICS
Mechanism of Action: Inhibits viral replication of CMV as well as herpes simplex (HSV-1 and HSV-2), Epstein Barr, and varicella zoster. **Peak Serum Level:** 1 hr. **Distribution:** Preferential distribution into CMV infected cells. Good ocular concentration. Limited data suggests concentration in the kidneys as well as significant levels in the lungs. Poor CNS penetration. 1%–2% plasma protein binding. **Metabolism/Elimination:** Minimal hepatic metabolism since conversion occurs within the viral cells. Primarily eliminated unchanged (>90%) by glomerular filtration. Removed by hemodialysis (50%). **Half-Life:** 2.53–3.6 hr. Increased in renal impairment 13 hr from the vitreous humor.

INDICATIONS/DOSAGE
Reduce dosage and/or interval in renal impairment. Reduce dosage or discontinue therapy if severe bone marrow depression occurs.

In the Adverse Effects section, underline indicates most frequent; CAPS indicates life threatening.

Treatment of cytomegalovirus retinitis in immunocompromised patients

Adult:

Induction: 5 mg/kg every 12 hr for 14–21 days. **Maintenance:** 5 mg/kg/day for 7 days/week. **Alternate Regimen:** 6 mg/kg/day for 5 days/week. **If Disease Progression Occurs:** Retreatment with dosing every 12 hr may be necessary. **Dosage reductions based on creatinine clearance (Clcr):**

- Clcr 50–79 mL/min: 2.5 mg/kg every 12 hr.
- Clcr 25–49 mL/min; 2.5 mg/kg every 24 hr.
- Clcr < 25 mL/min: 1.25 mg/kg every 24 hr.

Hemodialysis: Administer dose after dialysis. Not to exceed 1.25 mg/kg/day. Monitor neutrophil/platelet counts daily.

Pediatric (unlabeled use):

Induction: 2.5 mg/kg/day every 8 hr. **Maintenance:** 6–6.5 mg/kg/day for 5–7 days/week. **If Disease Progression Occurs:** 5 mg/kg every 12 hr.

Extraocular CMV infections including GI infections, pneumonitis, hepatobiliary infections (*unlabeled use*)

Adult:

Induction: 5 mg/kg every 12 hr for 14–21 days. **Alternate Regimen:** 2.5 mg/kg every 8 hr. **Maintenance:** 5 mg/kg/day for 7 days a week. **Alternate Regimen:** 6 mg/kg/day for 5 days a week. **If Disease Progression Occurs:** Retreatment with dosing every 12 hr may be necessary.

CONTRAINDICATIONS/ PRECAUTIONS

Contraindicated in: Hypersensitivity to ganciclovir/acyclovir. **Use cautiously in:** Elderly, renal impairment, severe bone marrow depression. **Pregnancy/Lactation:** No well-controlled trials to establish safety. Benefits must outweigh risks. Animal studies demonsrate teratogenic effects. Discontinue breastfeeding during therapy and for up to at least 72 hr following the last dose. **Pediatrics:** Safety and efficacy not established. Limited experience with use. Benefits must outweigh risks of potential long-term effects.

PREPARATION

Availability: 500 mg in 10 mL vials. **Reconstitution:** Dilute each 500 mg vial with 10 mL sterile water for injection (preservative free) for a final concentration of 50 mg/mL. **Infusion:** Further dilute dose in at least 100 mL (not to exceed 10 mg/mL concentration) compatible IV solution sufficient to infuse over 1 hr.

STABILITY/STORAGE

Vial: Store at room temperature. Reconstituted vial stable for 12 hr at room temperature. DO NOT REFRIGERATE. **Infusion:** Stable for 24 hr at room temperature and refrigerated.

ADMINISTRATION

General: Handle drug with care and adhere to institutional guidelines for the handling of chemotherapeutic/cytotoxic agents. Administer into veins with rapid IV flow to avoid phlebitis. Administer dose after hemodialysis. **Intermittent Infusion:** Infuse over at least 1 hr via infusion pump to avoid increased risk of renal toxicity.

COMPATIBILITY

Solution: Dextrose solutions, lactated Ringer's, Ringer's injection, sodium chloride solutions.

In the Adverse Effects section, underline indicates most frequent; CAPS indicates life threatening.

247

INCOMPATIBILITY
Solution: Bacteriostatic saline/water. **Y-site:** Foscarnet, ondansetron.

ADVERSE EFFECTS
CNS: Coma, abnormal dreams, ataxia, confusion, dizziness, headache, nervousness, paresthesia, pyschosis, somnolence, tremor. **Ophtho:** Retinal detachment. **CV:** dysrhythmia, hypertension, hypotension. **Resp:** Dyspnea. **GI:** Abdominal pain, abnormal liver function tests, anorexia, diarrhea, hemorrhage, nausea, vomiting. **GU:** Hematuria. **Renal:** Increased BUN/serum creatinine. **Derm:** Alopecia. **Endo:** Hypoglycemia. **Fld/Lytes:** Edema. **Heme:** Anemia, GRANULOCYTOPENIA, MYELOSUPPRESSION, THROMBOCYTOPENIA. **Hypersens:** Eosinophilia, rash, pruritus, urticaria. **Other:** Chills, fever, infections, malaise, phlebitis.

TOXICITY/OVERDOSE
Signs/Symptoms: Bone marrow depression, extension of adverse effects. **Treatment:** Supportive, hemodialysis (removes 50% drug) and hydration may be beneficial.

DRUG INTERACTIONS
Cytotoxic drugs: Increase bone marrow depression and toxic effects. **Imipenem:** Increased seizure potential. **Probenecid:** Reduced ganciclovir renal elimination and increased toxicity. **Zidovudine:** Increased granulocytopenia.

NURSING CONSIDERATIONS
Assessment
General:
Intake/output ratio, hydration status.

Physical:
Neurologic/mental status, cardiopulmonary status, integumentary system.
Lab Alterations:
Monitor BUN, serum creatinine, CBC with differential and platelet count.

Intervention/Rationale
Adequate hydration should be administered concurrently to enhance renal elimination. ● Neutrophil and platelet counts should be monitored every 2 days initially and weekly once maintenance therapy has begun. ● If prior history of ganciclovir-bone marrow suppression, monitor counts daily. Severe neutropenia (ANC < 500) or thrombocytopenia (< 25,000) require interruption of therapy until recovery is observed (ANC ≥ 750). ● If renal impairment is identified, dosage adjustment should be done. ● Assess skin and mucosal lesions for improvement/change. ● Evaluate mental status, assessing for confusion, nervousness, and/or psychoses.

Patient/Family Education
Treatment is not a cure for CMV; use is reserved for immunocompromised patients only. Regular ophthalmic examinations are necessary to minimize progression of the disease. Maintain good oral fluid intake/hydration. Avoid persons with known infections and crowds. Notify physician/nurse of signs of decreased WBC counts and/or infection (fever, sore throat, fatigue) and bleeding (increased bruising, nose-

In the Adverse Effects section, underline indicates most frequent; CAPS indicates life threatening.

bleeds, bleeding gums, melena). Instruct patient to use a soft toothbrush and electric razor to minimize bleeding tendency. Check oral temperatures daily. Caution male and female patients of teratogenic potential effects and to use contraceptive measures during therapy and for up to 4 months following treatment.

GENTAMICIN

(jen-ta-mye′-sin)
Trade Name(s): Cidomycin ♣, Garamycin
Classification(s): Aminoglycoside antibiotic
Pregnancy Category: D

PHARMACODYNAMICS/KINETICS
Mechanism of Action: Bactericidal, blocks bacterial protein synthesis, exhibits some neuromuscular blocking action. **Peak Serum Level:** Within 30 minutes of infusion completion. **Therapeutic Serum Levels:** Peak 4–8 mcg/mL. Trough < 2 mcg/mL. **Distribution:** Widely distributed in extracellular fluids. Lower serum concentrations result in expanded extracellular fluid volume. **Metabolism/Elimination:** Excreted unchanged via glomerular filtration in kidneys. **Half-Life:** 2 hr. Extended in renal failure (up to 24–60 hr).

INDICATIONS/DOSAGE

Treatment of gram-negative organisms/combination therapy in severe immunocompromised patients

Dosage interval may need to be adjusted in renal impairment. Adjust dosage based on serum levels.

Adult: Load 2 mg/kg followed by 3 mg/kg/day in divided doses every 8 hr. Not to exceed 5 mg/kg/day. Intrathecal dose 4–8 mg/day every 24 hr.

Pediatric: 6.0–7.5 mg/kg/day in divided doses every 6–8 hr. Intrathecal dose 1–2 mg/day every 24 hr.

Neonate: 7.5 mg/kg/day in divided doses every 6–8 hr. Premature or ≤ 1 week: 5 mg/kg/day in divided doses every 12 hr.

CONTRAINDICATIONS/PRECAUTIONS
Contraindicated in: Known hypersensitivity. **Use cautiously in:** Neuromuscular disorders (myasthenia gravis, Parkinson's disease, infant botulism). Newborns of mothers receiving high doses of magnesium sulfate. Concurrent administration of neuromuscular blocking agents. **Pregnancy/Lactation:** No well-controlled trials to establish safety. Benefits must outweigh risks. Crosses placenta. **Pediatrics:** Caution in premature infants/neonates due to renal immaturity and prolonged half-life.

PREPARATION
Availability: 10 mg/mL, 2 mL. 40 mg/mL in 1.5, 2, 10, 20 mL vials. 60, 80, 100 mL piggyback units. **Intrathecal:** 2 mg/mL in 2 mL ampules without preservative. **Infusion: Adults:** Further dilute in 50–200 mL of compatible IV solution. **Pediatrics:** Further dilute in compatible solution to a volume sufficient to infuse over 20–30 min.

In the Adverse Effects section, <u>underline</u> indicates most frequent; CAPS indicates life threatening.

249

STABILITY/STORAGE
Vial: Store at room temperature. **Infusion:** Stable for 7 days at room temperature/refrigerated.

ADMINISTRATION
General: Avoid rapid bolus administration. Schedule first maintenance dose at a dosing interval apart from loading dose. Administer additional dose after hemodialysis. Schedule dosing of penicillins and aminoglycosides as far apart as possible to prevent inactivation of aminoglycosides. **Intermittent Infusion:** Infuse over at least 30–60 min.

COMPATIBILITY
Solution: Dextrose solutions, Ringer's injection, sodium chloride solutions. **Syringe:** Clindamycin, penicillin G sodium. **Y-site:** Acyclovir, atracurium, cyclophosphamide, enalaprilat, esmolol, famotidine, foscarnet, hydromorphone, labetalol, magnesium sulfate, meperidine, morphine, multivitamins, ondansetron, pancuronium, tolazoline, vecuronium, vitamin B with C, zidovudine.

INCOMPABILITY
Solution: Fat emulsion. **Syringe:** Ampicillin, heparin. **Y-site:** Furosemide, heparin, hetastarch, mezlocillin.

ADVERSE EFFECTS
CNS: Convulsions, confusion, disorientation, neuromuscular blockade, lethargy, depression, headache, numbness, nystagmus, pseudotumor cerebri. **CV:** Hypertension, hypotension, palpitations. **Resp:** Respiratory depression, pulmonary fibrosis. **GI:** Hepatic necrosis, hepatomegaly, anorexia, increased bilirubin/LDH/transaminase, nausea, salivation, stomatitis, vomiting. **GU:** Casts, hematuria. **Renal:** Azotemia, increased BUN/serum creatinine, oliguria, proteinuria. **MS:** Arthralgia. **Fld/Lytes:** Hyperkalemia, hypomagnesemia. **Heme:** Agranulocytosis (transient), anemia (transient), eosinophilia, leukocytosis, leukopenia, pancytopenia, reticulocyte count alterations, thrombocytopenia. **Hypersens:** Angioneurotic edema, exfoliative dermatitis, purpura, rash, urticaria. **Other:** Fever, ototoxicity (deafness, dizziness, tinnitus, vertigo).

TOXICITY/OVERDOSE
Signs/Symptoms: Increased serum levels with associated nephrotoxicity and ototoxicity (tinnitus, high frequency hearing loss). **Treatment:** Removed by peritoneal/hemodialysis. Hemodialysis is more efficient. Exchange transfusions may be used in neonates. **Antidote(s):** Ticarcillin (12–20 g/day) may be given to promote complex formation with aminoglycosides to lower elevated serum levels.

DRUG INTERACTIONS
Amphotericin B, bacitracin, cephalothin, cisplatin, methoxyflurane, potent diuretics, vancomycin: Increased potential for nephrotoxicity, neurotoxicity, ototoxicity. **Anesthetics, anticholinesterase agents, citrate anticoagulated blood, metocurine, neuromuscular blocking agents, pancuronium, succinylcholine, tubocurarine:** Increased neuromuscular blockade/respiratory paralysis. **Beta lactam antibiotics (penicillins, cephalosporins) especially ticar-**

In the Adverse Effects section, <u>underline</u> indicates most frequent; CAPS indicates life threatening.

cillin: Inactivation of aminoglycosides. **Cephalosporins, penicillins:** Synergism against gram-negative and enterococci.

NURSING CONSIDERATIONS

Assessment
General:
Maintain adequate hydration, superinfection/infectious disease status.
Physical:
CN VIII (acoustic) evaluation, renal function.
Lab Alterations:
Measure peak/trough levels. Beta lactam antibiotic (penicillins, cephalosporins) may cause in vitro inactivation of gentamicin.

Intervention/Rationale
Assess BUN and serum creatinine/creatinine clearance to determine presence of renal toxicity. Adequate hydration recommended to prevent renal toxicity. ● CN VIII evaluation important to assess presence of ototoxicity. ● Antibiotic use may cause overgrowth of resistant organisms; observe for (fever, change in vital signs, increased WBC, vaginal infection/discharge). ● Draw peak serum levels 30 min after the infusion is complete and trough 30 min prior to the next dose.

Patient/Family Education
Increase oral fluid intake in order to minimize chemical irritation of kidneys. Notify physician/nurse if tinnitus, vertigo, or hearing loss is noted.

GLUCAGON
(gloo′-ka-gon)
Classification(s): Glucose elevating agent, hormone
Pregnancy Category: B

PHARMACODYNAMICS/KINETICS
Mechanism of Action: Polypeptide hormone produced by alpha cells of pancreas. Accelerates liver glycogen formation by stimulating synthesis of cyclic AMP. Increases breakdown of glycogen to glucose, resulting in elevation of blood sugar. Relaxes musculature of the GI tract. **Onset of Action:** 1 min. **Duration of Action:** 9–17 min. **Distribution:** Widely distributed throughout plasma/tissues. **Metabolism/Elimination:** Extensively degraded in liver/kidneys. **Half-Life:** 3–6 min.

INDICATIONS/DOSAGE

Emergency treatment of pronounced hypoglycemia in patients with diabetes mellitus when glucose administration is inadequate

Adult: 0.5–1.0 mg. Not to exceed 1 mg per dose. If no response within 5–20 minutes an additional one to two doses may be given.

Pediatric: 0.03–0.1 mg/kg. May repeat in 20 min as needed.

Neonate: 0.3 mg/kg/dose every 4 hr as needed.

Termination of insulin coma

Adult: 0.5–1.0 mg given after 1 hr of induced coma; larger doses may be used. May be repeated. In deep comatose states administer with glucose for a more rapid effect.

In the Adverse Effects section, <u>underline</u> indicates most frequent; CAPS indicates life threatening.

Radiographic diagnosis of GI tract

Adult: 0.5 mg immediately prior to radiographic study.

CONTRAINDICATIONS/PRECAUTIONS

Contraindicated in: Hypersensitivity to beef or pork protein. Diluent contains glycerin and phenol; avoid use if hypersensitivity exists. **Use cautiously in:** History of insulinoma or pheochromocytoma. **Pregnancy/Lactation:** No well-controlled trials to establish safety. Benefits must outweigh risks. Distributed in breast milk. Exercise caution if used during lactation.

PREPARATION

Availability: 1 mg with 1 mL diluent and 10 mg with 10 mL diluent vials. **Reconstitution:** Dilute to a final concentration of 1 mg/mL (1:1 solution). Dilute each 1 mg with 1 mL of diluent. **Only diluent provided by manufacturer should be used.**

STABILITY/STORAGE

Vial: Store at room temperature prior to reconstitution. Stable after reconstitution for 48 hr if refrigerated or 24 hr at room temperature. Should be used immediately after reconstitution.

ADMINISTRATION

General: Dosage is expressed in terms of drug in USP units. 1 USP unit equals 1 mg. **IV Push:** 1 mg (1 unit) or less over 1 minute. May be given through Y-site or three-way stopcock.

COMPATIBILITY/INCOMPATIBILITY

Data not available.

ADVERSE EFFECTS

CV: Hypertension, hypotension. **GI:** Nausea, vomiting (dose related). **Endo:** Hyperglycemia (in excessive doses). **Hypersens:** Allergic manifestations.

DRUG INTERACTIONS

Epinephrine: Intensifies hyperglycemic effect. **Insulin, oral hypoglycemics:** Glucagon negates the usual response. **Oral anticoagulants:** Increased hypoprothrombinemia.

NURSING CONSIDERATIONS

Assessment
General:
Hydration status, intake/output ratio, nutritional status.
Physical:
Metabolic status, neurologic status.
Lab Alterations:
Monitor serum electrolytes/blood sugar prior to and following completion of therapy. Evaluate coagulation studies for increased hypoprothrombinemia.

Intervention/Rationale
Assess for signs/symptoms of hypoglycemia (cold sweat, headache, dizziness, irritability, anxiety). Monitor blood sugar carefully as insulin needs or oral hypoglycemic needs may vary while undergoing therapy. For successful treatment of hypoglycemic shock, liver glycogen stores must be avilable. Drug is of limited value in patients with chronic hypoglycemia or in those with hypoglycemia associated with adrenal insufficiency or starvation. IV dextrose must be given immediately for hypoglycemia if patient fails to respond to drug. ● Evaluate

In the Adverse Effects section, <u>underline</u> indicates most frequent; CAPS indicates life threatening.

nutritional status (weight, evaluation of caloric intake in relation to caloric needs, dietary history). ● Assess neurological status of patient in relation to hypoglycemic events, seizure potential, or aspiration potential. ● Evaluate patients for increased bleeding potential.

Patient/Family Education
Completely educate regarding the nature of diabetes and how to prevent and detect any potential complications. Frequent urine and/or fingerstick evaluation of serum/urine glucose levels will be required. Carefully instruct regarding the technique of preparation/administration of glucagon prior to an emergency situation.

GLYCOPYRROLATE

(glye-koe-pye'-roe-late)
Trade Name(s): Robinul
Classification(s): Anticholinergic, antimuscarinic
Pregnancy Category: B

PHARMACODYNAMICS/KINETICS
Mechanism of Action: Synthetic anticholinergic agent. Inhibits action of acetylcholine at postganglionic sites in smooth muscle, secretory glands, and CNS. **Onset of Action:** 1 min. **Duration of Action:** 2–3 hr. **Distribution:** Rapidly distributed throughout body. Does not readily penetrate CNS or eye. **Elimination:** Eliminated primarily in feces via biliary excretion and urine. **Half-Life:** Unknown.

INDICATIONS/DOSAGE

Peptic ulcer treatment
Adult: 0.1–0.2 mg three to four times per day.

Neuromuscular blockade reversal
Adult/Pediatric: 0.2 mg for each 1 mg neostigmine or 5 mg pyridostigmine.

Intraoperative to counteract drug-induced or vagal traction reflexes
Adult: 0.1 mg as needed. Repeat every 2–3 min. *Pediatric:* 0.004 mg/kg. Repeat every 2–3 min. Not to exceed 0.1 mg/dose.

Preoperative antisecretory
Adult: 0.004 mg/kg 0.5–1.0 min prior to anesthesia. *Pediatric:* 0.004–0.01 mg/kg/dose 0.5–1.0 min prior to anesthesia.

CONTRAINDICATIONS/ PRECAUTIONS
Contraindicated in: Hepatic disease, hypersensitivity, myasthenia gravis, myocardial ischemia, narrow-angle glaucoma, obstructive uropathy, paralytic ileus, tachycardia. **Use cautiously in:** Asthma, allergies, CHF, coronary artery disease, dysrhythmias, elderly, hypertension, hyperthyroidism, prostatic hypertrophy. **Pregnancy/Lactation:** No well-controlled trials to establish safety. Benefits must outweigh risks. Distributed into breast milk. **Pediatrics:** Safety and efficacy not established in children less than 12 years old for peptic ulcer treatment.

PREPARATION
Availability: 0.2 mg/mL in 1, 2, 5, and 20 mL vials.

G

In the Adverse Effects section, <u>underline</u> indicates most frequent; CAPS indicates life threatening.

253

STABILITY/STORAGE
Vial: Store at room temperature.

ADMINISTRATION
General: May be given undiluted via Y-site or three-way stopcock into an already infusing IV solution. **IV Push:** 0.2 mg or less over 1–2 min.

COMPATIBILITY
Solution: Dextrose solutions, Ringer's injection, sodium chloride solutions. **Syringe:** Atropine, benzquinamide, chlorpromazine, codeine, diphenhydramine, droperidol, fentanyl, hydromorphone, levorphanol, lidocaine, meperidine, morphine, neostigmine, oxymorphone, procaine, prochlorperazine, promethazine, propriomazine, pyridostigmine, scopolamine.

INCOMPATIBILITY
Syringe: Chloramphenicol, dexamethasone, diazepam, dimenhydrinate, methohexital, pentazocine, pentobarbital, secobarbital, sodium bicarbonate, thiopental.

ADVERSE EFFECTS
CNS: Confusion, dizziness, drowsiness, headache, insomnia. **Ophtho:** <u>Blurred vision</u>, dilated pupils. **CV:** Bradycardia, palpitations. **GI:** <u>Constipation</u>, <u>dry mouth</u>, epigastric distress, nausea, vomiting. **GU:** Impotence, <u>urinary hesitancy</u>, <u>urinary urgency</u>, <u>urinary retention</u>. **Hypersens:** Allergic manifestations, urticaria. **Other:** Burning at site of injection, fever, flushing.

TOXICITY/OVERDOSE
Signs/Symptoms: Anaphylactic reactions, pronounced muscular weakness. **Treatment:** Symptomatic/supportive therapy. **Antidote(s):** Neostigmine 1 mg for each 1 mg of drug administered.

DRUG INTERACTIONS
Amantadine, tricyclic antidepressant: Increased anticholinergic effects. **Atenolol, digoxin:** Increased pharmacologic effects. **Phenothiazines:** Decreased antipsychotic effectiveness.

NURSING CONSIDERATIONS
Assessment
General:
Vital signs, intake/output ratio.
Physical:
GI tract, GU tract.
Lab Alterations:
May cause falsely decreased uric acid levels in patients with gout.

Intervention/Rationale
Monitor all vital signs carefully. Observe closely for adverse effects to be manifested. ● Monitor intake/output closely as drug may cause urinary retention. Have patient void prior to the preoperative administration of the drug. ● Monitor bowel sounds and assess for abdominal distention; drug can cause decreased motility of the GI tract resulting in constipation or if severe, may result in paralytic ileus.

Patient/Family Education
Drug may cause drowsiness as well as blurred vision. Any activities requiring visual acuity or alertness should be avoided until adverse reactions have been assessed. May cause sudden changes in blood pressure; change positions slowly and gradually to avoid rapid blood

In the Adverse Effects section, <u>underline</u> indicates most frequent; CAPS indicates life threatening.

pressure shifts. Notify physician before taking over-the-counter medications that could interfere with therapy. Report any signs of urinary hesitancy, frequency, or urgency.

GONADORELIN
(go-nad'-o-ra-lin)
Trade Name(s): Factrel
Classification(s): Gonadotropin, in vivo diagnostic aid
Pregnancy Category: B

PHARMACODYNAMICS/KINETICS
Mechanism of Action: A synthetic leutenizing releasing hormone, demonstrates gonadotropin releasing effects on the anterior pituitary.

INDICATIONS/DOSAGE

Evaluation of functional capacity/ response of gonadotropes of anterior pituitary, testing of suspected gonadotropin deficiencies, evaluation of residual gonadotropic function of pituitary after surgical removal/radiation ablation
Adult: 100 mcg once.

CONTRAINDICATIONS/ PRECAUTIONS
Contraindicated in: Hypersensitivity. **Pregnancy/Lactation:** No well-controlled trials to establish safety. Benefits must outweigh risks.

PREPARATION
Availability: 100 mcg, 500 mcg powder for injection/vial. **Reconstitution:** Add 2 mL of included diluent to the 100 or 500 mcg vial. Prepare immediately prior to use.

STABILITY/STORAGE
Vial: Store unopened vial at room temperature. After reconstitution, store at room temperature and use within 24 hr. Discard any unused solution and diluent.

ADMINISTRATION
General: Should be administered on days 1–7 of the menstrual cycle (early follicular phase). **IV Push:** A single dose over 15–30 sec.

COMPATIBILITY/INCOMPATIBILITY
Data not available.

ADVERSE EFFECTS
CNS: Headache, lightheadedness. **GI:** Abdominal discomfort, nausea.

TOXICITY/OVERDOSE
Signs/Symptoms: Extension of adverse effects. **Treatment:** May be treated symptomatically with supportive and/or resuscitative therapy.

DRUG INTERACTIONS
Levodopa, spironolactone: May elevate gonadotropin levels. **Digoxin, oral contraceptives:** Suppresses gonadotropin levels. **Dopamine antagonists, phenothiazines:** Increased prolactin and decreased response to drug.

NURSING CONSIDERATIONS
Assessment
General:
Hypersensitivity reactions.
Lab Alterations:
Draw hormonal blood samples 15, 30, 45, 60 min, and 2 hr after administration of drug.

In the Adverse Effects section, <u>underline</u> indicates most frequent; CAPS indicates life threatening.

Intervention/Rationale
Assess for allergic manifestations; keep epinephrine readily available as immediate treatment for any hypersensitivity reaction.

Patient/Family Education
Consult with physician before taking any over-the-counter drug that may interfere with pituitary testing. Review purpose of testing and potential adverse effects.

HALOPERIDOL LACTATE
(hal-o-per′-a-doll)
Trade Name(s): Haldol
Classification(s): Antipsychotic agent
Pregnancy Category: C

PHARMACODYNAMICS/KINETICS
Mechanism of Action: Depresses CNS at subcortical level of brain, midbrain, and brain stem reticular formation system. Directly affects chemoreceptor trigger zone by blocking dopamine receptors. **Onset of Action:** Rapid. **Distribution:** Protein binding > 90–92%. Distributed in breast milk. **Metabolism/Elimination:** Primarily hepatically metabolized. Excreted via urine. Small percentage eliminated via bile. Not removed by hemodialysis. **Half-Life:** 10–19 hr.

INDICATIONS/DOSAGE

Acute psychotic disorder management (*unlabeled use*)
Adult: 0.5–2.0 mg. Repeat as needed every 0.5–1.0 hr. May require up to 25 mg/dose.

Treatment of intractable hiccoughs (*unlabeled use*)
Adult: 3–5 mg every 2 hr for five to seven doses.

CONTRAINDICATIONS/ PRECAUTIONS
Contraindicated in: Children < 3 years of age, coma, hypersensitivity, severe toxic CNS depression, parkinson's syndrome. Known history of seizures or EEG abnormalities, severe cardiovascular disorders, thyrotoxicosis. **Use cautiously in: NOT FDA APPROVED FOR IV USE but in health-care practice is being used throughout the United States. Pregnancy/Lactation:** No well-controlled trials to establish safety. Benefits must outweigh risks. Not recommended for use during lactation. **Pediatrics:** Safety and efficacy in children < 3 years of age has not been established.

PREPARATION
Availability: 5 mg/mL single dose vials and 10 mL multidose vials. 50 mg/mL in 1 mL ampules and 1 mL disposable syringes. **Infusion:** May be added to compatible IV solution.

STABILITY/STORAGE
Vial: Store at room temperature. Protect from light. May discolor after several hours. **Infusion:** Stable at room temperature for 24 hr.

ADMINISTRATION
General: All IV doses are investigational. DO NOT administer the *decanoate* form of drug IV. Decrease dose of narcotics and all CNS depressants by 25%–33% of usual dose before, during, and for 24 hr after IV administration of

In the Adverse Effects section, underline indicates most frequent; CAPS indicates life threatening.

drug. **IV Push:** Administer 5 mg over 1 min. Give through Y-site or three-way stopcock of IV infusion. Flush with 2 mL or more of 0.9% sodium chloride before/after administration of drug. **Intermittent Infusion:** Single dose over 30 min. May be added to 25–50 mL of compatible IV solution. **Continuous Infusion:** Infuse at physician specified rate. Not to exceed 5 mg/min or 25 mg/hr. Titrate to desired effect and patient response.

COMPATIBILITY
Solution: Dextrose solutions, sodium chloride solutions. **Y-site:** Ondansetron.

INCOMPATIBILITY
Syringe: Heparin. **Y-site:** Foscarnet, heparin.

ADVERSE EFFECTS
CNS: Dyskinesia, hyperreflexia, motor restlessness, neuroleptic malignant syndrome, parkinsonian symptoms (drooling, marked drowsiness, fixed stare, hypersalivation, lethargy). **CV:** Hypotension, tachycardia. **Resp:** BRONCHOSPASM, laryngospasm, bronchopneumonia. **GI:** Anorexia, diarrhea, dyspepsia, nausea, vomiting, jaundice. **Derm:** Alopecia, photosensitivity. **Heme:** Agranulocytosis, anemia, leukocytosis, leukopenia. **Hypersens:** Maculopapular and aceneiform reactions. **Other:** Hyperpyrexia.

TOXICITY/OVERDOSE
Signs/Symptoms: Severe extrapyramidal reactions, hypotension, sedation. Coma with respiratory depression and severe hypotension may occur. **Treatment:** Symptomatic/supportive care. **Antidote(s):** No specific antidote, anticholinesterase and antiparkinson drugs may be useful in controlling extrapyramidal reactions. Hemodialysis is not effective in overdose.

DRUG INTERACTIONS
Alcohol, analgesics, anesthesia, barbiturates, opiates, sedatives: Increased CNS depression. **Lithium:** May cause neurotoxicity (extrapyramidal, neuroleptic malignant syndrome). **Methyldopa:** May produce psychiatric symptoms (aggressiveness, assaultiveness, disorientation, irritability). **Propranolol:** May produce life-threatening hypotension and bradycardia.

NURSING CONSIDERATIONS
Assessment
General:
Vital signs, ECG monitoring (recommended).
Physical:
Neurologic status.

Intervention/Rationale
Use of drug should be confined to critical care units with constant monitoring capabilities. ● Evaluate for development of extrapyramidal effects.

Patient/Family Education
Drowsiness may be associated with use of drug. Observe caution when engaging in activities requiring alertness and psychomotor coordination until CNS effects decrease. Notify physician if muscle twitching, involuntary movements, or jerky movements occur (signs of

H

In the Adverse Effects section, underline indicates most frequent; CAPS indicates life threatening.

developing tardive dyskinesia). Avoid alcohol and other CNS depressants.

HEPARIN

(hep'-a-rin)
Trade Name(s): Lipohepin, Liquaemin
Classification(s): Anticoagulant
Pregnancy Category: C

PHARMACODYNAMICS/KINETICS

Mechanism of Action: Combines with antithrombin III to inhibit thrombosis by inactivating Factor X-a and inhibiting the conversion of prothrombin to thrombin. Prevents formation of stable fibrin clot by inhibiting the activation of Factor XIII. **Onset of Action:** Immediate. **Peak Effect:** 5–10 min. **Duration of Action:** 2–6 hr (dose dependent). **Distribution:** Protein binding. Extensively bound to low density lipoprotein, globulins, fibrinogen. **Metabolism/Elimination:** Partially metabolized by liver heparinase and reticular endothelial system. 50% excreted unchanged in urine. **Half-Life:** 60–90 min.

INDICATIONS/DOSAGE

Adjust dosage based on partial thromboplastin time (PTT).

Blood transfusion

Adult: Add 400–600 units/100 mL whole blood.

Alternate Dosage: 7500 units to 100 mL of 0.9% sodium chloride. Add 6–8 mL of solution to each 100 mL whole blood.

IV solution catheter patency, implanted access patency

Adult: 10–500 units diluted in adequate amounts of 0.9% sodium chloride to reach to the end of the catheter or access.

Low dose prophylaxis for postoperative thromboembolism

Adult:
Intermittent Injection: 10,000 units as loading dose, repeated every 4–6 hr, adjusted according to clotting time. **IV Infusion:** 20,000–40,000 units/24 hr, preceded by a loading dose of 5000 units.

Open heart surgery

Adult: 150–400 units/kg during surgical procedure. 300 units/kg is often used for surgical procedures < 60 min and 400 units/kg for procedures > 60 min.

Pediatric: Loading dose of 50 units/kg followed by maintenance dose of 100 units/kg every 4 hr or 20,000 units/m^2/24 hr via continuous infusion.

CONTRAINDICATIONS/PRECAUTIONS

Contraindicated in: Hypersensitivity, blood dyscrasias, patients who cannot receive regular clotting time laboratory studies, uncontrollable bleeding (except DIC), severe thrombocytopenia. **Use cautiously in:** Diabetes, hypertension, patients with indwelling urinary catheters, presence of mild hepatic or renal disease, women > 60 years of age. **Pregnancy/Lactation:** No well-controlled trials to establish safety. Benefits must outweigh risks. Excreted in breast milk.

In the Adverse Effects section, <u>underline</u> indicates most frequent; CAPS indicates life threatening.

PREPARATION
Availability: 1000, 5000, 10,000, 20,000, 40,000 units/mL in 1, 2, 4, 5, 10, and 30 mL ampules/vials. **Infusion:** Dilute in compatible IV solution to physician specified concentration. Adequately mix drug prior to beginning infusion.

STABILITY/STORAGE
Vial: Store at room temperature. **Infusion:** Stable at room tempeature for 24 hr. Slight discoloration of infusion does not alter potency.

ADMINISTRATION
General: To prevent incompatible reactions, flush IV line with 0.9% sodium chloride or sterile water for injection prior to and immediately after administration of drug. Administer via infusion device. **IV Push:** Test dose: 1000 units or less over 1 minute. Followed by 5000 units or less over 1 minute periods. **Intermittent Infusion:** Infuse over 4–24 hr depending on the dosage required and the amount of diluent used.

COMPATIBILITY
Solution: Amino acids 4.25%, dextrose 25%, dextrose solutions, fat emulsions 10%, lactated Ringer's, Ringer's injection, sodium chloride solutions. **Syringe:** Aminophylline, amphotericin B, ampicillin, atropine, bleomycin, cefamandole, cefazolin, cefoperazone, cefotaxime, cefoxitin, chloramphenicol, cimetidine, cisplatin, clindamycin, cyclophosphamide, diazoxide, digoxin, dimenhydrinate, dobutamine, dopamine, epinephrine, fentanyl, fluorouracil, furosemide, leucovorin calcium, lidocaine, methotrexate, metoclopramide, mezlocillin, mitomycin, moxalactam, nafcillin, naloxone, neostigmine, norepinephrine, pancuronium, penicillin G, phenobarbital, piperacillin, sodium nitroprusside, succinylcholine, trimethoprim-sulfamethoxazole, verapamil, vinblastine, vincristine. **Y-site:** Acyclovir, aminophylline, ampicillin, atracurium, atropine, betamethasone, bleomycin, calcium gluconate, cephalothin, cephaprin, chlordiazepoxide, chlorpromazine, cimetidine, cisplatin, cyanocobalamin, cyclophosphamide, dexamethasone, digoxin, diphenhydramine, dopamine, edrophonium, enalaprilat, epinephrine, esmolol, estrogens, ethacrynate, fentanyl, fluorouracil, foscarnet, furosemide, hydralazine, insulin—regular, isoproterenol, kanamycin, labetalol, leukovorin calcium, lidocaine, magnesium, meperidine, methicillin, methotrexate, methoxamine, methylergonovine, metoclopramide, minocycline, mitomycin, morphine, neostigmine, norepinephrine, ondansetron, oxacillin, oxytocin, pancuronium, penicillin G potassium, pentazocine, phytonadione, prednisolone, procainamide, prochlorperazine, propranolol, pyridostigmine, ranitidine, scopolamine, sodium bicarbonate, streptokinase, succinylcholine, trimethophan, vecuronium, vinblastine, vincristine, zidovudine.

INCOMPATIBILITY
Syringe: Amikacin, amiodarone, chlorpromazine, diazepam, doxorubicin, droperidol, erythromycin, gentamicin, haloperidol, meperidine, methicillin, netilmicin, pentazocine, promethazine, streptomycin, tobramycin, vancomycin. **Y-site:**

In the Adverse Effects section, underline indicates most frequent; CAPS indicates life threatening.

259

Amiodarone, alteplase, diazepam, doxorubicin, ergotamine, gentamicin, haloperidol, phenytoin, tobramycin.

ADVERSE EFFECTS

CNS: Headache. **CV:** Chest pain, hypertension, increased capillary permeability. **Resp:** Asthma, epistaxis, rhinitis. **GI:** Hepatitis. **GU:** Hematuria. **Derm:** Rash. **Heme:** HEMORRHAGE, <u>thrombocytopenia</u>, white clot syndrome. **Hypersens:** Anaphylactoid reactions, gasping syndrome (premature infants), pruritus, urticaria, vasospastic allergic reactions. **Metab:** Hyperlipidemia. **Other:** Chills, fever, hematoma formation, local irritation/mild pain at injection site, subcutaneous or cutaneous necrosis.

TOXICITY/OVERDOSE

Signs/Symptoms: Bleeding is the primary symptom of overdose. Nosebleeds, tarry stools, hematuria, as well as easy bruising and petechiae formation may be noted as impending danger signs of frank hemorrhage. **Treatment:** Discontinue drug. Notify physician. **Antidote(s):** Protamine sulfate (1% solution).

DRUG INTERACTIONS

Antihistamines, digoxin, nicotine: May partially counteract the anticoagulant effect of drug. **Aspirin, dipyridamole, dextran, nonsteroidal anti-inflammatory drugs:** Increased risk of bleeding (affects platelet function). **Cefamandole, cefoperazone, moxalactam, plicamycin, quinidine:** Increased bleeding with drugs (decreased prothrombin activity). **Diazepam:** Heparin may increase plasma lev-

els. **Nitroglycerine IV, propylene glycol:** May cause heparin resistance.

NURSING CONSIDERATIONS

Assessment
Physical:
Hematopoietic system, GI tract.
Lab Alterations:
Draw blood for partial thromboplastin time 30 min prior to dose if being administered intermittently. If administered via continuous infusion, draw blood sample 1–2 hr after initiating therapy. May cause decreased serum triglycerides/cholesterol levels and prolonged prothrombin time, false increase of serum thyroxine, AST (SGOT), and ALT (SGPT). In drawing arterial blood gas samples, if heparin comprises 10% or more of the total volume of the blood sample, errors in measurement of pCO_2, HCO_3, and base excess may occur.

Intervention/Rationale
Assess for bleeding (easy bruising, hematuria, occult blood in the stools or tarry stools). ● Venipuncture/injections may require prolonged application of site pressure to prevent bleeding and/or hematoma formation. ● Hematest stools/vomitus/urine for presence of occult blood.

Patient/Family Education
Wear a Medic Alert bracelet or carry an indentification card to alert medical personnel of bleeding potential if involved in a trauma. Observe for signs/symptoms of frank or occult blood (easy bruising, tarry stools, hematuria, gum bleeding, nosebleeds); notify physician at once if symptoms are noted.

In the Adverse Effects section, <u>underline</u> indicates most frequent; CAPS indicates life threatening.

HETASTARCH (HES)

(het′-a-starch)
Trade Name(s): Hespan
Classification(s): Volume
expander
Pregnancy Category: C

PHARMACODYNAMICS/KINETICS
Mechanism of Action: Colloidal properties resemble those of human albumin. Primary effect is volume expansion resulting from the colloidal osmotic effect of drug. **Onset of Action:** Rapid. **Duration of Action:** 24 hr or longer. **Metabolism/Elimination:** Eliminated rapidly by the kidney via glomerular filtration. **Half-Life:** Approximately 90% is eliminated with average half-life of 17 days. Remainder has a half-life of 48 days.

INDICATIONS/DOSAGE

Plasma volume expansion resulting from burns, hemorrhage, surgery, sepsis, or trauma

(total dosage and infusion rate dependent on volume of blood loss and resultant hemoconcentration).
Adult: 500–1000 mL, not to exceed 20 mL/kg/hr or 1500 mL/24 hr.

CONTRAINDICATIONS/ PRECAUTIONS
Contraindicated in: Bleeding disorders, especially thrombocytopenia, renal failure with oliguria and anuria, severe cardiac failure. **Use cautiously in:** Impaired renal clearance, conditions lacking oxygen carrying capacity or plasma proteins/coagulation factors, patients with increased risk of CHF or pulmonary edema. **Pregnancy/Lactation:** No well-controlled trials to establish safety. Benefits must outweigh risks. **Pediatrics:** Safety and efficacy has not been established.

PREPARATION
Availability: 6 g/100 mL of 0.9% sodium chloride in 500 mL infusion bottles. Contains 77 mEq sodium per 500 mL.

STABILITY/STORAGE
Vial: Store at room temperature.

ADMINISTRATION
General: Administer by IV infusion only. Not a substitute for blood/plasma. **Intermittent/Continuous Infusion:** In acute shock up to 20 mL/kg/hr may be infused. In burns or septic shock administer at slower rates.

COMPATIBILITY/INCOMPATIBILITY
Data not available.

ADVERSE EFFECTS
CNS: Headache. **CV:** Peripheral edema of lower extremities. **GI:** Submaxillary and parotid gland enlargement, vomiting. **Derm:** Itching. **Hypersens:** Chills, periorbital edema, urticaria, wheezing. **Other:** Mild influenza-like symptoms, temperature elevations.

NURSING CONSIDERATIONS
Assessment
General:
Hypersensitivity reactions, baseline/daily weight, intake/output ratio, vital signs.
Physical:
Cardiopulmonary status.

In the Adverse Effects section, underline indicates most frequent;
CAPS indicates life threatening.

261

Lab Alterations:
Monitor serum electrolytes frequently especially in patients prone to pulmonary edema and/or CHF (due to high sodium content); increased indirect bilirubin, sedimentation rate, and hemoglobin; decreased platelet count.

Intervention/Rationale
Observe vital signs regularly. ● Monitor daily weights in patients on long-term replacement therapy. ● Observe for anaphylactoid reactions including periorbital edema, urticaria, and wheezing. ● Monitor for circulatory overload (increased risk with impaired renal function); assessment includes CVP, intake/output, adventitious breath sounds, and presence of jugular venous distention.

Patient/Family Education
Note signs/symptoms of bleeding (easy bruising, tarry stools, bloody urine, or bleeding gums). Notify physician immediately if symptoms are noted.

HYDRALAZINE
(hy-dral′-a-zeen)
Trade Name(s): Apresoline
Classification(s): Antihypertensive, vasodilator
Pregnancy Category: C

PHARMACODYNAMICS/KINETICS
Mechanism of Action: Alters cellular calcium metabolism and interferes with movement of calcium in the vascular smooth muscles that are responsible for initiating and maintaining a contractile state. Increases renin activity in plasma resulting in the production of angiotensin II causing stimulation of aldosterone and reabsorption of sodium. **Peak Effect:** 10–20 min. **Duration of Action:** 2–4 hr. **Distribution:** 87% protein bound. **Metabolism/Elimination:** Undergoes extensive metabolism by the liver. Excreted via urine as an active drug and metabolites. **Half-Life:** 2–7 hr.

INDICATIONS/DOSAGE

Management of moderate to severe hypertension in combination with diuretics. Treatment of CHF unresponsive to cardiac glycosides/diuretics
Adult: Usual dose 20–40 mg repeated as necessary. Reduce dosage in renal impairment.

Pediatric: 0.1–0.2 mg/kg/dose every 4–6 hr as needed.

Treatment of CHF, severe aortic insufficiency, and following valve replacement (*unlabeled use*)
Adult: Doses up to 800 mg three times in 24 hr.

CONTRAINDICATIONS/ PRECAUTIONS
Contraindicated in: Coronary artery disease, hypersensitivity, mitral valve/rheumatic heart disease. **Use cautiously in:** Cardiovascular or cerebrovascular disease, pulmonary hypertension, severe renal/hepatic disease. **Pregnancy/Lactation:** No well-controlled trials to establish safety. Benefits must outweigh risks. Use cautiously in lactating women. **Pediatrics:** Safety and efficacy not established in controlled

clinical trials although there is experience with drug use in children.

PREPARATION
Availability: 20 mg/mL in 1 mL ampules/vials.

STABILITY/STORAGE
Vial: Store at room temperature. Use as quickly as possible after drawing up with a needle into a syringe. Changes color after contact with a metal filter.

ADMINISTRATION
General: Use parenteral dose only if unable to tolerate oral form. Dosage should be adjusted to the lowest effective dose. **IV Push:** Slowly, at a rate not faster than 5 mg/min.

COMPATABILITY
Solution: Dextrose solutions, lactated Ringer's, Ringer's injection, sodium chloride solutions. **Y-site:** Heparin, hydrocortisone, potassium chloride, verapamil, vitamin B complex with C.

INCOMPATABILITY
Y-site: Aminophylline, ampicillin, diazoxide, furosemide.

ADVERSE EFFECTS
CNS: Dizziness, headache, numbness, peripheral neuritis as evidenced by paresthesia, tingling, tremors. **Ophtho:** Conjunctivitis, lacrimation. **CV:** Angina, hypotension, palpitations, tachycardia. **Resp:** Dyspnea, nasal congestion, hoarseness due to drug induced lupus. **GI:** Anorexia, constipation, diarrhea, hepatitis, nausea, paralytic ileus, vomiting. **GU:** Difficulty in micturition, impotence. **MS:** Muscle cramps. **Heme:** Agranulocytosis, decreased hemoglobin, decreased RBCs, leukopenia, lymphadenopathy, splenomegaly. **Hypersens:** Arthralgia, chills, eosinophilia, fever, purpura, pruritus, rash, urticaria. **Other:** Paradoxical pressor response, lupus-like syndrome.

TOXICITY/OVERDOSE
Signs/Symptoms: Headache, hypotension, tachycardia, and generalized flushing of the skin. Myocardial ischemia, possible MI, and cardiac dysrhythmias can develop. Profound shock can occur in severe overdose. **Treatment:** Cardiovascular support, treatment of shock with volume expanders and without pressors. If absolutely required, use a pressor least likely to increase tachycardia/cardiac dysrhythmias. Digitalis glycosides may be required.

DRUG INTERACTIONS
MAO inhibitors: Use with caution. **Nonsteroidal anti-inflammatory agents:** Decreased antihypertensive response. **Other parenteral antihypertensives:** Profound hypotension. **Sympathomimetics:** May induce tachycardia and angina.

NURSING CONSIDERATIONS
Assessment
General:
Vital signs, ECG monitoring (recommended), baseline/daily weight, intake/output ratio, neurologic status.
Physical:
Cardiopulmonary status, hematopoietic system.
Lab Alterations:
CBC, electrolytes, LE cell prep, ANA titer should be monitored before and during prolonged therapy.

In the Adverse Effects section, <u>underline</u> indicates most frequent; CAPS indicates life threatening.

Intervention/Rationale

Carefully evaluate patients with severe hypertension and uremia for development of neourological findings including mild to acute anxiety, severe depression, or coma. ● Assess for chest pain, ECG changes, palpitations, or dysrhythmias as a result of myocardial ischemia. ● Evaluate fluid status while observing for signs/symptoms of pulmonary edema/CHF. ● Monitor all vital signs with frequent blood pressure checks; blood pressure may begin to fall within a few minutes following parenteral injection (maximum blood pressure decrease occurs in 10–80 min). ● May produce a clinical picture similar to acute systemic lupus erythematosis (examples: arthralgia, myalgia, dermatoses, fever, anemia, splenomegaly, and rarely, necrotizing vasculitis); symptoms usually decrease when drug is discontinued.

Patient/Family Education

Weigh self and record daily. Assess for signs/symptoms of fluid retention (puffiness of hands/feet/fingers, edema of lower extremities, increased weight over a short time). May cause drowsiness; caution against driving or other activities that may require mental acuity. Inform physician immediately of chest pain, palpitations, paresthesias, tingling, or tremor development. Notify physician if general tiredness, fever, muscle/joint pain, rash, sore throat, pain, or weakness of hands or feet occur (symptoms of a lupus-like response to the drug).

HYDROCORTISONE SODIUM SUCCINATE

(hye-droe-kor′-ti-sone)

Trade Name(s): A-hydrocort, Solu-Cortef

Classification(s): Glucocorticoid

Pregnancy Category: Unknown

PHARMACODYNAMICS/KINETICS

Mechanism of Action: Primary hormone secreted by the adrenal cortex. Decreases inflammation by stabilizing the lysosomal membrane, suppresses immune response, stimulates bone marrow and effects on protein, carbohydrate, and fat metabolism.

Onset of Action: Rapid. **Peak Effect:** Unknown. **Duration of Action:** 1.0–1.5 days. **Distribution:** Widely distributed throughout the body. **Metabolism/Elimination:** Metabolized by the liver. Excreted via urine. Renal clearance is increased when plasma levels are increased. **Half-Life:** 8–12 hr.

INDICATIONS/DOSAGE

Medical management of adrenocortical insufficiency, control of inflammation and allergic conditions (asthma, ulcerative colitis) over a short-time period

Adult: 100–500 mg repeat every 1–6 hr as necessary.

Pediatric:

Infants: Loading dose: 1–2 mg/kg/24 hr. Maintenance dose: 25–150 mg/kg/24 hr. **Older Children:** 150–250 mg/kg/24 hr in divided doses.

In the Adverse Effects section, <u>underline</u> indicates most frequent; CAPS indicates life threatening.

Treatment of severe shock

Adult: 2 g or more every 2–4 hr. Use for no longher than 48–72 hr. Never give less than 25 mg/24 hr.

Anti-inflammatory

Adult/Pediatric: 0.8–4.0 mg/kg/24 hr in divided doses.

Status asthmaticus

Adult/Pediatric: 4–8 mg/kg/dose as one time dose. Followed by 2–4 mg/kg/dose every 6 hr over 5 days.

CONTRAINDICATIONS/ PRECAUTIONS

Contraindicated in: Hypersensitivity, systemic fungal infections, except for specific forms of meningitis. Administration of live virus vaccines to patients receiving steroids is clearly contraindicated. **Use cautiously in:** CHF, elderly, hypertension. Long-term therapy can lead to suppression of the adrenal glands. May alter signs of infection and new infections may appear with patients receiving steroids. Ulcerative colitis, thromboembolic disorders/ predisposition. **Pregnancy/Lactation:** No well-controlled trials to establish safety. Benefits must outweigh risks. Crosses the placenta. Found in breast milk. **Pediatrics:** Carefully assess infants born to mothers receiving substantial amounts of the drug during pregnancy for signs/ symptoms of hypoadrenalism. Chronic use in children may lead to suppression of growth.

PREPARATION

Availability: 100, 250, 500, and 1000 mg in 2, 4, and 8 mL vials and Mix-o-Vials. **Reconstitution:** Mix-o-Vial reconstitutes by pressing down the rubber stopper causing the diluent to flow into the lower vial. Agitate very gently and withdraw contents with a sterile needle. Reconstitute each 250 mg vial with 2 mL sterile water for injection. **Infusion:** Each 100 mg may be further diluted in a minimum of 100 mL and a maximum of 1000 mL of compatible IV solution.

STABILITY/STORAGE

Vial: Store at room temperature. After reconstitution solutions are stable for 24 hr at room temperature or below if protected from light. Heat labile/unstable: must not be autoclaved. **Infusion:** Stable for 24 hr at room temperature.

ADMINISTRATION

General: Dosage must be individualized according to the patient's needs and overall response to therapy. Maximal activity of adrenal cortex occurs between 2 AM–8 AM, with minimal activity between 4 PM–12 MN. Exogenous glucocorticoids suppress normal adrenocortical activity the least during the time of maximal adrenal activity. Administer drug prior to 9 AM if possible. **IV Push:** Not to exceed 500 mg over a 1 minute period. **Continuous/Intermittent Infusion:** May infuse over 15–30 min. Solution should be administered at physician prescribed rate and infused completely within a 24 hr period.

COMPATIBILITY

Solution: Dextrose solutions, fat emulsion: 10%, lactated Ringer's, Ringer's injection, sodium chloride

H

In the Adverse Effects section, underline indicates most frequent; CAPS indicates life threatening.

solutions. **Syringe:** Metoclopramide, thiopental. **Y-site:** Acyclovir, aminophylline, ampicillin, amrinone, atracurium, atropine, betamethasone, calcium gluconate, cephalothin, cephapirin, chlordiazepoxide, chlorpromazine, cyanocobalamin, deslanoside, dexamethasone, digoxin, diphenhydramine, dopamine, droperidol, edrophonium, enalaprilat, epinephrine, esmolol, estrogens, ethacrynate, famotidine, fentanyl, fluorouracil, foscarnet, furosemide, hydralazine, insulin–regular, isoproterenol, kanamycin, lidocaine, magnesium, menadiol, methicillin, methoxamine, methylergonovine, morphine, neostigmine, norepinephrine, ondansetron, oxacillin, oxytocin, pancuronium, penicillin G, pentazocine, phytonadione, prednisolone, procainamide, prochlorperazine, promethazine, propranolol, pyridostigmine, scopolamine, sodium bicarbonate, succinylcholine, trimethaphan, vecuronium.

INCOMPATIBILITY
Syringe: Doxapram. **Y-site:** Diazepam, ergotamine, phenytoin.

ADVERSE EFFECTS
CNS: <u>Depression</u>, euphoria, psychoses. **Ophtho:** Cataracts, increased intraocular pressure. **CV:** CHF, edema, hypertension, thromboembolism. **GI:** GI bleeding, pancreatitis, peptic ulceration, increased appetite, nausea, vomiting. **MS:** Aseptic necrosis of joints, myopathy, osteoporosis, weakness of muscles. **Derm:** Acne, depressed wound healing, ecchymoses, fragility of capillaries, <u>petechiae</u>. **Endo:**

<u>Adrenal suppression</u>, decreased growth (children), hirsutism, hyperglycemia, menstrual irregularities. **Fld/Lytes:** Hypocalcemia, <u>hypokalemia</u>, metabolic alkalosis, sodium retention. **Other:** Increased susceptibility to infection, Cushingoid appearance (moonface, buffalo hump).

TOXICITY/OVERDOSE
Signs/Symptoms: Two categories of toxicity: *Adrenal Insufficiency.* Caused by too rapid withdrawal of corticosteroids after long-term use. Withdrawal results in fever, myalgia, arthralgia, malaise, anorexia, orthostatic hypotension, faintness, dyspnea, and decreased blood sugar. *Induction of Cushingoid Changes.* Results from continuous use of large doses. These changes include moonface, central obesity, striae, hirsutism, acne, increased susceptibility to infection, hypertension, fluid and electrolyte imbalance.
Treatment: Tapering of all steroids should be gradual. Frequent laboratory tests and supplementation of steroids during periods of stress are treatment for toxicity.

DRUG INTERACTIONS
Amphotericin B, carbenicillin, mezlocillin, piperacillin, potassium depleting diuretics, ticarcillin: Increased hypokalemia. **Aspirin:** Steroids may reduce salicylate levels by increasing metabolism/clearance. **Cyclosporine:** Increased plasma levels of both drugs due to mutual inhibition of metabolism. **Insulin, oral hypoglycemic agents:** Increased requirements for diabetics receiving steroids. **Oral contraceptives, cyclophosphamide:** May block he-

H

In the Adverse Effects section, <u>underline</u> indicates most frequent; CAPS indicates life threatening.

patic metabolism. **Phenytoin, phenobarbital, rifampin:** May enhance the metabolic clearance of corticosteroids requiring increased dosage.

NURSING CONSIDERATIONS
Assessment
General:
Vital signs, intake/output ratio, baseline/daily weight, nutritional status.
Physical:
Cardiopulmonary status, infectious disease status, GI tract.
Lab Alterations:
Monitor lab studies prior to and throughout course of therapy, including blood sugar and electrolytes. Hematest stools for occult blood. Notify physician with positive findings. Suppresses reactions to allergy skin testing.

Intervention/Rationale
Monitor intake/output and daily weight. ● Evaluate nutritional status for negative nitrogen balance due to protein catabolism. ● Notify physician if signs/symptoms of CHF develop. Assess for weight increase, edema, hypertension, hypokalemia. ● Evaluate all vital signs including temperature to evaluate development of infections. ● Evaluate for signs/symptoms of adrenal insufficiency (fatigue, anorexia, nausea, vomiting, diarrhea, weight loss, weakness, dizziness, and low blood sugar); notify physician immediately if observed.

Patient/Family Education
While receiving steroids an identification bracelet or card should be carried at all times noting the fact that patient is receiving steroids. Stopping medication suddenly may be life threatening. Notify physician promptly if these signs and symptoms occur following dosage decrease or withdrawal of therapy: fatigue, anorexia, nausea, vomiting, diarrhea, weight loss, weakness, dizziness, decreased blood sugar.

HYDROMORPHONE HCL
(hye-droe-mor′-fone)
Trade Name(s): Dilaudid, Dilaudid HP
Classification(s): Narcotic agonist analgesic
Pregnancy Category: C
Controlled Substance Schedule: II

PHARMACODYNAMICS/KINETICS
Mechanism of Action: Binds with opiate receptors at various sites in CNS altering the perception of and emotional response to pain. Suppresses cough reflex by direct action on cough center in the medulla. **Onset of Action:** Rapid. **Peak Effect:** 0.5 hr. **Duration of Action:** 4–5 hr. **Metabolism/Elimination:** Metabolized by the liver. Excreted primarily via the urine. **Half-Life:** 2–3 hr.

INDICATIONS/DOSAGE

As a single agent or in conjunction with a nonnarcotic analgesic in the management of moderate to severe acute/chronic pain
Adult: 2–4 mg every 4–6 hr as needed. Patients may require higher doses.

In the Adverse Effects section, <u>underline</u> indicates most frequent; CAPS indicates life threatening.

267

CONTRAINDICATIONS/ PRECAUTIONS

Contraindicated in: Diarrhea caused by toxins, hypersensitivity, premature infants or during the labor/delivery of premature infants. **Use cautiously in:** Acute abdominal conditions, asthma, chronic obstructive pulmonary disease, head injuries, MAO inhibitor usage, narcotic analgesic that has abuse potential; dependency and tolerance can develop with repeated or prolonged use, renal/hepatic dysfunction. **Pregnancy/Lactation:** No well-controlled trials to establish safety. Benefits must outweigh risks. Crosses placenta. Present in breast milk. **Pediatrics:** Safety and efficacy not established.

PREPARATION

Availability: 1, 2, 3, 4, and 10 mg/mL in 1 mL amps/vials, 2 mL syringes (with 1 mL fill) and 20 mL vials. **Syringe:** Further dilute with 5 mL 0.9% sodium chloride or sterile water for injection.

STABILITY/STORAGE

Vial: Intact vials or ampules should not be stored under refrigeration due to possible precipitation or crystallization. Slight discoloration may develop but has not been associated with loss of drug potency.

ADMINISTRATION

General: IV route of administration is not always the first choice due to side effect potential. Rapid IV injection increases the incidence of adverse reactions. Do not administer IV unless a narcotic antagonist, emergency facilities, and skilled personnel for assisted/controlled ventilation are readily available. **IV Push:** 2 mg or less of a previously diluted solution over 4–5 min period. Administer via Y-site or three-way stopcock.

COMPATIBILITY

Solution: Amino acids, 8.5%, dextrose solutions, lactated Ringer's, Ringer's injection, sodium chloride solutions. **Syringe:** Atropine, chlorpromazine, cimetidine, diphenhydramine, fentanyl, glycopyrrolate, midazolam, pentazocine, pentobarbital, promethazine, ranitidine, scopolamine, thiethylperazine. **Y-site:** Acyclovir, amikacin, ampicillin, cefamandole, cefazolin, cefoperazone, ceforanide, cefotaxime, cefoxitin, ceftizoxime, cefuroxime, cephalothin, cephapirin, chloramphenicol, clindamycin, doxycycline, erythromycin, foscarnet, gentamicin, kanamycin, metronidazole, mezlocillin, moxalactam, nafcillin, ondansetron, penicillin G, piperacillin, tobramycin, trimethoprim-sulfamethoxazole, vancomycin.

ADVERSE EFFECTS

CNS: Coma, convulsions, agitation, anxiety, apathy, delirium, drowsiness, euphoria, headache, insomnia, mental confusion, mood changes, tremor. **CV:** ASYSTOLE, bradycardia, fainting, orthostatic hypotension, palpitations, peripheral vasodilation, tachycardia. **Resp:** APNEA, BRONCHOSPASM, respiratory arrest, respiratory depression: depressant effects begin by decreasing tidal volume, followed by a decreased respiratory rate as a result of decreased sensation of the respiratory center to carbon diox-

In the Adverse Effects section, underline indicates most frequent; CAPS indicates life threatening.

ide. **GI:** Anorexia, constipation, dry mouth. **GU:** Oliguria, reduced libido/potency, ureteral spasm, urinary retention/hesitancy. **Hypersens:** LARYNGOSPASM, pruritus, rash, urticaria. **Other:** Flushing, pain at injection site.

TOXICITY/OVERDOSE
Signs/Symptoms:
Overdose: Apnea, circulatory collapse, convulsions, cardiopulmonary arrest, and death may occur. Less severe toxic symptoms are CNS depression, miosis, and respiratory depression. Bradycardia, hypotension, hypothermia, pulmonary edema, pneumonia and shock occur in 40% or less of patients. **Treatment:** Maintain patent airway and institute assisted or controlled ventilation for apnea or severe respiratory depression/compromise. Hypotension may be treated with vasopressors. Fluid resuscitate as necessary. **Antidote(s):** Administer a narcotic antagonist, naloxone.

DRUG INTERACTIONS
Alcohol, antidepressants, antihistamines, sedatives, hypnotics: Exhibits additive CNS depression. **Buprenorphine, nalbuphine, pentazocine:** May decrease analgesic effect.

NURSING CONSIDERATIONS
Assessment
General:
Vital signs, pain control.
Physical:
Cardiovascular status, pulmonary status, GI tract.
Lab Alterations:
Increases serum amylase and lipase by increased biliary tract pressure.

Intervention/Rationale
Assess bowel function for hypoactivity resulting in constipation or paralytic ileus. ● Monitor blood pressure and heart rate before, during, and after administration of drug. ● Assess breath sounds and cough reflex (drug effects cough center by suppressing reflex), alter therapy if needed to prevent atelectasis or aspiration. ● May result in orthostatic hypotension—position patient or instruct patient to change positions gradually and slowly. ● Used concomitantly with a nonnarcotic analgesic may produce increased analgesic effects and allow lower doses of narcotic to be used.

Patient/Family Education
May cause dizziness/drowsiness. Avoid driving or engaging in any other activity that requires mental acuity until adverse effects have been determined. Avoid use of alcohol or other nervous system depressants while receiving this medication. Review all over-the-counter medications with physician prior to taking. May cause nausea, vomiting, or severe constipation; notify physician if symptoms become severe.

IDARUBICIN
(i-da′-roob-i-sin)
Trade Name(s): Idamycin
Classification(s): Anthracycline antineoplastic antibiotic
Pregnancy Category: D

PHARMACODYNAMICS/KINETICS
Mechanism of Action: Forms a complex with DNA causing inhibition

In the Adverse Effects section, underline indicates most frequent;
CAPS indicates life threatening.

269

of DNA synthesis. **Distribution:** Widely and rapidly distributed throughout body especially nucleated blood and bone marrow cells. Extensive tissue binding. Highly lipophilic resulting in increased cellular uptake. 95% protein binding that is concentration independent. **Metabolism/Elimination:** Extensive extrahepatic metabolism. Primarily eliminated as active metabolite (idarubicinol) via biliary tract and, to a lesser extent, by the kidneys. **Half-Life:** 22 hr, 45 hr idarubicinol.

INDICATIONS/DOSAGE

Treatment of acute myelogenous leukemia (as a combination regimen)

Adult: 12 mg/m²/day by slow injection for 3 days with ARA-C. Alternate dosage 25 mg/m² bolus followed by 200 mg/m²/day infusion for 5 days. If leukemia progression, a second course may be instituted. Delay repeat course and reduce dosage 25% if severe mucositis. Reduce dosage in hepatic/renal impairment. Avoid administraiton if serum bilirubin > 5 mg/dL.

CONTRAINDICATIONS/ PRECAUTIONS

Contraindicated in: Hypersensitivity. **Use cautiously in:** Myelosuppression from previous therapy or radiotherapy, previous CHF history, hepatic/renal impairment, patients with childbearing potential. **Pregnancy/ Lactation:** No well-controlled trials to establish safety. Embryotoxic/teratogenic effect demonstrated in rats. Benefits must outweigh risks. Discontinue breastfeeding prior to

drug administration. **Pediatrics:** Safety and efficacy not established.

PREPARATION

Availability: Lyophilized powder for injection in 5 mg and 10 mg single dose vials. **Reconstitution:** Dilute each 5 mg with 5 mL 0.9% sodium chloride for a final concentration of 1 mg/mL. Do not use bacteriostatic diluents. Contents under pressure; use caution. Avoid inhalation of aerosol. **Syringe:** No further dilution required. **Infusion:** Further dilute in physician specified volume of compatible IV solution.

STABILITY/STORAGE

Vial: Store at room temperature. Reconstituted solutions stable for 7 days refrigerated and 3 days room temperature. **Infusion:** Stable for 24 hr at room temperature.

ADMINISTRATION

General: Handle drug with care and adhere to institutional guidelines for the handling of chemotherapeutic/cytotoxic agents. Avoid inhalation of aerosolized powder/skin contact. Administer through rapidly flowing IV infusion into a large vein. Avoid extravasation. Notify physician immediately and elevate extremity/place intermittent ice packs (0.5 hr immediately then 0.5 hr four times per day for 3 days). **IV Push:** Give slowly over 10–15 min into tubing or Y-site of rapidly flowing compatible IV solution. **Intermittent/Continuous Infusion:** May infuse up to 24 hr as specified by physician.

COMPATIBILITY

Solution: Dextrose solutions, sodium chloride solutions.

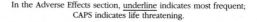

INCOMPATIBILITY
Syringe: Heparin. **Y-site:** Alkaline drugs.

ADVERSE EFFECTS
CV: CARDIAC TOXICITY/CARDIOMYOPATHY/CONGESTIVE HEART FAILURE (related to cumulative dose), DYSRHYTHMIAS, ECG abnormalities. **GI:** <u>Severe mucositis</u>, acute nausea/vomiting, diarrhea, increased liver enzymes (transient). **Renal:** Increased serum creatinine (transient). **Derm:** Alopecia. **Heme:** <u>MYELOSUPPRESSION</u>. **Nadir:** 10–14 days. **Hypersens:** Rash. **Other:** Chills, fever, tissue necrosis.

TOXICITY/OVERDOSE
Signs/Symptoms: Extension of adverse effects especially cardiac toxicity, myelosuppression, and GI toxicity. **Treatment:** Avoid cumulative doses. Symptomatic and supportive.

DRUG INTERACTIONS
Aminoglycosides, amphotericin B, nephrotoxic agents: Increased nephrotoxic potential. **Concomitant chemotherapy agents, immunosuppressants:** Increased myelosuppression. **Radiation therapy:** Increased cardiac toxicity.

NURSING CONSIDERATIONS
Assessment
General:
Vital signs, ECG (recommended), intake/output ratio, hypersensitivity reactions.
Physical:
Cardiopulmonary status, GI tract, infectious disease status, hematopoietic system.

Lab Alterations:
Assess CBC with differential and platelet count, BUN, serum creatinine, and liver function prior to and throughout course of therapy. Monitor serum uric acid.

Intervention/Rationale
Assess vital signs for signs/symptoms fluid/volume overload (drug may cause CHF). ● Assess for development of fever, chills, or other signs of infection and notify physician immediately. ● Maintain adequate hydration during therapy. Assess patient for development of bleeding (bleeding gums, easy bruising, hematest positive stools/urine/vomitus). ● Avoid intramuscular injections and rectal temperatures. ● Monitor uric acid levels throughout course of therapy and assure prophylactic allopurinol is prescribed.

Patient/Family Education
Hair loss may affect body image. Observe for signs of infection (fever, sore throat, fatigue) or bleeding (melena, hematuria, nosebleeds, easy bruising), especially 1 week following administration. Take and record oral temperature daily and report persistent elevation to physician. Use a soft toothbrush and electric razor to minimize bleeding tendency. Avoid crowded environments and persons with known infections. Use reliable contraception throughout the duration of therapy and 4 months following due to potential teratogenic and mutagenic effects of drug. Seek physician approval prior to receiving live virus vaccinations. Avoid over-the-counter products

---

In the Adverse Effects section, <u>underline</u> indicates most frequent; CAPS indicates life threatening.

containing aspirin or ibuprofen due to increased potential for bleeding. Report dizziness, unusual fatigue, or shortness of breath (drug may cause anemia).

IFOSFAMIDE
(i′-foss-fam-ide)
Trade Name(s): Ifex
Classification(s): Alkylating agent, antineoplastic
Pregnancy Category: D

PHARMACODYNAMICS/KINETICS
Mechanism of Action: Alkylating agent, following metabolic activation, interferes with tumor cell DNA synthesis, cell cycle nonspecific. **Metabolism/Elimination:** Extensively hepatically metabolized with saturation of metabolic pathways at high doses. Requires activation by microsomal enzymes for active metabolite formation. Active metabolites primarily eliminated by the kidneys. **Half-Life:** At doses 1.6–2.4 g/m²/day, 7 hr. At doses 3.8–5 g/m²/day, 15 hr.

INDICATIONS/DOSAGE

Combination therapy in germ cell testicular carcinoma
(in conjunction with mesna to prevent hemorrhagic cystitis).
Adult: 1.2 g/m²/day for 5 consecutive days. Repeat after 3 weeks or hematologic recovery.

CONTRAINDICATIONS/ PRECAUTIONS
Contraindicated in: Patients with severely depressed bone marrow, hypersensitivity to ifosfamide. **Use cautiously in:** Patients with immunosuppression, renal impairment, patients with fluid restrictions. **Pregnancy/Lactation:** No well-controlled trials to establish safety. Teratogenic potential is documented in males and females. Patients should avoid conception/pregnancy. Breastfeeding should be discontinued while receiving this agent. **Pediatrics:** Safety and efficacy has not been established.

PREPARATION
Availability: 1 g, 3 g single dose vials (as a combination pack that includes 200 and 400 mg of mesna, respectively). **Reconstitution:** Dilute each gram with 20 mL sterile water for injection or bateriostatic water for a final concentration of 50 mg/mL. **Infusion:** Further dilute to physician specified volume of compatible IV solution for a final concentration of 0.6–20.0 mg/mL.

STABILITY/STORAGE
Vial: Store at room temperature. Reconstituted vials with bacteriostatic water are stable for 1 week at room temperature or 3 weeks refrigerated. If sterile water for injection is used, refrigerate and use within 6 hr. **Infusion:** Stable for 1 week at room temperature or 6 weeks refrigerated.

ADMINISTRATION
General: Handle drug with care and adhere to institutional guidelines for the handling of chemotherapeutic/cytotoxic agents. Administer concurrently with mesna and at least 2 L of fluid per day to prevent bladder toxicities. **Intermittent/Continuous Infusion:** Administer as a slow

In the Adverse Effects section, <u>underline</u> indicates most frequent; CAPS indicates life threatening.

infusion over at least 30 minutes. May administer over 24 hr.

COMPATIBILITY

Solution: Dextrose solutions, lactated Ringer's, sodium chloride solutions. **Syringe:** Mesna. **Y-site:** Ondansetron.

ADVERSE EFFECTS

CNS: Seizures, polyneuropathy, <u>confusion</u>, depressive psychosis, dizziness, <u>hallucinations</u>, <u>somnolence</u>. **CV:** Cardiotoxicity, hypotension, hypertension. **Resp:** Pulmonary symptoms. **GI:** Anorexia, constipation, diarrhea, increased liver enzymes/bilirubin, liver dysfunction, <u>nausea</u>, salivation, stomatitis, <u>vomiting</u>. **GU:** Dysuria, hematuria, <u>ACUTE HEMORRHAGIC CYSTITIS</u>. **Renal:** Nephrotoxicity. **Derm:** <u>Alopecia</u>, dermatitis. **Heme:** Coagulopathy, <u>LEUKOPENIA</u>, <u>MYELOSUPPRESSION</u> (mild to moderate), <u>THROMBOCYTOPENIA</u>. **Nadir:** 7–14 days. **Hypersens:** Allergic reactions. **Metab:** Metabolic acidosis. **Other:** Phlebitis.

TOXICITY/OVERDOSE

Signs/Symptoms: Extension of adverse effects especially myelosuppression and concurrent infection. **Treatment:** Symptomatic and supportive.

DRUG INTERACTIONS

Concomitant chemotherapeutic agents, immunosuppressants: Increased myelosuppression.

NURSING CONSIDERATIONS

Assessment
General:
Vital signs, intake/output ratio.

Physical:
Infectious disease status, GU tract, GI tract, hematopoietic system, cardiopulmonary status, neurologic status.

Lab Alterations:
Monitor baseline and periodic renal/hepatic function, electrolytes, CBC with differential, and platelet count. Obtain urinalysis prior to each dose.

Intervention/Rationale
Maintain urine output at 100–200 mL/hr for 4 hr before initiating therapy and 24 hr following completion. Encourage patient to drink at least 2–3 L/day (adult) or 1–2 L/day (children) to promote adequate urine output and avoid hemorrhagic cystitis. Avoid administration in the evening to prevent accumulation in the bladder. ● Assess for development of fever, chills, or other signs of infection. ● Avoid all IM injections and rectal temperatures when platelet count is < 100,000 mm³. ● Assess for development of bleeding (bleeding gums, easy bruising, petechiae, hematest positive stools/vomitus/urine). ● Assure that proper antiemetic regimens are prescribed and given regularly to prevent nausea/vomiting. ● Assess for signs/symptoms of pulmonary toxicity with prolonged use (dyspnea, rales, crackles). ● Assess for signs and symptoms of cardiac toxicity that may occur early in therapy (characterized by symptoms of CHF). ● Assess for signs of neurologic changes (seizures, polyneuropathy).

In the Adverse Effects section, <u>underline</u> indicates most frequent; CAPS indicates life threatening.

273

Patient/Family Education

Review expected outcome and potential adverse effects of drug especially expected loss of hair. Observe for signs of infection (fever, sore throat, fatigue) or bleeding (hematuria, melena, bleeding gums, nosebleeds, easy bruising). Use a soft toothbrush and electric razor to minimize bleeding tendency. Take and record oral temperature daily and report persistent elevations to physician. Avoid crowded environments and persons with known infections. Use consistent and reliable contraception throughout the duration of therapy due to potential teratogenic and mutagenic effects of drug. Seek physician approval prior to receiving live virus vaccinations. Avoid over-the-counter products containing aspirin/ibuprofen throughout course of therapy due to increased potential for bleeding. IV fluids will be administered throughout the course of therapy in an effort to keep the kidneys flushed. Report dizziness, unusual fatigue, or shortness of breath (drug may cause anemia).

IMIPENEM-CILASTATIN

(i-me-pen'-em sye-la-stat'-in)
Trade Name(s): Primaxin
Classification(s): Broad spectrum antibiotic
Pregnancy Category: C

PHARMACODYNAMICS/KINETICS

Mechanism of Action: Bactericidal, interferes with bacterial cell wall synthesis. **Peak Serum Level:** End of infusion. **Distribution:** Widely distributed into saliva, sputum, aqueous humor, bone, bile, reproductive organs, myocardium, intestines, peritoneum, and wound fluids. 40% protein bound. **Metabolism/Elimination:** Cilastatin inhibits a renal enzyme responsible for metabolizing imipenem and increasing possible renal toxicity. Primarily eliminated unchanged (70%) by kidneys. Removed by hemodialysis. **Half-Life:** 0.85–1.3 hr. Cilastatin 0.83–1.1 hr.

INDICATIONS/DOSAGE

Treatment of serious infections of lower respiratory tract, urinary tract, intra-abdominal, gynecologic, septicemia, bone/joint, skin/skin structure, and endocarditis

Adult: Not to exceed 50 mg/kg/day or 4 g/day (whichever is less). Adjust dose/interval in renal impairment (based on creatinine clearance:

- Clcr 31–70 mL/min: 500 mg every 6–8 hr
- Clcr 21–30 mL/min: 500 mg every 8–12 hr
- Clcr 0–20 mL/min: 250–500 mg every 12 hr

If Clcr 0–5 mL/min, do not administer unless hemodialysis begins within 48 hr. Administer dose following hemodialysis and 12 hr later. **Mild Infections:** 250–500 mg every 6 hr. **Moderate Infections:** 500 mg–1 g every 6–8 hr. **Severe, Life Threatening:** 500 mg–1 g every 6 hr. **Uncomplicated UTI:** 250 mg every 6 hr. **Complicated UTI:** 500 mg every 6 hr.

Pediatric (unlabeled use): Safety and efficacy not established in children < 12 years old. 3–13 years old:

In the Adverse Effects section, underline indicates most frequent; CAPS indicates life threatening.

60–100 mg/kg/day in divided doses every 6 hr.

CONTRAINDICATIONS/ PRECAUTIONS

Contraindicated in: Patients hypersensitive to components. **Use cautiously in:** Hemodialysis patients, patients with renal impairment, patients with neurologic disorders, patients with a history of hypersensitivity to beta lactam/penicillin antibiotics and multiple allergens. **Pregnancy/Lactation:** No well-controlled trials to establish safety. Benefits must outweigh risks. **Pediatrics:** Safety and efficacy has not been established in children < 12 years old.

PREPARATION

Availability: 250 mg, 500 mg vials (containing 250 mg and 500 mg cilastatin, respectively). Contains 3.2 mEq sodium/g. **Reconstitution:** Dilute each vial with 10 mL sterile water or compatible diluent. Add to infusion solution. Then add additional 10 mL diluent to vial to ensure complete transfer. Reconstituted vials are not for direct administration. **Infusion:** Dilute 500 mg in at least 100 mL and 1 g in at least 250 mL compatible IV solution for a final concentration 5 mg/mL.

STABILITY/STORAGE

Vial: Store at room temperature. Stable 4 hr at room temperature and 24 hr refrigerated. **Infusion:** In dextrose, stable 4 hr at room temperature and 24 hr refrigerated. In sodium chloride, stable 10 hr at room temperature and 48 hr refrigerated.

ADMINISTRATION

General: Must be diluted prior to administration. Slow infusion rates are necessary to avoid nausea/vomiting. **Intermittent Infusion:** Administer 250–500 mg over at least 20–30 min and 1 g over at least 40–60 min.

COMPATIBILITY

Solution: Dextrose solutions (short stability), sodium chloride solutions. **Y-site:** Acyclovir, amikacin, famotidine, foscarnet, gentamicin, ondansetron, tobramycin, zidovudine.

ADVERSE EFFECTS

CNS: Seizures (especially with renal impairment), confusion, dizziness, headache, myoclonus, somnolence, tremor. **CV:** Hypotension, palpitations, tachycardia. **Resp:** Dyspnea, hyperventilation. **GI:** Hepatitis, pseudomembranous colitis, abdominal pain, diarrhea, increased liver enzymes, nausea, vomiting. **GU:** Anuria, oliguria. **Renal:** Increased serum creatinine/BUN. **MS:** Polyarthralgias. **Derm:** Candidiasis. **Fld/Lytes:** Hyponatremia, hyperchloremia, hyperkalemia. **Heme:** Anemia, eosinophilia, neutropenia, abnormal prothrombin time, thrombocytopenia. **Hypersens:** Pruritus, rash, urticaria. **Other:** Fever, transient hearing loss, erythema at injection site, phlebitis/thrombophlebitis.

TOXICITY/OVERDOSE

Signs/Symptoms: Seizures especially with high doses in renal impairment or patients on hemodialysis. **Treatment:** Symptomatic and supportive treatment. Hemodialysis may be helpful.

In the Adverse Effects section, underline indicates most frequent; CAPS indicates life threatening.

275

DRUG INTERACTIONS
Aminoglycosides: Synergistic effect against gram-positive organisms. **B-Lactam antibiotics:** Imipenem is a potent inducer of B-lactamase causing antagonism of antibacterial activity of beta lactams against some organisms. **Ganciclovir:** Potentiates seizure potential. **Probenecid:** Prolongs serum levels of imipenem.

NURSING CONSIDERATIONS
Assessment
General:
Vital signs, allergy history.
Physical:
GI tract, signs/symptoms superinfection (sore throat/stomatitis, vaginal discharge, perianal itching), infectious disease status.
Lab Alterations:
Monitor CBC, coagulation profile, renal/hepatic function, false-positive urine glucose with copper sulfate tests (Clinitest) (use glucose oxidase method).

Intervention/Rationale
Obtain careful history since patients with history of severe beta lactam sensitivity may also have imipenem sensitivity. Observe for signs/symptoms of anaphylaxis. ● Obtain cultures for sensitivity, first dose may be given while awaiting preliminary results. ● Assess neurologic function around scheduled time of infusion (may cause seizures with high doses in renal impairment). ● May cause pseudomembranous colitis (diarrhea, nausea/vomiting, fluid electrolyte disturbances), notify physician and obtain culture for *C. difficile* toxin).

Patient/Family Education
Complete course of therapy. Notify physician of any signs/symptoms of worsening infection (persistent fever/diarrhea) or signs of yeast infections (white patches or vaginal discharge).

IMMUNE GLOBULIN, INTRAVENOUS (IGIV, IVGG)
(im-myoon' glo'-byoo-lin)
Trade Name(s): Gamimune N, Gammagard, Gammar-IV, Iveegam, Sandoglobulin, Venoglobulin-I
Classification(s): Serum immune globulin
Pregnancy Category: C

PHARMACODYNAMICS/KINETICS
Mechanism of Action: In immunodeficiency, provides immediate IgG antibody levels. In other indications, exact mechanism unknown but may involve immunoregulation. **Onset of Action:** Immediate. **Distribution:** Widely distributed throughout body. **Metabolism/Elimination:** Eliminated via redistribution in extravascular fluid, tissue binding, or catabolism. **Half-Life:** 21–24 days.

INDICATIONS/DOSAGE

Treatment of immunodeficiency syndromes
Individualize treatment based on patient response.

In the Adverse Effects section, <u>underline</u> indicates most frequent; CAPS indicates life threatening.

Adult/Pediatric:
Gamimune N: 100–200 mg/kg/dose monthly. If response or desired IgG level is not achieved, increase the dose to 400 mg/kg or administer more frequently. **Gammagard:** 200–400 mg/kg/dose monthly. **Gammar-IV:** 100–200 mg/kg/dose every 3–4 weeks. **Iveegam:** 200 mg/kg/dose monthly. If response or desired IgG level is not achieved, the dose may be increased up to 800 mg/kg. **Sandoglobulin:** 200 mg/kg/dose monthly. If response or desired IgG level is not achieved, increase the dose to 300 mg/kg or administer more frequently. **Venoglobulin-I:** 200 mg/kg/dose monthly. If response or desired IgG level is not achieved, increase dose to 300–400 mg/kg or administer more frequently.

Idiopathic thrombocytopenic purpura (ITP)

Adult/Pediatric:
Gamimune-N: 400 mg/kg/day for 5 days. **Gammagard:** 1000 mg/kg. Additional doses may be administered based on clinical response/platelet counts. Up to three doses on alternate days may be given. **Sandoglobulin:** 400 mg/kg/day for 2–5 days. **Venoglobulin-I:** 500 mg/kg/day for 2–7 days. If patient responds, may discontinue. If platelet counts falls below 30,000 m³ or significant bleeding occurs, 500–2000 mg/kg may be given every 2 weeks or less to maintain platelet counts.

B-cell chronic lymphocytic leukemia

Adult:
Gammagard: 400 mg/kg every 3–4 weeks.

Kawasaki disease (*unlabeled use*)

Pediatric: 400 mg/kg/day for 3–5 days.

Autoimmune disorders (*unlabeled use*)

Adult/Pediatric: 400 mg/kg/day for 3–5 days or 1 g/kg/day for 2 days. Dosage will vary based on patient response.

CONTRAINDICATIONS/PRECAUTIONS

Contraindicated in: Patients allergic to gamma globulin or having IgA antibodies, patients with isolated IgA deficiency. **Use cautiously in:** Patients demonstrating prior sensitivity to any of these agents. **Pregnancy/Lactation:** No well-controlled trials to establish safety. Benefits must outweigh risks. No adverse fetal effects have been demonstrated.

PREPARATION

Availability: Gamimune-N: 5% in 10, 50, 100 mL vials. **Gammagard:** 50 mg/mL in 0.5, 2.5, 5, 10 g vials. **Gammar-IV:** 2.5 g/50 mL vials with diluent. **Iveegam:** 500 mg/10 mL, 1 g/20 mL, 2.5 g/50 mL, 5 g/100 mL vials with diluent. **Sandoglobulin:** 1 g, 3 g, 6 g vials with diluent. **Venoglobulin-I:** 2.5 g/50 mL, 5 g/100 mL vials with diluent.

Reconstitution: *Reconstitute with Provided Volume of Diluent:* Gammagard, Gammar-IV, Iveegam, Venoglobulin-I (sterile water), and Sandoglobulin (sodium chloride). **Gamimune N:** Ready to use. **Infusion:** Further dilute to physician specified final concentration in compatible IV solution.

In the Adverse Effects section, underline indicates most frequent; CAPS indicates life threatening.

277

STABILITY/STORAGE
Vial: Store at room temperature: Gammagard, Gammar-IV, Sandoglobulin, Venoglobulin-I. Store in refrigerator: Gamimune N, Iveegam. **Infusion:** Stable in refrigerator within 24 hr of preparation.

ADMINISTRATION:
General: Must be infused at indicated rates to minimize adverse effect incidence. If adverse effects occur, decrease infusion rate or discontinue the drug. **Intermittent/Continuous Infusion:** *Gamimune-N 5%:* 0.01–0.02 mL/kg/min for 30 min. May increase to 0.02–0.04 mL/kg/min (up to a maximum of 0.08 mL/kg/min) if no reaction. *Gammagard:* Initially, 0.5 mL/kg/hr. May increase up to 4 mL/kg/hr if no reaction. *Gammar-IV:* 0.01 mL/kg/min for 15–30 min. May increase to 0.02 mL/kg/min. Gradually increase to 0.03–0.06 mL/kg/min. *Iveegam 5%:* 1 mL/min. Not to exceed 2 mL/min. *Sandoglobulin:* Initial administration use 3% solution, 0.5–1.0 mL/min for 15–30 min. If no reaction, may increase to 1.5–2.5 mL/min. Administer subsequent infusions as 6% (or higher) concentrations at a rate of 2.0–2.5 mL/min. *Venoglobulin-I:* 0.01–0.02 mL/kg/min for the first 30 min. If no reaction, may increase to 0.04 mL/kg/min. May begin subsequent infusions at a higher rate.

COMPATIBILITY
Solution: Dextrose solutions, sodium chloride solutions.

ADVERSE EFFECTS
CNS: Headache. **CV:** Chest tightness, hypotension. **GI:** Nausea, vomiting. **MS:** Myalgia. **Hypersens:** ANAPHYLAXIS, urticaria. **Other:** Chills, fever, flushing, lethargy.

TOXICITY/OVERDOSE
Signs/Symptoms: Extension of adverse effects. **Treatment:** Symptomatic and supportive.

DRUG INTERACTIONS
Live Virus Vaccines: Do not administer 2 weeks prior or within 3 months after immune globulin administration because antibodies will interfere with immune response. If immune globulin must be administered within 2 weeks of live measles, mumps, rubella, repeat the vaccine at 3 months. This does not pertain to live polio virus or yellow fever vaccine.

NURSING CONSIDERATIONS
Assessment
General:
Vital signs.
Physical:
Signs/symptoms hypersensitivity reactions.
Lab Alterations:
Monitor platelet count (in ITP), immune globulin (in immunodeficiency).

Intervention/Rationale
Assess for allergic reaction; epinephrine should be available for treatment. ● Monitor vital signs especially during the first hour of infusion. Reduce flow rate or discontinue and notify physician if vital signs change significantly. ● Monitor appropriate parameters for disease states.

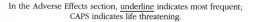

Patient/Family Education
Observe for early signs of allergic reaction (wheezing, chills, fever). Drug is pooled from human serum and risk of transmission of HIV/ Hepatitis B is present (however, advances in screening techniques reduce risk).

INDOMETHACIN
(in-doe-meth′-a-sin)
Trade Name(s): Indocin
Classification(s): Nonsteroidal anti-inflammatory agent

PHARMACODYNAMICS/KINETICS
Mechanism of Action: Inhibition prostaglandin synthesis, produces closure of patent ductus arteriosus (PDA). **Onset of Action:** Within 24–48 hr. **Distribution:** Widely distributed, 99% protein bound. **Metabolism/ Elimination:** Metabolized by liver to glucuronide conjugates and inactive metabolites that undergo enterohepatic recirculation. Eliminated via renal and biliary excretion. **Half-Life:** Varies inversely with postnatal age/weight: < 7 days: 20 hr; > 7 days: 12 hr. Mean: 12 hr.

INDICATIONS/DOSAGE

Closure of hemodynamically significant patent ductus arteriosus in premature infants weighing 500–1750 g, if, after 48 hr, medical management is ineffective.

Neonate: Age at first dose:
- < 48 hr: 0.2 mg/kg then 0.1 mg/kg for two doses every 12–24 hr.
- 2–7 days: 0.2 mg/kg for three doses every 12–24 hr.
- > 7 days: 0.2 mg/kg then 0.25 mg/kg for two doses every 12–24 hr.

If ductus closes or is significantly reduced within 48 hr after first course, no further doses are necessary. If it reopens, a second course of one to three doses may be given every 12–24 hr. If unresponsive to two courses, surgery may be necessary. Discontinue therapy if severe adverse effects result. If anuria or oliguria (< 0.6 mL/kg/hr) is evident at the second or third dose, do not give additional doses until lab results indicate normalized renal function.

Prophylaxis to reduce the incidence of symptomatic PDA in premature infants with a high probability of developing this condition.

Neonate: 0.2 mg/kg once 24 hr after birth.

CONTRAINDICATIONS/ PRECAUTIONS
Contraindicated in: Bleeding, especially intracranial hemorrhage or GI bleed, coagulation defects, congenital heart disease, necrotizing enterocolitis, proven/suspected untreated infection, renal impairment, thrombocytopenia. **Use cautiously in:** Patient with treated infections.

PREPARATION
Availability: 1 mg vials. **Reconstitution:** Dilute each vial with 1 mL or 2 mL sodium chloride or sterile water for injection (preservative free) for a final concentration of 0.1 mg/0.1 mL or 0.05 mg/0.1 mL, respectively.

STABILITY/STORAGE
Vial: Refrigerate vial. Prepare just prior to administration.

In the Adverse Effects section, underline indicates most frequent; CAPS indicates life threatening.

279

ADMINISTRATION
IV Push: Give over 5–10 sec.

COMPATIBILITY
Solution: Sodium chloride.

ADVERSE EFFECTS
Ophtho: Retrolental fibroplasia. **CV:** INTRACRANIAL BLEEDING, <u>pulmonary hypertension</u>, bradycardia. **Resp:** APNEA. **GI:** <u>GI bleed</u>, necrotizing enterocolitis, abdominal distention, transient ileus, vomiting. **GU:** <u>Oliguria</u>. **Renal:** <u>Elevated serum creatinine/BUN</u>, <u>reduced urine sodium</u>, <u>chloride</u>, <u>potassium osmolality</u>, <u>uremia</u>. **Fld/Lytes:** Fluid retention, <u>hyperkalemia</u>, hypoglycemia, <u>hyponatremia</u>. **Heme:** Bleeding, decreased platelet aggregation. **Metab:** ACIDOSIS, ALKALOSIS.

TOXICITY/OVERDOSE
Signs/Symptoms: Extension of adverse effects. **Treatment:** Symptomatic and supportive treatment.

DRUG INTERACTIONS
Aminoglycosides: Elevated peak/trough levels. **Digitalis:** Prolonged digitalis half-life. **Furosemide:** Blunted natriuretic effect.

NURSING CONSIDERATIONS
Assessment
General:
Vital signs, intake/output ratio.
Physical:
Cardiopulmonary status, GI tract.
Lab Alterations:
Monitor BUN/serum creatinine, platelet count, hemoglobin, arterial blood gases, and electrolytes.

Intervention/Rationale
Monitor cardiovascular and pulmonary status, including heart sounds and lung sounds routinely during course of therapy. ● Monitor urine output and report oliguria to physician immediately. ● Perform routine GI assessment and report abnormalities, including presence of diarrhea. ● Monitor for signs/symptoms of bleeding.

Patient/Family Education
Explain potential side effects and reason for therapy to parents.

INSULIN, REGULAR
(in′-su-lin)
Trade Name(s): Humulin, Iletin, Novolin, Velosulin
Classification(s): Hormone, insulin
Pregnancy Category: Unknown

PHARMACODYNAMICS/KINETICS
Mechanism of Action: Stimulates carbohydrate metabolism in skeletal/cardiac muscle and adipose tissue by facilitation of glucose transport into cells. Stimulates lipogenesis and protein synthesis. Promotes intracellular shift of potassium and magnesium in elevated serum levels. **Onset of Action:** 0.5–1.0 hr. **Peak Effect:** 2–3 hr. **Duration of Action:** 6–8 hr. **Distribution:** Rapidly distributed throughout extracellular fluids. **Metabolism/Elimination:** Rapidly metabolized by liver enzymes as well as (to a lesser extent) in the kidneys and muscle tissue. Glomerular filtrated with reabsorption (98%) at proximal tubule. Only small amount is excreted unchanged in urine. **Half-Life:** Few minutes, increased up to 13 hr in diabetic patients with antibody binding.

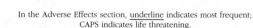
In the Adverse Effects section, <u>underline</u> indicates most frequent; CAPS indicates life threatening.

INDICATIONS/DOSAGE

Acute hyperglycemia/diabetic ketoacidosis

Adult: Adjust dose based on serum glucose level. Load: 100–200 units in two divided doses (50% dose should be IV push; if patient is in circulatory collapse, administer total dose as IV). Alternate dosage regimen load 2.4–7.2 units, then begin maintenance infusion at 2.4–7.2 units/hr.

Pediatric: Adjust dose based on serum glucose level. Load: 0.1 units/kg/dose IV push, then begin maintenance infusion 0.1 units/kg/hr. Decrease to 0.05–0.07 units/kg/hr if rate of increase of serum glucose exceeds 100 mg/dL per hour; increase to 0.14–0.2 units/kg/hr if rate of serum glucose decrease is less than 50 mg/dL/hr. Change to sliding scale or continue infusion at 0.02–0.06 units/kg/hr. Newly diagnosed patients in DKA with glucose < 800 mg/dL administer 50% initial loading and maintenance doses because sensitive to insulin. Alternate dosage load 0.5–2.0 units/kg/dose IV push or SC (50% dose should be IV push), then begin maintenance at 0.25–1.0 units/kg/dose every 2 hr or 0.5–2.0 units/kg/dose every 4–6 hr until glucose < 300 mg/dL and acidosis/ketosis resolving.

Hyperkalemia (after calcium gluconate/sodium bicarbonate)

Adult/Pediatric: 50% dextrose (0.5 mL/kg) and 1 unit insulin/4–5 g glucose administered.

Addition to hyperalimentation/IV fluids to assure proper glucose utilization and glycosuria reduction.

Adult/Pediatric: 5–40 units/infusion bag.

Provocative test for growth hormone secretion

Adult/Pediatric: 0.05–0.15 units/kg IV push following an overnight fast. Draw blood samples prior to, 30, 45, and 60 min after injection.

Glucose intolerance in premature infant

Neonate: After serum glucose has been stabilized at 45–130 mg/dL using dextrose, 0.025 units/kg/hr, increase the dextrose infusion rate and titrate insulin to maintain normoglycemia. Withdraw after several days of normoglycemia.

CONTRAINDICATIONS/PRECAUTIONS

Use cautiously in: Patients susceptible to hypoglycemia. **Pregnancy/Lactation:** Drug of choice in pregnancy for control of diabetes. Insulin does not pass into breast milk.

PREPARATION

Availability: 40 units/mL, 100 units/mL, 10 mL vials. **Iletin:** beef/pork, beef, pork. **Humulin, Novolin, Velosulin:** Human. **Infusion:** Add to volume of compatible IV solution suitable for administration for a final concentration of 0.2–1.0 unit/mL.

STABILITY/STORAGE

Vial: Unused vials should be stored in refrigerator. May be kept at room temperature while in use. **Syringe:** Prefilled syringes are stable for 1 week refrigerated. **Infusion:** Stable at room temperature/refrigerated for 48 hr.

In the Adverse Effects section, <u>underline</u> indicates most frequent; CAPS indicates life threatening.

281

ADMINISTRATION
General: Only regular insulin may be administered intravenously. Do not use U-500 insulin intravenously. Use appropriate insulin syringes to draw up dose. Binding to plastic tubing and bags may occur within 30–60 min especially with low concentrations. Prime tubing with IV solution containing insulin to saturate binding sites and prevent further adsorption. Human serum albumin may be added to infusion solutions to help reduce adsorption. Insulin requirements may be less with human products than pork, which is less than mixded beef–pork or beef. **IV Push:** May be given rapid IV push undiluted at a rate of 50 units/min. **Intermittent/Continuous Infusion:** Infuse over physician specified time or rate using an infusion control device.

COMPATIBILITY
Solution: Amino acids 4.25%/dextrose 25%, dextrose solutions, lactated Ringer's, sodium chloride. **Syringe:** Metoclopramide. **Y-site:** Dobutamine, famotidine, heparin, hydrocortisone, meperidine, morphine, pentobarbital, potassium chloride, sodium bicarbonate, vitamin B complex with C.

ADVERSE EFFECTS
Ophtho: Transient blurred vision. **Endo:** Hyperglycemic rebound (Somogyi), <u>HYPOGLYCEMIA</u> (blurred/double vision, confusion, fatigue, headache, hunger, hypothermia, loss of consciousness, muscle weakness, nausea, pallor, palpitations, perspiration, shallow breathing, tachycardia, tingling fingers, tremors), insulin resistance. **Hypersens:** ANAPHYLAXIS, angioedema, lymphadenopathy, urticaria.

TOXICITY/OVERDOSE
Signs/Symptoms: Extension of adverse effects especially hypoglycemia. **Treatment/Antidote:** If mild, oral administration of carbohydrates. If severe or comatose, dextrose 50%, 10–30 mL adults; 0.5–1.0 mL/kg children. If adequate glycogen stores, glucogon 1 unit.

DRUG INTERACTIONS
Alcohol, anabolic steroids, beta blockers, clofibrate, fenfluramine, guanethidine, monoamine oxidase inhibitors, phenylbutazone, salicylates, sulfinpyrazone, tetracycline: Increased hypoglycemia. **Beta blockers (especially nonselective):** Mask hypoglycemia symptoms except increased sweating. **Corticosteroids, dextrothyroxine, diazoxide, diltiazem, dobutamine, epinephrine, ethacrynic acid, furosemide, oral contraceptives, phenytoin (high doses), thiazide diuretics, thyroid hormones:** Decrease insulin's glucose lowering effect.

NURSING CONSIDERATIONS
Assessment
General:
Vital signs.
Physical:
Signs/symptoms of hyper/hypoglycemia.
Lab Alterations:
Obtain blood glucose prior to and during therapy.

Intervention/Rationale
Review time of peak effect and predictable times of hypoglycemic re-

actions prior to and during administration. Avoid large meals of high carbohydrate and fat content that increase serum glucose and decrease insulin's hypoglycemic effect. ● Evaluate vital signs for development of adverse effects.

Patient/Family Education

Review signs/symptoms of diabetes and the role of insulin in controlling, not curing the disease. Be aware of signs/symptoms of hypo/hyperglycemia and the treatments for each. Review dietary recommendations to combat hypoglycemia rather than administer additional insulin doses (use of complex carbohydrates). Insulin requirements may change with illnesses such as infections. Wear diabetic medical alert identification and carry small amounts of glucose products/complex carbohydrates. Review technique for drawing up insulin doses and the calibrations on the appropriate sized syringe and blood glucose (or urine) monitoring/interpretation of the prescribed method.

IRON DEXTRAN

(i'-ern dex'-tran)
Trade Name(s): InFeD
Classification(s): Antianemic, iron supplement
Pregnancy Category: B

PHARMACODYNAMICS/KINETICS

Mechanism of Action: Iron dextran circulates in plasma and enters reticuloendothelial system to split complex to provide iron for body stores. **Onset of Action:** Several days.

Peak Effect: 1–2 weeks. **Duration of Action:** Weeks to months. **Distribution:** Dextran complex distributed via plasma to liver, spleen, and bone marrow. Once released from dextran, bound to form hemoseridin ore ferritin, and to a lesser extent, transferrin. Iron dextran cleared from plasma by reticuloendothelial system. Dextran is metabolized and/or excreted. Iron is bound as body stores and eliminated through normal processes or blood loss. **Half-Life:** 6 hr.

INDICATIONS/DOSAGE

Treatment of iron deficiency anemia (when oral or IM administration is not feasible), iron replacement for blood loss

Adult/Pediatric (> 4 months):
Test Dose: 25 mg (0.5 mL) IV. If no adverse effects within 1 hr of test dose administration, may begin maintenance dose up to 100 mg/day; 50 mg/day < 10 kg; 25 mg/day < 5 kg (higher single doses have been given with increased risk of adverse effects) until total dose has been administered.

To restore hemoglobin and body iron stores

Adult/Pediatric (> 4 months):

$$\text{mg iron} = 0.3 \times \text{wgt (lb)} \times \left(100 - \frac{\text{observed hgb (mg/dl)} \times 100}{\text{desired hgb (mg/dl)}} \right)$$

Divide this result by 50, to calculate dose in milliliters. Administer this total amount as a single infusion or over a period of several days until total amount has been administered.

In the Adverse Effects section, <u>underline</u> indicates most frequent; CAPS indicates life threatening.

283

Replacement iron for blood loss

Adult/Pediatric (> 4 months):
mg iron = blood loss (mL) × hematocrit
Divide this result by 50, to calculate dose in milliliters.

CONTRAINDICATIONS/ PRECAUTIONS

Contraindicated in: Patients hypersensitive to iron dextran, anemias other than iron deficiency. **Use cautiously in:** Patients with serious liver/ renal impairment. **Pregnancy/Lactation:** Animal teratogenic potential has been identified with large doses. Benefits should outweigh risks. Small quantities pass into breast milk; use caution with breastfeeding. **Pediatrics:** Not recommended for infants less than 4 months of age.

PREPARATION

Availability: 50 mg/mL in 2 mL amps and 10 mL vials. **Syringe:** May give undiluted. **Infusion:** Dilute intermittent doses in at least 50–100 mL 0.9% sodium chloride (dextrose associated with increased pain and phlebitis). Single infusions may be diluted in 250–1000 mL 0.9% sodium chloride. Although not recommended, 1–8 mg/L has been added to parenteral nutrition solutions.

STABILITY/STORAGE

Vial: Store at room temperature. **Infusion:** Stable for 24 hr room temperature.

ADMINISTRATION

General: Administer only preparations for *IV* use. **IV Push:** Test doses should be administered over 5 min. Not to exceed 50 mg/min (1 mL/ min). **Intermittent/Continuous Infusion:** If no adverse effects 1 hr after initial test dose, may begin infusion over at least 1–6 hr. Flush with 10 mL 0.9% sodium chloride following administration.

COMPATIBILITY

Solution: Dextrose solutions (increased phlebitis), sodium chloride solutions.

ADVERSE EFFECTS

CNS: Convulsions, headache, paresthesia, syncope. **CV:** CARDIOVASCULAR COLLAPSE, chest pain, <u>hypotension</u>, shock, tachycardia. **Resp:** BRONCHOSPASM, dyspnea. **GI:** Abdominal pain, nausea, vomiting. **GU:** Hematuria. **MS:** Arthralgia, arthritis, myalgia. **Heme:** Leukocytosis, lymphadenopathy. **Hypersens:** ANAPHYLAXIS, rash, urticaria. **Other:** Chills, flushing, phlebitis, sweating.

TOXICITY/OVERDOSE

Signs/Symptoms: Long-term accumulation may lead to iron overload or hemosiderosis. **Treatment:** Symptomatic and supportive.

NURSING CONSIDERATIONS

Assessment
General:
Anaphylaxis potential, vital signs.
Physical:
Nutritional status.
Lab Alterations:
Monitor hemoglobin/hematocrit, reticulocyte counts, total iron binding capacity, and serum iron periodically. Prolongation of activated partial thromboplastin time (APTT)

In the Adverse Effects section, <u>underline</u> indicates most frequent; CAPS indicates life threatening.

if anticoagulant citrate dextrose solution used, falsely elevated serum bilirubin, falsely decreased serum calcium.

Intervention/Rationale
Evaluate for signs/symptoms of anaphylaxis and have treatment available at bedside prior to test dose administration. Monitor vital signs and watch for symptoms of anaphylaxis within 1 hr of test dose administration. ● Check vital signs prior to and after subsequent administration if no untoward effects have occurred. ● Within hours of administration with doses greater than 100 mg, a brownish coloration may be evident in serum.

Patient/Family Education
Explain therapeutic outcome of iron therapy and continuation of oral regimens/dietary supplements following this course of therapy. Instruct patient as to the possibility of adverse effects especially with initial administration; notify the physician if significant effects occur following treatment.

ISOPROTERENOL
(i-soe-proe-ter'-e-nole)
Trade Name(s): Isuprel
Classification(s):
Bronchodilator, vasopressor
Pregnancy Category: C

PHARMACODYNAMICS/KINETICS
Mechanism of Action: Beta adrenergic agonist activity resulting in positive inotropic/chronotropic effects and bronchodilation. Increases myocardial oxygen consumption/demand.

Onset of Action: Immediate. **Duration of Action:** < 1 hr. **Distribution:** Extensive tissue distribution. **Metabolism/Elimination:** Extensive hepatic metabolism. 50% excreted unchanged in urine.

INDICATIONS/DOSAGE

Adjunct in hypovolemia/hypoperfusion/CHF/cardiogenic shock
(Corrects hemodynamic imbalances in shock with low cardiac output and vasoconstriction that persists after adequate fluid replacement. Not useful if peripheral vascular dilation is present). Especially useful in the presence of bradycardia. Decreased efficiency in presence of CHF.
Adult: 0.5–5.0 mcg/min.

Diagnosis coronary artery lesions (*unlabeled use*)
Adult: 1–3 mcg/min.

Diagnosis mitral regurgitation (*unlabeled use*)
Adult: 4 mcg/min.

Management bronchospasm during anesthesia or acute asthma attacks unresponsive to inhalation therapy
Adult: Initial dose 0.01–0.02 mg. Repeat when necessary.

Treatment of cardiac dysrhythmias associated with AV block, cardiopulmonary resuscitation (advanced cardiac life support for immediate temporary control of atropine-resistant, hemodynamically significant, unstable bradycardia in patients with a pulse). Not indicated in patients with cardiac arrest

---

In the Adverse Effects section, <u>underline</u> indicates most frequent; CAPS indicates life threatening.

Adult: Initially 0.02–0.06 mg. Followed by 0.01–0.2 mg. Alternate dosage regimen 5 mcg/min.

Pediatric: 0.1 mcg/kg/min initially. Increase every 5–10 minutes to desired effect up to 0.1–1.0 mcg/kg/min.

Status Asthmaticus (*unlabeled use*)

Pediatric: 0.1–0.8 mcg/kg/min. Begin with 0.1 mcg/kg/min and increase by 0.1 mcg/kg/min at 15 min intervals until ventilation improves, heart rate exceeds 200 beats/min, or diastolic pressure falls below 40 mm Hg.

CONTRAINDICATIONS/ PRECAUTIONS

Contraindicated in: Angina pectoris, tachydysrhythmias, tachycardia or heart block associated with digitalis intoxication, ventricular dysrhythmias requiring inotropic therapy. **Use cautiously in:** Coronary artery disease, coronary insufficiency, diabetes, hyperthyroidism, patients sensitive to sympathomimetic agents, sulfite sensitive patients. **Pregnancy/ Lactation:** No well-controlled trials to establish safety. Benefits must outweigh risks.

PREPARATION

Availability: 0.2 mg/mL (1:5000) in 1 mL amp, 5 and 10 mL vials. **Syringe:** Dilute 1 mL to 10 mL with compatible IV solution for a final concentration of 0.02 mg/mL. **Infusion:** Further dilute each 5 mL in 250 mL (10 mL in 500 mL) compatible IV solution for a final concentration of 0.004 mg/mL.

STABILITY/STORAGE

Vial: Store at room temperature. **Infusion:** Stable at room temperature for 24 hr.

ADMINISTRATION

General: Must be diluted prior to administration. Do not use if pinkish to brownish in color. **IV Push:** May be given diluted (total volume 5 or 10 mL) rapid IV push. **Intermittent/ Continuous Infusion:** Infuse at physician specified rate.

COMPATIBILITY

Solution: Amino acids 4.25%/dextrose 25%, dextrose solutions, lactated Ringer's, Ringer's injection, sodium chloride solutions. **Syringe:** Ranitidine. **Y-site:** Amiodarone, amrinone, atracurium, bretylium, famotidine, heparin, hydrocortisone, pancuronium, potassium chloride, vecuronium, vitamin B complex with C.

INCOMPATIBILITY

Solution: Sodium bicarbonate.

ADVERSE EFFECTS

CNS: Dizziness, headache, nervousness, tremors, weakness. **CV:** VENTRICULAR DYSRHYTHMIAS, paradoxical Adams-Stokes syndrome, <u>palpitations</u>, <u>tachycardia</u>, angina, hypertension, hypotension. **Resp:** PULMONARY EDEMA. **GI:** Nausea, vomiting. **Other:** Flushing, sweating.

TOXICITY/OVERDOSE

Signs/Symptoms: Angina, dysrhythmias, hypertension, hypotension, tachycardia. **Treatment:** Reduce rate of administration or discontinue therapy.

In the Adverse Effects section, <u>underline</u> indicates most frequent; CAPS indicates life threatening.

DRUG INTERACTIONS
Bretylium, guanethidine, sympathomimetic agents, tricyclic antidepressants: Potentiates vasopressor activity. **Ergot alkaloids:** Increased blood pressure. **Halogenated hydrocarbons:** Sensitizes myocardium to catecholamines. **Oxytocics:** Severe persistent hypertension. **Potassium depleting diuretics:** Increased incidence of dysrhythmias.

NURSING CONSIDERATIONS
Assessment
General:
Vital signs, ECG monitoring, hydration status, intake/output ratio.
Physical:
Cardiopulmonary status.

Intervention/Rationale
Monitor blood pressure, heart rate, respirations, and ECG frequently during administration and after therapy. Monitor for dysrhythmias; discontinue therapy and contact physician if patient develops ventricular tachycardia/fibrillation (patients with cardiogenic shock are more likely to develop dysrhythmias; may require DC countershock). In treatment of third degree AV block, drug may be used until temporary pacemaker can be inserted. ● Monitor hemodynamics and lung sounds frequently before and during administration. ● Monitor volume status and correct hypovolemia prior to administration. ● Maintain adequate fluid intake to liquify secretions for maximal bronchodilation effect.

Patient/Family Education
Inform physician if headaches, chest pain, dizziness, palpitations, or nervousness occurs. Notify physician if pulmonary symptoms are not relieved.

KETAMINE
(ket'-a-meen)
Trade Name(s): Ketalar
Classification(s): General anesthetic
Pregnancy Category: Unknown

PHARMACODYNAMICS/KINETICS
Mechanism of Action: Anesthetizes via blocking pain perception and spinal cord transmission. **Onset of Action:** 30 sec. **Duration of Action:** 5–10 min. **Distribution:** Rapidly distributes into CNS. **Metabolism/Elimination:** Hepatic metabolism to less active metabolite. **Half-Life:** 2.5 hr.

INDICATIONS/DOSAGE

Induction of anesthesia prior to other general anesthetics. General anesthetic for short procedures

Adult/Pediatric: Individualize dosage.
Induction: 1.0–4.5 mg/kg (average dose 2 mg/kg to produce 5–10 minutes surgical anesthesia). Alternate dosage 1–2 mg/kg at 0.5 mg/kg/min. **Maintenance:** 50%–100% induction doses may be repeated as needed. Alternate dosage 0.1–0.5 mg/min.

CONTRAINDICATIONS/PRECAUTIONS
Contraindicated in: Patients in whom elevated blood pressure would be hazardous, psychiatric disorders, hypersensitivity. **Use cautiously in:**

In the Adverse Effects section, <u>underline</u> indicates most frequent; CAPS indicates life threatening.

287

Patients with history of hypertension or cardiac decompensation. **Pregnancy/Lactation:** No well-controlled trials to establish safety. Use is not recommended.

PREPARATION

Availability: 10 mg/mL in 20, 25, and 50 mL vials. 50 mg/mL in 10 mL vials. 100 mg/mL in 5 mL vials. **Infusion:** Dilute 500 mg in 250–500 mL compatible IV solution for a final concentration of 2 mg/mL or 1 mg/mL, respectively.

STABILITY/STORAGE

Vial: Store at room temperature. **Infusion:** Stable at room temperature for 48 hr.

ADMINISTRATION

General: Administer slowly to prevent respiratory depression and enhanced pressor response. **IV Push:** Administer over at least 1 min. Do not use 100 mg/mL vials. **Intermittent/Continuous Infusion:** Induction: 0.5 mg/kg/min. Maintenance: 0.1–0.5 mg/min.

COMPATIBILITY

Solution: Dextrose solutions, sodium chloride solutions, sterile water for injection. **Syringe:** Benzquinamide.

INCOMPATIBILITY

Syringe: Barbiturates, diazepam, doxapram.

ADVERSE EFFECTS

CNS: Confusion, excitement, hallucinations, irrational behavior, tonic/clonic movements, vivid imagery. **Ophtho:** Diplopia, nystagmus, slight elevation intraocular pressure. **CV:** Bradycardia, dysrhythmias, <u>elevated blood pressure and heart rate</u>, hypotension. **Resp:** Apnea, respiratory depression. **GI:** Anorexia, hypersalivation, nausea, vomiting. **Derm:** Transient erythema. **Other:** Local pain.

TOXICITY/OVERDOSE

Signs/Symptoms: Respiratory depression. **Treatment:** Supportive ventilation.

DRUG INTERACTIONS

Barbiturates, narcotics: Prolonged recovery time. **Halothane:** Decreased cardiac output, blood pressure, heart rate. **Tubocurarine, nondepolarizing muscle relaxants:** Increased neuromuscular effects. **Thyroid hormones:** Hypertension and tachycardia.

NURSING CONSIDERATIONS

Assessment
General:
Vital signs.
Physical:
Cardiopulmonary status.

Intervention/Rationale
Administer by personnel experienced with emergency airway management with access to ventilatory equipment. ● Monitor vital signs throughout administration.

Patient/Family Education
Avoid operating machinery requiring alertness for 24 hr. Avoid alcohol and other CNS depressants for 24 hr. Educate regarding adverse effect potential.

In the Adverse Effects section, <u>underline</u> indicates most frequent; CAPS indicates life threatening.

LABETALOL

(la-bet'-a-lole)
Trade Name(s): Normodyne,
Trandate
Classification(s): Beta
adrenergic blocker
Pregnancy Category: C

PHARMACODYNAMICS/KINETICS

Mechanism of Action: Alpha-1 receptor blockade and nonselective beta adrenergic receptor blockade. **Onset of Action:** 2–5 min. **Peak Effect:** 5–15 min. **Duration of Action:** 2–4 hr (up to 24 hr). **Distribution:** Rapidly and widely distributed into extravascular space especially lungs, liver, and kidneys. 50% protein bound. **Metabolism/Elimination:** Extensive hepatic metabolism. Primarily glucuronide conjugation. Metabolites excreted via urine and bile. **Half-Life:** 5.5 hr.

INDICATIONS/DOSAGE

Control of severe hypertension

Adult: Individualize dosage. Initially, 20 mg. Additional injections of 40 and 80 mg (range: 20–80 mg) may be given at 10 minute intervals until desired supine BP is achieved or total dose of 300 mg is administered. Higher initial doses of 1–2 mg/kg have been given with increased incidence of adverse effects. Alternate dosage 2 mg/min. Adjust infusion rate according to BP response or up to a maximum total dose of 300 mg. Begin oral therapy when the diastolic BP begins to decline. Reduce dosage in severe renal/hepatic impairment if therapy is continued for prolonged periods.

Pheochromocytoma (*unlabeled use*)

Adult: Controlled hypotension during anesthesia.
With Halothane: 20 mg (range 10–25 mg) following anesthesia induction, then 5–10 mg (range 2.5–15.0 mg) additional doses if necessary. **With Other Anesthetics:** 30 mg, then 5–10 mg if necessary.

CONTRAINDICATIONS/ PRECAUTIONS

Contraindicated in: Bronchial asthma, overt cardiac failure, second or third degree heart block, cardiogenic shock, severe bradycardia, known hypersensitivity. **Use cautiously in:** Patients with history of heart failure, hepatic impairment, diabetic patient receiving oral hypoglycemics. **Pregnancy/Lactation:** No well-controlled trials to establish safety. Does not affect the course of labor. Benefits must outweigh risks. Small quantities are present in breast milk. Exercise caution with breastfeeding. **Pediatrics:** Safety and efficacy has not been established.

PREPARATION

Availability: 5 mg/mL in 20, 40, 60 mL vials. 4 mL, 8 mL syringes. **Syringe:** No further dilution required. **Infusion:** Dilute 200 mg in 160 mL compatible IV solution for a final concentration of 1 mg/mL. Alternate dilution 200 mg in 250 mL for a final concentration of 2 mg/3 mL.

STABILITY/STORAGE

Vial: Store at room temperature. **Infusion:** Stable at room temperature or refrigeration for 72 hr in all so-

In the Adverse Effects section, underline indicates most frequent; CAPS indicates life threatening.

289

lutions. Stable for 24 hr in sodium chloride.

ADMINISTRATION

General: Individualize dosage. Keep patient supine until evaluation of adverse reactions. **IV Push:** Give 20 mg over 2 min. **Intermittent/Continuous Infusion:** Titrate to blood pressure beginning with 2 mg/min.

COMPATIBILITY

Solution: Dextrose solutions, lactated Ringer's, Ringer's injection, sodium chloride solutions. **Y-site:** Amikacin, aminophylline, ampicillin, butorphanol, calcium gluconate, cefazolin, ceftazidime, ceftizoxime, chloramphenicol, cimetidine, clindamycin, dopamine, enalaprilat, erythromycin, famotidine, fentanyl, gentamicin, heparin, lidocaine, magnesium, metronidazole, morphine, oxacillin, penicillin G potassium, piperacillin, potassium chloride, potassium phosphate, ranitidine, sodium acetate, tobramycin, trimethoprimsulfamethoxazole, vancomycin.

INCOMPATIBILITY

Y-site: Cefoperazone, nafcillin.

ADVERSE EFFECTS

CNS: Dizziness, numbness, scalp/skin tingling, somnolence, vertigo, yawning. **CV:** VENTRICULAR DYSRHYTHMIAS, <u>bradycardia</u>, <u>postural hypotension</u>. **Resp:** Wheezing. **GI:** Dyspepsia, nausea, taste distortion, vomiting. **Renal:** Transient increase serum creatinine/BUN. **Hypersens:** Pruritus. **Other:** Flushing, increased sweating.

TOXICITY/OVERDOSE

Signs/Symptoms: Excessive bradycardia and hypotension. **Treatment:** Symptomatic and supportive. Manage excess bradycardia with atropine/epinephrine, cardiac failure with digitalis and diuretic or dopamine or dobutamine, hypotension with vasopressors (e.g., norepinephrine), bronchospasm with epinephrine or aerosolized beta-2 agonist, and seizures with diazepam. Manage severe beta blocker overdose (hypotension/bradycardia) with glucagon (5–10 mg over 30 sec then 5 mg/hr and reduce as patient improves).

DRUG INTERACTIONS

Antihypertensive agents, diuretics: Additive hypotension. **Beta adrenergic agonists:** Blunted bronchodilator effect in bronchospasm. **Glutethimide:** Decrease pharmacologic effects of labetalol. **Halothane:** Synergistic cardiovascular adverse effects. **Nitroglycerin:** Blunted reflex tachycardia.

NURSING CONSIDERATIONS

Assessment
General:
Vital signs.
Physical:
Cardiopulmonary status.
Lab Alterations:
Falsely increased urinary catecholamines.

Intervention/Rationale
Monitor vital signs for several hours following administration. Measure supine BP immediately before and at 5 and 10 min intervals after injection. ● Establish patient's ability to withstand an upright position before allowing ambulation.

Patient/Family Education
Educate about adverse effects and expected therapeutic outcome.

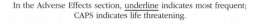

In the Adverse Effects section, <u>underline</u> indicates most frequent; CAPS indicates life threatening.

Continue all antihypertensive medications and avoid abrupt withdrawal. Slowly change positions when ambulating.

LEUCOVORIN CALCIUM (CITROVORUM FACTOR, FOLINIC ACID)

(loo-koe-vor'-in)
Trade Name(s): Wellcovorin
Classification(s): Folic acid derivative, antidote for folic acid antagonists
Pregnancy Category: C

PHARMACODYNAMICS/KINETICS

Mechanism of Action: Provides a reduced form of folic acid, tetrahydrofolic acid, necessary as a cofactor in biosynthesis of purines and pyrimidines of nucleic acids. By providing this form in overdose situations, "noncancer" cells, which do not need dihydrofolate reductase to convert the drug to the reduced form, are able to be "rescued." **Onset of Action:** Immediate. **Duration of Action:** 3–6 hr. **Distribution:** Distributed to all body tissues. **Metabolism/Elimination:** Liver maintains 50% body stores. Excreted as unused tetrahydrofolate derivatives via urine as dose exceeds 1 mg. **Half-Life:** 3.6 hr.

INDICATIONS/DOSAGE

Overdosage/rescue/folic acid antagonists

Adult/Pediatric: Various rescue schedules are employed. Within 24hr of methotrexate/folic acid an tagonist administration, 10 mg/m^2/dose every 6 hr for 72 hr or until methotrexate level falls below 10^{-8}M. If within 24 hr of antagonist administration, serum creatinine increases ≥ 50% above pretreatment, 100 mg/m^2/dose every 3 hr until serum methotrexate level is less than 5 × 10^{-8}M. Alternate dosage 40 mg/m^2 24 hr after administration, then 25 mg/m^2 every 6 hr for 72 hr—OR—6–15 mg/m^2 every 6 hr 2 hr after administration for 72 hr. If a large overdose or high doses are administered, up to 75 mg may be administered via infusion within 12 hr followed by 12 mg IM every 6 hr for four doses. If folic acid antagonist has less affinity for human dihydrofolate reductase (i.e., trimethoprim, pyrimethamine), 5–15 mg/day every 24 hr for 3 days or until blood counts return to normal (6 mg/day necessary if platelets < 100,000 mm^3) are adequate doses for hematologic toxicity reversal.

Concurrent administration with fluorouracil in metastatic colon carcinoma (increased response time/decreased progression)

Adult: 200 mg/m^2/day for 5 days.

Megaloblastic anemia

Adult/Pediatric: 1 mg daily.

Megaloblastic anemia associated with congenital deficiency

Adult/Pediatric: 3–6 mg/day.

CONTRAINDICATIONS/PRECAUTIONS

Contraindicated in: Pernicious anemia or megaloblastic anemia when

---

In the Adverse Effects section, <u>underline</u> indicates most frequent; CAPS indicates life threatening.

vitamin B_{12} is deficient. **Use cautiously in:** Pernicious/megaloblastic anemias untreated with B_{12} to avoid neurologic progression. **Pregnancy/Lactation:** No well-controlled trials to establish safety. Benefits must outweigh risks.

PREPARATION

Availability: 3 mg/mL in 1 mL amps. 5 mg/mL in 1 and 5 mL amps. 50, 100, and 350 mg vials.
Reconstitution: Use sterile water for injection for all doses greater than 10 mg/m^2; bacteriostatic water may be used for lower doses. Dilute 50 and 100 mg vials with 5 and 10 mL, respectively, of diluent for a final concentration of 10 mg/mL. Dilute 350 mg vial with 17 mL diluent for a final concentration of 20 mg/mL. **Syringe:** May give undiluted. **Infusion:** Further dilute required dose in volume (100–500 mL) of compatible IV solution sufficient to infuse over physician specified time.

STABILITY/STORAGE

Vial: Store at room temperature. Protect from light. Reconstituted vial should be used immediately if sterile water (no preservatives); if bacteriostatic water, stable for 7 days refrigerated. **Infusion:** Stable for 24 hr at room temperature.

ADMINISTRATION

General: Doses must be administered as per designated times to prevent significant hematologic toxicity. Doses greater than 25 mg must be administered parenterally. Do not exceed infusion rates because of calcium content. If inadvertent overdose is being treated, must be administered within 1 hr of overdose; ineffective after 4 hr de-

lay. **IV Push:** May be given undiluted IV push. Not to exceed 160 mg/min. **Intermittent/Continuous Infusion:** Infuse at physician specified rate. Not to exceed 160 mg/min.

COMPATIBILITY

Solution: Dextrose solutions, lactated Ringer's, Ringer's injection, sodium chloride solutions. **Syringe:** Bleomycin, cisplatin, cyclophosphamide, fluorouracil, furosemide, heparin, methotrexate, metoclopramide, mitomycin, vinblastine, vincristine. **Y-site:** Bleomycin, cisplatin, cyclophosphamide, doxorubicin, fluorouracil, furosemide, heparin, methotrexate, metoclopramide, mitomycin, vinblastine, vincristine.

INCOMPATIBILITY

Syringe: Droperidol. **Y-site:** Droperidol, foscarnet.

ADVERSE EFFECTS

Nontoxic in therapeutic doses. **Heme:** Thrombocytosis. **Hypersens:** Sensitization.

DRUG INTERACTIONS

Fluorouracil: Enhanced toxicity. **Folic acid antagonists:** Antagonize chemotherapeutic effect and hematotoxic effects. **Phenytoin:** Decrease in serum phenytoin concentration and increased seizure frequency. **Para-aminosalicyclic acid, phenytoin, primidone, sulfasalazine:** Decreased folate levels.

NURSING CONSIDERATIONS

Assessment
General:
Anaphylaxis
Lab Alterations:
Monitor creatinine clearance for dosage adjustment. Monitor meth-

otrexate serum levels, urine pH, serum folate levels, hemoglobin/hematocrit, and reticulocyte counts in megaloblastic anemia regimens.

Intervention/Rationale
Doses must be administered at specified times for efficacy and prevention of hematologic toxicity. ● Adhere to prescribed infusion rates. ● Assess patients for allergic reactions. ● Monitor methotrexate adverse reaction profile.

Patient/Family Education
Review importance of continuing additional therapies at the designated times to avoid toxicity. Maintain at least 2–3 L fluid intake during administration to avoid toxicity.

LEVORPHANOL TARTRATE
(le-vor'-fan-ole)
Trade Name(s): Levo-Dromoran
Classification(s): Narcotic agonist analgesic
Pregnancy Category: C (D for prolonged use or use of large doses at term)
Controlled Substance Schedule: II

PHARMACODYNAMICS/KINETICS
Mechanism of Action: Binds with opiate receptors at various sites in the CNS altering the perception of and emotional response to pain via an unidentified mechanism. **Onset of Action:** Immediate. **Peak Effect:** 30–60 min. **Duration of Action:** 4–8 hr. **Distribution:** Unknown. **Metabolism/Elimination:** Metabolized by the liver. Eliminated primarily via urine as glucuronide conjugate. **Half-Life:** 12–16 hr.

INDICATIONS/DOSAGE

Analgesic for relief of moderate to severe pain; severe intractable pain relief associated with terminal illness; preoperative sedation
Adult: 2–3 mg every 4–6 hr as needed.

CONTRAINDICATIONS/ PRECAUTIONS
Contraindicated in: Acute alcoholism, anoxia, bronchial asthma, diarrhea associated with a toxin, hypersensitivity, increased intracranial pressure, premature infants or labor/delivery of premature infants, respiratory depression. **Use cautiously in:** Anticoagulant therapy, chronic obstructive pulmonary disease, elderly/debilitated, impaired hepatic/renal function, may precipitate apnea in the asthmatic, use extreme caution in craniotomy/head injury and increased intracranial pressure (respiratory depression/ intracranial pressure may be further increased), seizures in the presence of a history of convulsive disorders with a marked increase in dosage. **Pregnancy/Lactation:** No well-controlled trials to establish safety. Benefits must outweigh risks. Crosses the placenta. Present in breast milk. **Pediatrics:** Safety and efficacy has not been established.

PREPARATION
Availability: 2 mg/mL in 1 mL amps and 10 mL vials. **Syringe:** Each dose should be diluted with 5 mL sterile water or 0.9% sodium chloride.

In the Adverse Effects section, underline indicates most frequent; CAPS indicates life threatening.

293

STABILITY/STORAGE
Vial: Store at room temperature.

ADMINISTRATION
General: IV is not the route of choice (usually administered S.C.). May be given IV through Y-site or threeway stopcock. **IV Push:** 3 mg or less of diluted drug may be administered slowly over 4–5 min.

COMPABILITY
Syringe: Glycopyrrolate.

ADVERSE EFFECTS
CNS: <u>Confusion</u>, delirium, disorientation, dizziness, euphoria, hallucinations, <u>sedation</u>. **Ophtho:** Blurred vision, diplopia, miosis. **CV:** Cardiac dysrhythmias, hypotension, orthostatic hypotension, palpitations, syncope. **Resp:** APNEA, BRONCHOSPASM, respiratory depression. **GI:** Anorexia, biliary tract spasm, constipation, dry mouth, nausea, vomiting. **GU:** Decreased libido, oliguria, ureteral spasm, urinary retention/hesitancy. **Derm:** Skin rash. **Hypersens:** ANAPHYLAXIS, LARYNGOSPASM, pruritus, urticaria. **Other:** Flushing, local tissue irritation, sweating.

TOXICITY/OVERDOSE
Signs/Symptoms: Increased severity of side effects, such as apnea, circulatory collapse, convulsions, or evidence of overdose, such as respiratory depression, extreme somnolence increasing to stupor or coma, are suggestive of the need for discontinuation of drug followed by physician notification. **Treatment:** Supportive, maintain airway via controlled or assisted ventilation, fluid resuscitation as required for treatment of hypo-

tension. **Antidotes(s):** Naloxone will reverse serious degrees of respiratory depression.

DRUG INTERACTIONS
Anesthetics, CNS depressants (alcohol, anticholinergics, antihistamines, barbiturates, hypnotics, narcotic analgesics, neuromuscular blockades, sedatives, MAO inhibitors, psychotropic agents), phenothiazines: May cause respiratory depression, hypotension, profound sedation, or coma when used concomitantly. **Buprenorphine, nalbuphine, pentazocine:** May decrease analgesic effect. **Cimetidine:** May cause CNS toxicity manifested by confusion, disorientation, respiratory depression with concomitant administration.

NURSING CONSIDERATIONS
Assessment
General:
Vital signs, ECG monitoring (recommended), pain assessment, tolerance/dependence potential.
Physical:
Pulmonary status, GI tract, neurologic status.
Lab Alterations:
May increase plasma amylase and lipase.

Intervention/Rationale
Assess respiratory rate and depth, cough and gag reflexes as this drug can cause depression of respiratory drive. Keep narcotic antagonist in close proximity. ● Assess blood pressure and heart rate prior to and during administration. ● Drug should be given in the smallest effective dose and as infrequently as possible in order to decrease the de-

In the Adverse Effects section, <u>underline</u> indicates most frequent; CAPS indicates life threatening.

velopment of tolerance and physicial dependence. ● Administer before intense pain occurs. Assess pain control/pain reduction after receiving medication in order to evaluate overall efficacy. ● Patient receiving IV administration should be lying down and must remain supine for 30–60 min after receiving the drug in order to decrease orthostatic changes. ● Evaluate heart rate for development of bradycardia/tachycardia. ● Turn, cough, and deep breathe at least every 2 hr in order to prevent atelectasis, especially in the postoperative period. ● Assess bowel sounds/function daily.

Patient/Family Education
Change positions slowly and gradually in order to minimize sudden drops in blood pressure. Alcohol and other CNS depressants must be avoided in order to prevent severe side effects. May cause drowsiness or dizziness; avoid driving and other activities that require mental acuity until adverse effects have been assessed.

LEVOTHYROXINE SODIUM (T4)
(le-voe-thye-rox'-een)
Trade Name(s): Levothroid, Synthroid
Classification(s): Thyroid hormone
Pregnancy Category: A

PHARMACODYNAMICS/KINETICS
Mechanism of Action: Stimulates the metabolism of all tissues in the body by increasing the rates of cellular level metabolism/oxidation. Increases the use and mobilization of glycogen stores. Stimulates protein synthesis. **Onset of Action:** 6–8 hr. **Peak Effect:** 24 hr. **Duration of Action:** Unknown. **Distribution:** Protein binding. 99% protein bound. Distributed throughout most body tissues. **Metabolism/Elimination:** Metabolized in the liver, via enterohepatic recirculation. Excreted in feces via bile. **Half-Life:** 6–7 days.

INDICATIONS/DOSAGE

Hypothyroidism
Adult: 50–100 mcg daily.
Pediatric:
■> 12 years: 2–3 mcg/kg/day.
■ 6–12 years: 4–5 mcg/kg/day.
■ 1–5 years: 5–6 mcg/kg/day.
■ 6–12 months: 6–8 mcg/kg/day.
■ 0–6 months: 8–10 mcg/kg/day.

Myxedema coma or stupor (without severe concomitant heart disease)
Adult: 200–500 mcg. If no response in 24 hr may give additional 100–300 mcg as indicated by patient response and serum protein bound iodine levels.

Cretinism
Neonate:
■ 6–12 months: 4.5–6.0 mcg/kg/day.
■ 0–6 months: 6.0–7.5 mcg/kg/day.

CONTRAINDICATIONS/ PRECAUTIONS
Contraindicated in: MI, thyrotoxicosis (except with antithyroid drugs), uncorrected adrenal insufficiency. **Use cautiously in:** Angina pectoris, arteriosclerosis, cardiovascular dis-

L

In the Adverse Effects section, <u>underline</u> indicates most frequent;
CAPS indicates life threatening.

295

ease, hypertension, ischemia, renal insufficiency, treatment of myxedema (patients are generally very sensitive to thyroid hormone). **Pregnancy/Lactation:** Does not readily cross placenta. No adverse fetal effects. Thyroid replacement should not be discontinued in hypothyroid women during pregnancy. Minute amounts are excreted in breast milk. Exercise caution when administering to pregnant women. **Pediatrics:** Potential hair loss may be experienced by children during the first few months of thyroid therapy.

PREPARATION

Availability: 200 and 500 mcg/vial in 6 and 10 mL vials. **Reconstitution:** Diluent usually provided with drug. Dilute each vial with 5 mL 0.9% sodium chloride. Shake well after reconstitution to dissolve lypholized powder completely. Administer reconstituted solution immediately after preparation; discard unused portion.

STABILITY/STORAGE

Vial: Store at room temperature. May acquire a pink color on exposure to light.

ADMINISTRATION

General: If parenteral route is required the IV route is preferred since absorption may be variable following IM admininstration. 0.1 mg (100 mcg) approximately equivalent to 65 mg (1 grain) thyroid. **IV Push:** Slowly over 1 minute via Y-site or threeway stopcock.

COMPATIBILITY/INCOMPATIBILITY

Data not available.

ADVERSE EFFECTS

CNS: Headache, <u>insomnia</u>, <u>irritability</u>, <u>nervousness</u>, tremors. **CV:** CARDIOVASCULAR COLLAPSE, angina, dysrhythmias, hypertension, hypotension, increased cardiac output, palpitations, <u>tachycardia</u>. **GI:** Cramps, diarrhea, nausea, vomiting. **GU:** Menstrual irregularities. **MS:** Accelerated bone maturation in children. **Derm:** Hair loss (children only). **Endo:** Menstrual irregularities. **Metab:** Heat intolerance, <u>weight loss</u>. **Other:** Fever, sweating.

TOXICITY/OVERDOSE

Signs/Symptoms: Toxicity is manifested as hyperthyroidism (tachycardia, chest pain, nervousness, insomnia, diaphoresis, tremors, weight loss). Massive overdose may demonstrate symptoms similar to thyroid storm (fever, CHF, hypoglycemia, massive fluid loss). **Treatment:** Withhold dose for 2–6 days. Supportive therapy and symptomatic treatment includes antiadrenergic drugs to control sympathetic overstimulation as well as oxygen and fever control as required.

DRUG INTERACTIONS

Digitalis glycosides: Decreased therapeutic effectiveness. **Imipramine, tricyclic antidepressants:** Increased antidepressant effect/sensitivity. **Insulin, oral hypoglycemic agents:** Increased dosage required for diabetic patients. **Ketamine:** May cause hypertension/tachycardia. **Oral anticoagulants:** Increased anticoagulant effect. **Sympathomimetic agents (amphetamines, vasopressors, decongestants):** Increased CNS and cardiac stimulation effects.

In the Adverse Effects section, <u>underline</u> indicates most frequent; CAPS indicates life threatening.

NURSING CONSIDERATIONS

Assessment:

General:

Vital signs, baseline/daily weight (including height in children).

Physical:

Metabolic status, GI tract.

Lab Alterations:

Thyroid function studies should be monitored prior to and throughout course of therapy.

Intervention/Rationale

Monitor blood sugars carefully; adjust insulin and oral hypoglycemic dosage in known diabetics accordingly. ● Assess heart rate and blood pressure before, during, and after drug administration, noting any tachydysrhythmias or chest pain. ● Evaluate development of changes in appetite, nausea, vomiting, weight, or diarrhea (occasionally associated with replacement therapy). ● In children monitor height, weight, and psychomotor development according to age.

Patient/Family Education

Notify physician immediately if chest pain, palpitations, sweating, nervousness, heat intolerance, or other signs of toxicity occur. Report unusual bleeding or bruising. Check pulse daily for at least 1 full minute; withhold dose and notify physician immediately if pulse is > 100 beats per minute. Avoid taking over-the-counter drugs that may interfere with thyroid replacement therapy (iodine-containing preparations). Medicine not to be stopped without physician directive.

LIDOCAINE HYDROCHLORIDE

(lye'-doe-kane)

Trade Name(s): Xylocaine, Xylocard ♣

Classification(s): Antiarrhythmic class 1B, local anesthetic

Pregnancy Category: B

PHARMACODYNAMICS/KINETICS

Mechanism of Action: Suppresses spontaneous depolarization of the ventricle during diastole by shifting flux of sodium across cell membranes. Suppresses the automaticity of conducting tissue of the heart. **Onset of Action:** 30–90 sec. **Peak Effect:** Immediate. **Duration of Action:** 10–20 min. **Therapeutic Serum Levels:** 1.5–6.0 mcg/mL. > 7 mcg/mL is usually toxic. **Distribution:** 40%–80% protein binding. Widely distributed throughout the body. Concentrated in adipose tissues. Crosses blood–brain barrier. **Metabolism/Elimination:** Extensively metabolized in the liver. Less than 3% excreted unchanged by the kidneys. **Half-Life:** Biphasic half-life. Distribution phase: 7–8 min. Terminal elimination phase: 60–120 min.

INDICATIONS/DOSAGE

Management of acute ventricular dysrhythmias

Adult:

Loading Dose:1 mg/kg. May be repeated at 0.5 mg/kg every 8–10 min for a maximum dose of 3 mg/kg as required. Followed by 1–4 mg/min infusion.

In the Adverse Effects section, underline indicates most frequent; CAPS indicates life threatening.

297

Pediatric: **Loading Dose:** 0.5–1.0 mg/kg. Followed by 20–50 mcg/kg/min infusion.

CONTRAINDICATIONS/PRECAUTIONS

Contraindicated in: Hypersensitivity to amide-type local anesthetics, severe degree of first, second, or third degree heart block without a functional temporary/permanent pacemaker, Stokes-Adams syndrome, Wolff-Parkinson-White (WPW) syndrome. **Use cautiously in:** CHF, excessive depression of cardiac conductivity (prolonged PR interval, widening of QRS complex, dysrhythmias), decreased cardiac output, digitalis toxicity, elderly/debilitated, heart block, hypovolemia, patients weighing < 50 kg, severe liver/renal disease, shock, untreated bradycardia. **Pregnancy/Lactation:** No well-controlled trials to establish safety. Benefits must outweigh risks. **Pediatrics:** Safety and efficacy for management of ventricular dysrhythmias in children has not been established.

PREPARATION

Availability: 10, 20, 40, 100, 200 mg/mL vials and prefilled syringes, premixed infusions of 1, 2, and 4 g in 250, 500 mL IV solution. **Infusion:** 1–2 g may be added to 250–1000 mL compatible IV solution. In children, 120 mg may be added to 100 mL compatible IV solution.

STABILITY/STORAGE

Vial: Store at room temperature. **Infusion:** Solution is stable for 24 hr at room temperature.

ADMINISTRATION

General: Avoid IV use of preparations containing preservatives or epinephrine. Containers of 1 g or more must be further diluted prior to administration. **IV Push:** May be given undiluted. Bolus Dose: Administer 50 mg or less over 1 minute. Too rapid administration may precipitate seizure activity.

Continuous Infusion: 1–4 mg/min titrated according to the rate of ventricular ectopy. **Must** be administered via infusion device.

COMPATIBILITY

Solution: Amino acids 4.25%, dextrose solutions, lactated Ringer's, Ringer's injection, sodium chloride solutions. **Syringe:** Glycopyrrolate, heparin, methicillin, metoclopramide, moxalactam, nalbuphine. **Y-site:** Alteplase, amiodarone, amrinone, cefazolin, dobutamine, dopamine, enalaprilat, famotidine, heparin, hydrocortisone sodium succinate, labetalol, nitroglycerin, potassium chloride, sodium nitroprusside, streptokinase, vitamin B with C.

INCOMPATIBILITY

Syringe: Ampicillin, cefazolin, dacarbazine.

ADVERSE EFFECTS

CNS: SEIZURES, convulsions, unconsciousness, apprehension, <u>confusion</u>, dizziness, <u>drowsiness</u>, euphoria, lightheadedness, slurred speech, tinnitus, tremors, twitching. **Ophtho:** Blurred vision, diplopia. **CV:** CARDIAC ARREST, bradycardia, cardiovascular collapse, hypotension, increased P-R interval

In the Adverse Effects section, <u>underline</u> indicates most frequent; CAPS indicates life threatening.

and QRS widening. **Resp:** Respiratory depression. **GI:** Nausea, vomiting. **Hypersens:** ANAPHYLAXIS, cutaneous lesions, edema, urticaria. **Other:** Malignant hyperthermia (tachycardia, tachypnea, metabolic acidosis, fever), venous thrombosis.

TOXICITY/OVERDOSE
Signs/Symptoms: Confusion, excitability, blurred vision, diplopia, nausea, vomiting, tinnitus, tremors, twitching, convulsions, dyspnea, severe dizziness, fainting, and decreased heart rate. **Treatment:** Discontinue infusion and monitor closely. For anaphylactic shock use epinephrine and corticosteroids. To correct CNS involvement use diazepam, short-acting barbiturates, and short-acting muscle relaxants. Maintain support of the patient; resuscitate as required.

DRUG INTERACTIONS
Beta-adrenergic blockers, cimetidine: Decreased metabolism and increased lidocaine toxic potential. **Phenytoin, procaine, propranolol, quinidine:** Additive cardiac depression and lidocaine toxic potential. **Tubocurarine:** Enhanced neuromuscular blockade.

NURSING CONSIDERATIONS
Assessment
General:
Vital signs, continuous ECG monitoring.
Physical:
Neurologic status, cardiopulmonary status.
Lab Alterations:
Monitor serum lidocaine levels and maintain therapeutic range between 1.5–5.0 mcg/mL. May in-crease creatine phosphokinase (CPK) levels. Monitor changes in fluid/electrolytes and acid-base balance during prolonged parenteral therapy.

Intervention/Rationale
Monitor ECG continuously throughout administration. ● Continuous infusion of drug should be gradually weaned over a specified period of time while monitoring ventricular ectopy rate and response to titration. Observe for signs of increased cardiac conductivity (sinus node dysfunction, prolongation of the PR interval, widening of QRS interval and complex, appearance or aggravation of dysrhythmias). ● Assess blood pressure and respiratory status frequently to observe for hypotension and respiratory depression. ● Assess neurological status frequently in order to identify and/or prevent CNS toxicity reactions.

Patient/Family Education
May cause drowsiness and occasional dizziness. Seek assistance with ambulatory activities. Notify nurse/physician if blurred or double vision is noted.

LORAZEPAM
(lor-az′-e-pam)
Trade Name(s): Ativan
Classification(s): Antianxiety agent, benzodiazepine, sedative/hypnotic
Pregnancy Category: D
Controlled Substance Schedule: IV

In the Adverse Effects section, underline indicates most frequent; CAPS indicates life threatening.

299

PHARMACODYNAMICS/KINETICS

Mechanism of Action: Depresses the CNS at the limbic/subcortical levels of the brain, probably potentiating gamma-aminobutyric acid (GABA) and other inhibitory transmitters. **Onset of Action:** Rapid. **Distribution:** Widely distributed throughout the body. Crosses the blood–brain barrier. **Metabolism/Elimination:** Metabolized by the liver. Excreted via urine in the form of oxidized and glucuronide-conjugated metabolites. **Half-Life:** 10–20 hr.

INDICATIONS/DOSAGE

Preoperative sedation

Adult: 0.044 mg/kg (not to exceed 2 mg) 15–20 min before surgery.

Surgical amnesia

Adult: Up to 0.05 mg/kg (not to exceed 4 mg). 2 mg is the **maximum** dose for patients > 50 years.

CONTRAINDICATIONS/ PRECAUTIONS

Contraindicated in: Acute narrow-angle glaucoma, hypersensitivity to benzodiazepines, chlordiazepoxide, glycols, or benzyl alcohol, psychoses. **Use cautiously in:** Elderly/debilitated, impaired liver/renal function, myasthenia, organic brain syndrome, patients with compromised pulmonary functions since underventilation and/or hypoxic cardiac arrest can occur. **Pregnancy/ Lactation:** Contraindicated in pregnancy, labor, delivery, and lactation as fetal toxicity can occur. **Pediatrics:**

Contraindicated in children. Safety and efficacy has not been established for children < 18 years of age.

PREPARATION

Availability: 2 and 4 mg/mL in 1 and 10 mL vials and 1 mL disposable cartridge units. **Reconstitution:** Dilute immediately prior to use with equal amounts of sterile water, 5% dextrose in water or 0.9% sodium chloride.

STABILITY/STORAGE

Vial: Parenteral form should be stored in the refrigerator in order to prolong shelf-life.

ADMINISTRATION

General: Rarely given IV. IM is the usual route of choice. Individualize dose for maximum benefits. **IV Push:** Each 2 mg or less over 1 min period may be administered direct IV via Y-site or threeway stopcock.

COMPATIBILITY

Solution: Dextrose solutions, sodium chloride solutions, sterile water for injection. **Syringe:** Cimetidine. **Y-site:** Acyclovir, atracurium, pancuronium, vecuronium, zidovudine.

INCOMPATIBILITY

Syringe: Buprenorphine. **Y-site:** Foscarnet, ondansetron.

ADVERSE EFFECTS

CNS: Ataxia, <u>dizziness</u>, <u>drowsiness</u>, headache, <u>lethargy</u>, mental depression, paradoxical excitation. **Ophtho:** Blurred vision, burning eyes. **CV:** Chest pain, hypotension, palpitations, tachycardia, transient hypotension. **Resp:** Respiratory depression, shortness of breath. **GI:** Abdominal discomfort, anorexia, constipation, diarrhea, dry mouth, nausea, taste alterations, vomiting.

In the Adverse Effects section, <u>underline</u> indicates most frequent; CAPS indicates life threatening.

Derm: Pruritus, rashes. **Heme:** Granulocytopenia, leukopenia. **Other:** Drug tolerance, flushing, physical dependence, psychological dependence, sweating.

TOXICITY/OVERDOSE
Signs/Symptoms: Toxicity or overdose is manifested by airway obstruction, possible apnea, delirium, hallucinations, drowsiness, restlessness. Hallucinations, horizontal nystagmus, and paradoxical reactions such as excitement, stimulation/hyperactivity are evidence of toxicity. **Treatment:** Supportive/symptomatic treatment including maintaining a patent airway and adequate ventilation/oxygenation. **Antidote(s):** Flumazenil IV as per physician order (reverses sedation or overdose). Physostigmine at 1 mg/min may reverse symptoms associated with anticholinergic overdose but may also cause seizures.

DRUG INTERACTIONS
Alcohol, other CNS depressants: Additive CNS depression. **Barbiturates, rifampin, valproic acid:** May increase metabolism and decrease effect of lorazepam. **Cimetidine:** Increases pharmacologic effect of lorazepam. **Levodopa:** May decrease efficacy of antiparkinson effect.

NURSING CONSIDERATIONS
Assessment
General:
Vital signs.
Physical:
Pulmonary status, neurologic status.
Lab Alterations:
Elevated LDH.

Intervention/Rationale
Assess anxiety level and how anxiety is manifested prior to and after receiving drug, in order to determine efficacy of drug and dosage. ● Assess respiratory rate and depth prior to and during administration. ● Patient should be maintained in a supine position for at least 8 hr after receiving the drug in order to prevent orthostatic effects. ● Evaluate neurological findings to determine development confusion, lack of concentration/coordination, and lethargy (manifestations of CNS adverse reactions—adjust dose accordingly). Consider withholding medication if coma or somnolence develops. ● Assess blood pressure prior to and following administration of drug to determine hypotensive effects.

Patient/Family Education
May cause drowsiness or dizziness. Avoid activities that require alertness or acute psychomotor coordination until CNS effects of the drug have dissipated. Seek assistance with ambulatory activities. Do not use drug in combination with alcohol or other CNS depressants. Disturbed nocturnal sleep may occur for the first few nights after discontinuance of the drug.

LYMPHOCYTE IMMUNE GLOBULIN
(lim'-foe-site e-mune' glob'-u-lin)
Trade Name(s): Atgam
Classification(s): Immune serum globulin
Pregnancy Category: C

In the Adverse Effects section, underline indicates most frequent; CAPS indicates life threatening.

301

PHARMACODYNAMICS/KINETICS

Mechanism of Action: Lymphocyte-selective immunosuppressant. May involve elimination of antigen-reactive T-lymphocytes or alter T-cell function. **Distribution:** Not fully known. Binds to circulating lymphocytes, granulocytes, platelets, bone marrow cells, and visceral tissues. Probably poorly distributed into lymphoid tissues (spleen, lymph nodes). **Metabolism/Elimination:** 1% of dose excreted unchanged in urine as equine IgG. **Half-Life:** 6 days.

INDICATIONS/DOSAGE

Adult dosage range 10–30 mg/kg/day. Pediatric dosage range 5–25 mg/kg/day (limited information available in children aged 3 months to 19 years).

Prevention of rejection of renal and skin allografts (used as adjunct to other immunosuppressants)

Adult/Pediatric: Usual dose 15 mg/kg/day for 14 days, followed by same dose every other day for 14 more days. Give first dose within 24 hr of transplantation.

Treatment of rejection of renal and skin allografts (used as adjunct to other immunosuppressants)

Adult/Pediatric: 10–15 mg/kg/day for 14 days. May follow with same dose every other day for another 14 days if necessary. Initiate therapy as soon as acute rejection is diagnosed.

Aplastic anemia

Adult/Pediatric: 10–20 mg/kg/day for 8–14 days, followed by same dose every other day for 14 days if necessary. May require prophylactic platelet transfusions.

Prevention/treatment of acute graft-vs-host disease in bone marrow transplant patients (*unlabeled use*)

Adult/Pediatric: 7–10 mg/kg/day every other day for six doses.

CONTRAINDICATIONS/PRECAUTIONS

Contraindicated in: Hypersensitivity elicited by systemic reaction to skin test. **Use cautiously in:** Local reaction to skin test. **Pregnancy/Lactation:** No well-controlled trials to establish safety. Benefits must outweigh risks. Probably crosses the placenta during the last 4 weeks of pregnancy. May be distributed into breast milk, since immunoglobulins are present in colostrum. **Pediatrics:** Limited safety and efficacy information. Has been safely given to a small number of pediatric renal transplant patients.

PREPARATION

Availability: 50 mg/mL in 5 mL amps. **Infusion:** Dilute in 250–1000 mL 0.45% or 0.9% sodium chloride. Final concentration not to exceed 1 mg equine IgG/mL. Invert IV solution container into which drug is added (solution is unstable in the presence of air). Gently rotate or swirl container after addition of drug to mix (do not shake).

STABILITY/STORAGE

Vial: Store in refrigerator. **Infusion:** Refrigerate diluted solutions if administration is delayed. Complete infusion within 12 hr of preparation.

In the Adverse Effects section, underline indicates most frequent; CAPS indicates life threatening.

ADMINISTRATION
General: Because of the risk of a severe anaphylactoid reaction, intradermal skin testing should be performed prior to administration. Test site should be observed for at least 1 hr for the appearance of a positive reaction. If a wheal/area of erythema greater than 10 mm, itching, or marked local swelling develops, infuse cautiously. A systemic reaction to the skin test such as generalized rash, tachycardia, dyspnea, hypotension, or anaphylaxis precludes further administration of the drug. **Infusion:** Administer with 0.2–1.0 micron in-line filter through a high-flow central vein, vascular shunt, or arteriovenous fistula to minimize risk of phlebitis and thrombosis. Infuse dose over at least 4 hr.

COMPATIBILITY
Solution: 0.45% or 0.9% sodium chloride.

INCOMPATIBILITY
Solution: Dextrose solutions, highly acidic solutions.

ADVERSE EFFECTS
CV: Hypotension. **Heme:** <u>Leukopenia</u>, <u>thrombocytopenia</u>. **Hypersens:** ANAPHYLAXIS, <u>erythema</u>, <u>rash</u>, <u>wheal</u>, <u>urticaria</u>. **Other:** Local/systemic infections, <u>febrile reactions</u>, serum sickness reactions.

DRUG INTERACTIONS
Immunosuppressants: Increased immunosuppressant effects.

NURSING CONSIDERATIONS
Assessment
General:
Vital signs, frequent temperatures.

Physical:
Hypersensitivity/anaphylaxis, infectious disease status.
Lab Alterations:
Monitor CBC periodically throughout therapy. Monitor platelet count in aplastic anemia patients to determine need for prophylactic platelet transfusions.

Intervention/Rationale
Observe continuously throughout skin testing period and duration of infusion for signs/symptoms of allergic reactions. Manage ATG-induced anaphylaxis with epinephrine, corticosteroids, assisted respiration, and other supportive measures. ● Patients have increased susceptibility to infection, lymphoma, and lymphoproliferative disorders, especially when used concomitantly with other immunosuppressants. To minimize or prevent febrile reaction, pretreat with an antipyretic, antihistamine, or corticosteroid. ● Discontinue therapy for severe leukopenia/thrombocytopenia.

Patient/Family Education
Educate regarding expected therapeutic outcome and side effects. Observe for early signs of allergic reaction (wheezing, chills, fever).

MAGNESIUM SULFATE
(mag-nee′-z-um sul′-fate)
Classification(s): Anticonvulsant, electrolyte
Pregnancy Category: B

PHARMACODYNAMICS/KINETICS
Mechanism of Action: Replaces/maintains magnesium level. As an anti-

In the Adverse Effects section, <u>underline</u> indicates most frequent; CAPS indicates life threatening.

303

convulsant, reduces muscle contractions by interfering with the release of acetylcholine at the myoneural junction. Acts peripherally to produce vasodilation. **Onset of Action:** Immediate. **Peak Effect:** Unknown. **Duration of Action:** 30 min. **Metabolism/Elimination:** Excreted by the kidneys at a rate proportional to plasma concentration and glomerular filtration rate.

INDICATIONS/DOSAGE

Hyperalimentation

Adult: 8–24 mEq daily added to hyperalimentation solution. *Pediatric > 6 years:* 2–10 mEq added to hyperalimentation solution.

Treatment of hypomagnesemia (severe)

Adult: 5 g or 50 mEq of 50% solution.

Preeclampsia/eclampsia

Adult: Loading dose: 2–4 g. Maintenance dose: 1–2 g daily as continuous infusion.

Convulsions

Adult: 1–4 g of 10% solution, repeat as necessary, infuse slowly.

CONTRAINDICATIONS/ PRECAUTIONS

Contraindicated in: Active labor, anuria, heart block, hypermagnesemia, hypocalcemia, myocardial damage. **Use cautiously in:** Any degree of renal insufficiency, patients receiving digitalis. **Pregnancy/Lactation:** Can cause fetal harm when administered to pregnant women. When administered during toxemia of pregnancy, the newborn is usually not compromised. Exercise considerable caution when administering to breastfeeding mothers. **Pediatrics:** Safety and efficacy not established.

PREPARATION

Availability: 10% (0.8 mEq/mL) solution in 10 and 20 mL amps and 20 and 50 mL vials. 12.5% (1 mEq/mL) solution in 8 and 20 mL vials. 25% (2 mEq/mL) solution in 150 mL vials. 50% (4 mEq/mL) solution in 2 mL amps, 2, 10, 20, 30, 50 mL vials and 5 and 10 mL syringes. **Syringe:** For IV injection a concentration of 20% (2 g/10 mL) or less should be used. **Infusion:** Dilute 4 g/ 250 mL compatible IV solution for anticonvulsant treatment. Add 5 g/ 1000 mL compatible IV solution for hypomagnesemia treatment.

STABILITY/STORAGE

Vial: Store at room temperature. Refrigeration may cause precipitation or crystallization. **Infusion:** Stable for 24 hr at room temperature.

ADMINISTRATION

General: Dosage should be individualized based on patient's needs and overall response to drug therapy. **IV Push:** Administer undiluted at a rate of 1.5 mL of a 10% solution (1 g/10 mL) over 1 min. **Intermittent Infusion:** *Anticonvulsant:* 4 g/250 mL IV solution at a rate not greater than 4 mL/min. *Hypomagnesemia:* 5 g/ 1000 mL over a 3 hr period of time. **Continuous Infusion:** Administer at physician prescribed rate. Use of infusion controlling device is required.

In the Adverse Effects section, <u>underline</u> indicates most frequent; CAPS indicates life threatening.

COMPATIBILITY

Solution: Dextrose solutions, sodium chloride solutions. **Syringe:** Metoclopramide. **Y-site:** Acyclovir, amikacin, ampicillin, cefamandole, cefazolin, cefoperazone, ceforanide, cefotaxime, cefoxitin, cephalothin, chloramphenicol, clindamycin, dobutamine, doxycycline, enalaprilat, erythromycin, esmolol, famotidine, gentamicin, heparin, hydrocortisone, labetalol, metronidazole, moxalactam, nafcillin, ondansetron, oxacillin, penicillin, piperacillin, potassium chloride, ticarcillin, tobramycin, trimethoprin-sulfamethoxazole, vancomycin, vitamin B with C.

INCOMPATIBILITY

Solution: Fat emulsion.

ADVERSE EFFECTS

CNS: Decreased deep tendon reflexes, drowsiness, flaccid paralysis. **CV:** Circulatory collapse, dysrhythmias, bradycardia, hypotension. **Resp:** Respiratory paralysis, depressed respiratory rate. **GI:** <u>Diarrhea</u>. **Fld/Lytes:** Hypocalcemia. **Other:** Flushing, hypothermia, sweating.

TOXICITY/OVERDOSE

Signs/Symptoms: Hypermagnesemia effects include: flushing, sweating, sharp drop in blood pressure, depression of reflexes, flaccid paralysis, hypothermia, circulatory collapse, depression of cardiac function, prolonged P-Q interval and widened QRS, CNS depression, and possible progression to fatal respiratory paralysis. **Treatment:** Discontinue drug and notify physician. Supportive/symptomatic treatment of patient is required. Administration of calcium gluconate to antagonize the effects of magnesium sulfate is a usual therapy: 5–10 mEq of calcium gluconate can reverse respiratory depression and heart block. Hypotension must be treated with vasopressors and fluid resuscitation. Maintain patent airway and support ventilation and oxygenation as indicated.

DRUG INTERACTIONS

Barbiturates, CNS depressants, general anesthetics, opiates: Additive CNS depression effects. **Neuromuscular blocking agents:** Prolonged respiratory depression with increased neuromuscular blocking effects.

NURSING CONSIDERATIONS

Assessment

General:
Intake/output ratio, vital signs, continuous ECG monitoring (recommended).
Physical:
Pulmonary status, neuromuscular reflex.
Lab Alterations:
Calcium, phosphorus, and magnesium balance should be monitored before, during, and after parenteral administration of the drug.

Intervention/Rationale

Maintain output > 100 mL during the 4 hr period before the drug is initiated. ● Assess vital signs at least every 15 min when administering drug for severe hypomagnesemia. ● Observe very closely for respiratory depression; should not be given with a respiratory rate of < 16/min. ● Monitor continuous ECG

In the Adverse Effects section, <u>underline</u> indicates most frequent; CAPS indicates life threatening.

305

for evidence of developing heart block. ● After use with toxemic mothers within 24 hr prior to delivery, observe the infant for signs/symptoms of magnesium toxicity including neuromuscular/respiratory depression. ● Patellar reflex should be tested prior to each parenteral dose; if reflex is absent, dose should be temporarily withheld until notification of physician has occurred.

Patient/Family Education
Notify physician/nurse if flushing occurs while receiving drug. Review therapeutic outcome and expected adverse effects.

MANNITOL
(man′-a-tol)
Trade Name(s): Osmitrol
Classification(s): Osmotic diuretic
Pregnancy Category: C

PHARMACODYNAMICS/KINETICS
Mechanism of Action: Increases osmotic pressure of glomerular filtrate; inhibits tubular reabsorption of water/electrolytes. Increases blood plasma osmolality causing increased flow of water into exracellular fluid. **Onset of Action:** 30–60 min. **Peak Effect:** 1 hr. **Duration of Action:** 6–8 hr. **Metabolism/Elimination:** Very slightly metabolized by liver. Freely filtered by the glomeruli with 90% excreted unchanged in urine. May be removed by hemodialysis. **Half-Life:** 15–100 min.

INDICATIONS/DOSAGE

Treatment of oliguria or inadequate renal function
Adult: Test dose of 200 mg/kg (50 mL of a 25% solution, 75 mL of a 20% solution or 100 mL of a 15% solution) is given over 3–5 min. If urine output does not increase, administer a second dose. If response is not adequate reevaluate patient. *Pediatric:* Test dose 200 mg/kg or 6 g/m² administered over 3–5 min. If urine output does not increase, administer a second dose of 2 g/kg or 60 g/m²/24 hr.

Oliguria treatment
Adult: 300–400 mg/kg of a 20% or 25% solution or up to 100 g of a 15%–20% solution.

Prevention of oliguria in acute renal failure
Adult: 50–100 g/24 hr as a 5%–25% solution.

Promote diuresis in drug toxicity
Adult: Up to 200 g titrated to maintain urine flow.

Reduction of intracranial pressure
Adult: 1.5–2.0 g/kg given as 15%, 20%, or 25% solution over a period of 30–60 min.

Reduction of intraocular pressure
Adult: 1.5–2.0 g/kg/24 hr as a 15%–20% solution over a 30 min period.

CONTRAINDICATIONS/PRECAUTIONS
Contraindicated in: Active intracranial bleeding, anuria caused by severe

renal disease, deyhdration, liver failure, pulmonary congestion, pulmonary edema, severe CHF, severe dehydration. **Pregnancy/Lactation:** No well-controlled trials to establish safety. Benefits must outweigh risks. Exercise caution when administering during lactation. **Pediatrics:** Dosage for patients < 12 years has not been established.

PREPARATION

Availability: 5% injection/1000 (50 g)/mL. 10% injection/1000 (100 g) and 500 (50 g) mL. 15% injection/150 (22.5 g) and 500 (75 g) mL. 20% injection/250 (50 g) and 500 (100 g) mL. 25% injection/50 (12.5 g) mL. Dosage equivalents: 1 g = approximately 5.5 mOsm.

Infusion: Add contents of two 50 mL vials (25%) to 900 mL sterile water for injection or compatible IV solution for a final concentration of 25 g/1000 mL. Concentrations > 15% have a tendency to crystallize. Must be diluted; may crystallize if added directly to an empty buretrol or IV bag.

STABILITY/STORAGE

Vial: Store at temperatures < 40° C, preferably between 15°–30° C. In concentrations of 15% or higher, may crystallize when exposed to low temperatures. If crystalization occurs solution should be autoclaved or warmed by carefully immersing in hot water (approximately 60° C) and periodically shaking vigorously; should not be used if all crystals cannot be completely dissolved. **Solution must be cooled to body temperature before using.**

ADMINISTRATION

General: Individualize concentration and rate of administration to maintain a urine flow of 30–50 mL/hr. In-line filter should be used for administration of drug. **IV Push:** A single dose of up to 3 g/kg over 30–90 min. **Intermittent Infusion:** A single dose should be administered over 90 minutes to several hr. **Continuous Infusion:** Administer at physician prescribed rate. Infusion device should be used.

COMPATIBILITY

Solution: Dextrose solutions, sterile water for injection. **Y-site:** Ondansetron.

ADVERSE EFFECTS

CNS: Convulsions, rebounding increase in intracranial pressure 8–12 hr after diuresis, confusion, dizziness, headache. **Ophtho:** Blurred vision. **CV:** Chest pain, CHF, edema, hypertension, hypotension, tachycardia, transient increase in plasma volume causing circulatory overload/pulmonary edema. **Resp:** Pulmonary congestion, rhinitis. **GI:** Diarrhea, nausea, vomiting. **GU:** Marked diuresis, urinary retention. **Renal:** Renal failure. **Fld/Lytes:** Hyperkalemia, hypokalemia, hypernatremia, hyponatremia, water intoxication. **Other:** Fever, phlebitis at IV site, thirst.

TOXICITY/OVERDOSE

Signs/Symptoms: Increased electrolyte excretion, hypotension, polyuria converting to oliguria, stupor, convulsions, hyperosmolality, and hyponatremia. **Treatment:** Discontinue infusion, notify physician. Fluid/electrolyte replacement as in-

In the Adverse Effects section, underline indicates most frequent; CAPS indicates life threatening.

307

dicated. Support patient as required.

DRUG INTERACTIONS
Lithium: Enhances excretion/decreases effectiveness of lithium.

NURSING CONSIDERATIONS

Assessment
General:
Vital signs, hemodynamic monitoring (recommended), intake/output ratio, baseline/daily weight.
Physical:
Neurologic status, integumentary status.
Lab Alterations:
Assess electrolytes, renal function studies, fluid balance, and urinary sodium content.

Intervention/Rationale
Monitor all vital signs hourly during administration with special emphasis on CVP and/or PWP and cardiac output. ● Assess intake/output hourly. Evaluate daily weights to verify positive/negative fluid status. Observe patient for signs/symptoms of pending dehydration (decreased skin turgor, increased thirst, dry mucous membranes). ● Monitor intracranial pressure and other neurological findings on an hourly basis if drug is being administered to decrease cerebral edema.

Patient/Family Education
Review rationale for medication administration as well as expected outcome and potential diuretic effect.

MECHLORETHAMINE (NITROGEN MUSTARD: HN$_2$)

(me-klor-eth′-a-meen)
Trade Name(s): Mustargen
Classification(s): Antineoplastic alkylating agent
Pregnancy Category: D

PHARMACODYNAMICS/KINETICS
Mechanism of Action: Alkylating agent that interferes with DNA replication and transcription of RNA, resulting in disruption of nucleic acid function. Inhibits rapidly proliferating cells. Palliative, not curative in its overall effect. **Metabolism/Elimination:** Extensively metabolized by the liver. Less than 0.01% of active drug is recovered in the urine. > 50% of inactive metabolites are excreted in the urine in the first 24 hr.

INDICATIONS/DOSAGE

Suppression of neoplastic growth in Hodgkin's disease (Stages III/IV), lymphosarcoma, bronchogenic cancer, specific types of chronic leukemia, polycythemia vera, mycosis fungoides

Adult: **Narrow margin of safety;** considerable care should be exercised with dosage determination. Dosage based on ideal dry body weight. 0.4 mg/kg as single dose or 0.1–0.2 mg/kg/day in divided dosages. Allow 3–6 weeks between courses of chemotherapy.

In the Adverse Effects section, <u>underline</u> indicates most frequent; CAPS indicates life threatening.

CONTRAINDICATIONS/ PRECAUTIONS

Contraindicated in: Hypersensitivity, infectious diseases. **Use cautiously in:** Anemia, bone marrow infiltrated with malignant cells, males/females of childbearing age, other chemotherapeutic agents, radiation therapy, severe leukopenia, thrombocytopenia. **Pregnancy/Lactation:** No well-controlled trials to establish safety. Benefits must outweigh risks. Known to cause fetal harm. Pregnancy should be avoided. **Pediatrics:** Safety and efficacy not established.

PREPARATION

Availability: 10 mg/vial. **Reconstitution:** Very unstable solution. Should be prepared immediately prior to use. Should not be used if droplets of water are visible within the vial or if the solution is not colorless. Reconstitute vial with 10 mL sterile water for injection or 0.9% sodium chloride for a final concentration of 1 mg/mL. With the needle in the rubber stopper, shake the vial several times to dissolve; **decomposes in 15 min from preparation time.** Unused solution should be neutralized with equal volumes of 5% sodium bicarbonate and 5% sodium thiosulfate prior to discarding.

STABILITY/STORAGE

Vial: Store at room temperature.

ADMINISTRATION

General: Handle drug with care and adhere to institutional guidelines for chemotherapeutic/cytotoxic agents. Drug is a potent **vesicant** and will cause painful inflammation; must be given directly into a vein, into a tubing of a running IV, or into a body cavity. Night time administration is preferred because of potential need for sedation to control side effects. In order to decrease the possibility of extravasation and minimize the reaction between drug/solution, injection into the rubber/plastic tubing of a free flowing IV is the preferred method of administration. If extravasation occurs, discontinue infusion and infiltrate affected area promptly with isotonic thiosulfate 1% or lidocaine and apply ice compresses to the affected area. **IV Push:** Extreme care should be taken to avoid extravasation of the drug. Total daily dose should be equally distributed over a 3–5 min time period.

COMPATIBILITY

Solution: Dextrose solutions, sodium chloride solutions. **Y-site:** Ondansetron.

ADVERSE EFFECTS

CNS: Seizures, headache, tinnitus, vertigo, weakness. **GI:** Anorexia, diarrhea, <u>nausea</u>, <u>vomiting</u>. **GU:** Delayed menses, gonadal suppression. **Derm:** Alopecia, erythema multiforme. **Heme:** <u>Granulocytopenia</u>, <u>hemolytic anemia</u>, <u>hyperuricemia</u>, <u>leukopenia</u>, <u>thrombocytopenia</u>. **Nadir:** 7–10 days (may last up to 3 weeks). **Hypersens:** Rash. **Other:** <u>Tissue necrosis with extravasation</u>, diminished hearing, metallic taste (immediately after dose), reactivation of herpes zoster, thrombosis, thrombophlebitis.

M

In the Adverse Effects section, <u>underline</u> indicates most frequent; CAPS indicates life threatening.

309

TOXICITY/OVERDOSE

Signs/Symptoms: Bleeding, bone marrow depression, hemolytic anemia, hyperuricemia, leukopenia, sustained nausea and vomiting, weakness, and death. **Treatment:** Discontinue drug; use supportive therapy, including blood transfusion as required to maintain patient throughout the toxic stage.

DRUG INTERACTIONS

Other antineoplastic agents: Increased myelosuppression activity.

NURSING CONSIDERATIONS

Assessment

General:
Hydration/nutritional status, intake/output ratio, baseline/daily weight.

Physical:
Hematopoietic system, GI status, infectious disease status.

Lab Alterations:
Increased AST (SGOT), ALT (SGPT), LDH, bilirubin, BUN, creatinine, and uric acid. Carefully monitor CBC/differential for signs/symptoms of bone marrow depression.

Intervention/Rationale

Assess fluid status; monitor intake/output and daily weights to determine negative/positive fluid balance. Maintain adequate hydration; force fluids as required. ● Alkalinize urine to increase uric acid excretion. ● Assess nutritional intake—strict recording of intake/output and calorie count. Adjust diet in accordance with manifestations of side effects. ● Administer antiemetics 30–40 min prior to therapy and around the clock for 24 hr as required. ● Assess daily for development of systemic infections (temperature elevation, elevated WBC). Hematest stools, vomitus, other drainage for presence of occult blood.

Patient/Family Education

Watch closely for signs/symptoms of infection (fever, sore throat, fatigue); bleeding (easy bruising, melena, petechiae, nosebleeds, bleeding gums). Take oral temperatures daily and record; notify physician if deviations from normal temperature occur. Immediately notify physician if fever or chills develop. Use consistent and reliable contraception throughout the duration of therapy due to potential teratogenic and mutagenic effects of the drug. Review hair loss potential, discuss methods of dealing with loss of personal identity. Instruct patient not to drink alcoholic beverages while undergoing therapy because of decreased effectiveness of the drug. Women of childbearing potential should be counseled to avoid becoming pregnant while undergoing drug therapy because of potential hazards to the fetus.

MEPERIDINE

(me-per′-a-deen)
Trade Name(s): Demerol
Classification(s): Narcotic agonist analgesic
Pregnancy Category: B (D for higher dosages/long-term use)
Controlled Substance Schedule: II

In the Adverse Effects section, underline indicates most frequent; CAPS indicates life threatening.

PHARMACODYNAMICS/KINETICS

Mechanism of Action: Binds with opiate receptors at various sites in the CNS, altering perception of and response to pain, via an unidentified mechanism. **Onset of Action:** Immediate. **Peak Effect:** 30 min. **Duration of Action:** 2–4 hr. **Distribution:** Widely distributed throughout tissues in the body. **Metabolism/Elimination:** Metabolized by the liver to an active metabolite, normeperidine. 5% excreted unchanged by kidneys. **Half-Life:** 3–4 hr.

INDICATIONS/DOSAGE

Preoperative medications; relief of moderate to severe pain; restoration of uterine tone/contractions affected by oxytocics

Adult: Dose should be individualized based on patient's needs. Usual dose: 10–50 mg. May be repeated every 2–4 hr.

Support of anesthesia

Adult: Individualize dose. Administer by slow IV injection or continuous IV infusion at 1 mg/min until desired effects are obtained.

CONTRAINDICATIONS/ PRECAUTIONS

Contraindicated in: Hypersensitivity, patients receiving MAO inhibitors 2 weeks prior to receiving this drug. **Use cautiously in:** Acute abdominal conditions, Addison's disease, alcohol use, asthma, CNS depression, chronic obstructive pulmonary disease, elderly/debilitated, glaucoma, head injury, hepatic/renal diseases, hypothyroidism, increased CSF pressure, prostatic hypertrophy, respiratory depression, seizures, shock, supraventricular tachycardia, urethral strictures. **Pregnancy/Lactation:** No well-controlled trials to establish safety. Benefits must outweigh risks. Crosses the placenta. **Pediatrics:** Use with extreme caution in children < 12 years.

PREPARATION

Availability: 50 and 100 mg/mL multidose vials. 10, 25, 50, 75, and 100 mg/mL single dose ampules, vials, and syringes. **IV Push:** Must be diluted with at least 5 mL sterile water for injection or 0.9% sodium chloride. **Infusion:** May be added to compatible IV solutions to form a concentration of 1 mg/mL. For anesthesia support dilute to 10 mg/mL with compatible IV solution.

STABILITY/STORAGE

Vial: Store at room temperature. Protect from light. **Infusion:** Stable for 24 hr at room temperature.

ADMINISTRATION

General: Do not administer IV unless a narcotic antagonist is immediately available. **IV Push:** A single diluted dose should be administered slowly over a 4–5 min period. **Continuous Infusion:** Infuse at physician specified rate. Infusions are based on the patient's needs/overall response to the drug. Drug titration occurs based on symptom relief as well as vital signs and respiratory rate and depth.

COMPATIBILITY

Solution: Dextrose solutions, lactated Ringer's, Ringer's injection, sodium chloride solutions. **Syringe:**

In the Adverse Effects section, underline indicates most frequent; CAPS indicates life threatening.

311

Atropine, benzquinamide, butorphanol, chlorpromazine, cimetidine, dimenhydrinate, diphenhydramine, droperidol, fentanyl, glycopyrrolate, metoclopramide, midazolam, pentazocine, perphenazine, prochlorperazine, ranitidine, scopolamine. **Y-site:** Acyclovir, amikacin, ampicillin, ampicillin-sulbactam, cefamandole, cefazolin, cefotaxime, cefotetan, cefoxitin, ceftizoxime, cefuroxime, cephalothin, chloramphenicol, clindamycin, doxycycline, erythromycin, gentamicin, heparin, insulin, metronidazole, moxalactam, ondansetron, oxacillin, oxytocin, penicillin, piperacillin, ranitidine, ticarcillin, ticarcillin-clavulanate, tobramycin, trimethoprim-sulfamethoxazole, vancomycin.

INCOMPATIBILITY
Syringe: Heparin, morphine, pentobarbital. **Y-site:** Cefoperazone, mezlocillin, nafcillin.

ADVERSE EFFECTS
CNS: Seizures, confusion, delirium, euphoria, hallucinations, headache, lethargy, unusual dreams, sedation. **Ophtho:** Blurred vision, diplopia, miosis. **CV:** CARDIAC ARREST, circulatory depression, dysrhythmias, bradycardia, hypotension, palpitations, postural hypotension, syncope, tachycardia. **Resp:** APNEA, BRONCHOSPASM, respiratory arrest, respiratory depression. **GI:** Anorexia, biliary tract spasm, constipation, nausea, vomiting. **GU:** Oliguria, reduced libido/potency, ureteral spasm, urinary retention. **Hypersens:** Allergic reactions, LARYNGOSPASM, pruritus, urticaria. **Other:** Flushing, sweating, psychological dependence, physical dependence, tolerance.

TOXICITY/OVERDOSE
Signs/Symptoms: Increased severity of minor signs/symptoms or development of major side effects such as allergic reactions, apnea, cardiac arrest, and shock. **Treatment:** Discontinue drug; notify physician. Treat signs/symptoms with supportive therapy based on manifestations. Monitor airway via controlled or assisted respirations. Resuscitate as required. **Antidote(s):** Naloxone will reverse respiratory depression.

DRUG INTERACTIONS
Alcohol, CNS depressants: Additive depressive effects. **Barbiturates, isoniazid, MAO inhibitors:** CNS excitation/depression. **Cimetidine:** CNS toxicity manifested by confusion, disorientation, seizures. **Phenytoin:** Decreases blood levels of phenytoin; decreases analgesic effect.

NURSING CONSIDERATIONS
Assessment
General:
Vital signs, continuous ECG monitoring (recommended), pain management.
Physical:
Cardiopulmonary status, neurologic status.
Lab Alterations:
Monitor for increased toxic effect especially seizures in patients with impaired renal function as evidenced by elevated BUN and creatinine.

In the Adverse Effects section, underline indicates most frequent; CAPS indicates life threatening.

Intervention/Rationale

Protect airway and maintain patency at all times. If used for post-operative pain management, assess breath sounds, respiratory rate, chest excursion; do not give if respiratory rate < 12/min. Encourage deep breathing and coughing in order to prevent atelectasis. ● Monitor circulatory status, including vital signs, to assess for hypotension, bradycardia. ● Observe patient frequently to prevent orthostatic changes with IV push administration. ● Assess pain control; for improved analgesia give medication before intense pain occurs. Adjust dosage scheduling according to needs/response of the patient. ● Keep narcotic antagonist available when administering the drug IV in order to counteract/correct respiratory depression.

Patient/Family Education

May cause drowsiness, dizziness; seek assistance with ambulation or repositioning activities. Avoid driving or otherwise engaging in activities requiring mental alertness. Avoid alcohol or other CNS depressants while taking the drug in order to prevent increased adverse effects. Change positions slowly and gradually in order to decrease significant and rapid shifting of blood pressure.

MESNA

(mez′-na)

Trade Name(s): Mesnex, Uromitexan ♣

Classification(s): Antidote for ifosfamide, detoxification agent

Pregnancy Category: B

PHARMACODYNAMICS/KINETICS

Mechanism of Action: Prevents ifosfamide-induced hemorrhagic cystitis by binding to urotoxic metabolites. **Onset of Action:** Rapid. **Duration of Action:** 4 hr. **Distribution:** Unknown. **Metabolism/Elimination:** Rapidly oxidized in bloodstream to its only metabolite, mesna disulfide. 33% eliminated in the urine as metabolite within 24 hr. **Half-Life:** 2 hr (drug). 1.17 hr (metabolite).

INDICATIONS/DOSAGE

Prevention of ifosfamide-induced hemorrhagic cystitis

Adult: 240 mg/m^2. Dose equal to 20% ifosfamide dose at same time as ifosfamide as well as 4 and 8 hr after ifosfamide dose. Repeat dosing schedule on each day that ifosfamide is administered.

CONTRAINDICATIONS/PRECAUTIONS

Contraindicated in: Hypersensitivity. **Pregnancy/Lactation:** No well-controlled trials to establish safety. Benefits must outweigh risks.

PREPARATION

Availability: 100 mg/mL in 2, 4, and 10 mL amps. **Infusion:** Add 4 mL (400 mg) to at least 16 mL of compatible IV solution to provide a final concentration of 20 mg/mL.

STABILITY/STORAGE

Vial: Store at room temperature. Decomposes quickly to an inactive compound; after ampule opened any unused drug should be discarded. **Infusion:** Diluted solutions are stable for 24 hr at room temper-

M

In the Adverse Effects section, <u>underline</u> indicates most frequent; CAPS indicates life threatening.

313

ature; should be refrigerated after preparation and used within 6 hr.

ADMINISTRATION

General: Must be administered with each dose of ifosfamide. **IV Push:** Single dose administered in bolus form over 2 minutes. **Intermittent Infusion:** Infuse in physician prescribed volume/rate.

COMPATIBILITY

Solution: Dextrolse solutions, lactated Ringer's, sodium chloride solutions. **Syringe:** Ifosfamide. **Y-site:** Ondansetron.

ADVERSE EFFECTS

CNS: Headache. **CV:** Hypotension. **GI:** Altered taste perception, diarrhea, nausea, soft stool, vomiting. **Other:** Fatigue.

NURSING CONSIDERATIONS

Assessment
General:
Intake/output ratio, hydration status.
Physical:
Genitourinary status.
Lab Alterations:
False-positive test for determination of urinary ketones, urinalysis for occult blood/cell count, BUN/creatinine for determination of altered renal state.

Intervention/Rationale
Maintain adequate hydration in order to increase drug excretion. Monitor intake and output; assess urine for occult and frank blood. Not effective in preventing hematuria from other causes.

Patient/Family Education
An unpleasant taste may accompany IV administration. Review adverse effects and expected outcome of therapy.

METARAMINOL
(me-ta-ram'-i-nole)
Trade Name(s): Aramine
Classification(s): Adrenergic agent, vasopressor
Pregnancy Category: Unknown

PHARMACODYNAMICS/KINETICS

Mechanism of Action: Stimulates alpha-beta-adrenergic receptors producing vasoconstriction and cardiac stimulation (positive inotropic effect). **Onset of Action:** 1–2 min. **Duration of Action:** 20 min to 1 hr. **Distribution:** Unknown; does not cross blood–brain barrier. **Metabolism/Elimination:** Metabolized in the liver. Metabolites eliminated via bile and kidneys.

INDICATIONS/DOSAGE

Hypotension treatment

Adult: 15–100 mg/500 mL IV fluid titrated to maintain desired blood pressure. *Pediatric:* 0.4 mg/kg or 12 mg/m^2 per IV fluid titrated to maintain desired blood pressure.

Severe shock

Adult: 0.5–5.0 mg IV push followed by infusion. *Pediatric:* 0.01 mg/kg or 0.3 mg/m^2.

CONTRAINDICATIONS/PRECAUTIONS

Contraindicated in: Cyclopropane or halogenated hydrocarbon anesthe-

In the Adverse Effects section, <u>underline</u> indicates most frequent; CAPS indicates life threatening.

sia, hypersensitivity, hypercapnia, hypoxia, peripheral or mesenteric thrombosis. **Use cautiously in:** Concurrent acidosis, coronary artery disease, diabetes mellitus, history of malaria, hypertension, hyperthyroidism, peripheral vascular disease, severe liver disease. **Pregnancy/Lactation:** No well-controlled trials to establish safety. Benefits must outweigh risks.

PREPARATION
Availability: 10 mg/mL in 1 and 10 mL vials. **Infusion:** Add 15–100 mg to 500 mL compatible IV solution.

STABILITY/STORAGE
Vial: Store at room temperature. **Infusion:** Stable at room temperature for 24 hr.

ADMINISTRATION
General: Allow 10 minutes between dosage increases. If extravasation occurs infiltrate area with 10–15 mL saline solution containing 5–10 mL phentolamine (in accordance with physician notification/order). **IV Push:** Single dose over at least 1 min. **Continuous Infusion:** Infuse at physician specified rate/volume.

COMPATIBILITY
Solution: Amino acid 4.25%, dextrose solutions, lactated Ringer's, Ringer's injection, sodium chloride solutions. **Y-site:** Amiodarone, amrinone.

ADVERSE EFFECTS
CNS: Apprehension, anxiety, dizziness, faintness, headache, nervousness, tremors. **CV:** Bradycardia, dysrhythmias, hypertension, hypotension, precordial pain, vaso-

constriction. **Resp:** Respiratory distress. **GI:** Nausea, vomiting. **GU:** Decreased urinary output. **Metab:** Hyperglycemia. **Other:** Flushing, pallor, sweating, tissue necrosis/sloughing at injection site with extravasation.

TOXICITY/OVERDOSE
Signs/Symptoms: Overdose symptoms include severe hypertension, dysrhythmias, convulsions, and/or cerebral hemorrhage. **Treatment:** For development or increased severity of adverse effects, decrease overall rate of infusion or temporarily discontinue infusion. **Antidote(s):** Phentolamine may be administered for blood pressure that does not respond to temporary discontinuance of infusion.

DRUG INTERACTIONS
Guanethidine: Partial or total reversal of antihypertensive of drug. **Halogenated hydrocarbon anesthetics:** May sensitize the myocardium to the effects of catecholamines resulting in serious dysrhythmias. **MAO inhibitors:** May cause severe hypertensive crisis or dysrhythmias. **Oxytocic drugs:** May cause severe persistent hypertention. **Tricyclic antidepressants:** Decreased pressor response requiring higher dosages of metaraminol.

NURSING CONSIDERATIONS
Assessment
General:
Vital signs, hemodynamic monitoring (recommended), intake/output ratio.
Physical:
Cardiac status, integumentary status.

In the Adverse Effects section, <u>underline</u> indicates most frequent; CAPS indicates life threatening.

315

Lab Alterations:
Hypercapnia, hypoxia, acidosis may decrease the effect of the drug or increase the number and severity of adverse effects. Assess electrolytes and ABGs throughout therapy.

Intervention/Rationale
Observe patient closely for adverse reactions. ● Monitor blood pressure and other vital signs even after discontinuation of the drug. Monitoring of CVP or PWP may be required to detect and successfully treat hypovolemia. ● Assess fluid status every hour by measuring output and calculating intake.

Patient/Family Education
Review therapeutic outcome and expected adverse effects.

METHICILLIN
(meth-i-sill′-in)
Trade Name(s): Staphcillin
Classification(s): Antibiotic (semisynthetic penicillin derivative)
Pregnancy Category: B

PHARMACODYNAMICS/KINETICS
Mechanism of Action: Bactericidal antibiotic, interferes with bacterial cell wall synthesis. **Peak Serum Level:** 30–60 min. **Distribution:** Distributed in synovial, pleural, pericardial, and ascitic fluids. Also found in bone and bile. Low concentrations found in CSF. 30%–50% bound to serum plasma proteins. **Metabolism/Elimination:** Primarily excreted unchanged in urine within 12 hr (30%–80%). Minimally removed by

hemo/peritoneal dialysis. **Half-Life:** 0.4–0.5 hr. Anuria 4–6 hr.

INDICATIONS/DOSAGE

Treatment of infections caused by penicillinase-producing staphylococci
Adult: 1–2 g every 4–6 hr. Reduce dosage in renal impairment. *Pediatric:* 100–300 mg/kg/day in divided doses every 4–6 hr.

CONTRAINDICATIONS/ PRECAUTIONS
Contraindicated in: Hypersensitivity to penicillins or cephalosporins. **Use cautiously in:** Renal impairment, hepatic failure. **Pregnancy/Lactation:** No well-controlled trials to establish safety. Benefits must outweigh risks. Crosses the placenta. Distributed into breast milk in low concentrations. May cause diarrhea, candidiasis, or allergic reactions in nursing infant.

PREPARATION
Availability: 1, 4, and 6 g vials. 1 g piggyback units. 10 g bulk packages. Contains 3 mEq sodium/g. **Reconstitution:** Add 1.5, 5.7, or 8.6 mL sterile water for injection or sodium chloride injection to 1, 4, and 6 g vials, respectively (resulting concentration is 500 mg/mL). Add 100, 50, or 20 mL sterile water for injection or 0.9% sodium chloride injection to 1 g piggyback units (provides solution containing 10, 20, or 50 mg/mL, respectively). **Infusion:** Further dilute each gram with 50 mL 0.45% or 0.9% sodium chloride injection (final concentration 2–20 mg/mL).

In the Adverse Effects section, underline indicates most frequent; CAPS indicates life threatening.

STABILITY/STORAGE
Vial: Store at room temperature. Reconstituted 500 mg/mL solutions are stable for 24 hr at room temperature or 4 days refrigerated. **Infusion:** Stable for 8 hr at room temperature or 24 hr refrigerated.

ADMINISTRATION
General: If possible, discontinue other IV solutions flowing through a common infusion site while methicillin is administered. **IV Push:** Give slow IV push at a rate of 10 mL/min. **Intermittent Infusion:** Infuse over 20–30 min.

COMPATIBILITY
Solution: Amino acids 4.25%/dextrose 25%, dextrose solutions, lactated Ringer's, sodium bicarbonate, sodium chloride solutions. **Syringe:** Chloramphenicol, erythromycin lactobionate, gentamicin, polymyxin B. **Y-site:** Heparin, hydrocortisone, potassium chloride, verapamil, vitamin B complex with C.

INCOMPATIBILITY
Solution: Dextran 40 (dextrose and saline), Ringer's injection. **Syringe:** Heparin, kanamycin, lincomycin.

ADVERSE EFFECTS
GI: Pseudomembranous colitis, black or hairy tongue, diarrhea, increased alkaline phosphatase, AST, and ALT (transient), nausea, stomatitis. **GU:** Hemorrhagic cystitis (high doses). **Renal:** <u>Interstitial nephritis</u>. **Heme:** Agranulocytosis, transient granulocytopenia, leukopenia, neutropenia, and thrombocytopenia. **Hypersens:** Rash, urticaria. **Other:** Phlebitis/thrombophlebitis (especially in elderly).

DRUG INTERACTIONS
Aminoglycosides: Inactivation of aminoglycoside. **Probenecid:** Higher and prolonged methicillin serum concentrations.

NURSING CONSIDERATIONS
Assessment
General:
Determine history of allergic or hypersensitivity reactions to penicillins/cephalosporins. Obtain specimens for organism susceptibility prior to initiation of therapy (first dose may be given while awaiting results). Infectious disease status (signs/symptoms of superinfection/bacterial/fungal overgrowth especially in elderly, debilitated, or immunosuppressed).
Physical:
GI tract, GU tract, signs/symptoms of anaphylaxis.
Lab Alterations:
Monitor CBC with differential, urinalysis, serum creatinine, BUN, AST (SGOT), and ALT (SGPT) periodically during therapy. Obtain frequent urinalysis to monitor for the presence of interstitial nephritis. False-positive urinary and serum protein, falsely increased uric acid concentrations, falsely increased urinary steroids, positive direct antiglobulin (Coombs'), falsely decreased serum aminoglycoside assays, false-positive reaction with copper-sulfate urine glucose tests (Clinitest).

Intervention/Rationale
Hypersensitivity reactions may be immediate and severe in penicillin-sensitive patients with a history of allergy, asthma, hay fever, or ur-

M

In the Adverse Effects section, <u>underline</u> indicates most frequent; CAPS indicates life threatening.

317

ticaria. ● Monitor frequency, quality, and character of stools for signs/symptoms of pseudomembranous colitis.

Patient/Family Education
Notify physician/nurse if skin rash, itching, hives, severe diarrhea, or signs of superinfection occurs.

METHOCARBAMOL

(metho-oh-karb'-a-mol)
Trade Name(s): Robaxin
Classification(s): Skeletal muscle relaxant
Pregnancy Category: C

PHARMACODYNAMICS/KINETICS

Mechanism of Action: CNS depressant with sedative and skeletal muscle relaxant effects. Does not depress neuronal conduction, neuromuscular transmission, or muscle excitability. **Onset of Action:** Rapid. **Distribution:** Widely distributed with highest concentrations in the kidney and liver. **Metabolism/Elimination:** Extensively metabolized, probably by the liver. Rapidly excreted in the urine. **Half-Life:** 0.9–1.8 hr.

INDICATIONS/DOSAGE

Relief of discomfort associated with acute, painful muscle conditions (adjunctive therapy along with rest, physical therapy, analgesics, etc.)
Adult: 1 g every 8 hr. Not to exceed 3 g per day for more than 3 consecutive days. If necessary, 1–2 g may be readministered after a drug-free interval of 2 days.

Control of neuromuscular manifestations of tetanus (not to replace debridement, tetanus antitoxin, penicillin, and other supportive therapies)
Adult: Initial dose 1–3 g followed by 1–2 g every 6 hr until nasogastric tube can be inserted and drug can be given orally. *Pediatric:* 60 mg/kg/24 hr in four divided doses. Maximum dose 1.8 g/m^2 daily for 3 consecutive days.

CONTRAINDICATIONS/ PRECAUTIONS

Contraindicated in: Hypersensitivity to orphenadrine, glaucoma, pyloric or duodenal obstruction, stenosing peptic ulcers, prostatic hypertrophy, bladder neck obstruction, cardiospasm, myasthenia gravis, impaired renal function. **Pregnancy/ Lactation:** No well-controlled trials to establish safety. Benefits must outweigh risks. **Pediatrics:** Not recommended for use in children < 12 years old, except for the treatment of tetanus.

PREPARATION

Availability: 100 mg/mL in 10 mL vials.

STABILITY/STORAGE

Vial: Store at room temperature. **Infusion:** Stable for 24 hr at room temperature.

ADMINISTRATION

General: Avoid extravasation (injection is hypertonic). **IV Push:** Administer undiluted at maximum rate of 300 mg/min (3 mL/min). **Intermittent Infusion:** Dilute 1 g with a maximum volume of 250 mL compatible IV solution.

In the Adverse Effects section, <u>underline</u> indicates most frequent; CAPS indicates life threatening.

COMPATIBILITY
Solution: Dextrose solutions, sodium chloride solutions.

ADVERSE EFFECTS
CNS: <u>Dizziness</u>, <u>drowsiness</u>, headache, <u>lightheadedness</u>, mild muscle incoordination, nystagmus, syncope. **Ophtho:** Blurred vision, conjunctivitis with nasal congestion. **CV:** Bradycardia, hypotension. **GI:** Metallic taste, nausea. **GU:** Hemolysis, increased hemoglobin and RBCs in urine. **Heme:** Leukopenia (rare). **Hypersens:** Rash, skin eruptions, pruritus, urticaria. **Other:** Fever; thrombophlebitis, sloughing, or pain at injection site.

DRUG INTERACTIONS
Alcohol and other CNS depressants: Additive depressant effects.

NURSING CONSIDERATIONS
Assessment
General:
Vital signs:
Physical:
Neurologic status, ophthalmologic status.
Lab Alterations:
Drug-induced color interference in urine screening tests for 5-hydroxindoleacetic (5-HIAA) and vanillymandelic acid (VMA).

Intervention/Rationale
Monitor blood pressure prior to and following administration. Patient should be recumbent for 10–15 min following administration. ● Monitor for neurologic/visual disturbances during therapy.

Patient/Family Education
Drug may cause drowsiness, dizziness, or lightheadedness; exercise caution with driving or performing other activities requiring alertness. Avoid alcohol or other CNS depressants. Urine may darken to brown, black, or green. Notify physician/nurse if skin rash, itching, fever, or nasal congestion occurs.

METHOHEXITAL
(metho-o-hex′-it-tal)
Trade Name(s): Brevital, Brietal ♥
Classification(s): General anesthetic, barbiturate
Pregnancy Category: C
Controlled Substance Schedule: IV

PHARMACODYNAMICS/KINETICS
Mechanism of Action: Ultra short-acting barbiturate. Produces CNS depression that results in hypnosis and anesthesia without analgesia; does not possess muscle relaxant properties. **Onset of Action:** Rapid. **Duration of Action:** 5–7 min. **Distribution:** Highly lipid-soluble. Quickly crosses blood–brain barrier. Rapidly distributed first to heart, kidneys, and liver, then to muscle and fatty tissues. **Metabolism/Elimination:** Oxidized and demethylated in the liver. **Half-Life:** 3–8 hr.

INDICATIONS/DOSAGE

Induction of anesthesia or as a supplement to other anesthetic agents; sole anesthetic in short, minimally painful procedures; used in conjunc-

In the Adverse Effects section, <u>underline</u> indicates most frequent; CAPS indicates life threatening.

319

tion with gaseous anesthetics for longer procedures

Adult: Individualize dosage. Induction dose 5–12 mL of a 0.1% solution (50–120 mg). Maintain anesthesia with intermittent injection 2–4 mL (20–40 mg) every 4–7 minutes (0.1% solution). A 0.2% solution may also be given by continuous drip at a rate of 1 drop/second.

CONTRAINDICATIONS/ PRECAUTIONS

Contraindicated in: Known hypersensitivity to barbiturates, latent or manifest porphyria, severe cardiovascular disease, shock, severe hepatic dysfunction, myxedema, absence of suitable veins for IV administration. **Use cautiously in:** Status asthmaticus, debilitated patients, respiratory, circulatory, renal, hepatic, or endocrine dysfunction, obstructive pulmonary disease, severe hypotension or hypertension, CHF, obsesity, increased intracranial pressure, myasthenia gravis. **Pregnancy/Lactation:** No well-controlled trials to establish safety. Benefits must outweigh risks. **Pediatrics:** Safety and efficacy not established.

PREPARATION

Availability: 500 mg in 50 mL vials. 2.5 and 5 g ampules. 2.5 and 5 g in 250 and 500 mL vials, respectively. **Reconstitution/Infusion:** Dilute with the following amounts to make a 0.1% solution (10mg/mL): 500 mg vial: 50 mL; 2.5 g vial: 250 mL; 2.5 g ampule: 15 mL to ampule, dilute to 250 mL; 5 g vial: 500 mL; 5 g ampule: 30 mL to ampule, dilute to 500 mL. Use sterile water as diluent (dextrose or sodium chloride may

also be used). Do not use bacteriostatic diluents. Solution is yellow when initial diluent is added. When further diluted to make a 0.1% solution, it should become clear and colorless.

STABILITY/STORAGE

Vial: Store at room temperature. Stable in sterile water for 6 weeks at room temperature (recommended to discard after 24 hr; contains no preservatives). **Infusion:** Stable for 24 hr in dextrose and sodium chloride at room temperature.

ADMINISTRATION

General: Do not use solutions that are not colorless after dilution to 0.1% or 0.2%. **IV Push:** Give slowly. **Continuous Infusion:** Infuse at a rate of 1 drop/second via infusion device.

COMPATIBILITY

Solution: Dextrose solutions, sodium chloride solutions.

INCOMPATIBILITY

Solution: Lactated Ringer's. **Syringe:** Atropine, glycopyrrolate, succinylcholine.

ADVERSE EFFECTS

CNS: Seizures, anxiety, emergence delirium, headache, restlessness. **CV:** CARDIORESPIRATORY ARREST, circulatory depression, hypotension, peripheral vascular collapse. **Resp:** APNEA, LARYNGOSPASM, RESPIRATORY DEPRESSION, BRONCHOSPASM, coughing, dyspnea, hiccoughs. **GI:** Abdominal pain, nausea, salivation, vomiting. **MS:** Muscle twitching, postanesthetic shivering. **Hypersens:** Acute allergic reaction, erythema, pruritus, rhinitis, urticaria. **Other:** In-

In the Adverse Effects section, <u>underline</u> indicates most frequent; CAPS indicates life threatening.

jury to nerves adjacent to injection site, pain at injection site, thrombophlebitis.

TOXICITY/OVERDOSE

Signs/Symptoms: (occur secondary to too rapid or repeated injections): Alarming fall in blood pressure, possibly to shock levels, apnea, laryngospasm, coughing and other respiratory difficulties. **Treatment:** Discontinue drug. Maintain or establish patent airway. Administer oxygen and assist ventilation if necessary.

DRUG INTERACTIONS

Alcohol-CNS depressants: Additive depressant effects.

NURSING CONSIDERATIONS

Assessment
General:
Vital signs, hypersensitivity/acute allergic reaction.
Physical:
Cardiopulmonary status.

Intervention/Rationale
Should only be given by those personnel trained in the administration of anesthetic agents/airway management. Additional agents must be given if skeletal muscle relaxation is required. ● Tolerance may develop with repeated use. ● Frequently assess for patency of airway.

Patient/Family Education
Educate about side effects/risks of receiving anesthesia. Avoid use of alcohol or other CNS depressants for 24 hr following administration.

METHOTREXATE
(metho-o-trex'-ate)
Trade Name(s): Amethopterin, Folex, Folex PFS, Mexate
Classification(s): Antimetabolite, antineoplastic agent
Pregnancy Category: X

PHARMACODYNAMICS/KINETICS

Mechanism of Action: Interferes with DNA synthesis and cell reproduction, cell cycle specific. **Peak Serum Concentration:** 0.5–2.0 hr. **Distribution:** Actively transported across cell membranes and widely distributed into body tissues (highest concentrations in kidneys, gallbladder, spleen, liver, and skin). Does not enter into CNS tissues unless given intrathecally. **Metabolism/Elimination:** Retained for weeks in the kidneys and for months in the liver. Approximately 50% bound to plasma proteins. Not appreciably metabolized. Excreted primarily by the kidneys; small amounts excreted in feces. **Half-Life:** 2–4 hr.

INDICATIONS/DOSAGE

Dosage schedules, route of administration, and duration of treatment vary according to individual patient, disease process, and physician. Institute leucovorin rescue based on methotrexate serum levels. If bilirubin between 3 and 5 mg/dL or AST > 180 units/mL, reduce dose by 25%.

Lymphoblastic leukemia

Adult/Pediatric: 2.5 mg/kg every 14 days. Used in conjunction with prednisone.

In the Adverse Effects section, <u>underline</u> indicates most frequent;
CAPS indicates life threatening.

321

Severe, recalcitrant, disabling psoriasis

Adult: 10–25 mg/week in a single dose until adequate response is achieved. Maximum weekly dose should not exceed 50 mg. Use lowest dose possible after optimal dose is achieved and resume conventional therapy as soon as possible.

Osteosarcoma (*unlabeled use*)

Adult/Pediatric: 12 g/m^2 as a 4 hr infusion in combination with other antineoplastic agents and leucovorin rescue (leucovorin rescue is used to prevent or decrease severe hematopoietic toxicity of massive doses of methotrexate).

CONTRAINDICATIONS/ PRECAUTIONS

Contraindicated in: Hypersensitivity, severely impaired renal function. **Use cautiously in:** Documented infection, peptic ulcer, ulcerative colitis, debilitated/elderly, malignant disease with preexisting liver damage, impaired hepatic function. **Pregnancy/Lactation:** Do not give to pregnant women or women of childbearing potential until the possibility of pregnancy has been excluded. Fetal deaths, abortion, and/or congenital anomalies have occurred in fetuses exposed to methotrexate. Distributed into breast milk and may cause serious adverse effects in nursing infant.

PREPARATION

Availability: 2.5 mg/mL in 2 mL vials. 25 mg/mL in 2, 4, 8, and 10 mL vials. 20, 50, 100, 250 mg and 1 g vials. **Reconstitution:** Reconstitute immediately prior to use with 2–20 mL sterile water, sodium chlo-

ride, or bacteriostatic water for injection. Discard any unused portions. **Infusion:** Further dilute reconstituted solution with sodium chloride or dextrose.

STABILITY/STORAGE

Vial: Store at room temperature. Prepare just prior to use. **Infusion:** Stable for 24 hr at room temperature.

ADMINISTRATION

General: Handle drug with care and adhere to institutional guidelines for the handling of chemotherapeutic/cytotoxic agents. **IV Push:** Give at a rate of 10 mg/min. May be given into a Y-site or threeway stopcock of a free-flowing IV. **Intermittent/Continuous Infusion:** Give via infusion device. Give high doses over 4–6 hr.

COMPATIBILITY

Solution: Amino acids 4.25%/dextrose 25%, dextrose solutions. **Syringe:** Bleomycin, cisplatin, cyclophosphamide, doxapram, doxorubicin, fluorouracil, furosemide, leucovorin, mitomycin, vinblastine, vincristine. **Y-site:** Bleomycin, cisplatin, cyclophosphamide, doxorubicin, fluorouracil, furosemide, heparin, leucovorin, metoclopramide, mitomycin, ondansetron, vinblastine, vincristine.

INCOMPATIBILITY

Syringe: Droperidol, metoclopramide, ranitidine. **Y-site:** Droperidol.

ADVERSE EFFECTS

CNS: Drowsiness, headache. **Ophtho:** Blurred vision, eye discomfort. **Resp:** PULMONARY TOXICITY. **GI:** ACUTE/CHRONIC HEPATOTOXICITY, abdominal distress, anorexia, bleeding/ulcerations of

In the Adverse Effects section, underline indicates most frequent; CAPS indicates life threatening.

mucous membranes, gingivitis, hematemesis, melena, <u>nausea</u>, pharyngitis, <u>ulcerative stomatitis</u>. **GU:** Cystitis, dysuria. **MS:** Myalgia, osteoporosis. **Derm:** Acne, alopecia, depigmentation/hyperpigmentation, ecchymoses, erythematous rashes, folliculitis, petechiae, photosensitivity. **Heme:** <u>LEUKOPENIA</u>, thrombocytopenia, PANCYTOPENIA, anemia, hemorrhage, hyperuricemia. **Nadir:** Hemoglobin 6–13 days, reticulocytes 2–7 days, leukocytes 4–7 days and 12–21 days, platelets 5–12 days. **Hypersens:** Pruritus, urticaria. **Other:** <u>Chills</u>, <u>fever</u>, <u>undue fatigue</u>, tinnitus, <u>malaise</u>.

TOXICITY/OVERDOSE

Signs/Symptoms: Bone marrow depression (WBC count < 1500, neutrophil count < 200, platelet count < 7500), serum bilirubin level > 1.2 mg/dL, ALT level > 450 units, presence of mucositis, and the presence of a persistent pleural effusion. **Treatment:** Delay further treatment until blood counts recover, mucositis is healed, and pleural effusion is resolved. Leucovorin rescue may be used to decrease severe hematopoietic toxicity and prevent death when massive doses of methotrexate have been given.

DRUG INTERACTIONS

Alcohol or hepatotoxic agents: Increased risk of hepatotoxicity. **Live virus vaccines:** Disseminated vaccinia infection. **Nonsteroidal anti-inflammatory agents with high dose methotrexate therapy** (indomethacin, ibuprofen): Severe methotrexate toxicity. **Other bone marrow depressants/**

radiation therapy: Increased bone marrow depression. **Aminobenzoic acid, chloramphenicol, phenytoin, phenylbutazone, salicylates, sulfonamides, sulfonylureas, tetracyclines:** Increased methotrexate toxicity. **Salicylates:** Delayed renal excretion of methotrexate. **Warfarin:** Increased anticoagulant activity/risk of hemorrhage.

NURSING CONSIDERATIONS

Assessment
General:
Vital signs, baseline and periodic weight, nutritional status, intake/output ratio, infectious disease status.
Physical:
GI status, hematopoietic status.
Lab Alterations:
Monitor total and differential leukocyte counts, platelet count, hematocrit, BUN, creatinine, ALT (SGPT), AST (SGOT), bilirubin, LDH, and uric acid prior to initiation of therapy and periodically during therapy (frequency depends on patient's clinical state and drug dose). Bone marrow aspiration and liver biopsy may be done periodically during course of therapy. Additional monitoring measures for patients receiving high dose methotrexate with leucovorin rescue include creatinine clearance (prior to dose initiation), serum creatinine prior to and 24 hr after each dose, plasma/serum methotrexate levels (12–24 hr after therapy), and urine pH determinations prior to each dose and every 6 hr during treatment (urine pH > 7.0 minimizes risk of methotrexate nephropathy).

In the Adverse Effects section, <u>underline</u> indicates most frequent;
CAPS indicates life threatening.

323

Intervention/Rationale

Adjust dietary intake as needed to prevent weight loss/electrolyte imbalance. Encourage increased fluid intake. ● Administer antiemetic as needed to prevent/combat nausea/vomiting. ● Examine patient's mouth before each dose and periodically during treatment course for presence of ulcerations/stomatitis. ● Assess for signs/symptoms of infection, abdominal pain, diarrhea, or bleeding tendencies and report to physician.

Patient/Family Education

Avoid alcoholic beverages, salicylate-or ibuprofen-containing products. Patient and others in household should avoid immunizations unless approved by physician. Avoid exposure to persons with known bacterial or viral infections, especially during periods of low blood counts. Inform physician immediately of suspected infection. Increase fluid intake and observe for subsequent increase in urine output to prevent nephrotoxicity. Inspect oral mucosa for ulcerations/bleeding. Report signs of bleeding/unusual bruising to physician. Proper oral hygiene is important, including avoidance of hard toothbrushes, toothpicks, dental floss, and mouthwashes containing alcohol. Use electric razor. Potential hair loss may have an effect on body image. Patients of childbearing age should use reliable contraceptives to prevent teratogenic and mutagenic effects of drug (during and at least 8 weeks after discontinuation of therapy). Avoid fresh fruits and vegetables during times of neutropenia. Use sunscreen and wear protective clothing when outdoors. Follow up with physician visits and lab work.

METHYLDOPATE

(meth-ill-doe'-pate)
Trade Name(s): Aldomet
Classification(s):
Antihypertensive (centrally acting antiadrenergic agent)
Pregnancy Category: B

PHARMACODYNAMICS/KINETICS

Mechanism of Action: Lowers arterial blood pressure by central stimulation of alpha-adrenergic receptors. May also reduce plasma renin activity. **Onset of Action:** 4–6 hr. **Duration of Action:** 10–16 hr. **Distribution:** Weakly bound to plasma proteins. Crosses the blood–brain barrier. **Metabolism/Elimination:** Metabolized in the liver and GI tract. Excreted largely unchanged in urine. Delayed excretion and accumulation of metabolites occurs with renal insufficiency. Removed by hemodialysis. **Half-Life:** 1.7 hr.

INDICATIONS/DOSAGE

Hypertension

(moderate to severe), reduce dose in impaired renal function and elderly.

Adult: 250–500 mg every 6 hr. Maximum dose 1 g every 6 hr (adjust dose to individual patient response and tolerance). *Pediatric:* 20–40 mg/kg/day or 0.6–1.2 g/m^2/day in equally divided doses every 6 hr. Maximum dose 65 mg/kg/

In the Adverse Effects section, <u>underline</u> indicates most frequent; CAPS indicates life threatening.

day, 2 g/m^2/day, or 3 g daily, whichever is less.

CONTRAINDICATIONS/ PRECAUTIONS

Contraindicated in: Hypersensitivity, active hepatic disease (acute hepatitis, active cirrhosis), pheochromocytoma, liver abnormalities or positive direct Coombs' associated with previous methyldopa therapy. **Use cautiously in:** Previous liver disease or dysfunction, renal failure, elderly. **Pregnancy/Lactation:** Crosses the placenta. No adverse reactions or obvious teratogenic effects seen in widespread use; however, fetal injury cannot be excluded. Benefits must outweigh risks. Neonates have slightly decreased blood pressure for approximately 2 days after delivery. Generally safe with careful physician management. Distributed into breast milk. Use with caution in breastfeeding mothers.

PREPARATION

Availability: 250 mg/5 mL in 5 and 10 mL vials. **Infusion:** Add 250 or 500 mg to 100 mL dextrose.

STABILITY/STORAGE

Vial: Store at room temperature. Protect from light. **Infusion:** Stable for 24 hr at room temperature.

ADMINISTRATION

General: Other agents may be preferred when rapid blood pressure reduction is required, as in hypertensive crisis (drug has slow onset of action). **Intermittent Infusion:** Give over 30–60 min.

COMPATIBILITY

Solution: Amino acids 4.25%/dextrose 25%, dextran, dextrose solutions, Ringer's injection, sodium chloride solutions. **Y-site:** Esmolol.

ADVERSE EFFECTS

CNS: Dizziness, lightheadedness, sedation. **CV:** Aggravation of angina pectoris, bradycardia, CHF, MYOCARDITIS, <u>orthostatic hypotension</u>, edema (sodium retention). **Resp:** Nasal congestion. **GU:** <u>Decreased libido/impotence</u>. **Derm:** Eczema, hyperkeratosis. **Heme:** HEMOLYTIC ANEMIA, positive direct antiglobulin (Coombs') test. **Hypersens:** Rash, urticaria. **Other:** Fever, lupus-like syndrome.

TOXICITY/OVERDOSE

Signs/Symptoms: Acute hypotension, excessive sedation, weakness, bradycardia, dizziness, lightheadedness, constipation, GI distention, flatus, diarrhea, nausea, vomiting. **Treatment:** Supportive therapy and symptomatic care. Keep patient supine. Monitor cardiac rhythm, administer IV fluids, treat electrolyte imbalance, use norepinephrine or dopamine with caution if aforementioned measures are inadequate.

DRUG INTERACTIONS

Diuretic/other hypotensive agents, levodopa: Increased hypotensive effect of methyldopa. **General anesthesia:** Increased hypotensive effects (reduce anesthetic dosage). **Haloperidol:** Adverse mental symptoms (dementia and high incidence of sedation). **Phenothiazines or tricyclic antidepressants:** Reduction in hypotensive effect.

In the Adverse Effects section, <u>underline</u> indicates most frequent; CAPS indicates life threatening.

NURSING CONSIDERATIONS

Assessment

General:
Monitor blood pressure and heart rate prior to initiation of therapy, periodically, during, and 4–6 hr after dose; daily weight; intake/output ratio.

Lab Alterations:
Monitor renal/hepatic function and CBC periodically during course of therapy. Possible interference with serum creatinine analysis. Falsely elevated urinary catecholamines.

Intervention/Rationale
Assess for signs and symptoms of edema related to sodium retention.

Patient/Family Education
Change positions slowly to avoid orthostatic hypotension. Treatment for hypertension is not a cure and medications/dietary changes may be necessary long-term. Monitor blood pressure at home. Follow up with physician at periodic intervals.

METHYLENE BLUE
(meth′-a-leen bloo)
Classification(s): Antidote, thiazine dye
Pregnancy Category: Unknown

PHARMACODYNAMICS/KINETICS
Mechanism of Action: In low concentrations, increases the conversion of methemoglobin to hemoglobin. When used in cyanide toxicity in high concentrations, oxidizes the ferrous iron of reduced hemoglobin to the ferric state, which changes methemoglobin to hemoglobin (prevents further reactions that interfere with cellular respiration). Also reverses intracellular acidosis. Possesses weak antiseptic and tissue-staining properties. **Metabolism/Elimination:** Excreted in urine and bile.

INDICATIONS/DOSAGE

Treatment for idiopathic and drug-induced methemoglobinemia, cyanide poisoning, chronic urolithiasis (alone or in combination with ascorbic acid)

Adult: 1–2 mg/kg. May repeat in 1 hr if needed.

CONTRAINDICATIONS/ PRECAUTIONS
Contraindicated in: Known hypersensitivity, severe renal impairment. **Use cautiously in:** Glucose-6-phosphate dehydrogenase deficiency. **Pregnancy/Lactation:** No well-controlled trials to establish safety. Benefits must outweigh risks.

PREPARATION
Availability: 10 mg/mL in 1 and 10 mL amps.

STABILITY/STORAGE
Vial: Store at room temperature.

ADMINISTRATION
General: Subcutaneous injection or extravasation may result in a necrotic abscess. **IV Push:** Give slowly over several minutes.

ADVERSE EFFECTS
CNS: Dizziness, headache, mental confusion. **CV:** Cyanosis, hypertension, precordial pain. **GI:** Blue-green feces, abdominal pain, nau-

In the Adverse Effects section, <u>underline</u> indicates most frequent; CAPS indicates life threatening.

sea, vomiting. **GU:** Blue-green urine. **Derm:** Skin stains (may be removed with hypochlorite solution). **Heme:** Marked anemia (long-term use), HEMOLYSIS (young infants). **Other:** Fever, methemoglobin formation (large doses), profuse sweating.

NURSING CONSIDERATIONS

Assessment
General:
Hypertension, ECG monitoring (recommended).
Physical:
GI tract, cardiovascular status.
Lab Alterations:
Monitor hemoglobin with long-term use. Interferes with hematesting of stools/vomitus for occult blood.

Intervention/Rationale
Evaluate for development of hypertension, precordial pain, or dysrhythmias (associated with cyanide toxicity).

Patient/Family Education
Drug may impart a blue color to stool/urine. Report pain or irritation at injection site to nurse immediately.

METHYLERGONOVINE
(meth-ill-er-goe-noe'-veen)
Trade Name(s): Methergine
Classification(s): Oxytocic
Pregnancy Category: C

PHARMACODYNAMICS/KINETICS
Mechanism of Action: Directly stimulates contraction of uterine smooth muscle. Increases amplitude and frequency of uterine contractions and tone, which impedes uterine blood flow. **Onset of Action:** 40 sec. **Duration of Action:** 45 min. **Distribution:** Distributes rapidly into plasma, extracellular fluid, and tissues. **Metabolism/Elimination:** Primarily metabolized in liver. Excreted in feces. Only a small amount excreted in urine. Elimination may be prolonged in neonates.

INDICATIONS/DOSAGE

Prevention and treatment of postpartum and postabortal hemorrhage due to uterine atony or subinvolution
(not for long-term or chronic use)

Adult: 0.2 mg. May repeat every 2–4 hr for a maximum of five doses (IV use limited to patients with severe uterine bleeding or other life-threatening complications of pregnancy).

CONTRAINDICATIONS/PRECAUTIONS
Contraindicated in: Known hypersensitivity or idiosyncratic reactions, induction of labor, threatened spontaneous abortion, obstetrical patient prior to placental delivery. **Use cautiously in:** Essential hypertension, heart disease, venoatrial shunts, mitral valve stenosis, occlusive peripheral vascular disease, sepsis, renal or hepatic impairment, coronary artery disease, toxemia of pregnancy, pregnancy-induced hypertension, hypocalcemia. **Pregnancy/Lactation:** Should not be administered prior to delivery of placenta (captivation of placenta may oc-

M

In the Adverse Effects section, <u>underline</u> indicates most frequent;
CAPS indicates life threatening.

327

cur). High doses given prior to delivery may cause problems in infant (hypoxia, intracranial hemorrhage). Use only when surgical and intensive care facilities are immediately available. Distributed into breast milk. May cause ergotism in infant.

PREPARATION
Availability: 0.2 mg/mL in 1 mL amps.

STABILITY/STORAGE
Vial: Store at room temperature away from direct heat and light. Do not use if discolored.

ADMINISTRATION
IV Push: Give slowly over 1 min. May be diluted to a 5 mL volume with sodium chloride before injection.

COMPATIBILITY
Solution: Sodium chloride solutions. **Y-site:** Heparin, hydrocortisone, potassium chloride, vitamin B complex with C.

ADVERSE EFFECTS
CNS: Dizziness, headache. **CV:** Hypertension, palpitations, temporary chest pain. **GI:** Nausea, vomiting. **Resp:** Dyspnea. **Derm:** Diaphoresis. **Other:** Tinnitus.

TOXICITY/OVERDOSE
Signs/Symptoms: Nausea, vomiting, abdominal pain, numbness, tingling of the extremities, rise in blood pressure, in severe cases may cause hypotension, respiratory depression, hypothermia, convulsions, coma. **Treatment:** Symptomatic, maintain patent airway and provide assisted ventilation if necessary. Correct hypotension with

vasopressors if needed. Warmth to extremities may help control peripheral vasospasms.

NURSING CONSIDERATIONS
Assessment
General:
Monitor blood pressure, pulse rate, and uterine response prior to and frequently during and after administration.
Physical:
Uterine assessment.

Intervention/Rationale
Report sudden vital sign changes. ● Observe and record character of vaginal bleeding. Report frequent periods of uterine relaxation.

Patient/Family Education
May experience strong uterine cramping. Educate regarding expected therapeutic outcome and adverse effects.

METHYLPREDNISOLONE
(meth-ill-pred-niss′-oh-lone)
Trade Name(s): A-MethaPred, Medrol, Solu-Medrol
Classification(s): Adrenal cortical steroid
Pregnancy Category: C

PHARMACODYNAMICS/KINETICS
Mechanism of Action: Diffuses across cell membranes and complexes with specific receptors in cytoplasm. Decreases inflammation, suppresses the immune response, promotes protein catabolism, gluconeogenesis, and redistribution of fat from peripheral to central areas

In the Adverse Effects section, <u>underline</u> indicates most frequent; CAPS indicates life threatening.

of the body. Reduces intestinal absorption and increases renal excretion of calcium. **Onset of Action:** Rapid. **Distribution:** Widely and rapidly distributed to muscles, liver, skin, intestines, and kidneys. **Metabolism/Elimination:** Metabolized primarily in the liver to biologically inactive compounds that are excreted primarily by the kidneys. **Half-Life:** 80–190 minutes.

INDICATIONS/DOSAGE

Used principally as an anti-inflammatory or immunosuppressant agent in a wide variety of diseases

(includes autoimmune, hematologic, organ transplantation, neoplastic, and other disorders). Dose varies according to type and severity of disorder being treated and the patient's response.

Adult/Pediatric: Dosage range 10 mg to 1.5 g daily, with a usual dose of 10–250 mg given up to six times daily. High doses are used for the treatment of severe shock states (up to 30 mg/kg/dose every 4–6 hr may be given—do not continue beyond 48–72 hr). In children, dosages are based on the severity of the condition being treated and the patient's response rather than strict adherence to dosage by age and body surface area or weight (do not give less than 0.5 mg/kg of body weight every 24 hr—maximum dose 30 mg/kg).

Acute spinal cord injury (*unlabeled use*)

Adult: Loading dose 30 mg/kg over 15 minutes followed by an infusion of 5.4 mg/kg/hr in sterile water over 23 hr. Must give within 8 hr of injury.

CONTRAINDICATIONS/ PRECAUTIONS

Contraindicated in: Hypersensitivity, systemic fungal infections. **Use cautiously in:** Hypertension, thromboembolic tendencies, myasthenia gravis, metastatic carcinoma, osteoporosis, Cushing's syndrome, tuberculosis, chronic active hepatitis B, ocular herpes simplex, renal insufficiency, acute glomerulonephritis, chronic nephritis, peptic ulcer disease, elderly (may require dose reduction). **Pregnancy/Lactation:** No well-controlled trials to establish safety. Benefits must outweigh risks. Large doses of cortisol given to animals early in pregnancy have caused cleft lip/palate, stillborn fetuses, and decreased fetal size. Distributes into breast milk and potentially causes suppressed infant growth, disturbances in endogenous corticosteroid production, or other undesirable effects in infants. Advise mothers taking corticosteroids not to breastfeed. **Pediatrics:** Prolonged therapy may result in retarded growth and development. A fatal "gasping sydrome" has resulted in some premature infants given corticosteroid products containing benzyl alcohol.

PREPARATION

Availability: 40, 125, 500, or 1000 mg in 1, 2, 3, 8, 20, and 50 mL vials and Mix-O-Vials. **Reconstitution:** Reconstitute conventional vials with sterile water for injection (use bacteriostatic water without preservatives for use in neonates). Reconstitute Mix-O-Vial using provided diluent.

M

In the Adverse Effects section, <u>underline</u> indicates most frequent; CAPS indicates life threatening.

329

Infusion: Dilute reconstituted drug with dextrose or sodium chloride to physician specified volume.

STABILITY/STORAGE
Vial: Store at room temperature. **Infusion:** Stable for 24 hr at room temperature.

ADMINISTRATION
General: Doses ordered once daily should be given in early morning to coincide with the body's normal cortisol secretion. **IV Push:** Give lower doses (< 500 mg) over at least 1 min. Massive doses should be given over a period of 3–15 min. **Continuous Infusion:** Massive doses may be given continuously every 12 hr for 24–48 hr following initial IV push dose.

COMPATIBILITY
Solution: Amino acids 4.25%/dextrose 25%, dextrose solutions, sodium chloride solutions. **Syringe:** Metoclopramide. **Y-site:** Acyclovir, amrinone, enalaprilat, famotidine.

INCOMPATIBILITY
Solution: Dextrose in sodium chloride (concentration dependent), lactated Ringer's. **Syringe:** Doxapram. **Y-site:** Ondansetron, potassium chloride, vitamin B complex with C.

ADVERSE EFFECTS
CNS: INCREASED INTRACRANIAL PRESSURE WITH PAPILLEDEMA, convulsions, depression, euphoria, headache, insomnia, neuritis, paresthesias, steroid psychosis, vertigo. **CV:** CARDIAC ARREST (after too rapid administration of large doses), dysrhythmias/ECG changes (from potassium deficiency),

thromboembolism/fat embolism. **GI:** Abdominal distention, increased appetite, nausea, peptic ulcer with perforation, weight gain, ulcerative esophagitis, vomiting. **GU:** Decreased motility or number of spermatozoa, postmenopausal bleeding. **MS:** Aseptic necrosis of joints, loss of muscle mass, muscle weakness, osteoporosis, spontaneous fractures. **Derm:** Angioneurotic edema, ecchymosis, impaired wound healing, thin fragile skin, petechiae, suppression of skin test reactions. **Endo:** Amennorrhea, Cushingoid appearance (moon face, buffalo hump), growth suppression (children), glycosuria, hyperglycemia, negative nitrogen balance. **Fld/Lytes:** Hypocalcemia, hypokalemia, metabolic acidosis, sodium/fluid retention. **Hypersens:** Urticaria. **Other:** Aggravation/masking of infections.

TOXICITY/OVERDOSE
Signs/Symptoms: Acute adrenal insufficiency from too rapid withdrawal after long-term use (fever, myalgia, malaise, anorexia, nausea, orthostatic hypotension, dizziness, desquamation of skin, dyspnea, hypoglycemia, fainting). Cushingoid changes from continued use of large doses (moon face, central obesity, acne, hirsutism, osteoporosis, hypertension, striae, ecchymoses, myopathy, sexual dysfunction, diabetes, hyperlipidemia, peptic ulcer, increased susceptibility to infection, fluid and electrolyte imbalance). **Treatment:** Recovery of normal adrenal and pituitary function may take up to 9 months. Steroids should be withdrawn gradually under the direct supervision of

In the Adverse Effects section, underline indicates most frequent; CAPS indicates life threatening.

a physician. Steroid supplementation may be required during times of stress (illness, surgery, injury). Management for large, acute overdoses is supportive.

DRUG INTERACTIONS
Amphotericin B, potassium-depleting diuretic: Increased chance of hypokalemia. **Attenuated-virus vaccines:** Enhanced virus replication with severe reactions. **Coumarin anticoagulants:** Reduced anticoagulant effects. **Cyclosporine:** Increased plasma levels of both drugs. **Cyclophosphamide:** Inhibition of cyclophosphamide metabolism. **Digitalis glycosides:** Enhanced potential for digitalis toxicity. **Erythromycin:** Inhibited corticosteroid metabolism. **Insulin, oral hypoglycemic agents:** Increased insulin/oral agent requirements. **Isoniazid:** Decreased antitubercular effectiveness. **Oral contraceptives:** Inhibited corticosteroid metabolism. **Phenytoin, phenobarbital, rifampin, ephedrine:** Decreased corticosteroid levels. **Salicylates:** Reduced salicylate levels. **Somatrem:** Inhibition of growth promoting effects.

NURSING CONSIDERATIONS
Assessment
General:
Vital signs, ECG monitoring (recommended with high doses), daily weight, intake/output ratio.
Physical:
Infectious disease status, endocrine/adrenal status, GI tract.
Lab Alterations:
False-negative nitroblue-tetrazolium test for bacterial infection. Monitor WBC, potassium, calcium, blood/urine glucose, serum so-

dium, serum cholesterol/lipids, hematologic values, and electrolytes periodically, especially during long-term therapy.

Intervention/Rationale
Monitor for signs/symptoms of infection (immunosuppressant effects of drug may mask signs). ● Assess patient for signs/symptoms of adrenal insufficiency periodically during course of therapy. ● Hematest all stools and report positive results immediately. ● Monitor blood pressure. If high dosages are used, continuous ECG monitoring is recommended.

Patient/Family Education
Educate about expected therapeutic outcome and side effects. Stopping medication may be life threatening. Notify physician if the following signs/symptoms occur during decrease or withdrawal of therapy: fatigue, anorexia, nausea, vomiting, diarrhea, weight loss, weakness, dizziness, decreased blood sugar.

METOCLOPRAMIDE
(met-oh-kloe-pra'-mide)
Trade Name(s): Maxeran ♣, Reglan
Classification(s): Antiemetic, GI stimulant
Pregnancy Category: B

PHARMACODYNAMICS/KINETICS
Mechanism of Action: Stimulates motility of the upper GI tract. Does not stimulate gastric, biliary, or pancreatic secretions. May sensitize tissues to the action of acetylcholine. Results in accelerated gastric empty-

In the Adverse Effects section, underline indicates most frequent; CAPS indicates life threatening.

331

ing and intestinal transit. **Onset of Action:** 1–3 min. **Duration of Action:** 1–2 hr. **Distribution:** Rapidly distributed to most tissues. Weakly protein bound (13%–22%). **Metabolism/Elimination:** Excreted primarily unchanged in the urine. Some conjugated in the bile. Removed by hemodialysis. **Half-Life:** 3–6 hr (impaired renal function—up to 24 hr).

INDICATIONS/DOSAGE

Reduce dosage in renal impairment.

Relief of gastric stasis

Adult: 10 mg IV push four times daily 30 min before meals and at bedtime.

Prevention of emesis associated with chemotherapy

Adult: 1–2 mg/kg 30 minutes before administration of chemotherapeutic agent. 2 mg/kg doses may be given at 3 hr intervals for three additional doses if needed.

Intubation of the small intestine

(when unable to pass tube through the pylorus) or radiographic examination of the upper GI tract (stimulates gastric emptying and intestinal transit of barium).

Adult: Single dose of 10 mg IV push.

Pediatric:
- Children 6–14 years of age: 2.5–5.0 mg IV push.
- Children younger than 6 years: 0.1 mg/kg.

CONTRAINDICATIONS/ PRECAUTIONS

Contraindicated in: Hypersensitivity, GI mechanical obstruction/perforation, pheochromocytoma, seizure disorder, patients receiving drugs likely to cause extrapyramidal reactions (phenothiazines). **Use cautiously in:** Renal impairment , mental depression, especially those with suicidal tendencies, Parkinson's disease, GI surgery with anastomosis/suture closure, sulfite sensitivity. **Pregnancy/Lactation:** No well-controlled trials to establish safety. No evidence of fetal harm in animal studies. Crosses the placenta. Benefits must outweigh risks. Readily distributes into breast milk. Caution when breastfeeding. **Pediatrics:** Use with caution due to ?increased incidence of extrapyramidal reactions.

PREPARATION

Availability: 5 mg/mL in 2, 10, 30, 50, and 100 mL vials. **IV Push:** May be given undiluted. **Infusion:** Dilute doses greater than 10 mg in 50 mL of compatible IV solution.

STABILITY/STORAGE

Vial: Store at room temperature. **Infusion:** Stable for 24 hr at room temperature.

ADMINISTRATION

IV Push: Give slowly over 1–2 min. **Intermittent Infusion:** Infuse over at least 15 min.

COMPATIBILITY

Solution: Amino acids 4.25%/dextrose 25%, dextrose solutions, lactated Ringer's, mannitol, sodium chloride solutions. **Syringe:** Aminophylline, ascorbic acid, atropine, benztropine, bleomycin, chlorpromazine, cisplatin, cyclophosphamide, cytarabine, dexamethasone,

In the Adverse Effects section, underline indicates most frequent; CAPS indicates life threatening.

dimenhydrinate, diphenhydramine, doxorubicin, droperidol, fentanyl, fluorouracil, heparin, hydrocortisone, hydroxyzine, insulin, leucovorin calcium, lidocaine, magnesium sulfate, meperidine, methylprednisolone, midazolam, mitomycin, morphine, pentazocine, perphenazine, prochlorperazine, promethazine, ranitidine, scopolamine, vinblastine, vincristine, vitamin B complex with C. **Y-site:** Acyclovir, bleomycin, cisplatin, cyclophosphamide, doxorubicin, droperidol, famotidine, fluorouracil, foscarnet, heparin, leucovorin calcium, methotrexate, mitomycin, ondansetron, vinblastine, vincristine, zidovudine.

INCOMPATIBILITY
Syringe: Ampicillin, calcium gluconate, cephalothin, chloramphenicol, furosemide, methotrexate, penicillin G potassium, sodium bicarbonate. **Y-site:** Furosemide.

ADVERSE EFFECTS
CNS: <u>Extrapyramidal reactions</u>, <u>drowsiness</u>, anxiety, dizziness, <u>fatigue</u>, headache, <u>lassitude</u>, parkinsonian-like reactions, <u>restlessness</u>. **CV:** Transient hypotension. **GI:** Diarrhea, nausea. **GU:** Nipple tenderness/gynecomastia in males, reversible amenorrhea. **Other:** Galactorrhea.

TOXICITY/OVERDOSE
Signs/Symptoms: Drowsiness, disorientation, and extrapyramidal reactions (are self-limiting, usually disappear within 24 hr). May also have muscle hypertonia, irritability, and agitation. **Treatment:** Extrapyramidal reactions may be controlled with anticholinergics or antiparkinson drugs or antihistamine with anticholinergic properties.

DRUG INTERACTIONS
Alcohol, sedatives/hypnotics, narcotics, tranquilizers: Additive sedative effects. **Anticholinergic drugs, narcotic analgesics:** Effects on GI motility antagonized. **Drugs absorbed from the stomach** (digoxin, cimetidine): Diminished absorption. **Drugs absorbed from the small bowel:** Accelerated absorption. **Ethanol:** Increased absorption. **Insulin:** May require dosage adjustment due to differences in food delivery to intestines. **Phenothiazine, butyrophenone, thioxanthines:** Potentiated extrapyramidal effects.

NURSING CONSIDERATIONS
Assessment
General:
Hydration status.
Physical:
GI tract, neurologic status.

Intervention/Rationale
Monitor for continued chemotherapy-induced emesis and provide adequate hydration. ● Perform complete abdominal assessment prior to therapy (presence of bowel sounds, abdominal distention, nausea, diarrhea, tenderness). Assess for extrapyramidal effects periodically during therapy.

Patient/Family Education
Drug may cause drowsiness. Avoid alcohol and other CNS depressants. Notify physician/nurse if involuntary movement of eyes, face, or limbs occurs.

M

In the Adverse Effects section, <u>underline</u> indicates most frequent; CAPS indicates life threatening.

333

METOPROLOL
(me-toe'-proe-lole)
Trade Name(s): Betaloc ♣,
Lopressor
Classification(s): Beta-adrenergic blocking agent (beta-1 selective)
Pregnancy Category: B

PHARMACODYNAMICS/KINETICS
Mechanism of Action: Selective inhibition of beta-1 adrenergic receptors in myocardium. Blocks beta-2 receptors in bronchial and vascular smooth muscle only at high doses.
Onset of Action: Rapid. **Distribution:** Widely distributed into body tissues with concentrations greater in the heart, liver, lungs, and saliva than in plasma. 11%–12% bound to albumin. Crosses the blood–brain barrier. **Metabolism/Elimination:** Metabolized in the liver by first-order kinetics. Excreted approximately 10% unchanged in urine via glomerular filtration. **Half-Life:** 3–4 hr.

INDICATIONS/DOSAGE

Reduces the risk of cardiovascular mortality in the early phase of hemodynamically stable MI
Adult: 15 mg given in three 5 mg injections at 2 min intervals (should follow with initiation of maintenance doses of oral metroprolol).

Control of ventricular rate in multifocal atrial tachycardia (*unlabeled use*)
Adult: 15 mg in three divided doses.

CONTRAINDICATIONS/PRECAUTIONS
Contraindicated in: Hypersensitivity, hypertension with bradycardia greater than first degree heart block, cardiogenic shock, overt cardiac failure, right ventricular failure secondary to pulmonary hypertension. **Use cautiously in:** Impaired myocardial function, well-compensated cardiac failure, sinus node dysfunction, major surgery using anesthetics that depress myocardial function, bronchospastic disease, diabetes mellitus, impaired hepatic function (reduce dose), AV conduction defects, cardiomegaly. **Pregnancy/Lactation:** No well-controlled trials to establish safety. Animal studies reveal increased miscarriages and decreased neonatal survival with high doses. Benefits must outweigh risks. Is distributed into breast milk. Use with caution and monitor infant for potential systemic effects. **Pediatrics:** Safety and efficacy not established.

PREPARATION
Availability: 1 mg/mL in 5 mL amp/syringes.

STABILITY/STORAGE
Vial: Store at room temperature.

ADMINISTRATION
IV Push: Give rapidly.

COMPATIBILITY/INCOMPATIBILITY
Data not available.

ADVERSE EFFECTS
CNS: Dizziness, headache, insomnia, nightmares, reversible mental depression, tiredness. **CV:** Hypotension, cold extremities, <u>bradycardia</u>, <u>dyspnea</u>, palpitations, Raynaud's

In the Adverse Effects section, <u>underline</u> indicates most frequent;
CAPS indicates life threatening.

phenomenon. **Resp:** Respiratory distress, bronchoconstriction, dyspnea, wheezing. **GI:** Abdominal pain, constipation, diarrhea, dry mouth, nausea. **MS:** Muscle aches. **Derm:** Dry skin, reversible alopecia, worsening of psoriasis. **Fld/Lytes:** Elevated serum transaminase and alkaline phosphatase, increased serum uric acid. **Heme:** Agranulocytosis, eosinophilia, nonthrombocytopenic purpura, thrombocytopenia purpura. **Hypersens:** LARYNGOSPASM, erythematous rash, pruritus, rash, sore throat. **Other:** Fever.

DRUG INTERACTIONS
Antiarrhythmic agents (disopyramide, lidocaine, quinidine, phenytoin, procainamide): Additive or antagonistic cardiac effects, additive toxic effects. **Cardiac glycosides:** Enhanced bradycardia. **Diuretics/other hypotensive agents:** Increased hypotensive effect. **Myocardial depressants, general anesthetics:** Increased risk of hypotension/heart failure. **Sympathomimetic agents:** Antagonized beta-1 adrenergic stimulating effects.

NURSING CONSIDERATIONS
Assessment
General:
Vital signs, daily weight, intake/output ratio. ECG monitoring (recommended).
Physical:
Cardiopulmonary status.
Lab Alterations:
Monitor serum glucose (diabetics).

Intervention/Rationale
Monitor vital signs prior to, frequently during, and after administration and check with physician before giving dose to patient with a pulse < 50. Abrupt withdrawal may result in myocardial ischemia or hypertension. Assess for signs and symptoms of cardiac failure. Monitor hemodynamic status closely in patients with MI (give atropine for bradycardia/heart block associated with decreased cardiac output; discontinue drug for atropine-refractory bradycardia and cautiously administer isoproterenol or prepare for insertion of temporary pacemaker). ● Pulmonary complications may occur in patients receiving high doses/history of asthma. Perform careful pulmonary assessment, especially in patients with documented bronchospastic disease. ● Drug may mask signs/symptoms of hypoglycemia. ● May mask signs/symptoms of hyperthyroidism. Monitor patients with thyrotoxicosis closely (abrupt withdrawal may precipitate thyroid storm).

Patient/Family Education
Educate regarding expected therapeutic outcome and side effects.

METRONIDAZOLE
(me-troe-ni′-da-zole)
Trade Name(s): Flagyl IV, Flagyl IV RTU, Metro IV
Classification(s): Anti-infective, antiamebic
Pregnancy Category: B

PHARMACODYNAMICS/KINETICS
Mechanism of Action: Bactericidal, amebicidal, and trichomonacidal. Effective against most anaerobic bacteria and many protozoa. Inactive against viruses and most aero-

In the Adverse Effects section, underline indicates most frequent; CAPS indicates life threatening.

335

bic bacteria. Disrupts DNA and inhibits nucleic acid synthesis. **Peak Serum Levels:** 1–3 hr. **Distribution:** Widely distributed into most body tissues (bone, bile, saliva, pleural fluid, peritoneal fluid, vaginal secretions, seminal fluid, CSF, cerebral and hepatic abscesses. Less than 20% bound to plasma proteins. **Metabolism/Elimination:** 30%–60% metabolized in the liver. Primarily excreted unchanged by the kidneys. Urine may be dark or reddish-brown in color. Removed by peritoneal/hemodialysis. **Half-Life:** 6–8 hr.

INDICATIONS/DOSAGE

Treatment of serious infections caused by anaerobic bacteria

Adult: Loading dose 15 mg/kg followed by a maintenance dose of 7.5 mg/kg every 6 hr. Maximum daily dose 4 g. Treat for a minimum of 7–10 days (serious infections may require treatment for 2–3 weeks).

Perioperative prophylaxis for contaminated or potentially contaminated colorectal surgery

Adult: 15 mg/kg over 30–60 min 1 hr prior to surgery, followed by 7.5 mg/kg at 6 and 12 hr intervals after initial dose. Alternatively, give 500 mg to 1 g, 1 hr prior to surgery, followed by 500 mg at 8 and 16 hr postoperatively.

CONTRAINDICATIONS/ PRECAUTIONS

Contraindicated in: Hypersensitivity. **Use cautiously in:** Blood dyscrasias, severe hepatic impairment (reduce dose). **Pregnancy/Lactation:** No well-controlled trials to establish safety.

Known tumorogenic potential in rats. Fetotoxicity has occurred when given intraperitoneally to pregnant mice. Use during first trimester pregnancy is contraindicated. Use during second and third trimesters only if benefits clearly outweigh risks. Distributed into breast milk. Breastfeeding should be interrupted for at least 24 hr after administration. **Pediatrics:** Safety and efficacy not established.

PREPARATION

Availability: 500 mg/vial powder for injection (must be neutralized prior to use). 500 mg/100 mL ready-to-use container. **Reconstitution:** Dilute powder for injection with 4.4 mL sterile water, bacteriostatic water, or sodium chloride for injection to a final concentration of 100 mg/mL. **Infusion:** Add reconstituted solution to 100 mL compatible IV solution. Final concentration not to exceed 8 mg/mL. Neutralize solution prior to administration with 5 mEq sodium bicarbonate for each 500 mg used. The addition of sodium bicarbonate generates carbon dioxide and may necessitate relieving the pressure in the container. Ready to use containers do not require neutralization.

STABILITY/STORAGE

Vial: Store at room temperature. Stable for 96 hr after reconstitution at room temperature. **Infusion:** Do not refrigerate. Use diluted and neutralized solutions within 24 hr.

ADMINISTRATION

Intermittent/Continuous Infusion: Give slowly over 60 minutes. Discontinue primary IV solution during infusion.

In the Adverse Effects section, <u>underline</u> indicates most frequent; CAPS indicates life threatening.

COMPATIBILITY
Solution: Dextrose solutions, Ringer's lactated, sodium chloride solutions. **Y-site:** Acyclovir, cyclophosphamide, enalprilat, esmolol, foscarnet, hydromorphone, labetalol, magnesium sulfate, meperidine, morphine, perphenazine.

INCOMPATIBILITY
Solution: Amino acids 10%.

ADVERSE EFFECTS
CNS: Seizures, ataxia, confusion, dizziness, <u>headache</u>, peripheral neuropathy, syncope. **GI:** Abdominal discomfort, anorexia, diarrhea, <u>nausea</u>, metallic taste, pseudomembranous colitis (rare), vomiting. **GU:** Dark or reddish-brown urine. **Heme:** BONE MARROW APLASIA (rare), leukopenia (mild, transient). **Hypersens:** Erythematous rash, pruritus. **Other:** Thrombophlebitis.

DRUG INTERACTIONS
Alcohol: Disulfiram-like reactions (confusional state, abdominal cramps, nausea, vomiting, headache, flushing). **Cimetidine:** Inhibited metronidazole metabolism. **Phenobarbital, phenytoin:** Decreased antimicrobial effectiveness. **Warfarin and other coumarin anticoagulants:** Potentiated anticoagulant effect.

NURSING CONSIDERATIONS
Assessment
General:
Intake/output ratio.
Physical:
Neurologic status, GI tract, infectious disease status, signs/symptoms of superinfection.

Lab Alterations:
Monitor total and differential leukocyte counts before and after treatment. Interference with values of AST (SGOT), ALT (SGPT), LDH, triglycerides, and hexokinase glucose.

Intervention/Rationale
Obtain specimens for culture and sensitivity prior to initiation of treatment (first dose may be given while awaiting results). ● Monitor frequency, quality, and character of stools. ● Assess for the development of peripheral neuropathy/seizures. ● Evaluate fluid status to determine hydration replacement needs.

Patient/Family Education
Avoid alcohol for at least 1 day following administration. Drug may impart a reddish-brown color to urine. Notify physician with any of the following: vaginal/rectal itching, vaginal discharge, foul-smelling urine, tingling/burning hands or feet.

MEZLOCILLIN
(mez-loe-sill'-in)
Trade Name(s): Mezlin
Classification(s): Antibiotic (synthetic extended-spectrum penicillin)
Pregnancy Category: B

PHARMACODYNAMICS/KINETICS
Mechanism of Action: Bactericidal antibiotic against susceptible organisms, inhibits cell wall mucopeptide synthesis. **Peak Serum Level:** 30 minutes. **Distribution:** 16%–42% bound to serum proteins. Distributed into ascitic, pleural, peritoneal, and

In the Adverse Effects section, <u>underline</u> indicates most frequent; CAPS indicates life threatening.

337

wound fluids, also into bile, heart, prostatic tissue, bronchial secretions, tonsils, muscle, gallbladder, adipose tissue, bone, and gynecologic tissue. Low concentrations found in CSF (higher concentrations found in inflamed meninges). **Metabolism/Elimination:** 15% of dose metabolized to microbiologically inactive substances. Drug and its metabolites excreted primarily by the kidneys and partially by bile. Removed by hemodialysis. **Half-Life:** 0.96–1.2 hr.

INDICATIONS/DOSAGE

Treatment of serious gram-negative infections (especially Pseudomonas aeruginosa)

Adjust dosage in renal impairment.

Adult: 200–300 mg/kg/day in four to six divided doses. Usual dose 3 g every 4 hr (18 g/day) or 4 g every 6 hr (16 g/day).

Pediatric (infants > 1 month of age and children up to age 12 years): 50 mg/kg every 4 hr (300 mg/kg/day).

Neonate:
- ■< 7 days of age: 75 mg/kg every 12 hr (150 mg/kg/day).
- ■ < 2000 g and > 7 days of age: 75 mg/kg every 8 hr (225 mg/kg/day).
- ■ > 2000 g and > 7 days: 75 mg/kg every 6 hr (300 mg/kg/day).

CONTRAINDICATIONS/ PRECAUTIONS

Contraindicated in: Hypersensitivity to penicillins or cephalosporins. **Use cautiously in:** Renal impairment. **Pregnancy/Lactation:** No well-controlled trials to establish safety. Benefits must outweigh risks. Mice and rats given two times the usual adult dose in reproductive studies reveal no evidence of harm to the fetus. Distributed into breast milk. Use with caution in breastfeeding mothers. **Pediatrics:** Limited safety and efficacy data available.

PREPARATION

Availability: 1, 2, 3, and 4 g vials. 20 g bulk vials. Contains 1.85 mEq sodium/g. **Reconstitution:** Dilute each gram with at least 10 mL of compatible IV solution. Shake vigorously. **Infusion:** Further dilute to a volume of 50 or 100 mL.

STABILITY/STORAGE

Vial: Store at room temperature. Solution is clear and white to pale yellow after reconstitution. Powder and reconstituted product may darken slightly when stored (potency of drug not affected). **Infusion:** If refrigerated, stable for 7 days in sodium chloride and dextrose or 48 hr in D_5 0.45 NS. Stable for 48 hr at room temperature.

ADMINISTRATION

General: If concurrently given with aminoglycosides, administer in separate infusions as far apart as possible. **IV Push:** Give slowly over 3–5 min. To avoid venous irritation, concentration of drug should not exceed 10%. **Intermittent Infusion:** Give over 30 min.

COMPATIBILITY

Solution: Dextrose solutions, sodium chloride solutions. **Syringe:** Heparin. **Y-site:** Cyclophosphamide, famotidine, hydromorphone, morphine, perphenazine.

In the Adverse Effects section, <u>underline</u> indicates most frequent; CAPS indicates life threatening.

INCOMPATIBILITY
Y-site: Ciprofloxacin, meperidine, ondansetron, verapamil.

ADVERSE EFFECTS
CNS: Dizziness, headache, lethargy, seizures. **CV:** CHF. **GI:** Diarrhea. **Renal:** Interstitial nephritis, nephropathy. **Fld/Lytes:** Hypokalemia, hypernatremia. **Heme:** Anemia, eosinophilia, granulocytopenia, leukopenia, transient neutropenia, thrombocytopenia, thrombocytopenic purpura (hematopoietic symptoms are usually reversible with discontinuation of therapy and are believed to be evidence of hypersensitivity), abnormalities of coagulation (prolonged clotting and prothrombin times). **Hypersens:** DEATH, VASCULAR COLLAPSE, hypersensitivity myocarditis, angioneurotic edema, BRONCHOSPASM, dermatitis, hypotension, LARYNGOSPASM, pruritis, sneezing, wheezing, urticaria. **Other:** Pain at injection site, phlebitis.

DRUG INTERACTIONS
Aminoglycosides: Synergistic effect. **Bacteriostatic antibiotics** (erythromycin, tetracycline): Diminished bactericidal effect of penicillins with concurrent use. **Chloramphenicol:** Decreased penicillin effect, increased chloramphenicol half-life. **Heparin, oral anticoagulants:** Altered coagulation and increased bleeding risks with high doses. **Probenecid:** Prolonged penicillin blood levels.

NURSING CONSIDERATIONS
Assessment
General:
Hypersensitivity.

Physical:
Infectious disease status, signs/symptoms of superinfection (especially in elderly, debilitated, or immunosuppressed).

Lab Alterations:
Assess coagulation studies (bleeding time, prothrombin time, platelet aggregation) prior to and throughout course of therapy. Evaluate electrolytes (especially sodium and potassium). False-positive urine protein levels.

Intervention/Rationale
Question patient about prior use of penicillins or cephalosporins and hypersensitivity reactions prior to initiation of therapy. Hypersensitivity reactions may be immediate and severe in penicillin-sensitive patients with a history of allergy, asthma, hay fever, or urticaria. ● Obtain specimens for culture and sensitivity before therapy is initiated (first dose may be given while awaiting results). ● Assess patient for signs and symptoms of infection prior to, during, and at completion of therapy.

Patient/Family Education
Notify physician/nurse if skin rash, itching, hives, severe diarrhea, or signs of superinfection occurs.

MICONAZOLE
(mi-kon′-a-zole)
Trade Name(s): Monistat IV
Classification(s): Antifungal agent
Pregnancy Category: C

In the Adverse Effects section, underline indicates most frequent;
CAPS indicates life threatening.

339

PHARMACODYNAMICS/KINETICS
Mechanism of Action: Antifungal against most pathogenic fungi. Alters cellular membranes, interferes with intracellular enzymes. **Distribution:** Distributes into most body tissues. Low concentration found in brain and CSF. 91%–93% bound to plasma proteins. **Metabolism/Elimination:** Metabolized primarily by the liver. 14%–22% of drug excreted in the urine as inactive metabolites. **Half-Life:** 20–25 hr.

INDICATIONS/DOSAGE

Treatment of severe systemic fungal infections and fungal meningitis
Adult: 200–3600 mg/day. Dosage and duration of therapy vary with diagnosis and affecting organism.

CONTRAINDICATIONS/ PRECAUTIONS
Contraindicated in: Hypersensitivity. **Use cautiously in:** Drugs containing cremophor-type vehicles (PEG 40, castor oil), hepatic insufficiency. **Pregnancy/Lactation:** No well-controlled trials to establish safety. Benefits must outweigh risks. Animal studies have not revealed evidence of harm to the fetus. **Pediatrics:** Safety and efficacy not established for children under the age of 1 year. Do not use in pediatric population unless benefits clearly outweigh potential risks.

PREPARATION
Availability: 10 mg/mL in 20 mL amps. **Infusion:** Dilute in 200 mL compatible IV solution.

STABILITY/STORAGE
Vial: Store at room temperature. Do not use darkened solutions. **Infusion:** Diluted solution stable at room temperature for 48 hr.

ADMINISTRATION
Intermittent Infusion: Give over 30–60 min (rapid injection may produce dysrhythmias or tachycardia).

COMPATIBILITY
Solution: Dextrose solutions, sodium chloride solutions. **Y-site:** Foscarnet, ondansetron.

ADVERSE EFFECTS
CNS: Anxiety, dizziness, drowsiness, headache. **Ophtho:** Dry eyes. **CV:** CARDIAC ARREST, cardiac dysrhythmias, transient tachycardia. **Resp:** RESPIRATORY ARREST. **GI:** Anorexia, bitter taste, diarrhea, nausea, vomiting. **GU:** Increased libido. **Fld/Lytes:** Hyponatremia. **Heme:** Thrombocytopenia, thrombocytosis, transient decrease in hemoglobin and anemia. **Hypersens:** ANAPHYLACTIC REACTION, pruritus. **Metab:** Hyperlipidemia, increased serum triglycerides. **Other:** Febrile reactions, phlebitis.

DRUG INTERACTIONS
Amphotericin B: Decreased antifungal effect of both drugs. **Coumarin drugs:** Enhanced anticoagulant effect. **Cyclosporine:** Increased cyclosporine levels. **Rifampin:** Reduced miconazole levels. **Phenytoin:** Altered metabolism of one or both drugs.

NURSING CONSIDERATIONS
Assessment
General:
Hypersensitivity.

In the Adverse Effects section, underline indicates most frequent; CAPS indicates life threatening.

Physical:
GI tract.
Lab Alterations:
Monitor blood counts, electrolytes, hepatic function, and lipids prior to, during, and following therapy.

Intervention/Rationale
Obtain specimens for fungal culture, serology, and histopathology prior to therapy to identify causative organism. Because of the risk of hypersensitivity/anaphylactic reactions, administer initial dose under supervision of a physician. ● Reducing dose, slowing infusion rate, and/or administering antiemetics before each dose may reduce nausea/vomiting.

Patient/Family Education
Educate regarding expected therapeutic outcome and side effects.

MIDAZOLAM
(mye-daze'-oh-lam)
Trade Name(s): Versed
Classification(s): Sedative/hypnotic (short-acting benzodiazepine)
Pregnancy Category: D
Controlled Substance Schedule: IV

PHARMACODYNAMICS/KINETICS
Mechanism of Action: Exact site and mode of action unknown. Appears to act on limbic, thalamic, and hypothalamic areas of the CNS to produce anxiolytic, sedative, hypnotic, skeletal muscle relaxant, and anticonvulsant effects. **Onset of Action:** 1–5 min. **Duration of Action:** Averages less than 2 hr. Effects may persist up to 6 hr in some patients. **Distribution:** Rapidly and widely distributed, with highest concentrations in liver, kidneys, lungs, fat, and heart. Crosses blood–brain barrier and distributes in CSF. Approximately 94%–97% bound to plasma proteins. **Metabolism/Elimination:** Metabolized extensively in the liver. Metabolites conjugated with glucuronic acid. Excreted in urine almost entirely as unchanged conjugated metabolite. **Half-Life:** 1–4 hr.

INDICATIONS/DOSAGE

Conscious sedation prior to short diagnostic procedures
Adult: Individualize dosage based on age, physical condition and concomitant medications. Total dose range of up to 0.05–0.15 mg/kg is adequate in average healthy adults (some patients may respond to as little as 1 mg). In rare cases, a total dose of up to 0.2 mg/kg may be necessary. Additional maintenance doses may be given in increments of 25% of the initial dose to maintain the desired level of sedation. Lower dosage by 25%–30% if narcotic premedication or other CNS depressants are used.

Induction of general anesthesia
Adult:
Unpremedicated Patients: 0.3–0.35 mg/kg (maximum dose of 0.6 mg/kg will prolong recovery). **Premedicated Patients:** 0.15–0.35 mg/kg. Titrate dose to individual patient's response. Dosage is variable, particularly when narcotic premedication is not used.

In the Adverse Effects section, underline indicates most frequent; CAPS indicates life threatening.

CONTRAINDICATIONS/ PRECAUTIONS

Contraindicated in: Hypersensitivity, acute narrow-angle glaucoma, depressive neurosis or psychotic reaction without anxiety, alcohol intoxication, shock, coma. **Use cautiously in:** Elderly (reduce dosage), suicidal tendencies, hepatorenal disease, severe fluid and electrolyte imbalance. **Pregnancy/Lactation:** Studies suggest increased risk of congenital malformation when used in the first trimester of pregnancy. Do not use in pregnancy. Distributed into breast milk. Use with caution in breastfeeding women. **Pediatrics:** Safety and efficacy not established in children under 18 years of age.

PREPARATION

Availability: 1 mg/mL in 2, 5, and 10 mL vials. 5 mg/mL in 1, 2, 5, and 10 mL vials and 2 mL Tel-E-Ject syringes.

STABILITY/STORAGE

Vial: Store at room temperature. **Infusion:** Stable at room temperature for 24 hr.

ADMINISTRATION

IV Push: For conscious sedation, dose may be diluted with sodium chloride or dextrose and injected over 2 or more minutes at intervals of 2 min (titrate slower in patients over the age of 60 and in those with chronic debilitating disease). For induction of anesthesia, inject dose over 20–30 sec and give supplemental doses at 2 min intervals. **Continuous Infusion (*Unlabeled route*):** Dilute to a 1:1 concentration and give via infusion device (250 mg in 250 mL).

COMPATIBILITY

Solution: Dextrose solutions, lactated Ringer's, sodium chloride solutions. **Syringe:** Atropine, benzquinamide, buprenorphine, butorphanol, chlorpromazine, cimetidine, diphenhydramine, droperidol, fentanyl, glycopyrrolate, hydromorphone, meperidine, metoclopramide, morphine, nalbuphine, promethazine, scopolamine. **Y-site:** Atracurium, famotidine, pancuronium, vecuronium.

INCOMPATIBILITY

Syringe: Dimenhydrinate, pentobarbital, perphenazine, prochlorperazine, ranitidine. **Y-site:** Foscarnet.

ADVERSE EFFECTS

CNS: Involuntary tonic/clonic movements, agitation, anxiety, combativeness, confusion, dizziness, drowsiness, euphoria, headache, hyperactivity, nightmares, oversedation, retrograde amnesia, restlessness. **Ophtho:** Blurred vision, diplopia. **CV:** CARDIAC ARREST, dysrhythmias, hypotension, vasovagal episode. **Resp:** APNEA, RESPIRATORY ARREST, respiratory depression, BRONCHOSPASM, dyspnea, hyperventilation. **GI:** Nausea, vomiting. **MS:** Muscle tremors, weakness. **Other:** Hiccoughs, induration, redness, pain, and phlebitis at injection site.

TOXICITY/OVERDOSE

Signs/Symptoms: Sedation, somnolence, confusion, impaired coordination/reflexes, coma, untoward effects on vital signs. **Treatment:** Maintain patent airway, monitor respiration, heart rate, and blood pressure, use supportive measures, treat hypotension with IV fluids, re-

In the Adverse Effects section, underline indicates most frequent; CAPS indicates life threatening.

positioning, and careful use of vasopressor agents. Value of peritoneal or hemodialysis unknown. **Antidote(s):** Flumazenil IV as per physician order (reverses sedation or overdose effects). Physostigmine 0.5–4.0 mg at a rate of 1 mg/min may reverse symptoms resembling central anticholinergic overdose (confusion, delirium, hallucinations, memory disruption, visual disturbances).

DRUG INTERACTIONS
Alcohol, barbiturates, CNS depressants: Increased risk of hypoventilation and prolonged drug effect. **Droperidol, fentanyl, narcotics, secobarbital:** Enhanced hypnotic effect of midazolam. Reduced thiopental dose required for anesthesia induction. **Inhalation anesthetics:** Reduce anesthetic dose if midazolam used for premedication.

NURSING CONSIDERATIONS
Assessment
General:
Vital signs.
Physical:
Neurologic status, cardiopulmonary status.

Intervention/Rationale
Monitor respirations, blood pressure, and heart rate prior to and during administration/procedure and during recovery period. ● Geriatric patients, those patients with underlying chronic disease states, and those receiving other CNS depressants are most at risk for complications and adverse effects. ● Consider withholding medication if somnolence develops. ● Patients that develop involuntary movements, hyperactivity/combativeness, or cerebral hypoxia during or after administration should be evaluated before proceeding. ● Emergency equipment for the administration of oxygen and control of respiration should be readily available during and immediately following administration.

Patient/Family Education
Pharmacological effects of this drug and the duration of effects vary. Drug may cause drowsiness; avoid engaging in tasks requiring mental alertness. Seek assistance with ambulatory activities. Avoid alcohol or other CNS depressants for 24 hr following administration.

MITOMYCIN
(mi-toe-mye′-sin)
Trade Name(s): Mutamycin
Classification(s): Antineoplastic antibiotic
Pregnancy Category: Unknown

PHARMACODYNAMICS/KINETICS
Mechanism of Action: Antineoplastic antibiotic. Active against gram-positive bacteria and some viruses, but its cytoxicity precludes its use as an anti-infective agent. Antineoplastic mechanism similar to that of alklylating agents. Causes cross-linking of DNA. May inhibit RNA and protein synthesis. **Distribution:** In animal studies, highest concentrations found in kidneys, muscles, eyes, lungs, intestines, and stomach. Not found in liver, spleen, or brain. Higher concentrations of drug found in cancer tissues than in

In the Adverse Effects section, underline indicates most frequent; CAPS indicates life threatening.

343

normal tissues. **Metabolism/Elimination:** Rapidly inactivated by microsomes in the liver and enzymes in kidneys, spleen, brain, and heart. Less than 10% excreted in urine as active drug. Small amount excreted in bile. **Half-Life:** 50 min.

INDICATIONS/DOSAGE

Palliative treatment of disseminated adenocarcinoma of the stomach or pancreas
(Use in combination with other chemotherapeutic agents—not recommended as single-agent therapy.)

Adult: Individualize dose based on clinical/hematological response, patient tolerance, and whether or not adjunctive myelosuppressive therapy is being used. Initial dose 20 mg/m^2 as a single treatment every 6–8 weeks. Adjust subsequent doses according to patient's hematological response to previous dose. Give additional doses after leukocyte count and platelet counts have returned to 3000/mm^3 and 75,000/mm^3, respectively. Discontinue drug if disease progresses after two courses of therapy, as response will be minimal. Adjust doses following initial dose; see table, this page.

CONTRAINDICATIONS/ PRECAUTIONS

Contraindicated in: Hypersensitivity or idiosyncratic reaction to mitomycin; primary therapy as a single agent or to replace surgery or radiotherapy; thrombocytopenia, coagulation disorder, or increased bleeding tendencies due to other causes; platelet count < 75,000 mm^3, leukocyte count < 3000/mm^3 or serum creatinine > 1.7 mg%; active chicken pox or herpes zoster. **Use cautiously in:** Renal impairment, bone marrow depression, infection. **Pregnancy/Lactation:** No well-controlled trials to establish safety. Animal studies have shown teratogenic effects. Benefits must outweigh risks. Do not give to breast-feeding women because of potential harmful effects on infant. **Pediatrics:** Safety and efficacy not established.

PREPARATION
Availability: 5, 20, and 40 mg vials. **Reconstitution:** Add 10, 40, or 80 mL of sterile water to vials containing 5, 20, or 40 mg of drug, respectively. Resultant concentration is approximately 0.5 mg/mL. Shake vial to enhance dissolution. If powder does not dissolve immediately, allow to stand at room temperature until completely dissolved.

Nadir after Prior Dose (cells/mm^3)		% of Prior Dose To Be Given
Leucocytes	Platelets	
> 4000	> 100,000	100
3000–3999	75,000–99,999	100
2000–2999	25,000–74,999	70
< 2000	< 25,000	50

In the Adverse Effects section, underline indicates most frequent; CAPS indicates life threatening.

STABILITY/STORAGE
Vial: Store at room temperature. Reconstituted vial at a concentration of 0.5 mg/mL is stable for 14 days refrigerated or 7 days at room temperature.

ADMINISTRATION
General: Handle drug with care and adhere to institutional guidelines for the handling of chemotherapeutic/cytotoxic agents. In the event of a spill, use sodium hypochlorite 5% (household bleach) or potassium permanganate 1% to inactivate mitomycin. Assure patency of IV site and closely assess site for signs and symptoms of infiltration or extravasation. Extravasation may cause necrosis and sloughing of surrounding tissue. **IV Push:** Administer slowly through the tubing of an IV infusion.

COMPATIBILITY
Solution: Lactated Ringer's, sodium chloride solutions. **Syringe:** Bleomycin, cisplatin, cyclophosphamide, doxorubicin, droperidol, fluorouracil, furosemide, heparin, leucovorin calcium, methotrexate, metoclopramide, vinblastine, vincristine. **Y-site:** Bleomycin, cisplatin, cyclophosphamide, doxorubicin, droperidol, fluorouracil, furosemide, heparin, leucovorin calcium, methotrexate, metoclopramide, ondansetron, vinblastine, vincristine.

INCOMPATIBILITY
Solution: Dextrose solutions.

ADVERSE EFFECTS
CNS: Drowsiness, headache, syncope. **Ophtho:** Blurred vision. **Resp:** PULMONARY TOXICITY, pulmonary infiltrates, dyspnea, nonproductive cough. **GI:** <u>Anorexia</u>, diarrhea, <u>nausea</u>, stomatitis, <u>vomiting</u>. **Renal:** Renal failure, rise in serum creatinine. **Derm:** Alopecia. **Heme:** BONE MARROW TOXICITY (thrombocytopenia/leukopenia: 2–4 weeks), HEMOLYTIC UREMIC SYNDROME (syndrome of microangiopathic hemolytic anemia, thrombocytopenia, renal failure, and hypertension). **Nadir:** 6 weeks. **Other:** Necrosis and tissue sloughing (with extravasation), cellulitis at injection site, fever, thrombophlebitis.

DRUG INTERACTIONS
Bone marrow depressants, radiation therapy: Increased bone marrow suppression. **Doxorubicin:** Increased cardiotoxicity with concomitant use. **Live virus vaccines:** Vaccine administration may cause rather than provide immunity against disease. **Vinca alkaloids:** Acute respiratory distress with previous or concomitant use of vinca alkaloids.

NURSING CONSIDERATIONS
Assessment
General:
Intake/output ratio, nutritional status, infectious disease status.
Physical:
GI tract, hematopoietic system, pulmonary status, GU tract.
Lab Alterations:
Monitor BUN, hemoglobin, and hematocrit, platelet count, ALT (SGPT), AST (SGOT), bilirubin, creatinine, LDH, uric acid, total and differential leukocyte count prior to, during, and after completion of therapy (renal and hematologic

In the Adverse Effects section, <u>underline</u> indicates most frequent; CAPS indicates life threatening.

345

function should be followed for several months following completion of therapy).

Intervention/Rationale
Nausea and vomiting may occur within 1–2 hr following administration—antiemetics given 30 minutes prior to administration may provide some relief. Nausea may continue for 2–3 days. ● Assess patient for signs of infection due to leukopenia (sore throat, fever) and bleeding due to thrombocytopenia (bleeding gums, bruising, petechiae, hematemesis, hematest positive stools). ● Assess pulmonary status prior to administration and periodically during therapy. ● In patients receiving long-term therapy, monitor for signs/symptoms of hemolytic uremia syndrome (thrombocytopenia, microangiopathic hemolytic anemia, renal failure, hypertension). ● Assess for development of fever, chills, or other signs of infection. ● Avoid IM injections and rectal temperatures when platelet count < 100,000.

Patient/Family Education
Inform of potential toxic effects, particularly bone marrow suppression. Notify physician of fever, chills, bleeding, sore throat, or signs of infection. Take and record oral temperature daily and report persistent elevations to physician. Avoid crowded environments and persons with known infections. Perform good oral care with a soft toothbrush and alcohol-free mouthwash. Use electric razor. Use consistent and reliable contraception throughout the duration of therapy due to potential terato-genic and mutagenic effects of drug. Do not drink alcohol or take over-the-counter medications containing aspirin or ibuprofen. Explore feelings and coping methods to deal with potential hair loss. Do not receive any vaccinations during therapy without the knowledge of the physician.

MITOXANTRONE
(mye-toe-zan′-trone)
Trade Name(s): Novantrone
Classification(s): Antineoplastic agent, antitumor antibiotic
Pregnancy Category: D

PHARMACODYNAMICS/KINETICS
Mechanism of Action: Synthetic antineoplastic agent. Has cytocidal effect on proliferating and nonproliferating cells. **Distribution:** Rapidly and extensively distributed to body tissues. 78% bound to plasma proteins. **Metabolism/Elimination:** Excreted in urine 65% unchanged. 25% excreted via bile. **Half-Life:** 5.8 days (2.3–13.0 days).

INDICATIONS/DOSAGE

Used in combination with other drugs for the initial treatment of acute nonlymphocytic leukemia (ANLL) in adults

(includes myelogenous, promyelocytic, monocytic, and erythroid acute leukemias).

Adult: 12 mg/m²/day on days 1–3. Second induction course may be given if complete remission does not occur.

CONTRAINDICATIONS/ PRECAUTIONS
Contraindicated in: Hypersensitivity. **Use cautiously in:** Cardiac disease, preexisting myelosuppression. **Pregnancy/Lactation:** No well-controlled trials to establish safety. May cause fetal harm. Low birth weight and retarded development seen in rat studies. Benefits must outweigh risks. Inform women becoming pregnant of the potential fetal risks. Because of potential risk to infant, discontinue breastfeeding before beginning treatment. **Pediatrics:** Safety and efficacy not established.

PREPARATION
Availability: 2 mg/mL in 10, 12.5, and 15 mL vials. **Infusion:** May be further diluted in at least 50 mL of compatible IV solution.

STABILITY/STORAGE
Vial: Store at room temperature. **Infusion:** Prepare just prior to administration.

ADMINISTRATION
General: Handle drug with care and adhere to institutional guidelines for the handling of chemotherapeutic/cytotoxic agents. In the event of a spill, use calcium hypochorite solution to inactivate mitoxantrone. Assure patency of IV, and avoid extravasation (tissue necrosis may occur). **IV Push:** Inject diluted solution slowly (over at least 3 minutes) into the tubing of a freely running IV. **Intermittent Infusion:** Infuse over physician specified time.

COMPATIBILITY
Solution: Dextrose solutions, sodium chloride solutions. **Y-site:** Ondansetron.

ADVERSE EFFECTS
CNS: Seizures, headache. **Ophtho:** Conjunctivitis, blue-green sclera. **CV:** CHF, dysrhythmias, ECG changes. **Resp:** Cough, dyspnea. **GI:** Abdominal pain, bleeding, diarrhea, <u>nausea</u>, <u>stomatitis</u>, <u>vomiting</u>. **GU:** Blue-green urine. **Renal:** Renal failure. **Derm:** Alopecia, ecchymosis. **Heme:** Hyperuricemia, sepsis/fungal infections, <u>SEVERE MYELOSUPPRESSION</u>. ***Nadir:*** 2 weeks. **Hypersens:** Petechiae. **Other:** Fever.

DRUG INTERACTIONS
Other myelosuppressants/radiotherapy: Increased bone marrow depression.

NURSING CONSIDERATIONS
Assessment
General:
Intake/output ratio, nutritional status, infectious disease status.
Physical:
Cardiopulmonary system, GI tract, hematopoietic system.
Lab Alterations:
Monitor BUN, hemoglobin, hematocrit, platelet count, ALT (SGPT), AST (SGOT), bilirubin, creatinine, LDH, uric acid, total and differential leukocyte count prior to, during, and after completion of therapy (renal and hematologic function should be followed for several months following completion of therapy).

Intervention/Rationale
Assess heart/lung sounds and monitor for signs/symptoms of CHF or cardiotoxicity. ● Nausea/vomiting may be treated with prophylactic

M

In the Adverse Effects section, <u>underline</u> indicates most frequent; CAPS indicates life threatening.

347

antiemetics 30 minutes prior to administration. ● Assess patient for signs of infection due to leukopenia (sore throat, fever) and bleeding due to thrombocytopenia (bleeding gums, bruising, petechiae, hematemesis, hematest positive stools). ● Assess oral mucosa frequently for presence of oral lesions/stomatitis.

Patient/Family Education

Drug will cause a blue-green colored urine for 24 hr after administration and also may cause bluish discoloration of the sclera. Inform of potential toxic effects, particularly bone marrow suppression. Notify physician of fever, chills, bleeding, sore throat, or signs of infection. Avoid crowded environments and persons with known infections. Perform good oral care with a soft toothbrush and alcohol-free mouthwash. Use electric razor. Use consistent and reliable contraception throughout the duration of therapy due to potential teratogenic and mutagenic effects of drug. Do not drink alcohol or take over-the-counter medications containing aspirin or ibuprofen. Explore feelings and potential coping mechanism in regard to possible hair loss. Do not receive any vaccinations during therapy without the knowledge of a physician.

MORPHINE
(mor'-feen)
Trade Name(s): Astramorph, Duramorph
Classification(s): Narcotic analgesic

Pregnancy Category: C
Controlled Substance Schedule: II

PHARMACODYNAMICS/KINETICS

Mechanism of Action: Binds to opiate receptors in the CNS. Alters perception of pain and produces analgesia. **Onset of Action:** Rapid. **Peak Effect:** 0.5 hr. **Duration of Action:** 3 hr. **Distribution:** Widely distributed to skeletal muscle, kidneys, liver, intestinal tract, lungs, spleen, and brain. **Metabolism/Elimination:** Metabolized primarily by the liver. Also metabolized to some degree by CNS, kidneys, lungs, and placenta. Excreted primarily in urine. Small amounts excreted in feces. **Half-Life:** 2–4 hr.

INDICATIONS/DOSAGE

Relief of moderate to severe acute and chronic pain; used preoperatively to sedate; reduce anxiety; facilitate anesthesia induction; and reduce anesthesia dosage

Adult: 2.5–15.0 mg IV push. Epidural: initial injection 5 mg with additional incremental doses of 1–2 mg (to a maximum dose of 10 mg/24 hr). If used as patient-controlled anesthesia device, adjust dose to severity of pain and response of the patient.

Severe, chronic cancer pain

(dose must be individualized according to response and tolerance of patient).

Adult: Loading dose of 15 mg, followed by a continuous infusion at 0.8–10.0 mg/hr and increase as necessary. *Pediatric:* Continuous infusion of 0.025–2.6 mg/kg/hr.

In the Adverse Effects section, <u>underline</u> indicates most frequent; CAPS indicates life threatening.

Severe pain associated with sickle cell crisis

Pediatric: 0.03–0.15 mg/kg/hr.

CONTRAINDICATIONS/ PRECAUTIONS

Contraindicated in: Biliary tract surgery, diarrhea caused by poisoning until toxic material eliminated, during labor and delivery of premature infant, hypersensitivity, premature infants. **Use cautiously in:** Acute asthma, cor pulmonale, debilitated patients, drug dependence, elderly, head injury/increased intracranial pressure, obstructive pulmonary disease, preexisting respiratory depression, hypoxia, or hypercapnia. **Pregnancy/Lactation:** No well-controlled trials to establish safety. Benefits must outweigh risks. Fetal withdrawal symptoms seen with illicit use. Distributed into breast milk; however, effects on infant may be insignificant. Wait 4–6 hr after administration to breastfeed infant.

PREPARATION

Availability: 2, 4, 8, 10, and 15 mg/mL. **Infusion:** Dilute to a concentration of 0.1–1.0 mg/mL in compatible IV solution.

STABILITY/STORAGE

Vial/prefilled syringes: Store at room temperature. **Infusion:** Stable at room temperature for 24 hr.

ADMINISTRATION

General: Rapid administration has caused anaphylactoid reaction, severe respiratory depression, hypotension, peripheral circulatory collapse, and cardiac arrest. Patients should be lying down during initial administration. **IV Push:** May dilute in 4–5 mL of sterile water and give slowly over 4–5 min. If undiluted, give slowly 1 mg/min. **Continuous Infusion:** Give via controlled infusion device at physician specified rate. **Epidural:** Use only preservative free preparation. Should be given only by those individuals familiar with the administration technique and management of potential patient problems.

COMPATIBILITY

Solution: Dextrose solutions, lactated Ringer's, Ringer's injection, sodium chloride solutions. **Syringe:** Atropine, benzquinamide, butorphanol, chlorpromazine, cimetidine, dimenhydrinate, diphenhydramine, droperidol, fentanyl, glycopyrrolate, heparin, metoclopramide, midazolam, pentazocine, perphenazine, ranitidine, scopolamine. **Y-site:** Acyclovir, amikacin, aminophylline, ampicillin, atracurium, calcium chloride, cefamandole, cefazolin, cefoperazone, ceforanide, cefotaxime, cefotetan, cefoxitin, ceftizoxime, cefuroxime, cephalothin, cephapirin, chloramphenicol, clindamycin, doxycycline, enalaprilat, erythromycin, esmolol, famotidine, foscarnet, gentamicin, heparin, hydrocortisone, insulin, labetalol, metronidazole, mezlocillin, moxalactam, nafcillin, ondansetron, oxacillin, pancuronium, penicillin G potassium, piperacillin, potassium chloride, ranitidine, sodium bicarbonate, ticarcillin, tobramycin, trimethoprim-sulfamethoxazole, vecuronium, vitamin B complex with C, zidovudine.

INCOMPATIBILITY

Y-site: Minocycline.

M

In the Adverse Effects section, underline indicates most frequent; CAPS indicates life threatening.

349

ADVERSE EFFECTS

CNS: Agitation, coma, dizziness, euphoria, <u>lightheadedness</u>, mental clouding/depression, restlessness, <u>sedation</u>. **Ophtho:** Visual disturbances. **CV:** CARDIOPULMONARY ARREST, bradycardia, hypotension, hypertension, orthostatic hypotension, tachycardia. **Resp:** APNEA, respiratory depression. **GI:** Biliary spasm or colic, constipation, <u>nausea</u>, <u>vomiting</u>. **GU:** Oliguria, urinary retention. **Derm:** Warmness of face, neck, and upper thorax. **Heme:** Thrombocytopenia. **Hypersens:** Pruritus, urticaria. **Other:** Flushing, <u>sweating</u>, pain at injection site.

TOXICITY/OVERDOSE

Signs/Symptoms: CNS depression (ranges from profound stupor to coma), miosis, respiratory depression, Cheyne-Stokes respiration, cyanosis, cold, clammy skin, hypothermia, flaccid skeletal muscles, bradycardia, hypotension, apnea, circulatory collapse, cardiopulmonary arrest. **Treatment:** Establish/maintain patent airway. Provide oxygen and assisted respiration if needed. **Antidote:** Naloxone is effective for circulatory and respiratory depression.

DRUG INTERACTIONS

Anticoagulants: Increased anticoagulant activity. **Chlorpromazine, methocarbamol:** Potentiated analgesic effect of morphine. **CNS depressants** (other opiate agonists, general anesthetics, tranquilizers, sedatives/hypnotics, alcohol): Additive CNS depression, respiratory and sedative effects. **Tricyclic antidepressants, MAO inhibitors:** Enhanced CNS depression.

NURSING CONSIDERATIONS

Assessment
General:
Vital signs, pain assessment (prior to and after administration).
Physical:
Pulmonary status, GI tract.

Intervention/Rationale
Administer pain medication before pain becomes too severe (analgesia is more effective when given on a regular basis). ● Oxygen, emergency airway equipment, and naloxone should be readily available (drug can cause respiratory depression). ● If receiving drug by epidural route, monitor respiratory status hourly while patient is receiving drug and for 24 hr after discontinuation (delayed respiratory depression may occur). ● Assess bowel function regularly. Administer stool softeners and laxatives when needed. Maintain hydration and increase bulk in diet when possible to combat constipation. ● Assess blood pressure, heart rate, and respiratory rate before, during, and following administration.

Patient/Family Education
Coordination or mental alertness may be affected; activities requiring mental alertness should be avoided. Call for help with ambulation, as drug may cause dizziness, drowsiness, and sedation. Ask for pain medication before pain becomes too severe. Change positions slowly to prevent orthostatic hypotension. Avoid concomitant use of other CNS depressants, including alcohol.

In the Adverse Effects section, <u>underline</u> indicates most frequent; CAPS indicates life threatening.

MOXALACTAM

(mox-a-lak'-tam)
Trade Name(s): Moxam
Classification(s): Cephalosporin antibiotic, third generation
Pregnancy Category: C

PHARMACODYNAMICS/KINETICS

Mechanism of Action: Bactericidal action, inhibition of bacterial cell wall synthesis. **Distribution:** Widely distributed to most tissues. Readily crosses into the CSF with inflammation. Concentrations in bone are usually adequate with higher doses. 57% protein binding. **Metabolism/Elimination:** Primarily eliminated via kidneys. **Half-Life:** 114–150 min. Prolonged in renal impairment.

INDICATIONS/DOSAGE

Treatment or prophylaxis of gram-positive and most gram-negative organisms

(provides greater gram-negative coverage than first and second generation cephalosporins) associated with respiratory tract, genitourinary tract, skin/skin structure, bone/joint, septicemia, and intra-abdominal infections. Dosage interval may need to be adjusted in renal impairment.

Adult: Administer prophylactic phytonadione 10 mg/week to all patients to prevent coagulopathy
▪ Mild skin/uncomplicated pneumonia: 500 mg every 8 hr.
▪ Mild uncomplicated UTI: 250–500 mg every 12 hr.
▪ Complicated UTI: 500 mg every 8 hr.
▪ Life-threatening infections: Up to 4 g every 8 hr. Not to exceed 12 g/day.

Pediatric: Administer prophylactic phytonadione to prevent coagulopathy. 150–200 mg/kg/day in divided doses every 6–8 hr. Not to exceed adult dosages or 10 g/day. Meningitis: 100 mg/kg then 150–200 mg/kg/day in divided doses every 6–8 hr. Not to exceed adult dosages or 12 g/day.

Neonate: Administer prophylactic phytonadione to prevent coagulopathy.
Meningitis: 100 mg/kg, then
▪ 0–1 week: 100 mg/kg/day in divided doses every 12 hr.
▪ 1–4 weeks: 150 mg/kg/day in divided doses every 8 hr.

CONTRAINDICATIONS/ PRECAUTIONS

Contraindicated in: Hypersensitivity to cephalosporins/penicillins, or related antibiotics. **Use cautiously in:** Impaired renal function. **Pregnancy/ Lactation:** No well-controlled trials to establish safety. Use only if benefits outweigh risk. Crosses placenta. Identified in breast milk in small quantities demonstrating potential infant bowel flora changes and pharmacologic effects. **Pediatrics:** Consider benefits and risks in young children because safety and efficacy has not been established. Neonates have demonstrated decreased elimination of cephalosporins.

PREPARATION

Availability: 1 g, 2 g vials and 10 g bulk package. Contains 3.8 mEq sodium/g. **Reconstitution:** Dilute each gram with at least 10 mL sterile wa-

M

In the Adverse Effects section, underline indicates most frequent; CAPS indicates life threatening.

351

ter for injection or compatible diluent to a maximum concentration of 50–100 mg/mL. **Intermittent infusion:** Dilute to a final volume of 50–100 mL compatible solution or final concentration of 10–20 mg/mL

STABILITY/STORAGE
Vial: Store at room temperature. Reconstituted vial/solution stable 24 hr at room temperature and 4 days refrigerated.

ADMINISTRATION
IV Push: Give slowly over at least 3–5 min. **Intermittent Infusion:** Infuse over at least 15–30 min.

COMPATIBILITY
Solution: Dextrose solutions, lactated Ringer's, Ringer's injection, sodium chloride solutions, sterile water for injection. **Syringe:** Heparin. **Y-site:** Cyclophosphamide, hydromorphone, magnesium sulfate, meperidine, morphine, perphenazine.

ADVERSE EFFECTS
CNS: Seizures (especially with high doses in renal impairment), confusion, dizziness, fatigue, headache, lethargy, paresthesia. **CV:** Hypotension. **Resp:** BRONCHOSPASM, interstitial pneumonitis. **GI:** Pseudomembranous colitis, anorexia, cholestasis, diarrhea, dysguesia, dyspepsia, elevated alkaline phosphatase, bilirubin, LDH, liver enzymes (AST, ALT, GGTP), gallbladder sludge, glossitis, nausea, vomiting. **GU:** Dysuria, genital moniliasis, genitoanal pruritus, hematuria, pyuria, vaginitis. **Renal:** Interstitial nephritis, decreased creatinine clearance, transient elevations

in BUN and serum creatinine. **Heme:** Decreased platelet function, hypoprothrombinemia, leukopenia, transient neutropenia, thrombocytopenia, agranulocytosis, anemia, aplastic anemia, bleeding, eosinophilia, lymphocytosis. **Hypersens:** ANAPHYLAXIS, angioedema, Stevens-Johnson syndrome, chest tightness, edema, eosinophilia, exfoliative dermatitis, joint pain, maculopapular rash, morbilliform eruptions, myalgias, pruritus, rash, urticaria. **Other:** Cellulitis, chills, diaphoresis, fever, flushing, inflammation, local swelling.

TOXICITY/OVERDOSE
Signs/Symptoms: High doses in renal impairment may cause seizures. **Treatment:** Discontinue agent when seizures begin. Administer anticonvulsant therapy and consider hemodialysis.

DRUG INTERACTIONS
Aminoglycosides: Potentiation of nephrotoxicity potential. **Bacteriostatic antibiotics (i.e., chloramphenicol):** Potential interference with cephalosporin bactericidal action. **Ethanol:** Consumption of alcohol with or up to 72 hr after therapy may result in disulfiram-like reaction beginning within 30 min of alcohol ingestion and lasting for several hours. **Oral anticoagulants:** Increased hypoprothrombinemic effects of anticoagulants.

NURSING CONSIDERATIONS
Assessment
General:
Allergy history, anaphylaxis.

In the Adverse Effects section, underline indicates most frequent; CAPS indicates life threatening.

Physical:
GI tract, signs/symptoms of super-infection (sore throat/stomatitis, vaginal discharge, perianal itching), infectious disease status.

Lab Alterations:
Monitor CBC, coagulation profile, renal, and hepatic function, false-positive direct Coombs', especially in azotemia, false-positive urine glucose with copper sulfate (Clinitest) (use Tes-Tape), false elevation urinary 17-ketosteroid values.

Intervention/Rationale
Observe for signs/symptoms of anaphylaxis. Patients with history of severe penicillin sensitivity may also have cephalosporin sensitivity (5%–10%). ● Obtain cultures for sensitivity, first dose may be given while awaiting preliminary results. ● May cause pseudomembranous colitis (diarrhea, nausea, vomiting, fluid/electrolyte disturbances; notify physician and obtain culture for *C. difficile* toxin).

Patient/Family Education
Complete course of therapy. Notify physician if there are any signs/symptoms of worsening infection (persistent fever/diarrhea) or signs of yeast infections (white patches in the mouth or vaginal discharge). Avoid alcohol during or up to 72 hr after stopping therapy (may result in acute alcohol intolerance that begins 30 min after alcohol ingestion and subsides 30 min to several hours afterwards; the reaction may occur up to 3 days after receiving the last dose). Patients may require weekly doses of phytonadione (vitamin K) to prevent bleeding.

MULTIVITAMIN INFUSION
Trade Name(s): MVC 9 + 3, MVI-12, MVI-Pediatric
Classification(s): Vitamins, multiple
Pregnancy Category: A

PHARMACODYNAMICS/KINETICS
Mechanism of Action: Multiple vitamin solution containing fat and water soluble vitamins in an aqueous solution. **Distribution:** Widely distributed, readily absorbed throughout body. **Metabolism/Elimination:** Used for various biological processes. Excess amounts of water soluble vitamins are excreted unchanged by the kidney.

INDICATIONS/DOSAGE

Prevention/correction of vitamin deficiencies due to inadequate diets/increased daily requirements, addition to parenteral nutrition
Adult: 5–10 mL/24 hr.

CONTRAINDICATIONS/PRECAUTIONS
Contraindicated in: Known hypersensitivity to components. **Pregnancy/Lactation:** No well-controlled trials to establish safety. Benefits must outweigh risks. Crosses placenta. Found in breast milk.

PREPARATION
Availability: 10 mL amps. 5 mL concentrate/vials. 10 mL two-chambered vials. **Infusion:** Never administer undiluted. Each dose must be diluted in a minimum of 500–1000 mL of compatible IV fluid. Solution is bright yellow and will color IV solution.

In the Adverse Effects section, underline indicates most frequent; CAPS indicates life threatening.

353

STABILITY/STORAGE
Vial: Keep refrigerated. Store in light-resistant containers. **Infusion:** Stable for 24 hr at room temperature.

ADMINISTRATION
General: Do not use if any crystals have formed in the vial/ampule. **Continuous Infusion:** Administer at physician prescribed rate of infusion.

COMPATIBILITY
Solution: Amino acids 4.25%/dextrose 25%, dextrose solutions, fat emulsion, lactated Ringer's, sodium chloride solutions. **Y-site:** Acyclovir, ampicillin, cefazolin, cephalothin, cephapirin, erythromycin, gentamicin.

INCOMPATIBILITY
Solution: Alkaline solutions.

ADVERSE EFFECTS
CV: Dizziness. **Hypersens:** ANAPHYLAXIS. **Other:** Fainting.

DRUG INTERACTIONS
Levodopa: Large amounts of pyridoxine (vitamin B_6) may interfere with beneficial effects.

NURSING CONSIDERATIONS
Assessment
General:
Nutritional status, dietary intake/needs assessment.
Physical:
Integumentary/body fat status.
Lab Alterations:
Evaluate total protein, albumin-globulin (A-G) ratio to determine deficiencies/supplementary requirements.

Intervention/Rationale
Higher than recommended doses of vitamins should not be used as a dietary supplement. Supervision/dietary assessment is important when preparation is administered. • Assess patient for alcoholism, hyperthyroidism, severe illness or injury, cachexia, malabsorption syndrome; all conditions that require increased vitamin intake.

Patient/Family Education
A single diagnosed vitamin deficiency usually coexists with other deficiencies. After the initial deficiency states are corrected, reinforce the necessity of adequate nutritional and multivitamin supplementation. After discontinuation of parenteral therapy, when taking oral vitamin supplements, stress the hazards of self-administration of megadoses of vitamins. Review adverse effects associated with fat-soluble vitamin ingestion not within recommended daily requirements.

MUROMONAB - CD3
(myoor-oh-mon'-ab)
Trade Name(s): Orthoclone OKT3
Classification(s): Immunosuppressive agent, murine monoclonal antibody
Pregnancy Category: C

PHARMACODYNAMICS/KINETICS
Mechanism of Action: Reverses graft rejection by blocking T-cell function that plays a primary role in acute graft rejection. **Onset of Action:** 3.3 days. **Duration of Action:** 7 days.

M

Distribution: Unknown. **Metabolism/ Elimination:** Unknown. **Half-Life:** 18 hr.

INDICATIONS/DOSAGE

Treatment of acute allograft rejection in renal transplantation

Adult: 5 mg/day for 10–14 days. Begin treatment as soon as acute rejection has been established. Reduce or discontinue concurrent immunosuppressive agents (may resume 3 days prior to OKT3 discontinuation).

CONTRAINDICATIONS/ PRECAUTIONS

Contraindicated in: Fluid overload, fever > 37.8° C, herpes zoster, hypersensitivity, chicken pox or recent exposure to chicken pox. **Use cautiously in:** Chronic debilitative diseases; induces the development of antibodies, use with extreme caution if a second course of therapy is required; males/females of childbearing age. **Pregnancy/Lactation:** No well-controlled trials to establish safety. Benefits must outweigh risks. **Pediatrics:** Safety and efficacy has not been established.

PREPARATION

Availability: 5 mg/mL in 5 mL ampules. **Syringe:** Does not require dilution. Must be withdrawn from vial via low protein binding 0.2–0.22 micron filter. Discard filter and attach needle for direct IV administration. **Do not shake.**

STABILITY/STORAGE

Vial: Store unopened vials under refrigeration. May have some fine translucent particles observable in vial (does not affect drug potency); use of filter will clear most particulate matter.

ADMINISTRATION

General: Drug administration should take place in a facility where patient can be monitored continuously. Do not administer by IV infusion or in conjunction with any other drugs. Patient's temperature should not exceed 37.8° C prior to the administration of the first dose. First dose reactions may be minimized by the use of steroids, cooling blanket, and an antipyretic regimen before/after dosage. **IV Push:** Single dose as a bolus over 1 min or less.

COMPATIBILITY/INCOMPATIBILITY

Data not available.

ADVERSE EFFECTS

CNS: Aseptic meningitis, <u>tremors</u>. **CV:** <u>Severe pulmonary edema, chest pain</u>. **Resp:** <u>Dyspnea</u>, wheezing. **GI:** Diarrhea, <u>nausea, vomiting</u>. **Heme:** Lymphomas. **Hypersens:** ANAPHYLAXIS, serum sickness. **Other:** Fever, chills, malaise, <u>infection</u> (i.e., cytomegalovirus, herpes simplex, staphylococcus epidermidis, pneumocystis carinii, Legionella, cryptococcus, serratia).

TOXICITY/OVERDOSE

Signs/Symptoms: Anaphylaxis, chest pain, severe pulmonary edema symptoms. **Treatment:** Most adverse effects may be treated symptomatically. Use antipyretics, steroids, and antihistamines as required; decrease drug or discontinue; change drug to another immunosuppressive agent.

In the Adverse Effects section, <u>underline</u> indicates most frequent; CAPS indicates life threatening.

355

DRUG INTERACTIONS
Other immunosuppressants: Additional immunosuppression.

NURSING CONSIDERATIONS

Assessment

General:
Baseline/daily weights, intake/output ratio, infectious disease potential, anaphylaxis prevention/treatment.

Physical:
Cardiopulmonary status.

Lab Alterations:
Monitor CBC/differential, circulating T-cells as CD3 antigen and 24 hr trough values (0.9 mcg/mL) of drug must be closely observed.

Intervention/Rationale
Assess patient for signs/symptoms of fluid overload prior to initiation of therapy. ● Evaluate patient regularly for development of increasing dyspnea, rales, rhonchi, or other symptoms of pulmonary edema. ● Immunosuppressive therapy may cause an increased susceptibility to infection. ● Must have a clear chest x-ray within 24 hr of administration and have gained < 3% above baseline weight within 7 days prior to receiving drug. Treat any fever > 37.8° C with antipyretics to decrease fever before administering any single dosage. Administer antipyretic before administration of drug in order to lower incidence of fever/chills. Corticosteroids may be administered prior to the first dose in an effort to decrease incidence of adverse reactions. Methylprednisolone sodium succinate (1 mg/

kg) preinjection; followed by hydrocortisone sodium succinate (100 mg) 30 minutes postinjection have been recommended to decrease the severity of first dose reaction. Use of a cooling blanket and acetaminophen is also recommended in an effort to prevent and/or treat severe fever/chills.

Patient/Family Education
Review expected adverse reactions. Severity of side effects will be less severe as treatment progresses. Should not receive any immunization and avoid contact with persons receiving oral polio vaccines unless approved by physician.

NAFCILLIN
(naf-sill′-in)
Trade Name(s): Nafcil, Nallpen, Unipen
Classification(s): Antibiotic, penicillinase-resistant penicillin
Pregnancy Category: B

PHARMACODYNAMICS/KINETICS
Mechanism of Action: Exhibits bactericidal effect against microorganisms by inhibiting cell wall synthesis during active phase of replication. Bacteria resist drug by producing penicillinases (enzymes that hydrolyze the drug). **Distribution:** Bound to plasma proteins. Distributed throughout most body tissues and fluids, including CSF. **Metabolism/Elimination:** Hepatically inactivated and excreted in bile. **Half-Life:** < 1 hr.

In the Adverse Effects section, <u>underline</u> indicates most frequent; CAPS indicates life threatening.

INDICATIONS/DOSAGE

Treatment of various types of infections caused by penicillinase-producing staphylococci

Adult: 500–1000 mg every 4 hr. Not to exceed 12 g/day. *Pediatric (> 1 month):* 50–200 mg/kg/24 hr in divided doses every 4–6 hr. Not to exceed 200 mg/kg/24 hr or 12 g/day.

CONTRAINDICATIONS/PRECAUTIONS

Contraindicated in: Known hypersensitivity to penicillin or cephalosporins. **Use cautiously in:** Bleeding disorders. **Pregnancy/Lactation:** No well-controlled trials to establish safety. Benefits must outweigh risks. Crosses the placenta. Secreted in breast milk; use cautiously in lactating women. Use during breastfeeding may cause diarrhea, candidiasis, or allergic reaction in infants. **Pediatrics:** Not recommended in infants < 1 month old.

PREPARATION

Availability: 500 mg, 1, 1.5, 2, 4, and 10 g vials and piggyback vials. 10 g bulk package. 2.9 mEq sodium/g. **Reconstitution:** Each 500 mg is diluted with 1.7 mL sterile water for injection providing a solution of 250 mg/mL. **Infusion:** Further dilute each 500 mg of reconstituted solution with 50 mL of compatible IV fluid.

STABILITY/STORAGE

Vial: Store at room temperature. Refrigerate unused medication after initial dilution; stable for 7 days. **Infusion:** Stable in compatible IV solutions at concentrations of < 40 mg/mL for 24 hr at room temperature and 96 hr with refrigeration.

ADMINISTRATION

General: Rapid administration may result in seizures. If concurrently given with aminoglycosides, administer in separate infusions as far apart as possible. Used for short-term therapy (24–48 hr) because of high incidence of thrombophlebitis especially in elderly. **IV Push:** Each 500 mg or less of diluted drug is to be administered over 5–10 min. **Intermittent Infusion:** Infuse over at least 30–60 min. **Continuous Infusion:** May be given over 24 hr or at physician specified volume/rate.

COMPATIBILITY

Solution: Dextrose solutions, lactated Ringer's, Ringer's solution, sodium chloride solutions. **Syringe:** Cimetidine, heparin. **Y-site:** Acyclovir, atropine, cyclophosphamide, diazepam, enalaprilat, esmolol, famotidine, fentanyl, hydromorphone, magnesium sulfate, morphine, zidovudine.

INCOMPATIBILITY

Y-site: Droperidol, labetalol, nalbuphine, pentazocine, verapamil.

ADVERSE EFFECTS

CNS: Seizures (high doses). **GI:** Hepatitis, diarrhea, nausea, vomiting. **Renal:** Interstitial nephritis. **Heme:** Anemia, bleeding tendencies, blood dyscrasias. **Hypersens:** ANAPHYLAXIS, exfoliative dermatitis, pruritus, skin rash, urticaria, wheezing. **Other:** Phlebitis, serum sickness (chills, fever, edema, arthralgia, myalgia, malaise), tissue

In the Adverse Effects section, underline indicates most frequent; CAPS indicates life threatening.

357

necrosis associated with extravasation.

TOXICITY/OVERDOSE

Signs/Symptoms: Myocarditis may occur at any time throughout course of treatment, initially exhibiting as rash, fever, eosinophilia. Second stage includes sinus tachycardia, ST changes, and slight increase in cardiac enzymes. **Treatment:** Notify physician, and, for severe manifestations of allergic reactions, discontinue drug and treat symptoms with antihistamines, epinephrine, and corticosteroids. Hemodialysis and peritoneal dialysis are only minimally effective in toxicity or overdose.

DRUG INTERACTIONS

Aminoglycosides: Inactivation of aminoglycosides. **Bacteriostatic antibiotics:** Slows the rapidity of bacterial growth and may decrease the bactericidal effects of nafcillin. **Beta-adrenergic blocking agents:** Increase potential risk/severity of anaphylactic reactions. **Chloramphenicol:** May decrease the effect of nafcillin and increase half-life of chloramphenicol. **Heparin, other anticoagulants:** May cause increased bleeding tendencies.

NURSING CONSIDERATIONS

Assessment

General:

Signs/symptoms of superinfection/bacterial/fungal overgrowth (especially in elderly, debilitated, or immunosuppressed). History of allergic/hypersensitivity reactions to penicillins/cephalosporins. Signs/symptoms of infection (prior to, during, and at completion of therapy).

Physical:

Hematopoietic system, anaphylactic potential.

Lab Alterations:

May cause positive direct Coombs' test. Monitor renal, hepatic, hematopoietic function during prolonged therapy. False-positive reaction with copper-sulfate urine glucose tests (Clinitest).

Intervention/Rationale

Assess for early signs of allergic manifestations especially in patients with a history of sensitivity to other drugs. ● Evalute regularly for increased bleeding tendencies. ● Therapy may be initiated prior to obtaining culture/sensitivity results when there is reason to believe the causative organism may be susceptible to the drug. ● Adjust drug and/or dosage accordingly once results are confirmed.

Patient/Family Education

Observe and report any signs of superinfection (loose, foul-smelling stools; vaginal itching or discharge; black furry overgrowth noted on tongue). Notify physician/nurse if skin rash, itching, hives, severe diarrhea, or signs of superinfection occur.

NALBUPHINE HYDROCHLORIDE

(nal'-byoo-feen)

Trade Name(s): Nubain

Classification(s): Narcotic agonist/antagonist analgesic

Pregnancy Category: C

In the Adverse Effects section, <u>underline</u> indicates most frequent; CAPS indicates life threatening.

PHARMACODYNAMICS/KINETICS
Mechanism of Action: Binds with opiate receptors at several sites in the CNS, altering perception of and emotional response to pain via an unidentified mechanism. Does not increase pulmonary artery pressure, systemic vascular resistance, or cardiac work unlike other narcotic agonist–antagonist analgesic drugs. **Onset of Action:** 2–3 min. **Peak Effect:** 30 min. **Duration of Action:** 3–6 hr. **Distribution:** Distributed throughout the body. Crosses the placenta. **Metabolism/Elimination:** Metabolized by the liver. Eliminated in feces via biliary excretion, approximately 7% is excreted unchanged in the urine. **Half-Life:** 5 hr.

INDICATIONS/DOSAGE

Relief of moderate to severe pain, preoperative analgesia
Adult: Dosage adjusted according to severity of pain. Usual dose 10 mg every 3–6 hr. Up to 20 mg can be given in a single dose if required. Maximum total daily dose is 160 mg.

CONTRAINDICATIONS/ PRECAUTIONS
Contraindicated in: Hypersensitivity. **Use cautiously in:** Biliary tract surgery, emotionally unstable patients, head injury, history of narcotic abuse, impaired respiratory status (other medications, asthma, uremia, severe infection, respiratory obstruction), increased intracranial pressure, may precipitate withdrawal symptoms if stopped too quickly after protracted use or if patient has been on opiates, MI with accompanying nausea/vomiting, renal/hepatic impairment. **Pregnancy/Lactation:** No well-controlled trials to establish safety. Benefits must outweigh risks. Has been used during labor but may cause respiratory depression in the newborn. Should be used with extreme caution in women delivering premature infants. **Pediatrics:** Safety and efficacy has not been established in children < 18 years of age.

PREPARATION
Availability: 10 and 20 mg/mL in 1 and 10 mL vials, 1 mL amps, and 1 mL disposable syringes.

STABILITY/STORAGE
Vial: Store at room temperature. Protect from excessive light.

ADMINISTRATION
General: Titrate drug according to symptomatic relief as well as respiratory rate and depth. Narcotic dependent patients may demonstrate withdrawal symptoms with nalbuphine administration. **IV Push:** Give each 10 mg or less over 3–5 min.

COMPATIBILITY
Solution: Dextrose solutions, lactated Ringer's, sodium chloride solutions. **Syringe:** Atropine, cimetidine, diphenhydramine, droperidol, glycopyrrolate, lidocaine, midazolam, prochlorperazine, ranitidine, scopolamine.

INCOMPATIBILITY
Syringe: Diazepam, pentobarbital. **Y-site:** Nafcillin.

ADVERSE EFFECTS
CNS: Delusions, depression, dizziness, hallucinations, nervousness, sedation, vertigo. **Ophtho:** Blurred

In the Adverse Effects section, underline indicates most frequent; CAPS indicates life threatening.

359

vision, diplopia, miosis (high doses). **CV:** Hypertension, orthostatic hypotension, palpitations, tachycardia. **Resp:** <u>Respiratory depression</u>, asthma, dyspnea. **GI:** Bitter taste, cramps, constipation, <u>dry mouth</u>, dyspepsia, nausea, paralytic ileus, vomiting. **GU:** Urinary urgency. **Hypersens:** Burning, itching, urticaria. **Other:** Flushing, speech difficulty, sweating, warmth.

TOXICITY/OVERDOSE
Signs/Symptoms: Respiratory depression, sedation, euphoria. **Treatment:** Treatment is supportive and symptomatic. Respiratory support via controlled ventilation may be required. **Antidote(s):** Immediate IV administration of naloxone is used to reverse respiratory depression.

DRUG INTERACTIONS
Alcohol, antihistamines, sedative hypnotics: Additive CNS depression. **MAO inhibitors:** May potentiate unpredictable fatal reactions. **Narcotic analgesics:** Decreases analgesic effects.

NURSING CONSIDERATIONS
Assessment
General:
Vital signs, pain management/control.
Physical:
Pulmonary status, neurologic/emotional status.
Lab Alterations:
May increase amylase and lipase levels.

Intervention/Rationale
Assess respiratory status prior to IV administration; do not administer if respiratory rate < 12/min. Monitor vital signs before, during, and after administration of the drug. ● Assess pain management and overall relief of pain with prescribed dosage; evaluate need for dosage increase/decrease. Use cautiously for patients who are considered emotionally unstable and those with known narcotic dependence, as significant withdrawal symptoms may be experienced when administering nalbuphine. ● If previous analgesic used was codeine, morphine, meperidine, or other similar type drug, dosage of nalbuphine should be decreased by 25% initially; if signs of withdrawal are not evident, progressively increase nalbuphine dose at scheduled intervals until analgesia is obtained.

Patient/Family Education
Review mechanism for obtaining "as needed" pain medication and the rationale of pain management. Seek assistance for ambulation or repositioning activities, drug may cause drowsiness or dizziness. Immediately report signs of itching, wheezing, hives, or anaphylactic reactions as drug can cause allergic type reactions. Avoid alcohol use.

NALOXONE HYDROCHLORIDE
(nal-ox'-zone)
Trade Name(s): Narcan
Classification(s): Antidote, narcotic antagonist
Pregnancy Category: B

In the Adverse Effects section, <u>underline</u> indicates most frequent; CAPS indicates life threatening.

PHARMACODYNAMICS/KINETICS

Mechanism of Action: Precise mechanism of action is not known. May act as a competitive antagonist at various opiate receptor sites in the CNS. **Onset of Action:** 2 min. **Duration of Action:** 1–2 hr. **Distribution:** Rapidly distributed into body tissues and fluids. **Metabolism/Elimination:** Metabolized by the liver, primarily by glucuronide conjugation. Excreted via the urine. **Half-Life:** 30–90 min. 3 hr (neonates).

INDICATIONS/DOSAGE

Narcotic overdose treatment (known/suspected)

Adult: 0.4–2.0 mg. May repeat in 2–3 min intervals for three doses. May be repeated as necessary if effective. *Pediatric:* 0.01 mg/kg. May be repeated. An additional dose of 0.1 mg/kg may be indicated if above dose is not effective. American Association of Pediatrics recommends 0.1 mg/kg/dose for infants 20 kg/5 years; use adult doses for older patients.

Postoperative narcotic depression

Adult: 0.1–0.2 mg at 2–3 min intervals to the desired level of reversal. Repeat doses may be required within 1–2 hr time periods depending on duration since last narcotic dose. *Pediatric:* 0.005–0.01 mg at 2–3 min intervals to the desired level of reversal. *Neonate:* 0.01 mg/kg at 2–3 min intervals to the desired level of reversal.

CONTRAINDICATIONS/ PRECAUTIONS

Contraindicated in: Hypersensitivity. **Use cautiously in:** Cardiac disease, potentially cardiotoxic drug usage, known or suspected physical dependence on opiates (severe withdrawal symptoms can occur). **Pregnancy/Lactation:** No well-controlled trials to establish safety. Benefits must outweigh risks. Readily crosses placenta.

PREPARATION

Availability: 0.02, 0.4, and 1 mg/mL in 1 and 2 mL ampules, 1, 2, and 10 mL vials, and 1 mL disposable syringes. **Syringe:** May be given undiluted or diluted with equal parts of sterile water for injection. **Infusion:** May be added to compatible IV solution (2 mg/500 mL) to deliver a concentration of 0.004 mg/mL.

STABILITY/STORAGE

Vial: Store at room temperature. **Infusion:** Stable for 24 hr at room temperature. After 24 hr discard unused solution.

ADMINISTRATION

General: IV use is recommended in emergency situations. Duration of action of some narcotics may exceed that of naloxone. Larger doses may be required when used to antagonize effect of buprenorphine, butorphanol, nalbuphine, pentazocine, and propoxyphene. **IV Push:** Each 0.4 mg is administered over 15 sec. **Continuous Infusion:** Infusion is titrated according to patient response and at physician specified rate/volume.

N

In the Adverse Effects section, underline indicates most frequent; CAPS indicates life threatening.

COMPATIBILITY
Solution: Dextrose solutions, sodium chloride solutions. **Syringe:** Benzquinamide, heparin.

ADVERSE EFFECTS
CNS: Irritability (increased crying in the newborn), tremulousness. **CV:** HYPERTENSION, tachycardia. **GI:** Nausea, vomiting. **Heme:** Increased partial thromboplastin time. **Other:** Sweating.

TOXICITY/OVERDOSE
Signs/Symptoms: Overdose may result in excitement, hypertension, hypotension, reversal of analgesia, pulmonary edema, ventricular tachycardia, and ventricular fibrillation. **Treatment:** Symptomatic/supportive; use of oxygen and controlled ventilation may be required.

NURSING CONSIDERATIONS
Assessment
General:
Vital signs.
Physical:
Cardiopulmonary status.

Intervention/Rationale
Observe patient continuously following administration; monitor all vital signs frequently. Carefully assess respiratory rate, effort, pattern, and degree of excursion. Duration of narcotic action may exceed that of naloxone; be prepared to administer repeated doses of drug and/or support respiratory system immediately as indicated. Assess patient for degree of pain following administration when used to treat postoperative respiratory depression; decreases respiratory depression and reverses analgesia. Maintain a patent airway and provide oxygen/artificial ventilation, cardiac support, and vasopressor therapy as needed. Will precipitate acute withdrawal symptoms in narcotic addicts; use cautiously especially with newborns of narcotic dependent mothers.

Patient/Family Education
If drug is effective explain antagonistic effects. Assess pain relief if drug is administered for postoperative reversal of narcotics.

NEOSTIGMINE
(nee-oh-stig′-meen)
Trade Name(s): Prostigmin
Classification(s): Anticholinesterase muscle stimulator, cholinergic agent
Pregnancy Category: C

PHARMACODYNAMICS/KINETICS
Mechanism of Action: Inhibits destruction of acetylocholine released from parasympathetic/somatic efferent nerves. Acetylcholine accumulates promoting increased stimulation of receptors. Facilitates transmission of impulses across the myoneural junction. **Onset of Action:** 4–8 min. **Peak Serum Level:** 20–30 min. **Duration of Action:** 2–4 hr. **Distribution:** 15%–25% protein bound. **Metabolism/Elimination:** Metabolized by plasma cholinesterases and microsomal enzymes of the liver. 80% eliminated by the urine within 24 hr (50% as unchanged drug/30% as metabolites). **Half-Life:** 47–60 min.

INDICATIONS/DOSAGE

Symptomatic control of myasthenia gravis

Adult: 1 mL of 1:2000 solution (0.5 mg). Subsequent dosages must be individualized. *Pediatric:* 0.01–0.04 mg/kg every 2–3 hr as needed.

Antidote for nondepolarizing neuromuscular blocking agents

Adult: 0.5–2.0 mg with 0.6–1.2 mg atropine sulfate and repeat as required. Only in exceptional cases should the dosage exceed 5 mg. *Pediatric:* 0.07–0.08 mg/kg with 0.008–0.025 mg/kg atropine sulfate.

CONTRAINDICATIONS/ PRECAUTIONS

Contraindicated in: Hypersensitivity to cholinergics or bromide, peritonitis. **Use cautiously in:** Bradycardia, bronchial asthma, cardiac dysrhythmias, epilepsy, hyperthyroidism, mechanical intestinal or urinary tract obstruction, peptic ulcer disease, recent coronary occlusion. **Pregnancy/Lactation:** No well-controlled trials to establish safety. Benefits must outweigh risks. May cause uterine irritability near term. Newborns may display muscle weakness. Does not appear to cross placenta or into breast milk. **Pediatrics:** Safety and efficacy has not been established.

PREPARATION

Availability: 1:1000 (1 mg/mL) solution in 10 mL vials. 1:2000 (0.5 mg/mL) solution in 1 mL amp/10 mL vial. 1:4000 (0.25 mg/mL) solution in 1 mL amps.

STABILITY/STORAGE

Vial: Store at room temperature. Protect from light.

ADMINISTRATION

General: May be administered via Y-site or three way stopcock of compatible IV solution. **IV Push:** Each 0.5 mg over 1 min.

COMPATIBILITY

Solution: Dextrose solutions, lactated Ringer's, Ringer's injection, sodium chloride solutions. **Syringe:** Glycopyrrolate, heparin, pentobarbital, thiopental. **Y-site:** Heparin, hydrocortisone sodium succinate, potassium chloride, vitamin B complex with C.

ADVERSE EFFECTS

CNS: <u>Seizures</u>, loss of consciousness, dizziness, drowsiness, headache, mental confusion, jitters. **Ophtho:** Diplopia, miosis, lacrimation, visual changes. **CV:** CARDIAC ARREST, <u>bradycardia</u>, hypotension, syncope. **Resp:** Respiratory depression, bronchoconstriction, BRONCHOSPASM, dyspnea, increased tracheobronchial secretions. **GI:** <u>Abdominal cramps</u>, <u>diarrhea</u>, dysphagia, increased gastric, salivary, and intestinal secretions, increased peristalsis, <u>nausea</u>, <u>vomiting</u>, <u>salivation</u>. **GU:** Incontinence, urinary frequency, urinary urgency. **MS:** Fasiculations, muscle cramps, muscle weakness, weakness. **Hypersens:** Allergic reactions, ANAPHYLAXIS, rash, urticaria. **Other:** Diaphoresis, flushing, sweating.

TOXICITY/OVERDOSE

Signs/Symptoms: Overdose signs/symptoms (cholinergic crisis) include increased respiratory secre-

---

In the Adverse Effects section, <u>underline</u> indicates most frequent; CAPS indicates life threatening.

363

tions and salivation, abdominal cramps, bradycardia, nausea, vomiting, diarrhea, diaphoresis, subjective symptoms of internal trembling, and severe anxiety. Tensilon test (edrophonium chloride) may be used to determine overdosage from underdosage. **Treatment:** Narrow margin of safety. If side effects occur discontinue drug and notify physician. Treat allergic manifestations with epinephrine; maintain adequate respirations using controlled ventilation if necessary. **Antidote(s):** Atropine sulfate 1–4 mg IV repeated every 3–10 min. Pralidoxime chloride (PAM) 2 g IV followed by 250 mg every 5 min may be needed to reactivate cholinesterase and reverse paralysis.

DRUG INTERACTIONS
Aminoglycosides, depolarizing muscle relaxants, succinylcholine: Increased neuromuscular blocking effect. **Anticholinesterase drugs:** Increased/worsening of myasthenic symptoms. **Corticosteroids:** Decreased anticholinesterase effect. **Local anesthetics, general anesthetics, antiarrhythmics:** Interfere with neuromuscular transmission requiring neostigmine dosage increase. **Magnesium:** Direct depressant effect on skeletal muscle, may antagonize beneficial effects of neostigmine.

NURSING CONSIDERATIONS
Assessment
General:
Vital signs, ECG monitoring (recommended).
Physical:
Pulmonary status, GI tract.

Intervention/Rationale
Assess vital signs frequently with special emphasis on respiratory pattern/rate. Maintain patent airway and keep well-oxygenated and ventilated until complete recovery of normal respiratory status is ascertained. ● Observe closely for improvement in muscle strength, vision, and ptosis 45–60 min after each dose. ● Epinephrine should always be available when drug is being administered in order to immediately counteract hypersensitivity reactions. ● Evaluate for development of cholinergic crisis as manifested by increased GI stimulation with epigastric distress, abdominal cramps, vomiting, diarrhea, muscle fasiculation followed by paralysis. ● Use of peripheral nerve stimulator may be required to exactly titrate the required dosage in severe cardiac disease/severely ill patients.

Patient/Family Education
Drug will relieve ptosis, double vision, difficulty in chewing and swallowing, trunk and limb weakness when used for treatment of myasthenia gravis. Wear an identification bracelet to indicate myasthenia gravis condition requiring a specialized medicine regimen. Take medicine exactly as ordered when converted from IV to the oral form of drug.

NETILMICIN
(ne-till-mye′-sin)
Trade Name(s): Netromycin
Classification(s): Aminoglycoside antibiotic
Pregnancy Category: D

In the Adverse Effects section, <u>underline</u> indicates most frequent;
CAPS indicates life threatening.

PHARMACODYNAMICS/KINETICS
Mechanism of Action: Bactericidal, blocks bacterial protein synthesis, exhibits some neuromuscular blocking action. **Peak Serum Level:** Within 30 minutes of infusion completion. **Therapeutic Serum Levels:** Peak 0.5–10.0 mcg/mL. Trough < 4 mcg/mL. **Distribution:** Widely distributed in extracellular fluids. Lower serum concentrations result with expanded extracellular fluid volume. **Metabolism/Elimination:** Excreted unchanged via glomerular filtration in kidneys. **Half-Life:** 2–3 hr. Prolonged in renal impairment (up to 24–60 hr).

INDICATIONS/DOSAGE

Treatment of gram-negative organisms/combination therapy in severe immunocompromised patients

Dosage interval may need to be adjusted in renal impairment. Adjust dosage based on serum levels.

Adult: 3–4 mg/kg/day in divided doses every 8–12 hr. Not to exceed 6.5 mg/kg/day. *Pediatric:* 3.6–5.4 mg/kg/day in divided doses every 8–12 hr. Not to exceed 6.5 mg/kg/day. *Neonate:* 4.0–6.5 mg/kg/day in divided doses every 12 hr.

CONTRAINDICATIONS/ PRECAUTIONS
Contraindicated in: Known hypersensitivity. **Use cautiously in:** Neuromuscular disorders (myasthenia gravis, Parkinson's disease, infant botulism), newborns of mothers receiving high doses of magnesium sulfate, concurrent administration of neuromuscular blocking agents.

Pregnancy/Lactation: No well-controlled trials to establish safety. Benefits must outweigh risks. Crosses placenta. **Pediatrics:** Caution in premature infants/neonates due to renal immaturity and prolonged half-life.

PREPARATION
Availability: 10 mg/mL, 2 mL; 25 mg/mL, 2 mL; 100 mg/mL, 1.5 mL vials. **Infusion:** *Adults:* Further dilute in 50–200 mL of compatible IV solution. *Pediatrics:* Further dilute in compatible solution to a volume sufficient to infuse over 20–30 min.

STABILITY/STORAGE
Vial: Store at room temperature. **Infusion:** Stable for 24 hr at room temperature and 3 days refrigerated.

ADMINISTRATION
General: Avoid rapid bolus administration. Schedule first maintenance dose at a dosing interval apart from loading dose. Administer additional dose after hemodialysis. Schedule dosing of penicillins and aminoglycosides as far apart as possible to prevent inactivation of aminoglycosides. **Intermittent Infusion:** Infuse over at least 30–60 minutes.

COMPATIBILITY
Solution: Amino acids, dextrose solutions, lactated Ringer's, Ringer's injection, sodium bicarbonate, sodium chloride solutions. **Syringe:** Doxapram. **Y-site:** Aminophylline, calcium gluconate.

INCOMPATIBILITY
Syringe: Heparin. **Y-site:** Furosemide, heparin, mezlocillin.

In the Adverse Effects section, underline indicates most frequent; CAPS indicates life threatening.

365

ADVERSE EFFECTS

CNS: Convulsions, confusion, disorientation, neuromuscular blockade, lethargy, depression, headache, numbness, nystagmus, pseudotumor cerebri. **CV:** Hypertension, hypotension, paliptations. **Resp:** Respiratory depression, pulmonary fibrosis. **GI:** Hepatic necrosis, hepatomegaly, increased bilirubin/LDH/transaminase, nausea, salivation, stomatitis, vomiting, anorexia. **GU:** Casts, hematuria. **Renal:** Azotemia, increased BUN/serum creatinine, oliguria, proteinuria. **MS:** Arthralgia. **Fld/Lytes:** Hyperkalemia, hypomagnesemia. **Heme:** Agranulocytosis (transient), anemia (transient), eosinophilia, leukocytosis, leukopenia, pancytopenia, reticulocyte count alterations, thrombocytopenia. **Hypersens:** Angioneurotic edema, exfoliative dermatitis, purpura, rash, urticaria. **Other:** Fever, ototoxicity (deafness, dizziness, tinnitus, vertigo).

TOXICITY/OVERDOSE

Signs/Symptoms: Increased serum levels with associated nephrotoxicity and ototoxicity (tinnitus, high frequency hearing loss). **Treatment:** Removed by peritoneal/hemodialysis. Hemodialysis is more efficient. Exchange transfusions may be used in neonates. **Antidote(s):** Ticarcillin (12–20 g/day) may be given to promote complex formation with aminoglycosides to lower elevated serum levels.

DRUG INTERACTIONS

Amphotericin B, bacitracin, cephalothin, cisplatin, methoxyflurane, potent diuretics, vancomycin: Increased potential for nephrotoxicity, neurotoxicity,

ototoxicity. **Anesthetics, anticholinesterase agents, citrate anticoagulated blood, metocurine, neuromuscular blocking agents, pancuronium, succinylcholine, tubocurarine:** Increased neuromuscular blockade/respiratory paralysis. **Beta lactam antibiotics (penicillins, cephalosporins) especially ticarcillin:** Inactivation of aminoglycosides. **Cephalosporins, penicillins:** Synergism against gram-negative and enterococci.

NURSING CONSIDERATIONS

Assessment
General:
Maintain adequate hydration, superinfection/infectious disease status.

Physical:
CN VIII (acoustic) evaluation, renal function.

Lab Alterations:
Measure peak/trough levels. Beta lactam antibiotic (penicillins, cephalosporins) may cause in vitro inactivation of gentamicin.

Intervention/Rationale
Assess BUN and serum creatinine/creatinine clearance to determine presence of renal toxicity. Adequate hydration recommended to prevent renal toxicity. ● Draw peak serum levels 30 min after the infusion is complete and trough 30 min prior to the next dose. ● Antibiotic use may cause overgrowth of resistant organisms; observe for (fever, change in vital signs, increased WBC, vaginal infection/discharge). ● CN VIII evaluation important to assess presence of ototoxicity.

In the Adverse Effects section, <u>underline</u> indicates most frequent; CAPS indicates life threatening.

Patient/Family Education
Increase oral fluid intake in order to minimize chemical irritation of kidneys. Notify physician/nurse if tinnitus, vertigo, or hearing loss is noted.

NITROGLYCERIN
(nye-tro-gli′-ser-in)
Trade Name(s): Nitro-Bid IV, Tridil
Classification(s): Antianginal coronary vasodilator
Pregnancy Category: C

PHARMACODYNAMICS/KINETICS
Mechanism of Action: Decreases cardiac oxygen demand by decreasing left ventricular end diastolic pressure (preload) and to a lesser degree, systemic vascular resistance (afterload). Increases blood flow via collateral coronary vessels. **Onset of Action:** 1–2 min. **Duration of Action:** 3–5 min. **Distribution:** Approximately 60% bound to plasma protein. **Metabolism/Elimination:** Metabolized by the liver and liver enzymes. **Half-Life:** 1–4 min.

INDICATIONS/DOSAGE

Treatment of angina pectoris, CHF, and acute MI, blood pressure control in perioperative period
Adult: 5 mcg/min, increase by 5 mcg/min every 3–5 min to 20 mcg/min. If no response noted increase by 10 mcg/min every 3–5 min, dosage dependent on hemodynamic parameters. No fixed patient dose.

CONTRAINDICATIONS/PRECAUTIONS
Contraindicated in: Constrictive pericarditis, hypersensitivity, hypotension, inadequate cerebral circulation, increased intracranial pressure, pericardial tamponade, uncorrected hypovolemia. **Use cautiously in:** Hypertrophic cardiomyopathy, liver/renal impairment, normal or decreased pulmonary capillary wedge pressure. **Pregnancy/Lactation:** No well-controlled trials to establish safety. Benefits must outweigh risks. May cause compromise in maternal/fetal circulation. **Pediatrics:** Safety and efficacy not established.

PREPARATION
Availability: 0.5 mg/mL in 10 mL amps. 0.8 mg/mL in 10 mL amps. 5 mg/mL in 1, 5, 10, and 20 mL vials and 10 mL amps. 10 mg/mL in 5 and 10 mL vials. **Infusion:** Must be diluted in compatible IV solution with a final concentration of 20–40 mcg/mL.

STABILITY/STORAGE
Vial: Store at room temperature. **Infusion:** Stable for up to 24 hr at room temperature. Do not use filters.

ADMINISTRATION
General: Standard IV infusion sets made of polyvinyl chloride plastic may absorb up to 40%–80% of the drug in solution. Use glass bottles only and specially designed tubing as per institutional policy. **Continuous Infusion:** Administer via infusion pump to ensure accurate rate delivery. Titrate in accordance with patient response and hemodynamics. Initiate infusion at 5 mcg/min, titrate carefully, and monitor closely.

N

In the Adverse Effects section, underline indicates most frequent; CAPS indicates life threatening.

367

COMPATIBILITY

Solution: Dextrose solutions, lactated Ringer's, sodium chloride solutions. **Syringe:** Heparin. **Y-site:** Amiodarone, amrinone, atracurium, dobutamine, dopamine, famotidine, lidocaine, pancuronium, ranitidine, sodium nitroprusside, streptokinase, vecuronium.

INCOMPATIBILITY

Y-site: Alteplase.

ADVERSE EFFECTS

CNS: Apprehension, <u>dizziness</u>, <u>headache</u>, lightheadedness, restlessness, weakness. **Ophtho:** Blurred vision. **CV:** <u>Orthostatic hypotension</u>, syncope, <u>tachycardia</u>. **GI:** Abdominal pain, nausea, vomiting. **MS:** Muscle twitching. **Derm:** Pallor. **Hypersens:** Anaphylactoid reactions, exfoliative dermatitis, oral mucosal/conjunctival edema. **Other:** Alcoholic intoxication (large doses only), flushing, perspiration, tolerance.

TOXICITY/OVERDOSE

Signs/Symptoms: Abdominal pain, angina, hypotension, postural hypotension, methemoglobinemia, shock, reflex paradoxical bradycardia, constrictive pericarditis, pericardial tamponade, decreased organ perfusion, and death. **Treatment:** Notify physician of all side effects. For accidental overdose with severe hypotension and reflex tachycardia and/or decreased pulmonary wedge pressure, decrease rate or temporarily discontinue infusion until symptoms are reduced. Place patient in Trendelenberg position, fluid resuscitate as needed. Use of an alpha-adrenergic agonist (methoxamine or phenylephrine) is sometimes required. Epinephrine and dopamine are contraindicated. Methemoglobinemia may be treated with methylene blue 0.2 mL/kg IV. Treat anaphylaxis; resuscitate as needed.

DRUG INTERACTIONS

Alcohol: Concomitant use may result in severe hypotension/cardiovascular collapse. **Calcium channel blockers:** Increased orthostatic hypotension. **Heparin:** Decreased pharmacologic effects of heparin.

NURSING CONSIDERATIONS

Assessment
General:
Vital signs, ECG monitoring (recommended), hemodynamic monitoring, hydration status.
Physical:
Cardiopulmonary status.
Lab Alterations:
May cause a false report of decreased serum chloresterol levels.

Intervention/Rationale
Monitor systolic blood pressure, heart rate, pulmonary wedge pressure, and intensity/duration of response to drug. Continually assess hemodynamic parameters; titrate infusion in accordance with patient response and hemodynamic response. ● Evaluate fluid status and adequately hydrate patient to prevent hypovolemic hypotension.

Patient/Family Education
Drug may cause headache; may be treated with acetaminophen or aspirin. May cause orthostatic hy-

In the Adverse Effects section, <u>underline</u> indicates most frequent; CAPS indicates life threatening.

potension; change to upright position slowly and gradually. Notify physician if blurred vision, dry mouth, or persistent headache occurs. Avoid alcohol use.

NITROPRUSSIDE SODIUM
(nye-trow-pruss'-ide)
Trade Name(s): Nipride, Nitropress
Classification(s): Hypotensive agent, vasodilator
Pregnancy Category: C

PHARMACODYNAMICS/KINETICS
Mechanism of Action: Produces peripheral vasodilation by direct action on venous and arteriolar smooth muscle. **Onset of Action:** 30–60 sec. **Duration of Action:** 1–10 min. **Metabolism/Elimination:** Rapidly metabolized in RBCs and tissues to cyanide and subsequently, by the liver to thiocyanate. Excreted via urine, feces. Exhaled via air primarily as metabolites. **Half-Life:** 3–4 days.

INDICATIONS/DOSAGE

Treatment of hypertensive emergencies, cardiogenic shock; controlled hypotension during surgery

Adult: 3 mcg/kg/min. Not to **exceed** 10 mcg/kg/min. If 10 mcg/kg/min does not reduce blood pressure adequately within 10 min, infusion should be changed to another agent for hypertensive management. Do not allow blood pressure to drop too rapidly. *Pediatric:* 1.4 mcg/kg/min, titrated slowly according to individual response.

CONTRAINDICATIONS/PRECAUTIONS
Contraindicated in: Compensatory hypertension as noted in arteriovenous shunt/coarctation of the aorta, decreased cerebral perfusion, emergency surgery in moribund patients, hypersensitivity. **Use cautiously in:** Elderly/debilitated, hypothyroidism, known hypertensive patients, poor surgical risk patients, severe renal/hepatic impairment. **Pregnancy/Lactation:** No well-controlled trials to establish safety. Benefits must outweigh risks.

PREPARATION
Availability: 50 mg in 2 and 5 mL vials. **Reconstitution:** Add 2–3 mL of 5% dextrose in water or sterile water for injection (without preservatives) to a 50 mg vial. **Infusion:** Add reconstituted drug to 250–1000 mL compatible IV solution. Must be administered as a continuous infusion. Freshly prepared infusion solution has a very faint brownish tint, if it is highly colored it should be discarded. Immediately after preparing infusion, wrap infusion bag/bottle in aluminum foil to protect from light.

STABILITY/STORAGE
Vial: Store at room temperature. Sensitive to and should be protected from light, heat, and moisture. **Infusion:** Stable for 24 hr at room temperature. No other drug or preservative should be added to the drug infusion.

ADMINISTRATION
General: Tachyphylaxis may occur during administration, particularly with rates higher than 10 mcg/kg/min. If noted, discontinue infusion

N

In the Adverse Effects section, underline indicates most frequent; CAPS indicates life threatening.

369

immediately. Use of an infusion controlling device is required in order to ascertain safety and accuracy. **IV Push:** Not for direct IV injection. **Intermittent/Continuous Infusion:** Use flow rate to decrease blood pressure gradually to desired preset parameters.

COMPATIBILITY
Solution: Dextrose solutions, sodium chloride solutions. **Syringe:** Heparin. **Y-site:** Amrinone, atracurium, dobutamine, dopamine, enalaprilat, famotidine, lidocaine, nitroglycerin, pancuronium, vecuronium.

ADVERSE EFFECTS
CNS: Loss of consciousness, ataxia, apprehension, <u>dizziness</u>, <u>headache</u>, increased intracranial pressure, restlessness. **Ophtho:** Blurred vision. **CV:** Bradycardia, ECG changes, palpitations, retrosternal discomfort, tachycardia. **Resp:** Dyspnea. **GI:** <u>Abdominal pain</u>, <u>nausea</u>, retching, vomiting. **MS:** Muscle twitching. **Fld/Lytes:** Acidosis. **Heme:** Methemoglobinemia, thrombocytopenia. **Metab:** Cyanide/thiocyanate toxicity. **Other:** Flushing, tinnitus.

TOXICITY/OVERDOSE
Signs/Symptoms: If severe hypotension occurs, drug effects are immediately reversed by decreasing the infusion rate or temporarily discontinuing the infusion. Plasma cyanide and thiocyanate levels should be monitored every 48–72 hr, levels should not exceed 100 mcg thiocyanate/mL or 3 micromoles of cyanide/mL. Side effects of thiocyanate toxicity include tinnitus, blurred vision, dyspnea, dizziness, headache, syncope, and metabolic acidosis. **Treatment:** Amyl nitrate inhalation and infusion of sodium nitrite and sodium thiosulfate are potential treatments.

DRUG INTERACTIONS
Ganglionic blocking agents, general anesthesia, other antihypertensives: Increased hypotensive reaction.

NURSING CONSIDERATIONS
Assessment
General:
Vital signs, hemodynamic monitoring (recommended), ECG monitoring (recommended).
Physical:
Cardiopulmonary status.
Lab Alterations:
Assess electrolytes and arterial blood gases; metabolic acidosis is the earliest and most reliable evidence of cyanide toxicity. May decrease bicarbonate concentration, PCO_2 and pH; may increase serum lactate levels; may cause increased serum cyanate and thiocyanate concentrations.

Intervention/Rationale
Assess blood pressure every 1 min until stabilized at desired level and every 5–15 min thereafter throughout therapy. Continuous monitoring is the preferred method of assessment. ● Keep patient supine when initiating or titrating this drug.

Patient/Family Education
Change positions slowly, gradually, and with assistance in order to prevent uncontrolled hypotension. Immediately report signs/symptoms of nausea, apprehension, head-

In the Adverse Effects section, <u>underline</u> indicates most frequent; CAPS indicates life threatening.

ache, and/or palpitations (all signs of pending toxicity).

NOREPINEPHRINE
(nor'-ep-a-nef-rin)
Trade Name(s): Levophed
Classification(s): Vasopressor
Pregnancy Category: C

PHARMACODYNAMICS/KINETICS
Mechanism of Action: Acts predominantly by a direct effect on alpha-adrenergic receptors and directly stimulates beta-adrenergic receptors of the heart causing vasoconstriction/cardiac stimulation. **Onset of Action:** Immediate. **Duration of Action:** 1–2 min. **Distribution:** Concentrates in sympathetic nervous tissue. Does not cross blood–brain barrier. **Metabolism/Elimination:** Rapidly metabolized by sympathetic nerve endings. Eliminated by the kidneys.

INDICATIONS/DOSAGE

Vasoconstriction and myocardial stimulation in shock treatment
Adult: 8–12 mcg/min initially, followed by 2–4 mcg/min infusion titrated according to overall blood pressure response. *Pediatric:* 2 mcg/m^2/min. Maintenance dose determined by blood pressure response. In severe hypotension during cardiac arrest, use initial dose of 0.1 mcg/kg/min with maintenance dose titrated accordingly.

CONTRAINDICATIONS/ PRECAUTIONS
Contraindicated in: General anesthesia with cyclopropane and halothane, hypercarbia, hypersensitivity, hypotension associated with volume deficits, mesenteric or peripheral vascular thrombosis, profound hypoxia. **Use cautiously in:** Hypovolemia, hyperthyroidism, severe cardiac diseases, sulfite sensitivity. **Pregnancy/Lactation:** Contraindicated in pregnancy/lactation as fetal anoxia can occur. Readily crosses the placenta.

PREPARATION
Availability: 1 mg/mL in 4 mL amp. **Infusion:** Dilute in 250–1000 mL of compatible IV solution.

STABILITY/STORAGE
Vial: Store at room temperature. **Infusion:** Stable for 24 hr at room temperature.

ADMINISTRATION
General: Care must be taken to avoid extravasation when administered peripherally, as local necrosis may result; infuse into a large vein. If extravasation occurs notify physician and in accordance with orders, infiltrate the area immediately with 10–15 mL sodium chloride containing 5–10 mg phentolamine in order to prevent sloughing/necrosis. Use infusion control device to assure accuracy of drug delivery. Correct blood volume depletion prior to initiating therapy. **Continuous Infusion:** Infuse at physician prescribed rate. Adjust infusion rate until adequate blood pressure/tissue perfusion is obtained and maintained. More or less of the drug may be added to each liter of diluent depending on the volume requirements of the patient.

N

In the Adverse Effects section, underline indicates most frequent; CAPS indicates life threatening.

COMPATIBILITY

Solution: Amino acids 4.25%/dextrose 25%, dextrose solutions, lactated Ringer's, sodium chloride solutions. **Syringe:** Glycopyrrolate. **Y-site:** Amiodarone, amrinone, famotidine, heparin, hydrocortisone, potassium chloride, vitamin B complex with C.

ADVERSE EFFECTS

CNS: Anxiety, dizziness, headache, insomnia, restlessness, tremor, weakness. **CV:** Bradycardia, dysrhythmias, increased peripheral vascular resistance, precordial pain. **Resp:** Apnea, respiratory difficulty. **GU:** Decreased urine output. **Endo:** Hyperglycemia. **Metab:** Metabolic acidosis.

TOXICITY/OVERDOSE

Signs/Symptoms: Overdose may result in severe hypertension, reflex bradycardia, increased peripheral vascular resistance, decreased cardiac minute output. Prolonged administration of vasopressors may result in plasma volume depletion. **Treatment:** Symptomatic/supportive therapy including discontinuation of the drug, fluid resuscitation, and full respiratory support as required.

DRUG INTERACTIONS

Alpha-adrenergic blocking agents: May antagonize drug effects. **Bretylium:** Potentiates the action of norepinephrine. **Doxapram, guanethidine, MAO inhibitors, methyldopa, tricyclic antidepressants:** Increased risk of hypertensive crisis. **Ergot alkaloids (ergotamine, methylergonovine, methsergide, oxytocin):** Concurrent use may produce increased vasoconstriction.

NURSING CONSIDERATIONS

Assessment

General:
Vital signs, hemodynamic monitoring (recommended).
Physical:
Neurovascular status.
Lab Alterations:
Periodic serum glucose monitoring, ABG evaluation.

Intervention/Rationale

Assess blood pressure every 2 min until stable then every 5 min. Check peripheral pulse rates, color/temperature/sensation/motion of extremities. ● Assess ECG, CVP, intra-arterial pressure, pulmonary artery pressure, pulmonary capillary wedge pressure, and cardiac output; consult with physician for parameters. ● When weaning drug, slow the infusion rate gradually in accordance with hemodynamic alterations observed.

Patient/Family Education

Instruct patient/family of frequency/rationale of vital sign monitoring. Discuss drug rationale and goals of therapy.

OCTREOTIDE

(ok-tree-oh'-tide)
Trade Name(s): Sandostatin
Classification(s): Somatostatin analogue
Pregnancy Category: B

PHARMACODYNAMICS/KINETICS

Mechanism of Action: Suppression of serotonin and gastroenteropancreatic peptides; suppression of

In the Adverse Effects section, underline indicates most frequent;
CAPS indicates life threatening.

growth hormone. **Peak Serum Level:** 0.4 hr. **Duration of Action:** Variable, extends up to 12 hr. **Distribution:** Rapid distribution, protein bound in plasma, lipoprotein (concentration-independent), and to a lesser extent, albumin. **Metabolism/ Elimination:** 32% excreted unchanged in urine. Reduced clearance in severe renal impairment. **Half-Life:** 1.5 hr. Prolonged in renal impairment.

INDICATIONS/DOSAGE

Symptomatic treatment of carcinoid tumors
Adult: 100–600 mcg/day in two to four divided doses (range 150–750 mcg/day).

Treatment of profuse diarrhea associated with vasoactive intestinal peptide (VIP) tumors
Adult: 200–300 mcg/day in two to four divided doses (range 150–750 mcg/day).

CONTRAINDICATIONS/ PRECAUTIONS
Contraindicated in: Hypersensitivity to drug or components. **Use cautiously in:** Hypothyroidism, severe renal impairment. **Pregnancy/Lactation:** No well-controlled trials to establish safety. No evidence of fetal harm. Exercise caution in breastfeeding mothers. **Pediatrics:** Limited data in children at doses of 1–10 mcg/kg.

PREPARATION
Availability: 0.05 mg, 0.1 mg, 0.5 mg in 1 mL amps. **Syringe:** No further dilution required.

STABILITY/STORAGE
Vial: Store in refrigerator. May be stored at room temperature for 24 hr prior to use.

ADMINISTRATION
General: Reserve IV administration for emergency use. **IV Push:** May be administered by rapid IV push.

COMPATIBILITY
Solution: Dextrose solutions, sodium chloride solutions.

INCOMPATIBILITY
Solution: Fat emulsion.

ADVERSE EFFECTS
CNS: Convulsions, anorexia, anxiety, decreased libido, depression, dizziness, drowsiness, headache, insomnia, syncope, vertigo. **Ophtho:** Burning eyes, visual disturbance. **CV:** Chest pain, CHF, hypertension, myocardial ischemia, orthostatic hypotension, palpitations. **Resp:** Rhinorrhea, shortness of breath. **GI:** Hepatitis, abdominal pain, cholelithiasis, constipation, diarrhea, fat malabsorption, flatulence, GI bleeding, heartburn, jaundice, liver enzyme elevation, nausea, rectal spasm, vomiting. **GU:** Oliguria, prostatitis, urine hyperosmolality. **MS:** Asthenia; back, muscle, joint, leg, shoulder pain; leg/muscle cramping; weakness. **Derm:** Hair loss, skin flaking. **Endo:** Galactorrhea, hyperglycemia, hypoglycemia, hypothyroidism. **Hypersens:** Pruritus, rash. **Other:** Chills, dry mouth, fatigue, fever, flushing, throat discomfort, thrombophlebitis.

TOXICITY/OVERDOSE
Signs/Symptoms: Hyper/hypoglycemia associated with neurologic and

In the Adverse Effects section, underline indicates most frequent; CAPS indicates life threatening.

373

mental disturbances. **Treatment:** Temporary withdrawal and symptomatic treatment.

DRUG INTERACTIONS
Cyclosporine: Decreased cyclosporine blood levels.

NURSING CONSIDERATIONS
Assessment
General:
Blood pressure prior to administration, hydration status.
Physical:
Neurologic status, GI tract, cardiopulmonary status.
Lab Alterations:
Monitor lipid profile, periodic 72 hr fecal fat and serum carotene. Monitor baseline total or free T4 levels with chronic therapy. Monitor biochemical markers for specific tumors: VIPoma—vasoactive intestinal peptide; Carcinoid—urinary 5-HIAA, plasma serotonin, and substance P.

Intervention/Rationale
Monitor neurologic symptoms such as dizziness, seizures. ● Evaluate for development of abdominal pain, diarrhea, and evidence of GI bleeding. Hematest stools/vomitus/drainage. ● Dietary fat absorption may be altered; periodic 72 hr fecal fat and serum carotene should be assessed. ● Evaluate blood pressure and heart rate prior to, throughout, and following administration.

Patient/Family Education
Educate patient regarding therapeutic outcome and adverse effects. Avoid changing positions quickly to avoid orthostatic hypotension. Notify physician/nurse

of chest pain, palpitations, and shortness of breath.

ONDANSETRON
(on-dan′-se-tron)
Trade Name(s): Zofran
Classification(s): Antiemetic
Pregnancy Category: B

PHARMACODYNAMICS/KINETICS
Mechanism of Action: Selective serotonin receptor antagonist to prevent nausea/vomiting. **Onset of Action:** 30 min. **Duration of Action:** 11–20 hr. **Distribution:** Distributed throughout body especially to central nervous system and in plasma (present in erythrocytes). 70%–75% protein bound. **Metabolism/Elimination:** Primarily hepatically metabolized via hydroxylation and glucuronidation. 5% of dose excreted unchanged in urine. **Half-Life:** 3.5–5.5 hr.

INDICATIONS/DOSAGE

Prevention of nausea/vomiting associated with emetogenic cancer chemotherapy regimens

Adult/Pediatric (4–18 years): 0.15 mg/kg three times beginning 30 minutes prior to chemotherapy, and 4 and 8 hr later.

CONTRAINDICATIONS/
PRECAUTIONS
Contraindicated in: Hypersensitivity. **Pregnancy/Lactation:** No well-controlled trials to establish safety. Benefits must outweigh risks. Excreted into breast milk of animals. **Pediatrics:** Limited data in children ≤ 3 years.

In the Adverse Effects section, underline indicates most frequent; CAPS indicates life threatening.

PREPARATION
Availability: 2 mg/mL in 20 mL multidose vials. **Infusion:** Dilute dose in 50 mL compatible IV solution.

STABILITY/STORAGE
Vial: Store at room temperature or refrigerate. Protect from light for prolonged storage. **Infusion:** Stable for 48 hr at room temperature/refrigerated.

ADMINISTRATION
General: Begin infusion prior to chemotherapy and at specified intervals to avoid emesis. **Intermittent Infusion:** Infuse over 15 min.

COMPATIBILITY
Solution: Dextrose solutions, Ringer's injection, sodium chloride solutions. **Y-site:** Amikacin, aztreonam, bleomycin, carboplatin, carmustine, cefazolin, ceforanide, cefotaxime, cefoxitin, ceftazidime, ceftizoxime, cefuroxime, chlorpromazine, cimetidine, cisplatin, clindamycin, cyclophosphamide, cytarabine, dacarbazine, dactinomycin, daunorubicin, dexamethasone, diphenhydramine, doxorubicin, doxycycline, droperidol, etoposide, famotidine, fluconazole, gentamicin, haloperidol, heparin, hydrocortisone, hydromorphone, ifosfamide, imipenem, magnesium sulfate, mannitol, mechlorethamine, meperidine, mesna, methotrexate, metoclopramide, miconazole, mitomycin, mitoxantrone, morphine, pentostatin, potassium chloride, prochlorperazine, promethazine, ranitidine, streptozocin, ticarcillin, ticarcillin-clavulante, vancomycin, vinblastine, vincristine, zidovudine.

INCOMPATIBILITY
Y-site: Acyclovir, aminophylline, amphotericin, ampicillin, ampicillin-sulbactam, amsacrine, cefoperazone, furosemide, ganciclovir, lorazepam, methylprednisolone, mezlocillin, piperacillin.

ADVERSE EFFECTS
CNS: Headache. **Resp:** BRONCHOSPASM. **GI:** Constipation, diarrhea, transient increases in AST (SGOT)/ALT (SGPT).

DRUG INTERACTIONS
Drugs inducing hepatic cytochrome P-450 enzymes: Increased ondansetron metabolism. **Drugs inhibiting hepatic cytochrome P-450 enzymes:** Decreased ondansetron metabolism resulting in increased serum levels.

NURSING CONSIDERATIONS
Assessment
General:
Hydration status.
Physical:
GI tract.
Lab Alterations:
Monitor baseline liver enzymes.

Intervention/Rationale
Monitor for continued chemotherapy-induced emesis and provide adequate hydration. ● Evaluate efficacy of drug and the need for additional doses/agents.

Patient/Family Education
Notify physician/nurse if nausea/vomiting is excessive. Drink plenty of fluids.

In the Adverse Effects section, <u>underline</u> indicates most frequent; CAPS indicates life threatening.

OXACILLIN
(ox-a-sill′-in)
Trade Name(s): Bactocill, Prostaphlin
Classification(s): Antibiotic, penicillinase-resistant penicillin
Pregnancy Category: B

PHARMACODYNAMICS/KINETICS
Mechanism of Action: Exhibits bactericidal effect against microorganisms by inhibiting cell wall synthesis during active phase of replication. Bacteria resist drug by producing penicillinases (enzymes that hydrolyze drug). **Distribution:** Distributed to all areas especially synovial, pleural, pericardial fluids; bone, lungs, sputum, bile. 89%–94% protein bound. **Metabolism/Elimination:** Partially metabolized to active and inactive metabolites. 40%–70% eliminated as unchanged drug and active metabolites in urine. **Half-Life:** 0.3–0.8 hr. Prolonged in renal impairment and neonates.

INDICATIONS/DOSAGE

Treatment of infections due to penicillinase-producing staphylococci

Adult/Pediatric (≥ 40 kg):
Mild to Moderate Upper Respiratory/Localized Skin/Soft Tissue: 250–500 mg every 4–6 hr. **Severe Infections (Lower Respiratory/Disseminated):** 1–2 g every 4–6 hr. Not to exceed 12 g/day.

Pediatric (< 40 kg):
Mild to Moderate Upper Respiratory/Localized Skin/Soft Tissue: 50 mg/kg/day in divided doses every 6 hr. **Se-**

vere Infections (Lower Respiratory/Disseminated): 100–200 mg/kg/day in divided doses every 4–6 hr. Not to exceed 200 mg/kg/day.

Neonate:
- < 7 days, < 2 kg: 50 mg/kg/day in divided doses every 12 hr.
- < 7 days, > 2 kg: 75 mg/kg/day in divided doses every 8 hr.
- > 7 days, < 2 kg: 100 mg/kg/day in divided doses every 8 hr.
- > 7 days, > 2 kg: 150 mg/kg/day in divided doses every 6 hr
- Not to exceed 200 mg/kg/day.

CONTRAINDICATIONS/PRECAUTIONS
Contraindicated in: Known hypersensitivity to penicillin or cephalosporins. **Use cautiously in:** Impaired hepatic/renal function, neonates. **Pregnancy/Lactation:** No well-controlled trials to establish safety. Benefits must outweigh risks. Appears safe for use in pregnancy. Crosses placenta. Secreted in low concentrations in breast milk. Potential infant bowel flora changes may result in diarrhea and candidiasis. **Pediatrics:** Limited data is available. Use cautiously.

PREPARATION
Availability: 250 mg, 500 mg, 1 g, 2 g, 4 g vials and 10 g bulk vial. Contains 2.8–3.1 mEq sodium/g. **Reconstitution:** Dilute each 250 mg with 5 mL sterile water for injection or sodium chloride injection. **Infusion:** Further dilute in at least 50–100 mL compatible IV solution to a final concentration 0.5–40.0 mg/mL.

STABILITY/STORAGE
Vial: Store at room temperature. Reconstituted solution stable for 3

days at room temperature and 7 days refrigerated. **Infusion:** Stable for 24 hr at room temperature and 7 days refrigerated.

ADMINISTRATION
General: If used concurrently with aminoglycosides, administer as separate infusions as far apart as possible. **IV Push:** Give slowly over at least 10 min. **Intermittent Infusion:** Infuse over 15–30 min.

COMPATIBILITY
Solution: Amino acids 4.25%/dextrose 25%, dextrose solutions, lactated Ringer's, Ringer's injection, sodium chloride solutions. **Y-site:** Acyclovir, cyclophosphamide, famotidine, foscarnet, heparin, hydrocortisone, hydromorphone, labetalol, magnesium sulfate, meperidine, morphine, perphenazine, potassium chloride, vitamin B complex with C, zidovudine.

INCOMPATIBILITY
Y-site: Verapamil.

ADVERSE EFFECTS
CNS: Neurotoxicity (high doses) (confusion, hallucinations, hyperreflexia, lethargy, myoclonus, seizures). **GI:** Diarrhea, nausea, pseudomembranous colitis, transient elevations AST (SGOT), ALT (SGPT), bilirubin, LDH, vomiting. **GU: Neonates:** Hematuria. **Renal:** Interstitial nephritis, nephropathy. **Neonates:** Transient azotemia, proteinuria. **Fld/Lytes:** Hypernatremia, hypokalemia. **Heme:** Agranulocytosis, anemia, eosinophilia, hemolytic, leukopenia, thrombocytopenia. **Hypersens:** ANAPHYLAXIS, rash, urticaria. **Other:** Thrombophlebitis.

TOXICITY/OVERDOSE
Signs/Symptoms: CNS excitation, seizures. **Treatment:** Supportive and symptomatic treatment.

DRUG INTERACTIONS
Aminoglycosides: Synergistic bactericidal action against *S. aureus*. Inactivation of aminoglycosides. **Bacteriostatic antibiotics** (chloramphenicol, erythromycin, tetracycline): Slows the rapidity of bacterial growth and may decrease the bactericidal effects of oxacillin. **Rifampin:** Dose dependent activity against *S. aureus*. Decreases emergence of rifampin resistant strains *S. aureus*. **Probenecid:** Produces higher and prolonged serum concentrations.

NURSING CONSIDERATIONS
Assessment
General:
Signs/symptoms of superinfection/bacterial/fungal overgrowth (especially in elderly, debilitated, immunosuppressed). History of allergic/hypersensitivity reaction to penicillins/cephalosporins. Signs/symptoms of infection (prior to, during, and at completion of therapy).
Physical:
Hematopoietic system, anaphylactic potential.
Lab Alterations:
False-positive urinary, CSF, or serum protein analysis using acetic acid, nitric acid, sulfosalicylic acid, or trichloroacetic acid (no interference with urine tests using bromphenol blue, i.e., Albustix, Albutest). May cause positive direct Coombs' test. False-positive reaction with copper-sulfate urine glucose tests (Clinitest).

In the Adverse Effects section, <u>underline</u> indicates most frequent; CAPS indicates life threatening.

377

Intervention/Rationale

Assess for early signs of allergic manifestations especially in patients with a history of sensitivity to related drugs. ● Evaluate regularly for increased bleeding tendencies. ● Obtain specimen for culture and sensitivity before initiation of therapy; first dose may be given while awaiting results. ● Monitor renal, hepatic, and hematopoietic function with prolonged use.

Patient/Family Education

Observe and report any signs of superinfection (loose, foul-smelling stools; vaginal itching or discharge; black furry overgrowth on tongue). Notify physician/nurse if skin rash, itching, hives, or severe diarrhea occurs.

OXYMORPHONE

(ox-i-mor′-fone)
Trade Name(s): Numorphan
Classification(s): Narcotic analgesic
Pregnancy Category: C
Controlled Substance Schedule: II

PHARMACODYNAMICS/KINETICS

Mechanism of Action: Binds to opiate receptors (mu, kappa, and sigma) in the CNS. Alters perception of pain and produces analgesia. **Onset of Action:** 5–10 min. **Peak Effect:** 0.5 hr. **Duration of Action:** 3–4 hr. **Distribution:** Distributes widely throughout body. **Metabolism/Elimination:** Primarily hepatically metabolized and undergoes conjugation. Excreted primarily in urine.

INDICATIONS/DOSAGE

Relief of moderate to severe acute and chronic pain; preoperative medication to sedate, reduce anxiety, facilitate anesthesia induction, and reduce anesthesia dosage

Adult: Initially, 0.5 mg. May repeat every 4–6 hr as needed. Increase dose cautiously until analgesia is obtained. Reduce doses in debilitated and elderly patients and severe liver impairment.

CONTRAINDICATIONS/PRECAUTIONS

Contraindicated in: Acute bronchial asthma, diarrhea caused by toxins, hypersensitivity to narcotics, upper airway obstruction. **Use cautiously in:** Head injuries, patients with abuse potential, patients susceptible to fluctuations in blood pressure, renal/hepatic impairment. **Pregnancy/Lactation:** No well-controlled trials to establish safety. Benefits must outweigh risks. Rapid placental transfer. Fetal withdrawal symptoms seen with illicit use. Following administration during labor, neonatal respiratory depression may occur. Crosses into breast milk; 4–6 hr should elapse prior to breastfeeding. **Pediatrics:** Safety and efficacy not established. Not recommended for use in < 12 years.

PREPARATION

Availability: 1 mg/mL in 1 mL amps. 1.5 mg/mL in 1 mL amps and 10 mL vials. **Syringe:** No further dilution required.

STABILITY/STORAGE

Vial: Store at room temperature.

In the Adverse Effects section, <u>underline</u> indicates most frequent; CAPS indicates life threatening.

ADMINISTRATION
General: Contains sulfites that may cause allergic reactions in susceptible patients. **IV Push:** Give by slow IV push.

COMPATIBILITY
Solution: Glycopyrrolate, ranitidine.

ADVERSE EFFECTS
CNS: COMA, convulsions, agitation, anxiety, <u>dizziness</u>, dysphoria, euphoria, hallucinations, headache, impaired mental/physical performance, increased intracranial pressure, insomnia, lethargy, <u>lightheadedness</u>, <u>sedation</u>, tremor. **Ophtho:** Blurred vision, diplopia, <u>miosis</u>. **CV:** Bradycardia, CARDIAC ARREST, CIRCULATORY COLLAPSE/DEPRESSION, dysrhythmia, hypertension, hypotension, palpitations, SHOCK, syncope, tachycardia. **Resp:** BRONCHOSPASM, RESPIRATORY ARREST/DEPRESSION, depression of cough reflex. **GI:** Abdominal pain, anorexia, biliary tract spasm, <u>constipation</u>, diarrhea, dry mouth, <u>nausea</u>, <u>vomiting</u>. **GU:** Oliguria, ureteral spasm, urinary retention. **Hypersens:** LARYNGOSPASM, edema, pruritus, urticaria. **Other:** Chills, flushing, physical/psychological dependence.

TOXICITY/OVERDOSE
Signs/Symptoms: CNS depression, miosis, respiratory depression; hypotension, bradycardia, hypothermia, pulmonary edema, pneumonia, shock; apnea, circulatory collapse, convulsions, cardiopulmonary arrest, death. **Treatment:** Symptomatic and supportive. **Antidote(s):** Naloxone is effective for circulatory and respiratory depression.

DRUG INTERACTIONS
Alcohol, antihistamines, barbiturate anesthetics, benzodiazepines, chlorpromazine: Increased CNS and respiratory depression. **Cimetidine:** Increased CNS toxicity. **Narcotic agonist–antagonists:** Decreased analgesic effect.

NURSING CONSIDERATIONS
Assessment
General:
Vital signs, pain assessment (prior to and after administration).
Physical:
Pulmonary status, GI tract, neurologic status.
Lab Alterations:
Increased biliary tract pressure produces unreliable increases in amylase/lipase for 24 hr after narcotic administration.

Intervention/Rationale
Administer pain medication before pain becomes too severe; analgesia is more effective when given on a regular basis. ● Oxygen, emergency airway equipment, and naloxone should be readily available (drug can cause respiratory depression). ● Assess bowel function regularly. Administer stool softeners and laxatives when needed. Maintain hydration and increase bulk in diet when possible to combat constipation. ● Evaluate blood pressure, heart rate, and respiratory status prior to, throughout, and following administration. Consider ECG monitoring for irregular and/or rapid and/or decreased heart rate.

Patient/Family Education
Coordination or mental alertness may be affected; activities requiring mental alertness should be

In the Adverse Effects section, <u>underline</u> indicates most frequent; CAPS indicates life threatening.

379

avoided. Call for help with ambulation, as drug may cause dizziness, drowsiness, and sedation. Ask for pain medication before pain becomes too severe. Change positions slowly to prevent orthostatic hypotension. Avoid concomitant use of other CNS depressants, including alcohol. Notify physician if vomiting/constipation become excessive or significant shortness of breath or difficulty breathing.

OXYTOCIN

(ox-i-toe′-sin)
Trade Name(s): Pitocin, Syntocinon
Classification(s): Oxytocic agent
Pregnancy Category: Unknown

PHARMACODYNAMICS/KINETICS
Mechanism of Action: Endogenous posterior pituitary hormone exhibiting uterine stimulant, vasopressive and weak antidiuretic effects. Unknown mechanism; primarily augments the number of contracting uterine myofibrils. **Onset of Action:** Immediate. **Peak Effect:** 40 min. **Duration of Action:** 1 hr. **Distribution:** Distributed throughout extracellular fluid. Small amounts to fetal circulation. **Metabolism/Elimination:** Rapidly destroyed in liver, kidneys, and functional mammary glands. Oxytocinase, enzyme produced early in pregnancy, inactivates oxytocin. Small amounts excreted unchanged in urine. **Half-Life:** 3–5 min.

INDICATIONS/DOSAGE

To initiate/augment uterine contractions or produce uterine contractions during third stage of labor

Adult: Dosage/rate of infusion are determined by uterine response. Decrease rate when labor established. **For Induction:** 0.001 units/min initially; increase by 0.001 units/min increments every 15 min until response observed. Additional increases of 0.001–0.002 units/min every 30 min until spontaneous labor pattern occurs. Higher infusion rates before term may be needed; at term, 0.009–0.01 units/min are rarely needed. **For Augmentation:** 0.002 units/min initially; increase slowly, to a maximum 0.02 units/min.

To control postpartum bleeding/hemorrhage:

Adult: 0.02–0.04 units/min after delivery (or after placenta delivery). Adjust rate to maintain uterine contraction and control atony for a total of 10 units.

Antepartum fetal heart rate testing (oxytocin challenge test) (*unlabeled use*)

Adult: 0.0005 units/min. Increase gradually at 15 min intervals to maximum 0.02 units/min. Discontinue infusion when three moderate uterine contractions occur within one 10 min interval. If no change in fetal heart rate, repeat test in 1 week.

To shorten induction-to-abortion time following prostaglandin or hypertonic abortifacients (*unlabeled use*)

Adult: 0.01–0.1 units/min. Cumulative dose 30 units/12 hr.

In the Adverse Effects section, <u>underline</u> indicates most frequent; CAPS indicates life threatening.

CONTRAINDICATIONS/ PRECAUTIONS

Contraindicated in: Significant cephalopelvic disproportion, unfavorable fetal positions that are undeliverable without conversion, obstetrical emergencies, fetal distress where delivery is not imminent, prolonged use in uterine inertia or toxemia, hypertonic/active uterine patterns, hypersensitivity. **Use cautiously in:** Cyclopropane anesthesia, first/second stage labor. **Pregnancy/Lactation:** Small quantities are found in breast milk. Breastfeeding should not begin until 24 hr after oxytocin discontinued for postpartum bleeding.

PREPARATION

Availability: 10 units/mL, 1 mL and 10 mL amps/vials. **Infusion:** *To Initiate/Augment Uterine Contractions during Third Stage of Labor:* Dilute 10 units (1 mL) in 1000 mL compatible IV solution for a final concentration of 0.01 units/mL. Physiologic electrolyte solution should be used for dilution. *To Control Postpartum Bleeding/Hemorrhage, to Shorten Induction-to-Abortion Time Following Prostaglandin or Hypertonic Abortifacients (unlabeled use):* Dilute 10 units (1 mL) in 500 mL compatible IV solution for a final concentration of 0.02 units/mL. *Antepartum Fetal Heart Rate Testing (Oxytocin Challenge Test) (unlabeled use):* Dilute 5–10 units (0.5–1.0 mL) in 1000 mL dextrose 5% for a final concentration 0.005–0.01 units/mL.

STABILITY/STORAGE

Vial: Store at room temperature. **Infusion:** Stable at room temperature for 24 hr.

ADMINISTRATION

General: Must be diluted prior to administration. An infusion control device must be used. Frequent monitoring of strength/frequency/duration of contractions, resting uterine tone, and fetal heart rate are necessary. **Intermittent/Continuous Infusion:** Infuse at physician prescribed rate.

COMPATIBILITY

Solution: Dextrose solutions, lactated Ringer's, Ringer's injection, sodium chloride solutions, sodium lactate 1/6M. **Y-site:** Heparin, hydrocortisone, meperidine, morphine, potassium chloride, vitamin B complex with C.

ADVERSE EFFECTS

CNS: *Maternal:* Coma, seizures. *Fetal:* PERMANENT CNS DAMAGE. **CV:** *Maternal/Fetal:* Dysrhythmia, premature ventricular contraction. *Fetal:* Bradycardia, hypotension. **GI:** Nausea, vomiting. **GU:** *Maternal:* Uterine rupture. **Fld/Lytes:** *Maternal:* WATER INTOXICATION, hypochloremia, hyponatremia. **Heme:** *Maternal:* FATAL AFIBRINOGENEMIA, increased blood loss, pelvic hematoma, postpartum hemorrhage, thrombocytopenia. **Hypersens:** *Maternal:* ANAPHYLAXIS. **Other:** Death

TOXICITY/OVERDOSE

Signs/Symptoms: Uterine rupture, cervical/vaginal lacerations, uteroplacental hypoperfusion, deceleration fetal heart rate, hypoxia, hypercapnia, and death, water intoxication. **Treatment:** Symptomatic and supportive. If water intoxi-

In the Adverse Effects section, <u>underline</u> indicates most frequent; CAPS indicates life threatening.

381

cated, discontinue drug, restrict fluid intake, initiate diuresis, correct fluid/electrolyte imbalance, administer hypertonic saline, control convulsions.

DRUG INTERACTIONS
Cyclopropane anesthesia: Increased hypotension, maternal sinus bradycardia, and abnormal AV rhythms. **Sympathomimetic agents:** Increased pressor effect and postpartum hypertension.

NURSING CONSIDERATIONS
Assessment
General:
Use external or internal fetal monitoring during administration. Monitor maternal blood pressure/heart rate before and during administration. Intake/output ratio. Labor progression status.
Physical:
Cardiovascular status, hematopoietic system.
Lab Alterations:
Monitor serum electrolytes to evaluate development of water intoxication.

Intervention/Rationale
Assess fetal maturity and presentation in augmentation/induction of labor. ● Assess character, duration, and frequency of contractions during administration. Follow physician orders for frequency of titration. Call physician for significant changes in fetal heart rate. ● Closely monitor for uterine hyperstimulation; if it occurs, reduce infusion rate or discontinue following notification of physician.

Patient/Family Education
Expect uterine contractions of varying intensity that will increase with intensity, frequency, and duration as drug is titrated. Educate patient regarding therapeutic outcome and adverse effects.

PANCURONIUM
(pan-cure-oh′-nee-yum)
Trade Name(s): Pavulon
Classification(s): Nondepolarizing neuromuscular blocking agent
Pregnancy Category: C

PHARMACODYNAMICS/KINETICS
Mechanism of Action: Causes partial paralysis by interfering with neural transmission at myoneural junction. Prevents acetylcholine from binding to receptors at muscle end plate. **Onset of Action:** 2–3 min (dose related). **Duration of Action:** 35–45 min (dose related). **Distribution:** Distributes rapidly throughout body. Variable protein binding to plasma proteins (87%), mainly gamma globulin and albumin, to a lesser extent. **Metabolism/Elimination:** Primarily eliminated unchanged in urine with small amounts metabolized. 40% unchanged drug and metabolites eliminated in urine. 11% in bile. **Half-Life:** 2 hr. Prolonged in severe renal/hepatic impairment.

INDICATIONS/DOSAGE
Individualize dosage based on patient response. Reduce dosage with concurrent inhalation anesthetic.

In the Adverse Effects section, <u>underline</u> indicates most frequent; CAPS indicates life threatening.

Adjunct to anesthesia to induce skeletal muscle relaxation and to facilitate mechanical ventilation

Adult/Pediatric: Initially, 0.04–0.1 mg/kg/dose. Increase by increments of 0.01 mg/kg. Repeat dose every 30–60 minutes. *Neonate:* Initially, a test dose of 0.02 mg/kg. Repeat 0.03–0.1 mg/kg/dose for two doses every 5–10 min as needed. Then 0.03–0.09 mg/kg/dose every 0.5–4.0 hr as needed.

To facilitate skeletal muscle relaxation for endotracheal intubation

Adult/Pediatric: 0.06–0.1 mg/kg/dose. Doses up to 0.16 mg/kg have been administered.

CONTRAINDICATIONS/ PRECAUTIONS

Contraindicated in: Hypersensitivity. **Use cautiously in:** Cardiovascular disease, edematous states, elderly, hepatic/biliary/renal disease, myasthenia gravis, neonates, neuromuscular disease. **Pregnancy/Lactation:** No well-controlled trials to establish safety. Benefits must outweigh risks. Reduce dosage in patients receiving magnesium for preeclampsia to avoid prolongation of effects. Crosses placenta in small amounts. Administer in close proximity to delivery to avoid significant placental transfer. **Pediatrics:** Neonates are particularly sensitive to effects; begin with lower doses.

PREPARATION

Availability: 1 mg/mL in 10 mL vials. 2 mg/mL in 2.5 and 5 mL amps. Contains benzyl alcohol. **Syringe:** No further dilution required. **Infusion:** Not recommended. Prepare as per physician order in compatible IV solution.

STABILITY/STORAGE

Vial: Store under refrigeration to prolong stability up to 2 years. Stable at room temperature for 6 months. **Infusion:** Stable for 48 hr at room temperature or refrigerate.

ADMINISTRATION

General: Unconsciousness must be established prior to administration to prevent patient distress. Administer only by trained personnel with the ability to provide ventilatory support. **IV Push:** Give by rapid direct IV push. **Intermittent Infusion:** Administer at physician prescribed rate. Infusions of 0.1 mg/kg/hr have been used.

COMPATIBILITY

Solution: Dextrose solutions, lactated Ringer's, sodium chloride solutions. **Syringe:** Heparin, hydrocortisone, meperidine, methohexital, neostigmine, promethazine, succinylcholine, thiopental, tubocurarine. **Y-site:** Aminophylline, cefazolin, cefuroxime, cimetidine, dobutamine, dopamine, epinephrine, esmolol, fentanyl, gentamicin, heparin, hydrocortisone, isoproterenol, lorazepam, midazolam, morphine, nitroglycerin, ranitidine, sodium nitroprusside, trimethoprim-sulfamethoxazole, vancomycin.

INCOMPATIBILITY

Syringe: Bariturates. **Y-site:** Diazepam.

ADVERSE EFFECTS

CNS: <u>Prolonged paralysis, skeletal muscle weakness.</u> **CV:** Increased

In the Adverse Effects section, <u>underline</u> indicates most frequent; CAPS indicates life threatening.

383

cardiac output, heart rate, mean arterial pressure; hypotension; tachycardia. **Resp:** APNEA, RESPIRATORY INSUFFICIENCY. **GI:** Salivation. **MS:** Prolonged neuromuscular blockade. **Heme:** METHEMOGLOBINEMIA (in premature infants). **Hypersens:** BRONCHOSPASM, transient rash. **Other:** Flushing.

TOXICITY/OVERDOSE

Signs/Symptoms: Prolonged skeletal muscle relaxation. **Treatment:** Symptomatic and supportive treatment. **Antidote(s):** Pyridostigmine, neostigmine, or edrophonium in conjunction with atropine or glycopyrrolate will antagonize pancuronium action. Concurrent administration of other neuromuscular blockers or impaired renal/hepatic function may not allow complete reversal.

DRUG INTERACTIONS

Aminoglycosides, bacitracin, clindamycin, inhalation anesthetics (enflurane, halothane, isoflurane), polymyxin B, lincomycin, magnesium sulfate, neuromuscular blocking agents (metocurine, tubocurarine), quinidine, quinine, tetracycline: Increased neuromuscular blockade and prolonged paralysis. **Azathioprine:** Neuromuscular blocking effect reversal. **Succinycholine:** Potentiation of neuromuscular blockade and prolonged paralysis. Delay pancuronium administration until succinylcholine effects subside. **Theophylline:** Resistance to or reversal of pancuronium effects. Cardiac arrhythmias may occur.

NURSING CONSIDERATIONS

Assessment

General:
Vital signs, ECG (recommended), continuous monitoring of respiratory rate.

Physical:
Cardiopulmonary status, neuromuscular status.

Lab Alterations:
Monitor electrolytes.

Intervention/Rationale

Produces apnea (use cautiously in patients with cardiovascular disease, severe electrolyte disorders, bronchogenic cancer, and neuromuscular diseases). Maintain patent airway. ● Monitor response to drug during intraoperative period by use of a peripheral nerve stimulator. ● Assess postoperatively for presence of any residual muscle weakness. Evaluate hand grip, head lift, and ability to cough in order to ascertain full recovery from residual effects of drug. ● Correct electrolyte deficiencies prior to surgery. ● Assess status of corneas; consider lubrication as needed. ● Assess need for sedation; obtain order and administer during use of paralytic agent. ● Monitor blood pressure, respiratory status, and ECG before and during administration.

Patient/Family Education

Discuss the rationale for hand grip, head lift, and cough demonstration in the immediate postoperative phase in order to assure patient cooperation. Inform patient and family that consciousness is unaffected by drug. Explain side effects to patient and family. Continue to ex-

In the Adverse Effects section, underline indicates most frequent;
CAPS indicates life threatening.

plain procedures and therapies to patient unless sedation is administered.

PAPAVERINE
(pa-pav′-er-een)
Trade Name(s): Papaverine
Classification(s): Peripheral vasodilator
Pregnancy Category: C

PHARMACODYNAMICS/KINETICS
Mechanism of Action: Direct relaxation of all smooth muscle tone especially when spasmodically contracted. Produces vasodilation secondary to increasing levels of intracellular cyclic AMP. Direct vasodilatory action on cerebral blood vessels. **Onset of Action:** Rapid. **Duration of Action:** 3 hr. **Distribution:** Distributed throughout body with a significant amount localized in fat deposits and in liver. 90% protein bound. **Metabolism/Elimination:** Undergoes rapid hepatic metabolism. Excreted in urine as inactive drug. **Half-Life:** Variable.

INDICATIONS/DOSAGE

Vascular spasm associated with acute MI, angina pectoris, peripheral/pulmonary embolism, peripheral vascular disease; cerebral angiospastic states; ureteral, biliary, GI colic spasms

Adult: 30 mg initially, then 30–120 mg every 3 hr as needed. *Pediatric (unlabeled use):* 6 mg/kg/day in four divided doses.

CONTRAINDICATIONS/ PRECAUTIONS
Contraindicated in: Complete AV heart block, hypersensitivity. **Use cautiously in:** Depressed cardiac conduction, glaucoma, impaired hepatic function. **Pregnancy/Lactation:** No well-controlled trials to establish safety. Benefits must outweigh risks. **Pediatrics:** Safety and efficacy not established.

PREPARATION
Availability: 30 mg/mL in 2 and 10 mL amps. **Syringe:** No further dilution required.

STABILITY/STORAGE
Vial: Stable at room temperature. Do not refrigerate. Use immediately after drawing into syringe.

ADMINISTRATION
General: IV route is recommended when immediate effect is desired. **IV Push:** Administer 30 mg slowly over 1–2 min.

COMPATIBILITY
Solution: Dextrose solutions, Ringer's injection, sodium chloride solutions. **Syringe:** Phentolamine.

INCOMPATIBILITY
Solution: Lactated Ringer's.

ADVERSE EFFECTS
CNS: Drowsiness, headache, excess sedation, vertigo. **CV:** Increased blood pressure, heart rate, and depth of respiration, hypotension. **Resp:** APNEA. **GI:** Abdominal distress, anorexia, constipation, diarrhea, hepatotoxicity (jaundice/altered liver function tests). **Heme:** Eosinophilia. **Hypersens:** Rash. **Other:** Flushing, malaise, sweating.

In the Adverse Effects section, underline indicates most frequent;
CAPS indicates life threatening.

385

TOXICITY/OVERDOSE

Signs/Symptoms: Vasomotor instability with nausea, vomiting, CNS depression, nystagmus, diplopia, diaphoresis, flushing, dizziness, sinus tachycardia, seizures, tachydysrhythmias, ventricular fibrillation **Treatment:** Symptomatic and supportive treatment.

DRUG INTERACTIONS

Levodopa: Decreased antiparkinson effectiveness.

NURSING CONSIDERATIONS

Assessment
General:
Vital signs, ECG (recommended).
Physical:
GI tract, cardiopulmonary status, neurologic status.
Lab Alterations:
Monitor liver enzymes periodically.

Intervention/Rationale
Monitor blood pressure and heart rate prior to and throughout course of therapy. Monitor ECG to assess for AV block—withhold drug if present. ● Evaluate neurologic status periodically for development of drowsiness and excess sedation. ● Assess patient for signs/symptoms of hepatotoxicity.

Patient/Family Education
May cause dizziness and drowsiness. Use caution with activities requiring acuity. Avoid alcohol. May cause flushing, sweating, headache, tiredness, jaundice, rash, nausea, anorexia, abdominal distress, constipation, diarrhea; notify physician if any of these occur.

PARALDEHYDE
(par-al′-de-hyde)
Trade Name(s): Paraldehyde
Classification(s): Anticonvulsant, sedative/hypnotic
Pregnancy Category: C
Controlled Substance Schedule: IV

PHARMACODYNAMICS/KINETICS

Mechanism of Action: Nonspecific, reversible CNS depression. **Onset of Action:** 5–15 min. **Duration of Action:** 8–12 hr. **Distribution:** Distributed extensively into CSF. **Metabolism/Elimination:** Primarily (70%–80%) hepatically metabolized. Small fractions (20%–30%) exhaled unchanged via the lungs. Negligible amount eliminated unchanged via urine. **Half-Life:** 7.5 hr (3.5–9.5 hr). Increased in hepatic impairment.

INDICATIONS/DOSAGE

Emergency treatment of tetanus, eclampsia, status epilepticus, and poisoning by convulsive drugs

Adult: 0.2–0.4 mL/kg/dose or 5 mL. *Pediatric:* 0.1–0.15 mL/kg/dose.

CONTRAINDICATIONS/PRECAUTIONS

Contraindicated in: Bronchopulmonary disease, hepatic insufficiency, hypersensitivity. **Use cautiously in:** Asthma, hepatic impairment. **Pregnancy/Lactation:** No well-controlled trials to establish safety. Benefits must outweigh risks. Crosses the placenta. Use during labor may cause neonatal respiratory depres-

In the Adverse Effects section, underline indicates most frequent; CAPS indicates life threatening.

sion. **Pediatrics:** Safety and efficacy not established.

PREPARATION

(Information from Mason N. Preparing intravenous paraldehyde. *Hosp Ther*, 1989; 14(3):22, 24–25) **Availability:** A parenteral dosage form is no longer available in the United States. It may be prepared by pharmacy for emergency situations. The final concentration is 4% solution (4 g/100mL). **Reconstitution:** Use an oral preparation that does not contain an antioxidant (i.e., resorcinol). Forest Pharmaceuticals (Paral) manufactures a pure preparation, 1 g/mL, 30 mL liquid. It should be sterilized by filtration using a hydrophilic solvent-resistant filter compatible with paraldehyde that has not oxidized. USP sterility and pyrogen testing standards should ensure conformity. **Infusion:** 4 g (4 mL) should be added via already specified filter to 100 mL sodium chloride solution. Adsorption to polyvinyl chloride bags may occur; glass bottles are recommended.

STABILITY/STORAGE

Liquid: Store at room temperature. **Infusion:** Prepare prior to administration. Discard after 24 hr.

ADMINISTRATION

General: Adsorption to IV tubing and equipment cannot be minimized; 10%–16% may be lost via adsorption. Do not administer if brownish color. **Intermittent/Continuous Infusion:** Infuse slowly at a rate not to exceed 1 mL/min.

COMPATIBILITY

Solution: Dextrose solutions, sodium chloride solutions.

ADVERSE EFFECTS

CNS: <u>Sedation</u>. **CV:** Cardiac failure, hypotension. **Resp:** Pulmonary edema, pulmonary hemorrhage, severe coughing. **GI:** Toxic hepatitis. **Derm:** <u>Mucous membrane irritation</u>. **Heme:** HEMOLYSIS. **Hypersens:** <u>Erythematous rash</u>. **Metab:** ACIDOSIS. **Other:** Strong, unpleasant breath, thrombophlebitis.

TOXICITY/OVERDOSE

Signs/Symptoms: Coma, severe hypotension, respiratory depression, pulmonary edema, cardiac failure. **Treatment:** Supportive and symptomatic treatment.

DRUG INTERACTIONS

CNS depressants (alcohol, antihistamines, barbiturates, narcotics): Additive CNS depressant effects. **Disulfiram:** Inhibits acetaldehyde dehydrogenase. Avoid concomitant use.

NURSING CONSIDERATIONS

Assessment
General:
Vital signs.
Physical:
Cardiopulmonary status, neurologic status.
Lab Alterations:
Monitor arterial blood gases, electrolytes, and CBC with differential.

Intervention/Rationale
Observe patient closely for evidence of respiratory depression. ● Monitor blood pressure; observe for hypotension. ● Assess patient for evidence of neurologic changes that may indicate potential seizure activity.

In the Adverse Effects section, <u>underline</u> indicates most frequent; CAPS indicates life threatening.

387

Patient/Family Education
Avoid alcohol/sedatives and avoid activities requiring alertness.

PENICILLIN G (PENICILLIN G POTASSIUM, PENICILLIN G SODIUM)
(pen-i-sill'-in)
Trade Name(s): Pfizerpen
Classification(s): Antibiotic
Pregnancy Category: B

PHARMACODYNAMICS/KINETICS
Mechanism of Action: Bactericidal, inhibition of cell wall mucopeptide biosynthesis. **Peak Serum Level:** Rapid. **Distribution:** Distributed throughout body. 45%–68% protein bound. **Metabolism/Elimination:** 60% eliminated as unchanged drug and active metabolites in urine; small amounts in bile. **Half-Life:** 30–60 min. Increased in renal impairment and neonates.

INDICATIONS/DOSAGE

Treatment of infections caused by susceptible organisms including gram-positive aerobes/anaerobes and susceptible gram-negative cocci/bacilli

Adult: (In divided doses): 100,000–250,000 units/kg/day in divided doses every 4–6 hr.
Actinomycosis: Cervicofacial: 1–6 million units/day. **Thoracic/Abdominal:** 10–20 million units/day.
Anthrax: 5–20 million units/day.
Clostridial Infection: 20 million units/day. **Diphtheria:** 300,000–400,000 units/day. **Gonococcal Infections: Dis-**

seminated: 10 million units/day.
Arthritis/Septicemia/Meningitis: 100,000 units/kg/day every 6 hr.
Gram-negative Bacillary Bacteremia: 20–30 million units/day. **Listeria Infections:** 15–20 million units/day.
Lyme Disease (*unlabeled use*): 20 million units/day. **Meningococcal Meningitis:** 20–30 million units/day continuous infusion or 200,000–300,000 units/kg/day every 6 hr.
Pneumococcal Infections: *Empyema:* 10–20 million units/day. **Meningitis:** 20–24 million units/day.
Suppurative arthritis, osteomyelitis, mastoiditis, endocarditis, peritonitis, pericarditis: 10–20 million unit/day.
Neurosyphilis: 12–24 million units/day every 4 hr.

Pediatric: 100,000–250,000 units/kg/day in divided doses every 4–6 hr. Up to 500,000 units/kg/day in divided doses for brain abscess. Not to exceed adult doses.

Neonate:
< 7 Days, < 2 kg: 50,000 units/kg/day every 12 hr.
Meningitis: 100,000 units /kg/day every 12 hr.
< 7 Days, ≥ 2 kg: 75,000 units/kg/day every 8 hr.
Meningitis: 150,000 units/kg/day every 8 hr.
> 7 days, < 2 kg: 75,000 units/kg/day every 8 hr.
Meningitis: 150,000 units/kg/day every 8 hr.
> 7 days, ≥ 2 kg: 100,000 units/kg/day every 6 hr.
Meningitis: 200,000 units/kg/day every 6 hr.
Congenital Syphilis: 50,000 units/kg/day every 12 hr. **Gonococcal Ophthalmia:** 100,000 units/kg/day every

In the Adverse Effects section, underline indicates most frequent; CAPS indicates life threatening.

6 hr. **Listeria:** 500,000–1,000,000 units/day.
Treatment of Infant Born to Mother with Gonococcal Infection: Full-term 50,000 units, low birth weight 20,000 units.

Prophylaxis of bacterial endocarditis in GI, biliary, or genitourinary surgery/instrumentation

Adult: 2 million units 30–60 min prior to procedure and 1 million units 6 hr later (if unable to take oral medication). *Pediatric:* 50,000 units/kg 30–60 min prior to procedure and 25,000 units/kg 6 hr later. Not to exceed adult doses.

CONTRAINDICATIONS/ PRECAUTIONS

Contraindicated in: Hypersensitivity to penicillin or cephalosporins. **Use cautiously in:** Hypersensitivity to monobactams/carbapenems, impaired renal function, neonates. **Pregnancy/Lactation:** No well-controlled trials to establish safety. Appears to be safe for use in pregnancy when benefits outweigh risks. Crosses placenta. Distributed in low concentrations in breast milk. Use during lactation may cause diarrhea, candidiasis, or allergic reaction in infant. **Pediatrics:** Use caution in neonates due to incomplete development of renal function.

PREPARATION

Availability: *Penicillin G potassium:* 200,000 units, 500,000 units, 1,000,000 units, 5,000,000 units, 10,000,000 units, 20,000,000 units per vial. Each mg equals 1355–1595 units. Contains 1.7 mEq potassium

and 0.3 mEq sodium/million units. *Penicillin G Sodium:* 5,000,000 units per vial. Each mg equals 1420–1667 units. Contains 2 mEq sodium/million units. **Reconstitution:** Dilute each vial with manufacturer specified amount of compatible diluent on each vial to result in respective final concentration. **Infusion:** Further dilute in 50–100 mL compatible IV solution for a final concentration of 100,000–500,000 units/mL. Large doses (i.e., 5 million units) may be added to 1 L volume of compatible IV solution.

STABILITY/STORAGE

Vial: Store at room temperature. Reconstituted solution stable for 7 days refrigerated. **Infusion:** Stable for 24 hr at room temperature and 7 days refrigerated.

ADMINISTRATION

General: Vials containing 10–20 million units are for intravenous administration. **Intermittent Infusion: Adults:** Administer over 30–120 min. **Pediatrics:** Administer over 15–30 min. **Continuous Infusion:** Administer over physician specified time (i.e., 12–24 hr).

COMPATIBILITY

Penicillin G Potassium: Solution: Amino acids 4.25%/dextrose 25%, dextrose solutions, lactated Ringer's, Ringer's injection, sodium chloride solutions, sterile water for injection. **Syringe:** Heparin. **Y-site:** Acyclovir, cyclophosphamide, enalaprilat, esmolol, foscarnet, heparin, hydrocortisone, hydromorphone, labetalol, magnesium sulfate, meperi-

In the Adverse Effects section, <u>underline</u> indicates most frequent;
CAPS indicates life threatening.

389

dine, morphine, perphenazine, potassium chloride, verapamil, vitamin B complex with C.

Penicillin G Sodium: *Solution:* Dextrose solutions, sodium chloride solutions. **Syringe:** Chloramphenicol, cimetidine, gentamicin, heparin, kanamycin, lincomycin, streptomycin.

INCOMPATIBILITY

Penicillin G Potassium: *Solution:* Fat emulsion. **Syringe:** Metoclopramide. **Penicillin G Sodium:** *Solution:* Fat Emulsion.

ADVERSE EFFECTS

CNS: Neurotoxicity (high doses) (confusion, hallucinations, hyperreflexia, lethargy, myoclonus), seizures. **CV:** Exacerbation CHF. **GI:** Pseudomembranous colitis, diarrhea, nausea, vomiting. **Renal:** Interstitial nephritis, nephropathy. **Fld/Lytes:** Hyperkalemia, hypernatremia, hypokalemia. **Heme:** Agranulocytosis, anemia, eosinophilia, hemolytic anemia, leukopenia, thrombocytopenia. **Hypersens:** ANAPHYLAXIS, Stevens-Johnson Syndrome, rash, serum sickness, urticaria. **Other:** Jarisch-Herxheimer reaction (in spirochete treatment) (headache, fever, chills, sweating, sore throat, arthralgia, increased heart rate, and blood pressure), thrombophlebitis.

TOXICITY/OVERDOSE

Signs/Symptoms: CNS excitation, seizures, hyperkalemia (Pen G K) characterized by hyperreflexia, convulsions, coma, cardiac arrhythmias, cardiac arrest, hypernatremia (Pen G Na), and exacerbation of CHF. **Treatment:** Supportive and symptomatic treatment. Hemodialysis may be effective in removal.

DRUG INTERACTIONS

Aminoglycosides: Synergistic bactericidal action against *S. aureus.* **Bacteriostatic antibiotics** (chloramphenicol, erythromycin, tetracycline): Decreased bactericidal effects. **Nonsteroidal anti-inflammatory (NSAIDs) agents/Sulfinpyrazone:** Increased penicillin half-life by decreasing renal elimination and protein displacement of penicillin. Increased adverse effects. **Potassium sparing diuretics:** Increased hyperkalemia risk. **Probenecid:** Produces higher and prolonged penicillin serum concentrations.

NURSING CONSIDERATIONS

Assessment

General:

Determine history of allergic or hypersensitivity reactions to penicillins/cephalosporins. Obtain specimen for culture and sensitivity before therapy is initiated (first dose may be given while awaiting results). Signs/symptoms of superinfection/bacterial/fungal overgrowth (especially in elderly, debilitated, or immunosuppressed).

Physical:

Signs/symptoms of anaphylaxis, neurologic status.

Lab Alterations:

Periodically evelate renal, hepatic, and hematologic systems. False-positive urinary, CSF or serum protein using acetic acid, nitric acid, sulfosalicylic acid, or trichloroacetic acid (no interference with urine tests using bromphenol blue, i.e.,

In the Adverse Effects section, underline indicates most frequent; CAPS indicates life threatening.

Albustix, Albutest). High penicillin concentrations interfere with albumin binding to dyes for serum albumin concentration. False-positive urine glucose with cupric sulfate tests (Clinitest). False increase serum uric acid concentrations with copper-chelate methods (phosphotungstate and uricase methods unaffected). Guthrie tests for PKU in neonates unreliable while receiving penicillin (sodium hydroxide and hydrochloric acid must be added to the sample to permit interpretation). False increase in urinary 17-ketogenic steroids and 17-ketosteroids. False decrease in in aminoglycoside concentrations because of inactivation. Decrease in excretion aminohippurate sodium (PAH) and phenolsulfonphthalein (PSP) (tests should not be done). False increases in aminolevulinic acid (ALA) (test should not be done unless a separation process is done). May interfere with HLA antigens and subsequent typing.

Intervention/Rationale
Hypersensitivity reactions may be immediate and severe in penicillin-sensitive patients with a history of allergy, asthma, hay fever, or urticaria. ● Observe for development of seizures with high doses.

Patient/Family Education
Notify physician/nurse if skin rash, itching, hives, severe diarrhea, or signs of superinfection (black overgrowth, vaginal itching/discharge, loose stools) occur. Discuss the importance of using antibiotic prophylaxis as prescribed for patients with rheumatic fever, history, or congenital heart disease.

PENTAMIDINE
(pen-tam'-i-deen)
Trade Name(s): Pentacarinat ♣, Pentam 300
Classification(s): Anti-infective, antiprotozoal
Pregnancy Category: C

PHARMACODYNAMICS/KINETICS
Mechanism of Action: Unknown. It may interfere with nuclear metabolism and inhibition of DNA, RNA, phospholipid, protein synthesis. **Distribution:** Extensive tissue binding. **Metabolism/Elimination:** ⅓ excreted unchanged in the urine in first 6 hr with small amounts in the remaining 6–8 hr. Accumulation may occur with renal impairment. **Half-Life:** 6.4 hr (5.1–7.7 hr). Increased in renal impairment.

INDICATIONS/DOSAGE

Treatment of *Pneumocystis carinii* pneumonia (PCP)
Adult/Pediatric: 4 mg/kg once daily for 14–21 days. Alternate pediatric doses of 150 mg/m^2 once daily for 5 days, then 100 mg/m^2 for the remainder of therapy. Reduce dosage, extend infusion time, or extend the dosing interval in renal impairment.

Treatment of *African trypanosomiasis* (*unlabeled use*):
Adult/Pediatric: 4 mg/kg once daily for 10 days.

Treatment of visceral leishmaniasis (*unlabeled use*):
Adult/Pediatric: 2–4 mg/kg daily or every other day for 15 doses.

P

In the Adverse Effects section, underline indicates most frequent; CAPS indicates life threatening.

391

CONTRAINDICATIONS/ PRECAUTIONS
Contraindicated in: Hypersensitivity. **Use cautiously in:** Anemia, hepatic/ renal dysfunction, hyperglycemia, hypertension, hypocalcemia, hypoglycemia, hypotension, leukopenia, pancreatitis, thrombocytopenia, ventricular tachycardia. **Pregnancy/Lactation:** No well-controlled trials to establish safety. Benefits must outweigh risks. Breastfeeding should be discontinued if possible (consider benefits versus risks).

PREPARATION
Availability: 300 mg vial. **Reconstitution:** Dilute each vial with 3–5 mL sterile water for injection or dextrose 5% for a final concentration of 60–100 mg/mL, respectively. **Infusion:** Further dilute desired dose in 50–250 mL compatible IV solution.

STABILITY/STORAGE
Vial: Stable at room temperature. Protect from light. Reconstituted vial stable at room temperature for 48 hr (manufacturer recommends discarding unused portions). **Infusion:** Stable at room temperature for 48 hr.

ADMINISTRATION
General: Avoid rapid IV administration. Patient should be supine to avoid hypotension. **Intermittent Infusion:** Administer over at least 60 minutes.

COMPATIBILITY
Solution: Dextrose solutions, sodium chloride solutions. **Y-site:** Zidovudine.

INCOMPATIBILITY
Y-site: Foscarnet.

ADVERSE EFFECTS
CNS: Confusion, hallucinations, neuralgia. **CV:** <u>Hypotension</u>, VENTRICULAR TACHYCARDIA. **Resp:** BRONCHOSPASM. **GI:** Anorexia, diarrhea, <u>elevated liver function tests</u>, nausea. **Renal:** Acute renal failure, <u>elevated serum creatinine</u>. **Endo:** Hyperglycemia, <u>HYPOGLYCEMIA</u>. **Fld/Lytes:** Hyperkalemia, hypocalcemia. **Heme:** <u>LEUKOPENIA</u>, THROMBOCYTOPENIA. **Hypersens:** Stevens-Johnson syndrome, rash. **Other:** <u>Fever</u>, phlebitis.

TOXICITY/OVERDOSE
Signs/Symptoms: Extension of adverse effects especially with rapid infusions. **Treatment:** Symptomatic and supportive.

DRUG INTERACTIONS
Aminoglycosides, amphotericin B, cisplatin, methoxyflurane, polymyxin B, vancomycin: Additive nephrotoxicity. **Antineoplastic agents, zidovudine:** Additive bone marrow depression.

NURSING CONSIDERATIONS
Assessment
General:
Vital signs, ECG (recommended).
Physical:
Neurologic status, hematopoietic system, renal status.
Lab Alterations:
Monitor the following before, during, and after therapy: daily BUN, serum creatinine, blood glucose, CBC, platelet count, liver function tests, serum calcium.

Intervention/Rationale
Monitor blood pressure closely during administration and several times after. ● Evaluate patient for signs/symptoms of hypoglyce-

In the Adverse Effects section, <u>underline</u> indicates most frequent; CAPS indicates life threatening.

mia. ● Assess neurologic status for development of hallucinations, confusion, and neuralgia. ● Evaluate need for ECG monitoring based on patient history and/or presence of rapid and/or irregular heart rate.

Patient/Family Education
Notify physician/nurse of fever, bleeding, sore throat, or signs of infection. Hypoglycemia may occur during administration. Complete entire cycle of drug therapy even if feeling better.

PENTAZOCINE
(pen-tax′-oh-seen)
Trade Name(s): Talwin
Classification(s): Narcotic agonist/antagonist analgesic
Pregnancy Category: C
Controlled Substance Schedule: IV

PHARMACODYNAMICS/KINETICS
Mechanism of Action: Competitive antagonist at mu receptor and agonist at kappa and sigma receptors (opiate receptors in the CNS that mediate analgesic activity). **Onset of Action:** 2–3 min. **Peak Effect:** 15 min. **Duration of Action:** 1 hr. **Distribution:** Widely distributed throughout body. 60% protein bound. **Metabolism/Elimination:** Primarily hepatically metabolized. Less than 13% excreted unchanged in urine. **Half-Life:** 2–3 hr.

INDICATIONS/DOSAGE

Relief of moderate to severe pain; preoperative or preanesthetic medication; supplement to surgical anesthesia

Reduce dosage in hepatic impairment.

Adult: 30 mg every 3–4 hr as needed for pain. Not to exceed 30 mg/dose or 360 mg/day. *Labor Patients:* 20 mg. May repeat for two to three doses at 2–3 hr intervals to provide adequate pain relief when contractions become regular.

CONTRAINDICATIONS/PRECAUTIONS
Contraindicated in: Hypersensitivity, narcotic dependent patients who have not been detoxified. **Use cautiously in:** Emotionally unstable patients, head injury, hepatic/renal impairment, accompanied with hypertension or left ventricular failure, patients with recent narcotic administration or history of drug abuse because of potential withdrawal effects, premature labor, respiratory depression, severe bronchial asthma. **Pregnancy/Lactation:** No well-controlled trials to establish safety. Benefits must outweigh risks. Crosses placenta. No adverse effects during labor have been identified. **Pediatrics:** Safety and efficacy not established.

PREPARATION
Availability: 30 mg/mL in 1, 1.5, 2, and 10 mL. **Syringe:** No further dilution required. May be diluted.

STABILITY/STORAGE
Vial: Store at room temperature.

ADMINISTRATION
General: Contains sulfites that may cause allergic reactions in susceptible patients. Narcotic dependent patients may demonstrate withdrawal symptoms. **IV Push:** Admin-

In the Adverse Effects section, underline indicates most frequent; CAPS indicates life threatening.

393

ister via direct IV push slowly over 1 minute.

COMPATIBILITY

Solution: Dextrose solutions, lactated Ringer's, Ringer's injection, sodium chloride solutions. **Syringe:** Atropine, benzquinamide, butorphanol, chlorpromazine, cimetidine, dimenhydrinate, diphenhydramine, droperidol, fentanyl, hydromorphone, meperidine, metoclopramide, morphine, perphenazine, prochlorperazine, promethazine, propiomazine, ranitidine, scopolamine. **Y-site:** Heparin, hydrocortisone, potassium chloride, vitamin B complex with C.

INCOMPATIBILITY

Syringe: Barbiturates, glycopyrrolate, heparin, pentobarbital. **Y-site:** Nafcillin.

ADVERSE EFFECTS

CNS: Confusion, depression, disorientation, disturbed dreams, <u>dizziness/lightheadedness</u>, <u>euphoria</u>, excitement, hallucinations, headache, insomnia, irritability, paresthesia, sedation, syncope, tinnitus, tremor, weakness. **Ophtho:** Blurred vision, difficulty focusing, diplopia, miosis, nystagmus. **CV:** Circulatory depression, decreased blood pressure, hypertension, hypotension, shock. **Resp:** RESPIRATORY DEPRESSION, dyspnea, transient neonatal apnea. **GI:** Abdominal distress, anorexia, constipation, cramps, diarrhea, dry mouth, <u>nausea</u>, taste alteration, <u>vomiting</u>. **GU:** Urinary retention: **MS:** Neuromuscular/psychiatric muscle tremors. **Heme:** Moderate transient eosinophilia, reversible granulocytopenia. **Hypersens:** ANAPHYLAXIS, toxic epidermal necrolysis, facial edema, pruritus, rash, urticaria. **Other:** Altered rate/strength uterine labor contractions, chills, diaphoresis, flushed skin, stinging on injection.

TOXICITY/OVERDOSE

Signs/Symptoms: Increased blood pressure, respiratory depression, tachycardia. **Treatment:** Symptomatic/supportive treatment. **Antidote(s):** Naloxone will reverse respiratory depression.

DRUG INTERACTIONS

Alcohol: Increased CNS depression. **Barbiturate anesthetics:** Increased CNS and respiratory depression.

NURSING CONSIDERATIONS

Assessment

General:
Vital signs, pain management/control.

Physical:
Pulmonary status, neurologic/emotional status, GI tract.

Lab Alterations:
Evaluate baseline and periodic CBC with differential.

Intervention/Rationale

Assess respiratory status prior to administration; do not administer if respiratory rate < 12/min. Monitor vital signs prior to, during, and after administration. ● Oxygen and emergency equipment and naloxone should be readily available. ● Perform pain assessment prior to and after administration. Administer pain medication before pain becomes too severe; analgesia is more effective when given on a regular basis. ● Administer stool softeners and laxatives when needed. ● Use

In the Adverse Effects section, <u>underline</u> indicates most frequent; CAPS indicates life threatening.

cautiously for patients emotionally unstable and with known narcotic dependence, as significant withdrawal symptoms may occur.

Patient/Family Education
Review mechanism for obtaining as needed (prn) pain medication and the rationale of pain management. Seek assistance for ambulation or repositioning activities. Drug may cause blurred vision, dizziness, drowsiness; avoid activities requiring mental acuity. Avoid alcohol and other CNS depressants. Notify physician if vomiting or constipation become excessive. Notify physician if there is significant shortness of breath or difficulty breathing. Notify physician if skin rash, confusion, or disorientation occurs.

PENTOBARBITAL
(pen-toe-bar'-bi-tal)
Trade Name(s): Nembutal
Classification(s): Barbiturate, sedative/hypnotic
Pregnancy Category: D
Controlled Substance Schedule: II

PHARMACODYNAMICS/KINETICS
Mechanism of Action: Central nervous system depression of sensory cortex, motor activity, and cerebellar function. **Onset of Action:** Immediate to 5 min. **Peak Effect:** 1 min. **Duration of Action:** 3–6 hr. **Therapeutic Serum Levels:** 25–40 mcg/mL (therapeutic coma). **Distribution:** Rapidly distributed to all tissues/fluids with high concentrations in brain/liver. 35%–45% bound to plasma proteins (due

to high lipid solubility). **Metabolism/ Elimination:** Primarily metabolized by the liver to an inactive metabolite. Eliminated by kidneys. **Half-Life:** 35–50 hr.

INDICATIONS/DOSAGE

Dosage should be individualized and titrated based on patient response. Reduce dosage for debilitated patients.

Preanesthetic sedative

Adult: 100 mg once (for 70 kg patient). Followed by additional doses in small increments at intervals of at least 1 minute, up to a total of 200–500 mg, if necessary. *Pediatrics:* Reduce dosage proportionally. 50 mg may be given initially.

Emergency control of acute convulsive episodes

Adult/Pediatrics: Keep IV dosage to a minimum to avoid excessive CNS depression following seizures.

Management of increased intracranial pressure by inducing therapeutic coma (*unlabeled use*):

Adult: Initially, 10–15 mg/kg, followed by 1–3 mg/kg/hr. *Pediatrics:* Initially, 3–5 mg/kg/dose, followed by 2–3.5 mg/kg/hr to maintain serum level 25–40 mcg/mL.

CONTRAINDICATIONS/ PRECAUTIONS
Contraindicated in: Barbiturate sensitivity, patients with porphyria or severe liver impairment, presence of severe acute/chronic pain. **Use cautiously in:** Severe respiratory distress when administering large doses. **Pregnancy/Lactation:** Known terato-

In the Adverse Effects section, underline indicates most frequent; CAPS indicates life threatening.

395

genic effects. May cause fetal damage/abnormalities. Benefits must outweigh risks. Readily crosses placenta. Full doses decrease the force and frequency of uterine contractions. Small amounts distributed into breast milk; drowsiness in infants reported. **Pediatrics:** May produce paradoxical irritability, excitability, and aggression. Hyperkinetic states may be induced/aggravated.

PREPARATION
Availability: 50 mg/mL in 1 mL, 2 mL tubexes and 20 mL, 50 mL vials. **Syringe:** No further dilution required. **Infusion:** Further dilute to physician specified volume in compatible IV solution to a final concentration not greater than 10 mg/mL (up to 12.5 mg/mL). 50 mg/mL has been used for intermittent administration.

STABILITY/STORAGE
Vial: Store at room temperature. **Infusion:** Prepare concentrated solutions just prior to administration. Stable for 12 hr.

ADMINISTRATION
General: Restrict IV use to conditions when other routes are not feasible. Patient should be on ventilator support with doses for therapeutic coma induction. Avoid perivascular extravasation or intra-arterial injection due to the highly alkaline nature of the drug. Use a separate IV line for concentrated infusions; avoid administration of any other drugs through that line. **IV Push:** May administer direct IV push at a rate not to exceed 50 mg/min. **Intermittent Infusion:** May infuse over 10–30 min. Not to exceed 50 mg/

min. **Continuous Infusion:** May infuse continuously at physician specified rate. Not to exceed 50 mg/min.

COMPATIBILITY
Solution: Dextrose solutions, lactated Ringer's, Ringer's injection, sodium chloride solutions. **Syringe:** Aminophylline, ephedrine, hydromorphone, neostigmine, scopolamine, sodium bicarbonate, thiopental. **Y-site:** Acyclovir, insulin.

INCOMPATIBILITY
Syringe: Benzquinamide, butorphanol, chlorpromazine, cimetidine, dimenhydrinate, diphenhydramine, droperidol, fentanyl, glycopyrrolate, meperidine, midazolam, nalbuphine, pentazocine, perphenazine, prochlorperazine, promethazine, ranitidine.

ADVERSE EFFECTS
CNS: <u>CNS depression</u>, agitation, ataxia, confusion, hallucinations, hyperkinesia, insomnia, lethargy, paradoxical excitement, <u>somnolence</u>. **CV:** Bradycardia, hypotension, syncope. **Resp:** APNEA, BRONCHOSPASM, hypoventilation, LARYNGOSPASM, respiratory depression. **GI:** Constipation, diarrhea, nausea, vomiting. **MS:** Arthritic/myalgic/neuralgic pain. **Heme:** Agranulocytosis, megaloblastic anemia, thrombocytopenia. **Hypersens:** Angioneurotic edema, morbilliform rash, rash. **Other:** Arterial spasm (with inadvertent arterial administration), thrombophlebitis.

TOXICITY/OVERDOSE
Signs/Symptoms: CNS and respiratory depression that may progress to Cheynes-Stokes respiration, areflexia, pupillary constriction, olig-

In the Adverse Effects section, <u>underline</u> indicates most frequent; CAPS indicates life threatening.

uria, tachycardia, hypotension, coma. **Treatment:** Symptomatic and supportive treatment, hemodialysis may be beneficial in severe intoxication, anuria, or shock.

DRUG INTERACTIONS

Acetaminophen, beta blockers, corticosteroids, digitoxin, doxycycline, oral anticoagulants, oral contraceptives, quinidine, rifampin, theophylline, tricyclic antidepressants: Pentobarbital decreases the effects of these agents. **Alcohol, anesthetics, antihistamines, chloramphenicol, CNS depressants, monoamine oxidase inhibitors, valproic acid:** Increased pentobarbital effects. **Phenytoin:** Unpredictable effect on phenytoin metabolism.

NURSING CONSIDERATIONS

Assessment
General:
Vital signs, signs/symptoms of hypersensitivity, history of chemical dependency.
Physical:
Mental status (especially children/elderly), cardiopulmonary status (respiratory depression/barbiturate toxicity/coma).
Lab Alterations:
Assess hematologic profile.

Intervention/Rationale
Respiratory depression can precede potentially fatal reactions requiring discontinuation. ● Monitor patient closely for development of symptomatic bradycardia. ● Prolonged use may result in physical dependency: Do not withdraw abruptly. ● Assure patient safety secondary to mental status changes (side rails raised, help with ambulation).

Patient/Family Education
Increased dreaming may be experienced when drug is discontinued. Avoid activities requiring mental alertness. Change positions gradually. Call for help with ambulation activities. Notify physician if any signs of fever, sore throat, mouth sores, easy bruising/bleeding occur. Avoid alcohol or other agents not prescribed by physician. Explain rationale/outcome of therapeutic pentobarbital coma.

PENTOSTATIN
(pen-toe-stat'-in)
Trade Name(s): Nipent
Classification(s): Antineoplastic antibiotic
Pregnancy Category: D

PHARMACODYNAMICS/KINETICS
Mechanism of Action: Unknown antitumor effect. Inhibits enzyme adenosine deaminase resulting in cytotoxic effect on tumor DNA and RNA. **Distribution:** Distributed to a large extent into kidneys. Little CNS penetration. 4% plasma protein bound. **Metabolism/Elimination:** Primarily excreted unchanged by kidneys. **Half-Life:** 5.7 hr. Prolonged in renal impairment.

INDICATIONS/DOSAGE

Treatment of alpha-interferon refractory hairy cell leukemia
Adult: 4 mg/m^2 every other week. Temporarily hold if absolute neutrophil count < 200 cells/mm^3; resume therapy when count returns to predose levels.

In the Adverse Effects section, underline indicates most frequent; CAPS indicates life threatening.

397

CONTRAINDICATIONS/ PRECAUTIONS

Contraindicated in: Hypersensitivity. **Use cautiously in:** Myelosuppression, renal impairment. **Pregnancy/Lactation:** Causes fetal harm. No well-controlled trials to establish safety. Benefits must outweigh risks. **Pediatrics:** Safety and efficacy in children/adolescents not established.

PREPARATION

Availability: 10 mg powder for injection vials. **Reconstitution:** Dilute each 10 mg vial with 5 mL sterile water for injection for a final concentration of 2 mg/mL. **Syringe:** No further dilution required. **Infusion:** May be diluted in 25–50 mL compatible IV solution.

STABILITY/STORAGE

Vial: Store at refrigerated temperatures. Reconstituted vials stable at room temperature for 8 hr. **Infusion:** Use within 8 hr (no preservative).

ADMINISTRATION

General: Hydrate with 500–1000 mL of IV solution prior to and an additional 500 mL following administration. **IV Push/Intermittent Infusion:** Give over 20–30 min.

COMPATIBILITY

Solution: Dextrose solutions, sodium chloride solutions.

ADVERSE EFFECTS

CNS: <u>Headache</u>, anxiety, confusion, depression, dizziness, somnolence. **Ophtho:** Eye pain, abnormal vision. **CV:** Abnormal ECG, dysrhythmias. **Resp:** PLEURAL EFFUSION, LUNG FIBROSIS, <u>cough</u>, <u>upper respiratory infection</u>, dyspnea, pneumo-

nia. **GI:** Hepatitis, <u>nausea</u>, <u>vomiting</u>, anorexia, diarrhea, stomatitis, elevated liver function tests (reversible). **GU:** Dysuria, hematuria, urinary hesitancy/frequency. **Renal:** Increased BUN/creatinine. **MS:** Arthralgia, myalgia. **Derm:** Alopecia, skin discoloration, herpes simplex/zoster. **Fld/Lytes:** Hyponatremia. **Heme:** <u>Leukopenia</u>, <u>anemia</u>, thrombocytopenia, hemorrhage. **Hypersens:** <u>Rash</u>. **Metab:** Metabolic acidosis. **Other:** <u>Fatigue</u>, <u>fever</u>, <u>chills</u>, peripheral edema, thrombophlebitis, weight loss.

TOXICITY/OVERDOSE

Signs/Symptoms: Death associated with severe CNS, hepatic, pulmonary, and renal toxicity. **Treatment:** Symptomatic and supportive.

DRUG INTERACTIONS

Allopurinol: Increased skin rash incidence. **Fludarabine:** Increased fatal pulmonary toxicity. **Vidarabine:** Increased adverse effects.

NURSING CONSIDERATIONS

Assessment

General:
Vital signs, intake/output ratio.
Physical:
Cardiopulmonary status, neurologic status, GI tract, hematopoietic system, infectious disease status.
Lab Alterations:
Assess CBC with differential and platelet count, BUN, serum creatinine and liver function prior to and throughout course of therapy.

Intervention/Rationale

Assess for development of fever, chills, or other signs of infection

In the Adverse Effects section, <u>underline</u> indicates most frequent; CAPS indicates life threatening.

and notify physician immediately. ● Maintain adequate hydration prior to and during therapy. ● Assess patient for development of bleeding (bleeding gums, easy bruising, hematest positive stools/ urine/vomitus). ● Avoid intramuscular injections and rectal temperatures. ● If nausea becomes a problem, antiemetics may be administered 0.5 hr prior to administration.

Patient/Family Education
Observe for signs of infection (fever, sore throat, fatigue) or bleeding (melena, hematuria, nosebleeds, easy bruising). Take and record oral temperature daily and report persistent elevation to physician. Use a soft toothbrush and electric razor to minimize bleeding tendency. Avoid crowded environments and persons with known infections. Use reliable contraception throughout the duration of therapy and 4 months following due to potential teratogenic and mutagenic effects of drug. Seek physician approval prior to receiving live virus vaccinations. Avoid over-the-counter products containing aspirin or ibuprofen due to increased potential for bleeding. Report dizziness, unusual fatigue, or shortness of breath (drug may cause anemia).

PERPHENAZINE
(per-fen′-a-zeen)
Trade Name(s): Trilafon
Classification(s): Antiemetic, phenothiazine antipsychotic
Pregnancy Category: Unknown

PHARMACODYNAMICS/KINETICS
Mechanism of Action: Blocks postsynaptic dopamine receptors in the brain. As antiemetic, inhibits the medullary chemoreceptor trigger zone. **Onset of Action:** Immediate. **Distribution:** Widely distributed into tissues/fluids with high concentrations in brain, lung, liver, kidneys, spleen. Highly bound to plasma proteins. **Metabolism/Elimination:** Extensively hepatically metabolized to inactive metabolites that are eliminated in urine and feces. **Half-Life:** 10–20 hr.

INDICATIONS/DOSAGE

Control of severe nausea and vomiting; relief of intractable hiccoughs
Adult: Fractional 1 mg doses administered at not less than 1–2 min intervals up to a total dose of 5 mg.

CONTRAINDICATIONS/ PRECAUTIONS
Contraindicated in: Blood dyscrasias, bone marrow depression, cerebral arteriosclerosis, comatose or severely depressed patients, coronary artery disease, high doses concurrent CNS depressants, liver damage, phenothiazine hypersensitivity, severe hypotension/hypertension. **Use cautiously in:** Patients predisposed to hypotension, seizure history, hepatic/renal impairment, elderly patients, sodium bisulfite sensitivity. **Pregnancy/Lactation:** No well-controlled trials to establish safety. Benefits must outweigh risks. No placenta transfer of drug. Use near term may cause maternal hypotension and/or neonatal extrapyramidal effects, hyper/hy-

P

In the Adverse Effects section, <u>underline</u> indicates most frequent; CAPS indicates life threatening.

399

poreflexia, jaundice. **Pediatrics:** Safety and efficacy is not established in children less than 12 years old.

PREPARATION
Availability: 5 mg/mL in 1 mL amps. **Syringe:** Dilute 1 mL with 9 mL 0.9% sodium chloride for a final concentration 0.5 mg/mL. **Infusion:** Dilute to physician specified volume of compatible IV solutions.

STABILITY/STORAGE
Vial: Store at room temperature. Protect from light. **Infusion:** Prepare just prior to administration. Protect from light. Slight yellow discoloration will not affect potency/efficacy (marked discoloration requires discarding the vial).

ADMINISTRATION
General: Reserve IV use for hospitalized, recumbent patients when alternative routes not feasible. Discontinue IV administration as soon as symptoms are controlled. **IV Push:** Administer not more than 1 mg per injection slowly. **Intermittent Infusion:** Infuse slowly at physician specified rate. Preferred route in the surgical patient.

COMPATIBILITY
Solution: Dextrose solutions, sodium chloride solutions. **Syringe:** Atropine, butorphanol, chlorpromazine, cimetidine, dimenhydrinate, diphenhydramine, droperidol, fentanyl, meperidine, metoclopramide, morphine, pentazocine, prochlorperazine, promethazine, ranitidine, scopolamine. **Y-site:** Acyclovir, amikacin, ampicillin, cefamandole, cefazolin, ceforanide, cefotaxime, cefoxitin, cefuroxime, cephalothin, cephapirin, chloramphenicol, clindamycin, doxycycline, erythromycin, famotidine, gentamicin, kanamycin, metronidazole, mezlocillin, moxalactam, nafcillin, oxacillin, penicillin G, piperacillin, ticarcillin, ticarcillin/clavulanate, tobramycin, trimethoprim-sulfamethoxazole, vancomycin.

INCOMPATIBILITY
Syringe: Midazolam, pentobarbital. **Y-site:** Cefoperazone.

ADVERSE EFFECTS
CNS: Ataxia, cerebral edema, dizziness, drowsiness, extrapyramidal effects (pseudoparkinsonism, dystonias, akathesia), headache, paresthesia, tardive dyskinesia, tremor. **Ophtho:** Blurred vision, glaucoma, lenticular opacities, miosis, mydriasis, photophobia. **CV:** CARDIAC ARREST, CIRCULATORY COLLAPSE, VENTRICULAR DYSRHYTHMIAS, CHF, bradycardia, hypertension, <u>hypotension</u>, syncope, tachycardia. **GI:** Constipation, dry mouth, jaundice, nausea, vomiting. **Derm:** Dry skin, eczema, hair loss, photosensitivity. **Endo:** Galactorrhea, hypo/hyperglycemia, syndrome of inappropriate antidiuretic hormone (SIADH). **Heme:** AGRANULOCYTOSIS, anemia, APLASTIC ANEMIA, eosinophilia, leukocytosis, leukopenia, PANCYTOPENIA, thrombocytopenia. **Hypersens:** Pruritus, urticaria. **Other:** Heat stroke, NEUROLEPTIC MALIGNANT SYNDROME, SUDDEN DEATH.

TOXICITY/OVERDOSE
Signs/Symptoms: CNS depression, hypotension, extrapyramidal symptoms. **Treatment:** Symptomatic and supportive treatment.

In the Adverse Effects section, <u>underline</u> indicates most frequent; CAPS indicates life threatening.

DRUG INTERACTIONS
Alcohol: Increased CNS depression. **Anticholinergics:** Decreased phenothiazine effects; increased anticholinergic effects. **Barbiturates:** Decreased phenothiazine pharmacologic effects. **Barbiturate anesthetics:** Increased neuromuscular excitation and hypotension. **Bromocriptine:** Inhibits bromocriptine efficacy. **Epinephrine, norepinephrine:** Decreased pressor effect and peripheral vasoconstrictive effects. **Guanethidine:** Inhibits hypotensive effect. **Lithium:** Increased disorientation, extrapyramidal effects. **Phenytoin:** Alteration in phenytoin serum levels. **Propranolol:** Increased plasma levels of both drugs. **Tricyclic antidepressants:** Increased TCA serum concentration.

NURSING CONSIDERATIONS
Assessment
General:
Lying/standing blood pressure, vital signs, ECG (recommended), intake/output ratio.

Physical:
Respiratory status, GI tract, neurologic status.

Lab Alterations:
Increased/altered liver function tests, false-positive/negative urine bilirubin, false-positive/negative urine pregnancy test, increased protein bound iodine (unrelated to increased thyroxine).

Intervention/Rationale
Maintain supine position during therapy. ● Drug may cause depressed cough/gag reflex. ● May cause constipation with prolonged use or mask diagnosis of intestinal obstruction. ● Evaluate patient for development of extrapyramidal symptoms (drooling, rigidity, shuffling gait, tremors) or symptoms of tardive dyskinesia (rhythmical involuntary movements of tongue, face, jaw or mouth, protrusion of the tongue, or chewing-like movements). ● After abrupt withdrawal of long-term therapy, assess for dizziness, feelings of warmth/cold, gastritis, headache, insomnia, nausea, sweating, tachycardia, and/or vomiting.

Patient/Family Education
Dry mouth occurs frequently and may be relieved by sugar free candy/gum or frequent oral care. Notify physician immediately if jaundice, fever, sore throat, cellulitis, or weakness becomes apparent (symptoms of developing blood dyscrasias). Report urinary retention and/or constipation. Wear sunscreen/protective clothing while outside to avoid photosensitivity reactions. Change positions slowly and seek assistance with ambulatory functions to prevent orthostatic hypotension. Avoid alcohol or other CNS depressants.

PHENOBARBITAL
(fee-noe-bar′-bi-tal)
Trade Name(s): Luminal
Classification(s): Barbiturate, sedative/hypnotic
Pregnancy Category: D
Controlled Substance Schedule: IV

In the Adverse Effects section, underline indicates most frequent; CAPS indicates life threatening.

401

PHARMACODYNAMICS/KINETICS

Mechanism of Action: Central nervous system depression of sensory cortex, motor activity, and cerebellar function. **Onset of Action:** 5 min. **Peak Effect:** 30 min. **Duration of Action:** 4–6 hr (hypnotic doses 6–10 hr). **Therapeutic Serum Levels:** 10–40 mcg/mL. **Distribution:** Rapidly distributed to all tissues/fluids with high concentrations in brain/liver. 20%–45% bound to plasma proteins (due to high lipid solubility). **Metabolism/Elimination:** Primarily metabolized by the liver to an inactive metabolite. 25% excreted in urine as unchanged drug, 75% as inactive metabolite. **Half-Life:** 2–6 days.

INDICATIONS/DOSAGE

Individualize dosage, reduce dosage for elderly and debilitated patients.

Sedation

Adult: 100–130 mg. Not to exceed 600 mg/24 hr. *Pediatric:* 2–3 mg/kg/dose (IV not recommended).

Anticonvulsant

Keep IV dosage to a minimum to avoid excessive CNS depression following seizures.

Adult: 200–300 mg initially. Repeat, if necessary, after 6 hr. Alternate dosage 300–800 mg initially, then 120–240 mg every 20 minutes as needed. Not to exceed 1–2 g/24 hr. *Pediatric:* 15–20 mg/kg; then 6 mg/kg every 20 minutes as needed. Alternate dosage 3–5 mg/kg/day every 12–24 hr. Not to exceed 40 mg/kg/24 hr. *Neonate:* 15–20 mg/kg. Then 4–5 mg/kg/day every 12–24 hr. Not to exceed 40 mg/kg/24 hr.

CONTRAINDICATIONS/PRECAUTIONS

Contraindicated in: Barbiturate sensitivity, patients with porphyria or severe liver impairment, presence of severe acute/chronic pain. **Use cautiously in:** Severe respiratory distress when administering large doses. **Pregnancy/Lactation:** Known teratogenic effects. May cause fetal damage/abnormalities. Benefits must outweigh risks. Readily crosses placenta. Full doses decrease the force and frequency of uterine contractions. Neonatal coagulation defects may occur within 24 hr of birth following maternal ingestion for convulsions. Small amounts distributed into breast milk; drowsiness in infants reported. **Pediatrics:** May produce paradoxical irritability, excitability, and aggression. Hyperkinetic states may be induced/aggravated.

PREPARATION

Availability: 30 mg/mL in 1 mL tubex. 60 mg/mL in 1 mL tubex. 65 mg/mL in 1 mL vial. 130 mg/mL in 1 mL vial/syringe. 120 mg sterile powder vial. **Reconstitution:** Dilute 120 mg sterile powder with at least 10 mL sterile water for injection. **Syringe:** No further dilution required. May dilute in an equal volume of compatible diluent. **Infusion:** May further dilute in small volume of compatible IV solution as per physician's order.

STABILITY/STORAGE

Vial: Store at room temperature. **Infusion:** Not generally considered sta-

In the Adverse Effects section, underline indicates most frequent; CAPS indicates life threatening.

ble in solution. Prepare just prior to administration.

ADMINISTRATION
General: Restrict IV use to conditions when other routes are not feasible. Patient should be under close supervision when administering. Avoid perivascular extravasation and intra-arterial injection due to the highly alkaline nature of the drug. **IV Push:** May administer undiluted or diluted by IV push. Not to exceed 60 mg/min in adults or 30 mg/min (or 2 mg/kg/min) in children. **Intermittent Infusion:** Not to exceed 60 mg/min in adults or 2 mg/kg/min in children.

COMPATIBILITY
Solution: Dextrose solutions, lactated Ringer's, Ringer's injection, sodium chloride solutions. **Syringe:** Heparin.

INCOMPATIBILITY
Syringe: Benzquinamide, ranitidine.

ADVERSE EFFECTS
CNS: Agitation, ataxia, <u>CNS depression</u>, confusion, hallucinations, hyperkinesia, insomnia, lethargy, paradoxical excitement, <u>somnolence</u>. **CV:** Bradycardia, hypotension, syncope. **Resp:** APNEA, BRONCHOSPASM, hypoventilation, LARYNGOSPASM, respiratory depression. **GI:** Constipation, diarrhea, nausea, vomiting. **MS:** Arthritic/myalgic/neuralgic pain. **Heme:** Agranulocytosis, megaloblastic anemia, thrombocytopenia. **Hypersens:** Angioneurotic edema, morbilliform rash, rash. **Other:** Arterial spasm (with inadvertent arterial administration), thrombophlebitis.

TOXICITY/OVERDOSE
Signs/Symptoms: CNS and respiratory depression that may progress to Cheyne-Stokes respiration, areflexia, pupillary constriction, oliguria, tachycardia, hypotension, coma. **Treatment:** Symptomatic and supportive treatment. Alkalinization of urine/increasing urinary flow will substantially increase the rate of excretion. Hemodialysis may be beneficial in severe intoxication, anuria, or shock.

DRUG INTERACTIONS
Acetaminophen, beta blockers, corticosteroids, digitoxin, doxycycline, oral anticoagulants, oral contraceptives, quinidine, rifampin, theophylline, tricyclic antidepressants: Phenobarbital decreases the effects of these agents. **Alcohol, anesthetics, antihistamines, chloramphenicol, CNS depressants, monoamine oxidase inhibitors, valproic acid:** Increased phenobarbital effects. **Phenytoin:** Unpredictable effect on phenytoin metabolism.

NURSING CONSIDERATIONS
Assessment
General:
Vital signs, signs/symptoms of hypersensitivity, history of chemical dependency.
Physical:
Mental status (especially children/elderly), pulmonary status (respiratory depression/barbiturate toxicity/coma).
Lab Alterations:
Assess hematologic profile.

Intervention/Rationale
Respiratory depression can precede potentially fatal reactions

P

In the Adverse Effects section, <u>underline</u> indicates most frequent; CAPS indicates life threatening.

403

requiring discontinuation. ● Prolonged use may result in physical dependency: Do not withdraw abruptly. ● Assure patient safety secondary to mental status changes (side rails raised, help with ambulation).

Patient/Family Education
Increased dreaming may be experienced when drug is discontinued. Avoid activities requiring mental alertness. Change positions gradually. Call for help with ambulation activities. Notify physician if any signs of fever, sore throat, mouth sores, easy bruising/bleeding occur. Avoid alcohol or other agents not prescribed by physician.

PHENTOLAMINE
(fen-tole'-a-meen)
Trade Name(s): Regitine, Rogitine ♣
Classification(s): Antihypertensive
Pregnancy Category: Unknown

PHARMACODYNAMICS/KINETICS
Mechanism of Action: Alpha adrenergic blockade of presynaptic and postsynaptic receptors. Acts on the arterial and venous systems resulting in lower total peripheral resistance and venous return. Competitive antagonism of endogenous and exogenous alpha-active agents. **Onset of Action:** Immediate. **Duration of Action:** 5–10 min. **Distribution:** Unknown. **Metabolism/Elimination:** 10% eliminated in urine as active drug; the remainder is unknonw. **Half-Life:** 19 min.

INDICATIONS/DOSAGE

Preoperative prevention/control of hypertensive episodes in pheochromocytoma
Adult: 2.5–5.0 mg. Repeat every 5 min if necessary until hypertension is controlled, then every 2–4 hr as needed. Alternate dosage 5 mg 1–2 hr prior to surgery and repeat if necessary. *Pediatric:* 1 mg or 0.05–0.1 mg/kg/dose. Repeat every 5 minutes if necessary until hypertension is controlled, then every 2–4 hr as needed. Alternate dosage 1 mg or 0.05–0.1 mg/kg/dose 1–2 hr prior to surgery; repeat if necessary.

Diagnosis of pheochromocytoma (not the method of choice)
Adult: 2.5 mg (less false-positive tests and hypotension) or 5 mg. If negative results with 2.5 mg, administer 5 mg. *Pediatric:* 1 mg or 0.1 mg/kg or 3 mg/m².

Prevention of dermal necrosis/sloughing from dopamine/norepinephrine
Adult/Pediatric: 10 mg/L may be added to dopamine/norepinephrine IV solution (pressor effect of agent is not affected).

Treatment of hypertensive crisis secondary to MAO inhibitors/sympathomimetic amines; rebound hypertension to clonidine, propranolol, other antihypertensives (*unlabeled use*)
Adult: 5–10 mg.

Treatment of left ventricular failure secondary to acute MI (*unlabeled use*)
Adult: 0.17–0.4 mg/min.

In the Adverse Effects section, <u>underline</u> indicates most frequent; CAPS indicates life threatening.

CONTRAINDICATIONS/ PRECAUTIONS

Contraindicated in: Angina/coronary artery disease evidence, hypersensitivity to phentolamine or related compounds, MI. **Pregnancy/Lactation:** No well-controlled trials to establish safety. Benefits must outweigh risks.

PREPARATION

Availability: 5 mg in 1 mL vial with 25 mg mannitol. **Reconstitution:** Dilute with 1 mL sterile water for injection or 0.9% sodium chloride for a final concentration of 5 mg/mL. For diagnosis of pheochromocytoma, dilute with 1 mL sterile water for injection. **Syringe:** No further dilution required. **Infusion:** For sloughing prevention, add to 1 L compatible IV solution for 0.01 mg/mL concentration.

STABILITY/STORAGE

Vial: Stable at room temperature. Reconstituted solution should be used immediately. Solutions are stable for 48 hr at room temperature and 1 week refrigerated. Stable for 24 hr at room temperature in syringe. **Infusion:** Prepare just prior to administration. Stable for 1 week at room temperature in 0.9% sodium chloride.

ADMINISTRATION

IV Push: Administer by direct IV push undiluted. For diagnosis of pheochromocytoma, insert needle into a vein and delay injection until pressor response has subsided (stabilized blood pressure taken every 10 min for 30 min); inject rapidly; record blood pressure at 30 sec intervals for first 3 min, then 60 sec intervals for the next 7 min.

COMPATIBILITY

Solution: Sodium chloride solutions. **Syringe:** Papaverine. **Y-site:** Amiodarone.

ADVERSE EFFECTS

CNS: Dizziness. **CV:** <u>Acute/prolonged hypotensive episodes</u>, dysrhythmias, orthostatic hypotension, <u>tachycardia</u>. **GI:** Diarrhea, nausea, vomiting. **Other:** Flushing, nasal stuffiness, weakness.

TOXICITY/OVERDOSE

Signs/Symptoms: Extension of adverse effects. **Treatment:** Symptomatic and supportive; epinephrine is contraindicated because of alpha/beta stimulation. **Antidote(s):** Norepinephrine to maintain normal blood pressure.

DRUG INTERACTIONS

Ephedrine, epinephrine: Vasoconstrive and hypertensive effects of these agents are antagonized by phentolamine.

NURSING CONSIDERATIONS

Assessment
General:
Vital signs.
Physical:
Cardiovascular system, GI tract.
Lab Alterations:
Evaluate urinary catecholamines (pheochromocytoma diagnosis).

Intervention/Rationale
Monitor blood pressure closely during administration. Keep patient in supine position.
For Diagnosis of Pheochromocytoma:
Withhold nonessential sedatives, analgesics and other medications

P

In the Adverse Effects section, <u>underline</u> indicates most frequent; CAPS indicates life threatening.

405

for 24 hr prior to testing. Withhold antihypertensives until blood pressure returns to untreated levels. Do not perform test on normotensive patients. Keep patient at rest in supine position throughout testing. Positive response is indicated by a drop in blood pressure of more than 35 mm Hg systolic and 25 mm Hg diastolic (usually 60 mm Hg systolic and 25 mm HG diastolic). Maximal blood pressure decrease evident within 2 min after injection. Return to preinjection blood pressure occurs within 15–30 min. Positive response must be confirmed by measurement of urinary catecholamines/metabolites or other diagnostic procedures.

Patient/Family Education
Maintain reclining position during treatment. Avoid rapid position changes following administration.

PHENYLEPHRINE
(fen-il-eff'-rin)
Trade Name(s): Neo-Synephrine
Classification(s): Vasopressor
Pregnancy Category: C

PHARMACODYNAMICS/KINETICS
Mechanism of Action: Direct postsynaptic alpha receptor stimulant resulting in peripheral vasoconstriction. Little effect on beta receptors. **Onset of Action:** Immediate. **Duration of Action:** 15–20 min. **Distribution:** Widely distributed into tissues. **Metabolism/Elimination:** Pharmacologic effects terminated in tissues. Primarily metabolized by liver and in intestines by monoamine oxidase. The final route of elimination has

not been determined. **Half-Life:** 2–3 hr.

INDICATIONS/DOSAGE

Treatment of mild to moderate hypotension
Adult: 0.2 mg (0.1–0.5 mg). Not to exceed an initial dose of 5 mg. Do not repeat more frequently than every 10–15 min. *Pediatric:* 5–20 mcg/kg/dose every 10–15 min. Do not repeat more frequently than every 10–15 min.

Treatment of severe hypotension or shock
Adult: 0.1–0.18 mg/min and titrate to desired effect. Usual maintenance dose of 0.04–0.06 mg/min is adequate when blood pressure is stabilized. *Pediatric:* 0.1–0.5 mcg/kg/min. Titrate to desired effect.

Emergency treatment of hypotension during spinal anesthesia
Adult: 0.2 mg. Subsequent doses should not exceed the preceding dose by more than 0.1–0.2 mg. Not to exceed 0.5 mg/dose.

Treatment of paroxysmal supraventricular tachycardia
Adult: 0.25–0.5 mg/dose. Subsequent doses should not exceed the preceding dose by more than 0.1–0.2 mg. Not to exceed 1 mg/dose. *Pediatric:* 5–10 mcg/kg/dose. Subsequent doses should not exceed the preceding dose by more than 0.05–0.1 mg. Not to exceed 1 mg/dose.

Prolongation of spinal anesthesia
Adult: 2–5 mg added to anesthetic solution.

In the Adverse Effects section, <u>underline</u> indicates most frequent;
CAPS indicates life threatening.

Vasoconstriction for regional anesthesia

Adult: 1 mg added to each 20 mL local anesthetics.

CONTRAINDICATIONS/ PRECAUTIONS

Contraindicated in: Hypersensitivity to phenylephrine, severe hypertension, ventricular tachycardia. **Use cautiously in:** Bradycardia, elderly patients, hyperthyroidism, myocardial disease, partial heart block, severe arteriosclerosis, patients sensitive to sodium bisulfite. **Pregnancy/ Lactation:** No well-controlled trials to establish safety. Benefits must outweigh risks. May cause uterine contractions and constriction uterine blood vessels.

PREPARATION

Availability: 1% (10 mg/mL) in 1 mL amps. **Syringe:** Dilute to 0.1–1.0 mg/mL with compatible IV solution. Dilute 1 mL 1% with 9 mL sterile water for injection. **Infusion:** Dilute to 0.02–0.1 mg/mL with compatible IV solution based on patient's individual requirements. Usually 10 mg (1 mL) added to 250 mL or 500 mL results in a final concentration of 1:25,000 or 1:50,000 solution, respectively. If prompt initial vasopressor response is not obtained, add additional increments of drug (10 mg or more) to infusion.

STABILITY/STORAGE

Vial: Store at room temperature. **Infusion:** Stable for 48 hr at room temperature.

ADMINISTRATION

General: Avoid extravasation. Ante-cubital fossa veins are preferred to minimize extravasation potential. **IV Push:** May administer direct IV push as diluted solution over 1 minute. For treatment of paroxysmal supraventricular tachycardia, give diluted solution over 20–30 sec. **Continuous Infusion:** Adjust flow rate until desired effect is obtained. **Adult:** Administer as per physician specified rate. **Pediatric:** To calculate the rate:

0.3 mg/kg × wt (kg)
equals mg added to 50 mL
-OR-
1.5 mg/kg × wt (kg)
equals mg added to 250 mL
Then infuse at 0.1 × mL/hr
equals mcg/kg/min.

COMPATIBILITY

Solution: Dextrose solutions, lactated Ringer's, Ringer's injection, sodium chloride solutions. **Y-site:** Amiodarone, amrinone, famotidine, zidovudine.

ADVERSE EFFECTS

CNS: Excitability, headache, restlessness, tremor. **CV:** Dysrhythmias, peripheral/visceral vasoconstriction, reflex bradycardia. **Resp:** RESPIRATORY DISTRESS. **Renal:** Decreased renal perfusion. **Derm:** Pallor, pilomotor response, tissue necrosis.

TOXICITY/OVERDOSE

Signs/Symptoms: Ventricular extrasystole, ventricular tachycardia, sensation of head fullness, tingling of extremities. **Treatment:** Symptomatic and supportive treatment. **Antidote(s):** Alpha adrenergic blocking agent (phentolamine) to relieve excess elevation of blood pressure. If extravasation, infiltrate site with

In the Adverse Effects section, underline indicates most frequent; CAPS indicates life threatening.

407

phentolamine, 5–10 mg in 10–15 mL saline within 12 hr.

DRUG INTERACTIONS
Alpha adrenergic blockers: Antagonizes vasopressor effects. **Atropine:** Blocks bradycardia from phenylephrine and enhances pressor effect. **Bretylium:** Potentiation of vasopressor action and arrhythmogenic potential. **Digitalis glycosides, halogenated hydrocarbon anesthetics:** Sensitizes myocardium to catecholamine effects. **Diuretics:** Decreased arterial responsiveness to pressors. **Ergot alkaloids, monoamine oxidase inhibitors:** Enhanced adrenergic effects phenylephrine and increased pressor response. **Guanethidine:** Increased pressor response and hypertension. **Oxytocin:** Produces severe persistent hypertension. **Tricyclic antidepressants:** Altered sensitivity to phenylephrine.

NURSING CONSIDERATIONS
Assessment
General:
Blood pressure (continuous during first 5 minutes, then every 3–5 min until stabilized), continuous ECG, respiratory rate, signs/symptoms of hypersensitivity, intake/output ratio.
Physical:
Cardiopulmonary status.
Lab Alterations:
Monitor baseline and periodic renal function studies.

Intervention/Rationale
Monitor blood pressure closely until stabilized and thereafter during IV administration. ● Evaluate quality and depth of respirations (base-line and periodic). ● Evaluate patient carefully for development of central/peripheral vasoconstrictive effects.

Patient/Family Education
Notify physician/nurse of headache, dizziness, difficulty breathing, or pain at IV infusion site.

PHENYTOIN
(fen'-i-toyn)
Trade Name(s): Dilantin
Classification(s): Antiarrhythmic, anticonvulsant
Pregnancy Category: Unknown

PHARMACODYNAMICS/KINETICS
Mechanism of Action: Inhibition of seizure activity transmission at the motor cortex. Stabilizes the threshold against hyperexcitability by promotion of sodium efflux from neurons. Prolongs the effective refractory period. **Therapeutic Serum Levels:** Within 1–2 hr. 10–20 mcg/mL. Free phenytoin 1–2 mcg/mL. **Distribution:** Unknown. 95% protein bound. Hepatic/renal impairment decreases binding and increases free phenytoin serum levels. **Metabolism/Elimination:** Primarily hepatically metabolized to an inactive metabolite (60%–75%) that undergoes enterohepatic circulation (subject to saturation producing significant increases in serum levels with small increases in dosage). **Half-Life:** 22 hr.

INDICATIONS/DOSAGE
Adjust dosage based on serum levels and in hepatic impairment.

In the Adverse Effects section, <u>underline</u> indicates most frequent; CAPS indicates life threatening.

408

Status epilepticus

Oral therapy should be instituted as soon as possible.

Adult: 15–20 mg/kg or 150–250 mg. Repeat 100–150 mg at 30 minute intervals. Not to exceed 1.5 g in 24 hr. *Pediatric/Neonate:* 15–20 mg/kg in divided doses of 5–10 mg/kg or 250 mg/m².

Seizure disorders

Adult: 15–18 mg/kg. Then 300–400 mg/day in divided doses every 12–24 hr. Not to exceed 1.5 g in 24 hr. *Pediatric:* 10–15 mg/kg. Then 4–7 mg/kg/day in divided doses every 12–24 hr. Not to exceed 20 mg/kg in 24 hr. *Neonate:* 15–20 mg/kg. Then 4–6 mg/kg/day in divided doses every 12–24 hr. Not to exceed 20 mg/kg in 24 hr.

Prophylactic control of seizures during neurosurgery

Adult: 100–200 mg at 4 hr intervals during surgery and the immediate postoperative period.

Cardiac dysrhythmias (refractory to conventional treatment or due to digitalis intoxication) (*unlabeled use*).

Adult: 50–100 mg. Repeat at 5 min intervals until dysrhythmia disappears, adverse effects occur, or a total of 1 g is given.

CONTRAINDICATIONS/ PRECAUTIONS

Contraindicated in: Adams-Stokes syndrome, hypersensitivity to hydantoins, second or third degree heart block, sinus bradycardia. **Use cautiously in:** Acute intermittent porphyria, hepatic impairment, SA node depression. **Pregnancy/Lactation:** No well-controlled trials to establish safety. Benefits must outweigh risks. Phenytoin may cause fetal damage; patients must be aware of the hazards of use and consider discontinuation during pregnancy. Serum levels should be monitored carefully (altered absorption and metabolism during pregnancy).

PREPARATION

Availability: 50 mg/mL in 2 mL and 5 mL amps/vials. Contains 46 mg phenytoin/mL and 0.2 mEq sodium/mL. Phenytoin sodium 100 mg is equivalent to 92 mg phenytoin. **Syringe:** No further dilution required. **Infusion:** Addition to IV solutions is not recommended due to lack of solubility and resultant precipitation. If necessary, further dilute in physician specified volume of sodium chloride only.

ADMINISTRATION

General: Flush needle or catheter with sodium chloride immediately before and after administration to avoid precipitation and irritation. **IV Push:** May be given undiluted IV push slowly at a rate not to exceed 50 mg/min in adults or 0.5 mg/kg/min in pediatrics. **Intermittent Infusion:** Not recommended. Not to exceed 50 mg/min or 0.5–1.5 mg/kg/min. An in-line filter may be used. Infusion should not last longer than 20–30 min. Assess the clarity of the infusion bag and tubing frequently for any precipitants.

COMPATIBILITY

Solution: Sodium chloride solutions (for a limited time/concentration

In the Adverse Effects section, underline indicates most frequent; CAPS indicates life threatening.

409

dependent). **Y-site:** Esmolol, famotidine, foscarnet.

INCOMPATIBILITY
Solution: Dextrose solutions, fat emlusion, lactated Ringer's. **Y-site:** Aminophylline, clindamycin, heparin, hydrocortisone, potassium chloride, vitamin B complex with C.

STABILITY/STORAGE
Vial: Store at room temperature. **Infusion:** Prepare just prior to administration. Stable for 20–30 min in sodium chloride (precipitation may still occur). A precipitate may form with refrigeration or freezing (dissolves when left at room temperature). A faint yellow discoloration may occur that has no effect on the potency.

ADVERSE EFFECTS
CNS: <u>Ataxia</u>, circumoral tingling, confusion, dizziness, <u>drowsiness</u>, dysarthria, <u>headache</u>, insomnia, motor twitching, nervousness, numbness, <u>nystagmus</u>, slurred speech, <u>tremor</u>, vertigo. **Ophtho:** Conjunctivitis, <u>diplopia</u>, photophobia. **CV:** VENTRICULAR FIBRILLATION, ATRIAL/VENTRICULAR CONDUCTION DEPRESSION, CARDIOVASCULAR COLLAPSE, chest pain, edema, <u>hypotension</u>. **Resp:** Acute pneumonitis, pulmonary fibrosis. **GI:** Toxic hepatitis, constipation, diarrhea, jaundice, nausea, vomiting. **MS:** Periarteritis nodosa, polyarthropathy. **Derm:** Alopecia, hirsutism. **Endo:** Hyperglycemia. **Heme:** AGRANULOCYTOSIS, anemia, eosinophilia, LEUKOPENIA, PANCYTOPENIA, THROMBOCYTOPENIA. **Hypersens:** Toxic epidermal necrolysis, <u>morbilliform</u> <u>rash</u>, urticaria. **Other:** Fever, gingival hyperplasia, weight gain.

TOXICITY/OVERDOSE
Signs/Symptoms: Nystagums, ataxia, dysarthria, comatose, pupils unresponsive, hypotension. **Treatment:** Symptomatic and supporting treatment, hemodialysis may be beneficial.

DRUG INTERACTIONS
Allopurinol, chloramphenicol, cimetidine, diazepam, disulfiram, ethanol, isoniazid, miconazole, phenylbutazone, succinimides, sulfonamides, trimethoprim, valproic acid: Increased phenytoin effect due to phenytoin metabolism inhibition. **Antineoplastics, folic acid, influenza virus vaccine, loxapine, nitrofurantoin, pyridoxine:** Decreased phenytoin effect. **Barbiturates, carbamazepine, diazoxide, ethanol (chronic), folic acid, theophylline:** Decreased phenytoin effect due to increased phenytoin metabolism. **Chlorpheniramine, ibuprofen, imipramine:** Increased phenytoin effect. **Corticosteroids, cyclosporine, dicumarol, digitoxin, disopyramide, doxycycline, estrogens, haloperidol, methadone, metyrapone, oral contraceptives, quinidine:** Increased metabolism by phenytoin. **Dopamine, furosemide, levodopa, metyrapone, sulfonylureas:** Decreased pharmacologic effect by phenytoin. **Lithium:** Increased lithium toxicity. **Meperidine:** Decreased analgesic effect; increased toxic effects. **Salicylates (dose dependent), valproic acid:** Increased phenytoin effect due to phenytoin displacement. **Tricyclic antidepressants:** Increased seizure potential.

In the Adverse Effects section, <u>underline</u> indicates most frequent; CAPS indicates life threatening.

NURSING CONSIDERATIONS

Assessment
General:
Vital signs, signs/symptoms of hypersensitivity reactions.

Physical:
Neurologic status, cardiopulmonary status, ophthalmologic status, dermatologic status, hematopoietic status.

Lab Alterations:
CBC with differential and platelet count. Phenytoin may interfere and produce lower than normal results with metyrapone and dexamethasone test: Avoid the use of phenytoin for 7 days prior to and during. Protein bound iodine may be suppressed by phenytoin without signs of hypothyroidism or low T3. Phenytoin may increase serum alkaline phosphatase or gamma glutamyl transferase. Phenytoin may cause slight decrease in urinary 17-hydroxycorticosteroids and 17-ketosteroids and increased 6-beta-hydroxycortisol excretion.

Intervention/Rationale
Monitor blood pressure before and after administration. Assess for the development of dysrhythmias (especially occurs with too rapid administration). ● Change to oral therapy as soon as possible. ● Assess for the development of diplopia, conjunctivitis, or photophobia. ● Evaluate neurologic status closely for the presence of ataxia, nystagmus, tremors, or headache. ● Periodically evaluate for the development of skin rash. ● Evaluate for bleeding tendencies, gingival hyperplasia, easy bruisability, and ecchymosis.

Patient/Family Education
Avoid activities requiring mental alertness. Avoid alcoholic beverages. Explain the importance of carrying identification describing medication usage and seizure type. May cause drowsiness, blurred vision, dizziness. Notify physician if any signs of rash, severe nausea/vomiting, swollen glands, bleeding/tender gums, sore throat, unexplained fever, unusual bleeding/bruising, headache, malaise, pregnancy. Do not take any other medications unless recommended by your physician.

PHYSOSTIGMINE
(fi-zoe-stig'-meen)
Trade Name(s): Antilirium
Classification(s): Anticholinesterase muscle stimulator, cholinergic agent
Pregnancy Category: Unknown

PHARMACODYNAMICS/KINETICS
Mechanism of Action: Inhibition of the destructive action of acetylcholinesterase on acetylcholine resulting in prolongation of peripheral and central acetylcholine effects. At high dosages, direct blocking action at autonomic ganglia and depolarization block. **Onset of Action:** 3–8 min. **Peak Effect:** 5 min. **Duration of Action:** 45–60 min (up to 5 hr). **Distribution:** Widely distributed throughout the body. Readily penetrates blood–brain barrier. **Metabolism/Elimination:** Rapidly hydrolyzed by cholinesterase. Small amounts excreted in urine. **Half-Life:** 15–40 min (up to 1–2 hr).

In the Adverse Effects section, underline indicates most frequent; CAPS indicates life threatening.

411

INDICATIONS/DOSAGE

Reversal of toxic CNS effects due to anticholinergic agents including tricyclic antidepressants, antihistamines, phenothiazine

Postanesthesia

Adult/Pediatric: Give twice the dose of atropine or scopolamine (on a weight basis) administered. *Adult:* 0.5–1.0 mg. Repeat at 10–30 min intervals if desired response is not obtained.

Overdosage of anticholinergic drugs

Adult: 0.5–2.0 mg. May repeat 1–4 mg at 30–60 min intervals if life-threatening signs such as dysrhythmia, convulsions, coma recur. *Pediatric:* Reserve usage for life-threatening situations. Not to exceed maximum total dose of 2 mg or 4 mg over 30 min. Repeat doses may be given until response occurs, adverse cholinergic effects, or maximum total dose is reached. 0.02 mg/kg; repeat at 5–10 min intervals. *Alternate Dosage:* 0.03 mg/kg or 0.9 mg/m² *Alternate Dosage:* 0.01–0.03 mg/kg/dose. May repeat once after 15–30 min if life-threatening signs such as dysrhythmia, convulsions, coma occur up to maximum total dose. *Alternate Dosage:* Test dose 0.5 mg. If toxic effects persist, 0.5 mg every 5 min. Maintenance Dose: Lowest effective dose or 0.02 mg/kg every 30–60 min if life-threatening signs/symptoms recur.

Stimulation peristalsis with postoperative intestinal atony (*unlabeled use*)

Adult: 0.5–2.0 mg.

CONTRAINDICATIONS/PRECAUTIONS

Contraindicated in: Asthma, cardiovascular disease, diabetes, gangrene, intestinal/urogenital obstruction, patients receiving choline esters or depolarizing neuromuscular blocking agents, vagotonic state. **Use cautiously in:** Bradycardia, epilepsy, parkinsonism, sodium bisulfite sensitivity. **Pregnancy/Lactation:** There have been no reports of congenital defects. Transient muscular weakness in neonates has been noted if mothers received treatment. Benefits must outweigh risks.

PREPARATION

Availability: 1 mg/mL in 1 mL syringe and 2 mL amps. Contains benzyl alcohol as preservative. **Syringe:** No further dilution required. If dilution is necessary, dose may be diluted further in 10 mL compatible IV solution.

STABILITY/STORAGE

Vial: Store at room temperature.

ADMINISTRATION

General: Must be given by slow IV push. Atropine should be available for use as an antidote. **IV Push:** May be given undiluted IV push slowly over 5 min at a rate not to exceed 1 mg/min adults or 0.5 mg/min children.

COMPATIBILITY

Solution: Dextrose solutions, sodium chloride solutions, sterile water for injection.

ADVERSE EFFECTS

CNS: Convulsions, ataxia (high doses), hallucinations, restlessness, tremor (high doses). **Ophtho:** Miosis. **CV:** Bradycardia, irregular heart rate, palpitations. **Resp:** RESPIRATORY PARALYSIS, BRONCHOSPASM, dyspnea, pulmonary edema. **GI:** Diarrhea, epigastric pain, nausea, vomiting. **MS:** Muscle weakness, twitching. **Other:** Lacrimation, salivation, sweating.

TOXICITY/OVERDOSE
Signs/Symptoms: Bradycardia, coma, confusion, diarrhea, hypertension, hypotension, miosis, muscle weakness, nausea, paralysis, excessive salivation, seizures, sweating, tachycardia, vomiting. **Treatment:** Mechanical ventilation with repeated bronchial aspiration, symptomatic and supportive. **Antidote(s):** Atropine sulfate every 3–10 min until control of cholinergic effects or atropine overdosage signs. Give 0.5 mg atropine for every 1 mg physostigmine **Adults:** 2–4 mg. **Children:** 1 mg. Pralidoxime may be useful for skeletal muscle and ganglionic effects of high doses if atropine is not effective.

DRUG INTERACTIONS
Choline esters, depolarizing neuromuscular blockers (decamethonium, succinylcholine): Antagonism of pharmacologic effect by physostigmine.

NURSING CONSIDERATIONS
Assessment
General:
Vital signs, ECG monitoring (recommended).
Physical:
Cardiopulmonary status, GI tract, neurologic status.

Intervention/Rationale
Assess vital signs frequently with special emphasis on respiratory pattern/rate. Maintain patent airway and keep well oxygenated/ventilated until complete recovery of normal respiratory status is ascertained. ● Observe closely for improvement in muscle strength, vision, and ptosis 45–60 min after each dose. ● Epinephrine should be available in order to counteract hypersensitivity. ● Evaluate for development of cholinergic crisis as manifested by increased GI stimulation with epigastric distress, abdominal cramps, vomiting, diarrhea, muscle fasiculation followed by paralysis. Atropine should be available as antidote. Discontinue drug if excessive salivation, emesis, frequent urination, or diarrhea occurs. Reduction of dosage may be necessary if excess sweating or nausea occurs. ● Evaluate for development of dysrhythmias and potential cardiopulmonary arrest.

Patient/Family Education
Notify physician if excess salivation, vomiting, diarrhea, or frequent urination occurs.

PHYTONADIONE
(fi-tone-a′-di-own)
Trade Name(s):
AquaMEPHYTON
Classification(s): Vitamin K
Pregnancy Category: C

PHARMACODYNAMICS/KINETICS
Mechanism of Action: Lipid soluble synthetic analogue of vitamin K that is responsible for synthesis of active prothrombin, proconvertin, plasma thromboplastin compo-

In the Adverse Effects section, <u>underline</u> indicates most frequent; CAPS indicates life threatening.

413

nent, and Stuart factor. **Onset of Action:** 3–6 hr (hemorrhage control), 12–14 hr (prothrombin normalized). Up to 8–24 hr. **Distribution:** Initially concentrated in the liver with little tissue accumulation. **Metabolism/Elimination:** Rapidly metabolized by the liver. Little is known of elimination.

INDICATIONS/DOSAGE

Reserve usage for situations where other routes of administration are not feasible and the risk of severe reactions is warranted. IM/SC routes preferred.

Anticoagulant-induced hypoprothrombinemia

(when bleeding is present or immediately threatened)

Adult: 10–50 mg (depending on bleeding severity). Repeat every 4 hr if needed.

Neonatal hemorrhagic disease prophylaxis

Adult: 1–5 mg to mother 12–24 hr before delivery. *Neonate:* 1500 g: 0.5 mg. > 1500 g: 1 mg.

Treatment of hemorrhagic disease

Pediatric: 1–5 mg/dose. *Neonate:* 1–2 mg/dose.

Treatment of hypoprothrombinemia due to malabsorption states or drug-induced (other than anticoagulants)

Adult: 2–25 mg. Repeat if necessary. Not to exceed 50 mg. *Pediatric:* Infants: 2 mg. Older children: 5–10 mg. Not to exceed 10 mg/dose.

Vitamin K deficiency

Pediatric: 1–2 mg/dose once.

CONTRAINDICATIONS/PRECAUTIONS

Contraindicated in: Hypersensitivity to any component. **Use cautiously in:** Impaired liver function. **Pregnancy/Lactation:** No well-controlled trials to establish safety. Benefits must outweigh risks. Crosses placenta. Distributes into breast milk.

PREPARATION

Availability: 2 mg/mL in 0.5 mL amps. 10 mg/mL in 1 mL amps, 2.5 and 5 mL vials. Contains 9 mg/mL benzyl alcohol as preservative (an amount considered safe by American Academy of Pediatrics when administered in neonates in recommended doses). Only the aqueous colloidal solution may be given intravenously (do not use the aqueous dispersion; IM use only). **Syringe:** No further dilution required. If desired, dilute with compatible IV solution prior to administration. **Infusion:** Dilute in physician specified volume of compatible IV solution.

STABILITY/STORAGE

Vial: Store at room temperature. Protect from light. **Infusion:** Administer immediately after preparation. Protect from light.

ADMINISTRATION

IV Push: May be given undiluted IV push slowly; not to exceed 1 mg/min. **Intermittent Infusion:** Administer over 15–30 min.

COMPATIBILITY

Solution: Dextrose solutions, lactated Ringer's, Ringer's injection, sodium chloride solutions. **Syringe:** Doxapram. **Y-site:** Ampicillin, epinephrine, famotidine, heparin, hydrocortisone, potassium chloride, tolazoline, vitamin B complex with C.

INCOMPATIBILITY
Y-site: Dobutamine.

ADVERSE EFFECTS
CNS: Convulsive movements, dizziness, dulled consciousness. **CV:** CARDIAC ARREST, CIRCULATORY COLLAPSE, cardiac irregularities, chest constriction, chest pain, hypotension, rapid, weak pulse, shock. **Resp:** RESPIRATORY ARREST, BRONCHOSPASM, dyspnea. **MS:** Cramplike pains. **Derm:** Cyanosis, hyperhydrosis. **Hypersens:** ANAPHYLAXIS (especially with initial administration), rash, urticaria. **Other:** DEATH, facial flushing, pain, swelling, tenderness.

TOXICITY/OVERDOSE
Signs/Symptoms: Extension of severe adverse effects. **Treatment:** Supportive and symptomatic treatment.

DRUG INTERACTIONS
Coumarin/indandione derivatives: Antagonism of pharmacologic effect by phytonadione.

NURSING CONSIDERATIONS
Assessment
General:
Vital signs, signs/symptoms of hypersensitivity.
Physical:
Cardiopulmonary status.
Lab Alterations:
Assess platelets and coagulation profile.

Intervention/Rationale
Measures for treatment of anaphylactic reactions should be available. ● Monitor vital signs closely. ● Evaluate patient for development of dysrhythmias and potential cardiac arrest.

Patient/Family Education
Explain therapeutic outcome and adverse effects. Notify physician of chest pain, dizziness, shortness of breath, or difficulty breathing.

PIPECURONIUM
(pip-a-cure'-o-nee-um)
Trade Name(s): Arduan
Classification(s): Long-acting nondepolarizing neuromuscular blocking agent
Pregnancy Category: C

PHARMACODYNAMICS/KINETICS
Mechanism of Action: Causes partial paralysis by interfering with neural transmission at myoneural junction. Prevents acetylcholine from binding to receptors at muscle end plate. **Onset of Action:** 2–3 min. **Peak Effect:** 5 min. **Duration of Action:** 35–45 min. **Distribution:** Rapidly distributed throughout body. **Metabolism/Elimination:** Primarily eliminated as unchanged drug (75%) by kidneys. **Half-Life:** 0.9–2.7 hr.

INDICATIONS/DOSAGE

Adjunct to general anesthesia for skeletal muscle relaxation for procedures ≥ 90 minutes, endotracheal intubation

---

In the Adverse Effects section, <u>underline</u> indicates most frequent; CAPS indicates life threatening.

Individualize dosage based on ideal body weight and clinical response.

Adult/Pediatric: 0.085–0.1 mg/kg/dose. Reduce dosage based on creatinine clearance. Children (3 months to 1 year) are less sensitive to doses than adults. **Endotracheal Intubation:** 0.07–0.085 mg/kg provides 1–2 hr of blockade. **Following Succinylcholine:** 0.05 mg/kg/dose provides 0.75 hr of blockade. **Maintenance:** 0.01–0.015 mg/kg/dose provides 50 minutes of blockade.

CONTRAINDICATIONS/PRECAUTIONS

Contraindicated in: Hypersensitivity. **Use cautiously in:** Bronchial asthma, myasthenia gravis, obese patients, patients undergoing C-section, renal impairment, severe electrolyte disturbances. **Pregnancy/Lactation:** No well-controlled trials to establish safety. Benefits must outweigh risks. Embryotoxic in lab animals. **Pediatrics:** Children 3 months to 1 year exhibit similar dose response as adults. Children 1–14 years are less sensitive than adults.

PREPARATION

Availability: 10 mg lyophilized powder in 10 mL vial. **Reconstitution:** Dilute with 5–10 mL sterile water or compatible IV solution. Bacteriostatic water may be used (avoid use in neonates; contains benzyl alcohol). **Syringe:** No further dilution required.

STABILITY/STORAGE

Vial: Store at room temperature or refrigerate. Protect from light. Reconstituted vial stable for 24 hr refrigerated; discard unused solution.

ADMINISTRATION

General: Unconsciousness must be established prior to administration to prevent patient distress. Contains no analgesic properties. Administer in facilities capable of maintaining mechanical ventilation/patent airways. **IV Push:** Give slowly over 30–60 sec.

COMPATIBILITY

Solution: Bacteriostatic water, dextrose solutions, lactated Ringer's, sodium chloride solutions, sterile water for injection.

ADVERSE EFFECTS

CNS: Hypesthesia, CNS depression. **CV:** Ventricular dysrhythmia, atrial fibrillation, bradycardia, cerebrovascular accident, hypertension, hypotension, myocardial ischemia. **Resp:** Atelectasis, dyspnea, increased bronchial secretions, respiratory depression. **GU:** Anuria. **Renal:** Increased serum creatinine. **MS:** Inadequate blockade, muscle atrophy, prolonged neuromuscular blockade. **Endo:** Hypoglycemia. **Fld/Lytes:** Hyperkalemia. **Hypersens:** Rash, urticaria. **Other:** Thrombosis.

TOXICITY/OVERDOSE

Signs/Symptoms: Apnea, airway closure, respiratory insufficiency. **Treatment:** Provide cardiovascular support. Assure patent airway and ventilation. Resuscitate as necessary. **Antidote(s):** Reverse blockade symptoms with anticholinesterase reversing agents (edrophonium, neostigmine, pyridostigmine) and anticholinergic agents (atropine, glycopyrrolate).

In the Adverse Effects section, <u>underline</u> indicates most frequent; CAPS indicates life threatening.

DRUG INTERACTIONS
Aminoglycosides, clindamycin, diuretics, general anesthetics (enflurane, isoflurane, halothane), lincomycin, lithium, magnesium sulfate, muscle relaxants, polypeptide antibiotics (bacitracin, polymyxin B), verapamil: Increased neuromuscular blockade.

NURSING CONSIDERATIONS
Assessment
General:
Vital signs.
Physical:
Cardiopulmonary status, neuromuscular status.
Lab Alterations:
Monitor electrolytes.

Intervention/Rationale
Produces apnea (use cautiously in patients with cardiovascular disease, severe electrolyte disorders, bronchogenic cancer, and neuromuscular disease). Maintain patent airway. ● Monitor response to drug during intraoperative period by use of a peripheral nerve stimulator. ● Assess postoperatively for presence of any residual muscle weakness. Evaluate hand grip, head lift, and ability to cough in order to ascertain full recovery from residual effects of drug. ● Correct electrolyte deficiencies prior to surgery. ● Eval-uate blood pressure and heart rate prior to, throughout, and following administration.

Patient/Family Education
Discuss the rationale for hand grip, head lift, and cough demonstration in the immediate postoperative phase in order to assure patient cooperation.

PIPERACILLIN
(pi-per′-a-sill-in)
Trade Name(s): Pipracil
Classification(s): Antibiotic (synthetic extended-spectrum penicillin)
Pregnancy Category: B

PHARMACODYNAMICS/KINETICS
Mechanism of Action: Bactericidal antibiotic against susceptible organisms. Inhibits bacterial cell wall synthesis. **Peak Serum Level:** Immediate. **Distribution:** Widely distributed to most tissues including pleural, peritoneal, synovial, and wound fluids. Readily crosses into CSF with inflammation. 16%–22% bound to plasma proteins including albumin and gamma globulin. **Metabolism/Elimination:** Rapidly excreted unchanged in urine by tubular secretion and glomerular filtration. Partly (10%–20%) excreted in bile. **Half-Life:** 0.6–1.3 hr (dosage dependent). Prolonged in renal impairment.

INDICATIONS/DOSAGE
Hemodialysis: Maximum dose 2 g every 8 hr on dialysis days; 6 g/day. Administer an additional 1 g dose after each dialysis. Not to exceed 500 mg/kg/day or 24 g/day.

Treatment of serious gram-negative infections (especially *Pseudomonas aeruginosa*)
Adjust dosage in renal impairment.

Serious infections
Adult: 12–18 g/day in divided doses every 4–6 hr. CrCl 20–40 mL/min:

In the Adverse Effects section, <u>underline</u> indicates most frequent; CAPS indicates life threatening.

417

12 g/day (4 g every 8 hr)CrCl < 20 mL/min: 8 g/day (4 g every 12 hr). *Pediatric:* 200–300 mg/kg/day in divided doses every 4–6 hr. Cystic Fibrosis: up to 300–600 mg/kg/day in divided doses every 4–6 hr.

Neonate (unlabeled use): 200 mg/kg/day in divided doses every 12 hr. **Meningitis:** 400 mg/kg/day in divided doses every 12 hr.

Complicated urinary tract infections

Adult: 8–16 g/day in divided doses every 6–8 hr. CrCl 20–40 mL/min: 9 g/day (3 g every 8 hr). CrCl < 20 mL/min: 6 g/day (3 g every 12 hr). *Pediatric:* 125–200 mg/kg/day in divided doses every 6–8 hr.

Uncomplicated urinary tract infections and community acquired pneumonia

Adult: 6–8 g/day in divided doses every 6–12 hr. CrCl < 20 mL/min: 6 g/day (3 g every 12 hr). *Pediatric:* 100–125 mg/kg/day in divided doses every 6–12 hr.

Surgical prophylaxis for certain perioperative and/or postoperative infections

Adult:
Intra-abdominal: 2 g just prior to surgery and 2 g during surgery and 2 g 6 hr postoperatively for no more than 24 hr. **Vaginal Hysterectomy:** 2 g just prior to surgery and 2 g 6 hr later and 2 g 12 hr after first dose. **Cesarean Section:** 2 g after cord clamped and 2 g every 4 hr after initial dose and 2 g 8 hr after first dose. **Abdominal Hysterectomy:** 2 g just prior to surgery and 2 g in recovery and 2 g after 6 hr.

CONTRAINDICATIONS/ PRECAUTIONS

Contraindicated in: Hypersensitivity to penicillins or cephalosporins. **Use cautiously in:** Impaired renal function, neonates. **Pregnancy/Lactation:** No well-controlled trials to establish safety. Benefits must outweigh risks. Crosses placenta. No evidence of harm to fetus in animal studies. Distributed into breast milk. May cause potential changes in neonate bowel flora and candidiasis. **Pediatrics:** Safety and efficacy in children less than 12 years old has not been established (dosing guidelines are available). Neonates have demonstrated decreased elimination.

PREPARATION

Availability: 2, 3, and 4 g vials and 40 g pharmacy bulk vial. Contains 1.85 mEq sodium/g. **Reconstitution:** Dilute each gram with at least 5 mL sterile water for injection or compatible diluent for a final concentration of 200–300 mg/mL. **Syringe:** No further dilution required. Not to exceed 300 mg/mL. **Infusion:** Further dilute to a final volume of 50–100 mL compatible IV solution for a final concentration of 10–20 mg/mL.

STABILITY/STORAGE

Vial/Infusion: Store vial at room temperature. Reconstituted vial/solution stable for 24 hr at room temperature and 1 week refrigerated. Slight darkening of solution does not indicate a loss of potency.

ADMINISTRATION

General: If concurrently given with aminoglycosides, administer in separate infusions as far apart as possible. **IV Push:** Give slowly over 3–5 min. **Intermittent Infusion:** Administer over 30–60 min.

COMPATIBILITY
Solution: Dextrose solutions, lactated Ringer's, sodium chloride solutions. **Syringe:** Heparin. **Y-site:** Acyclovir, ciprofloxacin, cyclophosphamide, enalaprilat, esmolol, famotidine, foscarnet, hydromorphone, labetalol, magnesium sulfate, meperidine, morphine, perphenazine, verapamil, zidovudine.

INCOMPATIBILITY
Syringe: Aminoglycosides. **Y-site:** Ondansetron.

ADVERSE EFFECTS
CNS: Seizures, hallucinations, lethargy, neuromuscular irritability, neurotoxicity (high doses). **CV:** CHF, myocarditis. **GI:** Pseudomembranous colitis, <u>diarrhea</u>, increased liver enzymes, nausea. **Fld/Lytes:** Hypokalemia, hypernatremia. **Heme:** Abnormal clotting times/prothrombin time, anemia, bleeding, LEUKOPENIA, GRANULOCYTOPENIA, THROMBOCYTOPENIA. **Hypersens:** ANAPHYLAXIS, rash, urticaria. **Other:** Pain at injection site, superinfection, thrombophlebitis.

TOXICITY/OVERDOSE
Signs/Symptoms: High doses in renal impairment may cause seizures and bleeding abnormalities. **Treatment:** Symptomatic and supportive treatment. Consider hemodialysis in significant overdosage.

DRUG INTERACTIONS
Aminoglycosides: Inactivation by piperacillin. **Bacteriostatic antibiotics:** Diminished bactericidal effect of piperacillin. **Beta adrenergic blockers:** Increased risk and severity of anaphylactic reactions. **Chloramphenicol:** Decreased piperacillin effect; increased chloramphenicol half-life. **Heparin/oral anticoagulants:** Altered coagulation/increased risk of bleeding. **Probenecid:** Prolonged piperacillin levels.

NURSING CONSIDERATIONS
Assessment
General:
Hypersensitivity.
Physical:
Infectious disease status, signs/symptoms of superinfection (especially in elderly, debilitated, or immunosuppressed).
Lab Alterations:
Periodically evalute renal, hepatic, and hematologic system with long-term use. Assess coagulation studies (bleeding time, prothrombin time, platelet aggregation) prior to and throughout course of therapy. Evaluate electrolytes (especially sodium and potassium). False-positive urine protein levels. Positive Coombs' test or direct antiglobulin test.

Intervention/Rationale
Obtain specimens for culture and sensitivity before therapy is initiated (first dose may be given while awaiting results). ● Assess patient for signs and symptoms of infection prior to, during, and at completion of therapy. ● Question patient about prior use of penicillins or cephalosporins and allergic or hypersensitivity reactions prior to initiation of therapy. Hypersensitivity

P

In the Adverse Effects section, <u>underline</u> indicates most frequent; CAPS indicates life threatening.

419

reactions may be immediate and severe in penicillin sensitive patients with a history of allergy, asthma, hay fever, or urticaria. ● Monitor serum electrolytes and cardiac status (assess for signs and symptoms of CHF due to high sodium content) periodically during therapy. ● Discontinue therapy and call physician if bleeding occurs.

Patient/Family Education
Notify physician/nurse if skin rash, hives, itching occur. Observe for signs/symptoms of worsening infection (persistent fever), persistent diarrhea, signs of yeast infections (white patches in the mouth or vaginal discharge).

PLASMA PROTEIN FRACTION

(plaz'-ma proe'-teen frak'-shun)
Trade Name(s): Plasmanate, Plasma-Plex, Plasmatein, Protenate
Classification(s): Plasma volume expander
Pregnancy Category: C

PHARMACODYNAMICS/KINETICS
Mechanism of Action: Maintains normal blood volume similar to albumin (ineffective in maintaining oncotic pressure). Causes a shift of fluid from interstitial spaces into circulation with slight increases in plasma proteins. **Distribution:** Distributed throughout plasma. **Metabolism/Elimination:** Unknown.

INDICATIONS/DOSAGE
Dosage depends on patient's condition and response to therapy. Not to exceed 250 g in 48 hr. If necessary, consider whole blood or plasma.

Treatment of hypovolemic shock (via plasma volume expansion)
Adult: 250–500 mL (12.5–25.0 g protein) initially. *Pediatric:* 6.6–33.0 mL/kg/dose initially.

Hypoproteinemia
Adult: 1000–1500 mL (50–75 g protein) per day. Higher doses may be needed in severe states with continued protein loss. Adjust rate based on clinical response. If edema is present or large amounts of protein continue to be lost, consider concentrated serum albumin 25%.

CONTRAINDICATIONS/PRECAUTIONS
Contraindicated in: Cardiac failure, history of allergic reaction to albumin, patients on cardiopulmonary bypass, presence of normal or increased intravascular volume, severe anemia. **Use cautiously in:** Hepatic failure, low cardiac reserve, patients without albumin deficiency, patients at risk of circulatory overload, renal failure. **Pregnancy/Lactation:** No well-controlled trials to establish safety. Benefits must outweigh risks.

PREPARATION
Availability: 5% ready-to-use preparation containing 83%–90% normal human albumin, ≤ 17% alpha and beta globulins and ≤ 1% gamma globulin with 130–160 mEq/L so-

In the Adverse Effects section, <u>underline</u> indicates most frequent; CAPS indicates life threatening.

dium and ≤ 2 mEq/L potassium. 25 g albumin provides osmotic equivalent to 500 mL (2 units) fresh frozen plasma or 2 units whole blood. 50 mL (without injection sets), 250 mL, and 500 mL vials with injection sets. Each vial includes an administration set. **Infusion:** Ready for use.

STABILITY/STORAGE

Vial: Store at room temperature. Solution is transparent, nearly colorless to slightly brownish. Do not use solution if turbid, frozen or containing sediment. **Infusion:** Discard unused portion (preparation does not contain preservative). Do not use solution if longer than 4 hr after connection of administration set.

ADMINISTRATION

General: May be administered without respect to patient's blood group or Rh factor. Monitor blood pressure during administration, slow or stop infusion if hypotension occurs suddenly. Consult manufacturer guidelines. Solutions with protein hydrolysates, alcohol, or amino acids must not be administered through the same infusion set. Administer at a site distant from area of infection or trauma. **Intermittent/ Continuous Infusion: Hypovolemia:** 5–10 mL/min. Not to exceed 10 mL/ min. **Hypoproteinemia:** Approaching normovolemia, not to exceed 5–8 mL/min.

COMPATIBILITY

Solution: Most intravenous solutions of carbohydrates/electrolytes. **Y-site:** Packed red blood cells, whole blood.

INCOMPATIBILITY

Y-site: Solutions containing protein hydrolysates, alcohol, amino acids.

ADVERSE EFFECTS

CNS: Headache. **CV:** Changes in blood presure/heart rate, hypotension (rapid infusion), tachycardia. **Resp:** Dyspnea, pulmonary edema (rapid infusion). **GI:** Nausea, vomiting. **MS:** Back pain. **Derm:** Erythema. **Hypersens:** Urticaria. **Other:** Chills, fever, flushing, hypersalivation.

TOXICITY/OVERDOSE

Signs/Symptoms: Hypotension and pulmonary edema with rapid administration, extension of adverse effects. **Treatment:** Symptomatic and supportive treatment; decrease or discontinue infusion if rate related.

NURSING CONSIDERATIONS

Assessment
General:
Vital signs, intake/output ratio.
Physical:
Cardiopulmonary status.
Lab Alterations:
False elevations alkaline phosphatase with albumin component from placental sources. Monitor hemoglobin/hematocrit.

Intervention/Rationale
Monitor for signs of volume overload. Consider RBC and plasma transfusions in patients who require greater than 250 g in 48 hr. Monitor normovolemic patients for signs of hypervolemia including dyspnea, pulmonary edema, abnormal rise in blood pressure, and central venous pressure. ● Monitor vital signs during administration;

In the Adverse Effects section, underline indicates most frequent; CAPS indicates life threatening.

421

hypotension may occur if infused too rapidly. Adjust rates based on clinical response. ● Concentrated normal serum albumin may be needed if continued large losses of protein. ● Antihistamines may be administered to prevent allergic reactions.

Patient/Family Education
Notify physician if any signs of difficulty in breathing, chest/back pain, palpitations. Make patient aware that this product is nonreactive for Hepatitis B surface antigen.

PLICAMYCIN
(plye-ka-mye′-sin)
Trade name(s): Mithracin
Classification(s): Antineoplastic antibiotic, hypocalcemic agent
Pregnancy Category: X

PHARMACODYNAMICS/KINETICS
Mechanism of Action: Unknown. Complexation with DNA and inhibition of cellular RNA and enzymatic RNA synthesis. Blocks hypercalcemic action of pharmacologic doses of vitamin D; acts on osteoclasts and blocks parathyroid action; decreased serum phosphate levels and urinary calcium excretion. **Onset of Action:** *Hypocalcemic:* 24–48 hr. **Duration of Action:** *Hypocalcemic:* 3–15 days.
Distribution: Throughout body especially in liver, renal tubules, areas of active bone resorption. Crosses the blood–brain barrier and persists in brain tissue longer than other tissues. **Metabolism/Elimination:** Rapidly cleared from blood and excreted.

40% excreted 15 hr after administration.

INDICATIONS/DOSAGE
Base daily dose on body weight; use ideal body weight if abnormal fluid retention.

Malignant testicular tumors
Adult: 25–30 mcg/kg/day for 8–10 days. Not to exceed ten daily doses or 30 mcg/kg/day. If tumor remains unchanged, may repeat courses at monthly intervals. If regression is significant, additional courses at monthly intervals are administered.

Paget's Disease (*unlabeled use*)
Adult: 15 mcg/kg/day for 10 days.

Hypercalcemia/hypercalciuria in symptomatic patients associated with advanced neoplasms
Adult/Pediatric: 25 mcg/kg/day for 3–4 days. Repeat at ≥ 1 week intervals to achieve or maintain desired results. Intermittent doses every 3–7 days may be needed. If there is significant renal/hepatic impairment, a single dose of 12.5 mcg/kg has been recommended.

CONTRAINDICATIONS/PRECAUTIONS
Contraindicated in: Coagulation disorders or increased bleeding susceptibility, hypersensitivity, impaired bone marrow function, thrombocytopenia, thrombocytopathy. **Use cautiously in:** Electrolyte imbalance, hepatic/renal impairment. **Pregnancy/Lactation:** May cause fetal harm. Patient must be aware of risk to fetus. Benefits must outweigh risks. Excretion in breast

In the Adverse Effects section, underline indicates most frequent; CAPS indicates life threatening.

milk is unknown. Breastfeeding should be discontinued.

PREPARATION

Availability: 2500 mcg/vial with 100 mg mannitol. **Reconstitution:** Dilute each vial with 4.9 mL sterile water for injection for a final concentration 500 mcg/mL. Discard unused solution (no preservative in vial). **Infusion:** Dilute daily dose in 1000 mL compatible IV solution.

STABILITY/STORAGE

Vial: Store in refrigerator. May be stored at room temperature for up to 3 months. Reconstituted solutions are stable for 24 hr at room temperature and 48 hr refrigerated. **Infusion:** Stable for 24 hr at room temperature.

ADMINISTRATION

General: Handle drug with care and adhere to institutional guidelines for the handling of chemotherapeutic/cytotoxic agents. Avoid rapid direct IV injection because of higher incidence of severe GI side effects. Avoid extravasation (moderate heat to area of extravasation may help disperse the drug and minimize discomfort and irritation). In the event of a spill, trisodium phosphate 10% should be added for 24 hr to inactivate the drug. **Intermittent/Continuous Infusion:** Administer as slow infusion over 4–6 hr.

COMPATIBILITY

Solution: Dextrose solutions, sodium chloride solutions.

ADVERSE EFFECTS

CNS: Depression, drowsiness, headache, lethargy, malaise, weakness. **GI:** Hepatotoxicity, <u>anorexia</u>, <u>diarrhea</u>, increased AST (SGOT), ALT (SGPT), LDH, alkaline phosphatase, bilirubin, ornithine carbamyl transferase, isocitric dehydrogenase, bromosulphalein reaction, <u>nausea</u>, <u>stomatitis</u>, <u>vomiting</u>. **GU:** Proteinuria. **Renal:** Increased BUN/serum creatinine. **Fld/Lytes:** Decreased serum calcium, phosphorus, potassium. **Heme:** <u>THROMBO-CYTOPENIA</u>, abnormal clot retraction, depressed clotting/bleeding time, depressed hemoglobin, NEUTROPENIA, depressed prothrombin. **Hypersens:** Rash. **Other:** Fever, flushing, thrombophlebitis.

TOXICITY/OVERDOSE

Signs/Symptoms: Exaggerated adverse effects especially hematologic effects. **Treatment:** Symptomatic and supportive treatment.

DRUG INTERACTIONS

Immunosuppressants: Increased myelosuppression.

NURSING CONSIDERATIONS

Assessment
General:
Vital signs, intake/output ratio, hypersensitivity reactions.
Physical:
Neurologic status, GI tract, infectious disease status, hematopoietic system.
Lab Alterations:
Assess CBC with differential and platelet count, BUN, serum creatinine, and liver function prior to and throughout course of therapy. Monitor serum electrolytes, especially calcium.

Intervention/Rationale
Assess for development of fever, chills, or other signs of infection

In the Adverse Effects section, <u>underline</u> indicates most frequent; CAPS indicates life threatening.

423

and notify physician immediately. ● Maintain adequate hydration during therapy. ● Assess patient for development of bleeding (bleeding gums, easy bruising, hematest positive stools,/urine/vomitus). ● Avoid intramuscular injections and rectal temperatures. ● If nausea becomes a problem, antiemetics may be administered 0.5 hr prior to administration.

Patient/Family Education
Observe for signs of infection (fever, sore throat, fatigue) or bleeding (melena, hematuria, nosebleeds, easy bruising) especially 1 week following administration. Take and record oral temperature daily and report persistent elevation to physician. Use a soft toothbrush and electric razor to minimize bleeding tendency. Avoid crowded environments and persons with known infections. Use reliable contraception throughout the duration of therapy and 4 months following due to potential teratogenic and mutagenic effects of drug. Seek physician approval prior to receiving live virus vaccinations. Avoid over-the-counter products containing aspirin or ibuprofen due to increased potential for bleeding. Report dizziness, unusual fatigue, or shortness of breath (drug may cause anemia).

POTASSIUM ACETATE
(poe-tass′-ee-um as′-sa-tate)
Classification(s): Potassium supplement
Pregnancy Category: C

PHARMACODYNAMICS/KINETICS
Mechanism of Action: Maintains osmotic pressure and ion balance on a cellular level. **Metabolism/Elimination:** 80%–90% excreted via urine with the remainder excreted in the stool/perspiration.

INDICATIONS/DOSAGE

Prevention/treatment potassium depletion

Adult: Must be individualized for each patient and usually expressed in mEq. **Replacement:** Less than 20 mEq/hr in concentrations of 40 mEq/L or less. Total 24 hr dose not to **exceed** 150 mEq.

Pediatric: **Replacement:** Total 24 hr dose not to exceed 3 mEq/kg.

CONTRAINDICATIONS/PRECAUTIONS
Contraindicated in: Acute dehydration, severe hemolytic reactions, severe renal impairment with oliguria, anuria, azotemia, untreated chronic adrenocortical insufficiency. **Use cautiously in:** Cardiac disease, immediate postoperative period until urine flow is determined, myotonia congenita, patients receiving potassium-sparing drugs. **Pregnancy/Lactation:** No well-controlled trials to establish safety. Benefits must outweigh risks. May cause fetal harm, administer only when clearly needed. Exercise caution when administering drug to breastfeeding women.

PREPARATION

Availability: 2 mEq potassium/acetate/mL and 4 mEq potassium/acetate/mL in 20, 30, 50, and 100 mL vials. 3.93 g potassium acetate equals 40 mEq potassium and acetate. **Infusion:** Avoid layering of drug by thoroughly agitating the prepared IV solution. Do not add drug to bottle/bag in the hanging position, can cause inadvertent bolusing of patient. Further dilute prescribed dose in 500–1000 mL compatible IV solution.

STABILITY/STORAGE

Vial: Store at room temperature. **Infusion:** Stable at room temperature for 24 hr following admixture preparation.

ADMINISTRATION

General: IV potassium acetate must be administered slowly as a dilute solution. Concentrated potassium solutions must not be given. Parenteral form of drug must be given by the continuous or intermittent infusion route. May **never** be given IV push without specific dilution or IM under any circumstances. Administer at physician prescribed rate with fluid volume in accordance with patient's requirements. **Intermittent/Continuous Infusion:** Usual dose of 10 mEq/hr. For **severe** metabolic states 40 mEq/hr may be administered **with extreme caution.**

COMPATIBILITY

Solution: Dextrose solutions, sodium chloride solutions.

INCOMPATIBILITY

Solution: Fat emulsion 10%.

ADVERSE EFFECTS

CV: Cardiac dysrhythmias, ECG changes (increased P-R interval, widened QRS, ST segment depression, tall tented T waves). **GI:** Abdominal discomfort, bowel ulceration, diarrhea, nausea, vomiting. **GU:** Oliguria. **Fld/Lytes:** Hyperkalemia. **Metab:** Metabolic alkalosis associated with excess administration. **Other:** Phlebitis/pain at site of injection/infusion.

TOXICITY/OVERDOSE

Signs/Symptoms: Paresthesia of the extremities, weakness or heaviness of legs, flaccid paralysis, mental confusion, cold skin, gray pallor, peripheral vascular collapse, hypotension, cardiac dysrhythmias, heart block. **Treatment:** Dependent on severity. In patients with severe hyperkalemia interventions that facilitate the shift of potassium into the cells, such as the administration of 50–100 mEq of sodium bicarbonate and/or 50% dextrose with or without insulin, have been recommended. Hemodialysis or peritoneal dialysis will decrease plasma potassium concentrations and may be required for patients with renal insufficiency.

DRUG INTERACTIONS

Angiotensin converting enzyme (ACE) inhibitor: May cause potassium retention as a result of decreased circulating aldosterone levels. **Digitalis glycosides:** Potassium administration in digoxin toxic patients may increase A-V conduction disturbances. **Other potassium products:** Concomitant administration can cause hyperkalemia.

In the Adverse Effects section, underline indicates most frequent;
CAPS indicates life threatening.

NURSING CONSIDERATIONS

Assessment

General:
Continuous ECG monitoring (recommended), hydration status, intake/output ratio.

Physical:
Cardiac status.

Lab Alterations:
Excess or prolonged administration of drug may result in metabolic alkalosis. Assessment of plasma potassium concentrations is essential throughout and following therapy.

Intervention/Rationale

Evaluate for development of various cardiac dysrhthmias associated with electrolyte status. ● Assess fluid status, correct dehydration prior to therapy. Monitor intake/output accurately. ● **DO NOT administer undiluted potassium.**

Patient/Family Education

Review the purpose of therapy. Be extremely observant of any burning or stinging at IV site and notify nurse/physician immediately if symptoms are experienced.

POTASSIUM CHLORIDE

(poe-tass′-ee-um klor-ide′)
Classification(s): Electrolyte, electrolyte supplement
Pregnancy Category: C

PHARMACODYNAMICS/KINETICS

Mechanism of Action: Major cation of intracellular fluid that is essential for the maintenance of acid-base balance, isotonicity, and serves as an activation mechanism for many enzymatic reactions. Transmits nerve impulses and assists in facilitating contraction of smooth, skeletal, and cardiac muscle. **Distribution:** Enters extracellular fluid; actively transfers into cells. **Metabolism/Elimination:** Excreted by the kidneys.

INDICATIONS/DOSAGE

Treatment of potassium depletion and specific dysrhythmia treatment for cardiac glycoside toxicity

Adult: 10–20 mEq/hr (not to exceed 150 mEq/24 hr maximum). In **urgent** cases as much as 40 mEq/hr up to 400 mEq/24 hr may be given. *Pediatric:* 2–3 mEq/kg/day or 40 mEq/m²/24 hr.

CONTRAINDICATIONS/PRECAUTIONS

Contraindicated in: Acute tissue trauma, hyperkalemia, postoperative oliguria, uncorrected adrenal cortex disease. **Use cautiously in:** Cardiac disease, impaired renal function. **Pregnancy/Lactation:** No well-controlled trials to establish safety. Benefits must outweigh risks. May cause fetal harm, administer only when clearly needed. Use cautiously in lactating women.

PREPARATION

Availability: 10, 20, 30, 40 mEq in 5, 10, 15, and 20 mL ampules, vials, and syringes. **Infusion:** Each single dose must be diluted and completely mixed in 100–1000 mL compatible IV solution. Not to exceed 40 mEq/100 mL.

In the Adverse Effects section, <u>underline</u> indicates most frequent; CAPS indicates life threatening.

STABILITY/STORAGE

Vial: Store at room temperature. Contains no preservatives and should be used within 24 hr after opening or discarded. **Infusion:** Stable at room temperature 24 hr after preparation.

ADMINISTRATION

General: IV potassium chloride must be administered slowly as a dilute solution. Concentrated potassium solutions must not be given. Parenteral form of drug must be given by the continuous or intermittent infusion route. May **never** be given IV push without specific dilution or IM under any circumstances. Administer at physician prescribed rate with fluid volume in accordance with patient's requirements. Use of IV infusion device is recommended. Avoid extravasation; if noted, contact physician, and inject area with 1% procaine and hyaluronidase via 27 gauge or 25 gauge needle in accordance with physician order. Follow by warm compresses for pain relief. **Intermittent/Continuous Infusion:** Usual dose of 10 mEq/hr. For **severe** metabolic states 40 mEq/hr may be administered **with extreme caution.**

COMPATIBILITY

Solution: Dextrose solutions, fat emulsion 10%, lactated Ringer's, Ringer's injection, sodium chloride solutions. **Y-site:** Acyclovir, aminophylline, amiodarone, ampicillin, atropine, betamethasone, calcium gluconate, cephalothin, cephapirin, chlordiazepoxide, chlorpromazine, deslanoside, dexamethasone, digoxin, diphenhydramine, dobutamine, dopamine, droperidol, endrophonium, enalaprilat, epinephrine, esmolol, estrogen, ethacrynate, famotidine, fentanyl, fluorouracil, furosemide, hydralazine, insulin, isoproterenol, kanamycin, labetalol, lidocaine, magnesium sulfate, methicillin, methoxamine, methylergonovine, minocycline, morphine, neostigmine, norepinephrine, ondansetron, oxacillin, oxytocin, penicillin G potassium, pentazocine, phytonadione, prednisolone, prochlorperazine, propranolol, pyridostigmine, scopolamine, sodium bicarbonate, succinylcholine, trimethaphan, zidovudine.

INCOMPATIBILITY

Y-site: Diazepam, phenytoin.

ADVERSE EFFECTS

CNS: Confusion, paralysis, paresthesias, restlessness. **CV:** ECG changes (increased P-R interval, ST segment depression, tall tented T-waves), dysrhythmias. **GI:** Abdominal discomfort, bowel ulceration, diarrhea, nausea, vomiting. **GU:** Oliguria. **Fld/Lytes:** Hyperkalemia **Other:** Pain at injection/infusion site, tissue necrosis with extravasation, weakness.

TOXICITY/OVERDOSE

Signs/Symptoms: Toxic symptoms are those of hyperkalemia, including fatigue, muscle weakness, paresthesia, confusion, dyspnea, widened QRS complex, cardiac dysrhythmias, including loss of P waves. **Treatment:** Discontinue drug. Use 50 g dextrose and 10 units of regular insulin to promote diffusion of potassium into the cells. Use calcium salts to reverse ECG effects in patients who are not digitalized. So-

P

In the Adverse Effects section, <u>underline</u> indicates most frequent; CAPS indicates life threatening.

427

dium bicarbonate can be given if acidosis is noted. Hemodialysis may be indicated if accompanied by renal impairment. Sodium polystyrene sulfonate orally or rectally via retention enema may be used to remove potassium from the body.

DRUG INTERACTIONS

Angiotensin converting enzyme (ACE) inhibitor: May cause potassium retention as a result of decreased circulating aldosterone levels. **Digitalis glycosides:** Potassium administration in digoxin toxic patients may increase A-V conduction disturbances. **Potassium-sparing diuretics, other potassium products:** May cause hyperkalemia with concomitant use.

NURSING CONSIDERATIONS

Assessment

General:
Continuous ECG monitoring (recommended), hydration status, intake/output ratio, vital signs.
Physical:
Cardiac status.
Lab Alterations:
Assessment of plasma potassium concentrations is essential throughout and following therapy. Monitor all serum electrolytes during and following therapy.

Intervention/Rationale

Assess for signs/symptoms of hypokalemia (fatigue, weakness, metabolic acidosis, polyuria, polydipsia) and hyperkalemia (paresthesia, listlessness, mental confusion, weakness, dysrhythmias). ● Continuous cardiac monitoring is preferred for infusions of over 10 mEq/hr. ● In the immediate

postoperative phase assess adequate urine output before administration of drug infusion. ● Monitor heart rate, blood pressure, and ECG periodically throughout administration of drug.

Patient/Family Education

Notify nurse/physician immediately if unusual fatigue, tingling of extremities, or burning at the site of administration occurs. Review the ultimate goal of potassium therapy including the need for periodic blood testing to ascertain appropriate levels. Potassium rich foods such as avocados, bananas, navy beans, prunes, and spinach can increase serum potassium.

POTASSIUM PHOSPHATE

(poe-tass'-ee-um foss'-fate)
Classification(s): Electrolyte modifier, potassium supplement
Pregnancy Category: C

PHARMACODYNAMICS/KINETICS

Mechanism of Action: Acts as a buffer to maintain acid-base balance. Buffer for renal excretion of hydrogen ions. Maintains calcium levels. **Distribution:** Enters extracellular fluid via active transport. **Metabolism/Elimination:** > 90% excreted by kidneys.

INDICATIONS/DOSAGE

Maintenance/replacement therapy

Adult: 10 mM phosphorus/day via IV infusion. TPN solution: 10–15 mM/L with larger doses as required. *Pediatric:* 1.5 mM of phosphorus/day via IV infusion.

In the Adverse Effects section, underline indicates most frequent; CAPS indicates life threatening.

CONTRAINDICATIONS/ PRECAUTIONS

Contraindicated in: Acute dehydration, hyperkalemia, hyperkalemic form of familial periodic paralysis, severe renal impairment with oliguria, anuria, azotemia, untreated Addison's disease. **Use cautiously in:** Cardiac disease, potassium-sparing diuretic therapy. **Pregnancy/Lactation:** No well-controlled trials to establish safety. Benefits must outweigh risks.

PREPARATION

Availability: 3 mM phosphorus and 4.4 mEq potassium/mL in 5, 10, 15, 20, 30, 40, 50, 150 mL vials. **Infusion:** Further dilute prescribed dose and thoroughly mix dosage in 250–1000 mL compatible IV solution.

STABILITY/STORAGE

Vial: Store at room temperature. Contains no preservatives, discard unused portion 12 hr after opening. **Infusion:** Stable at room temperature for 24 hr following admixture.

ADMINISTRATION

General: Administer via infusion only in dilute concentrations. No IM or IV push administration. Assess for extravasation; if noted, contact physician, and inject area with 1% procaine and hyaluronidase via 27 gauge or 25 gauge needle in accordance with physician order. Follow by warm compresses for pain relief. **Intermittent/Continuous Infusion:** Infuse slowly in accordance with physician rate/volume in order to avoid phosphate or potassium intoxication. Administration rate dependent on individual needs of the patient.

COMPATIBILITY

Solution: Amino acids 4.25%/dextrose 25%, dextrose solutions, sodium chloride solutions. **Y-site:** Esmolol, famotidine, labetalol.

INCOMPATIBILITY

Solution: Dextrose/Ringer's injection, dextrose/Ringer's lactate, lactated Ringer's, Ringer's injection.

ADVERSE EFFECTS

CNS: Listlessness, mental confusion, paresthesia. **CV:** Cardiac dysrhythmias, ECG changes, hypotension. **GI:** Abdominal pain, diarrhea, nausea, vomiting. **GU:** Oliguria. **MS:** Flaccid paralysis, muscle cramps (hyperkalemia), tremors (hypocalcemia). **Derm:** Cold skin. **Fld/Lytes:** Hyperkalemia, hyperphosphatemia, hypocalcemia, hypomagnesemia. **Other:** Irritation at IV site.

TOXICITY/OVERDOSE

Signs/Symptoms: Paresthesia of the extremities, flaccid paralysis, listlessness, confusion, weakness and heaviness of the legs, hypotension, cardiac dysrhythmias, heart block, ECG abnormalities. **Treatment:** Discontinue the infusion. Restore serum calcium with calcium gluconate or calcium chloride. Lower serum potassium with 50% dextrose and insulin to facilitate passage of potassium into the cells. Use of sodium polystyrene as a potassium exchange resin or hemodialysis may be required for patients with renal impairment.

DRUG INTERACTIONS

Angiotensin converting enzyme (ACE) inhibitor: May cause potassium retention as a result of lower circulat-

In the Adverse Effects section, <u>underline</u> indicates most frequent; CAPS indicates life threatening.

429

ing aldosterone levels. **Digitalis glycosides:** Can cause severe or complete heart block. **Potassium products:** Concomitant administration may cause hyperkalemia. **Potassium-sparing diuretics and salt substitutes:** May produce hyperkalemia with cardiac dysrhythmias and cardiac arrest.

NURSING CONSIDERATIONS

Assessment
General:
Continuous ECG monitoring (recommended), hydration status, intake/output ratio, vital signs.
Physical:
Cardiac status.
Lab Alterations:
Monitor serum calcium, potassium, chloride, phosphate, and sodium levels. Avoid rapid infusion of drug and assess for signs/symptoms of hypocalcemic tetany. Monitor urinary pH for patients receiving drug for urinary acidification. Hypocalcemia/tetany can result in high concentrations of phosphate.

Intervention/Rationale
Monitor heart rate, blood pressure, and ECG periodically throughout administration of drug. ● Assess for signs/symptoms of hypokalemia (fatigue, weakness, metabolic acidosis, polyuria, polydipsia) and hyperkalemia (paresthesia, listlessness, mental confusion, weakness, dysrhythmias). ● Continuous cardiac monitoring is preferred for infusions of over 10 mEq/hr. ● In the immediate postoperative phase assess adequate urine output before administration of drug infusion.

Patient/Family Education
Review the ultimate goal of the therapy including the need for periodic blood testing to ascertain appropriate levels. Notify nurse/physician if pain, burning, or redness occurs at the site of infusion. Potassium rich foods such as avocados, bananas, navy beans, prunes, and .spinach can increase serum potassium.

PRALIDOXIME
(pra-li-dox'-eem)
Trade Name(s): Protopam
Classification(s): Antidote/anticholinergic poisoning
Pregnancy Category: C

PHARMACODYNAMICS/KINETICS
Mechanism of Action: Primary effect is reactivation of cholinesterase that has recently been inactivated by phosphorylation, as a result of exposure to organophosphates. **Peak Effect:** 5–15 minutes. **Distribution:** Widely distributed throughout extracellular water. Does not enter CSF. Is not bound to plasma protein. **Metabolism/Elimination:** Metabolized by the liver. 80%–90% excreted unchanged by kidney. **Half-Life:** 1.7 hr.

INDICATIONS/DOSAGE

Organophosphate poisoning

Atropine 2–6 mg IV must be given concurrently after cyanosis disappears. With continued exposure and unrelieved symptoms additional atropine doses may be given. (Atropine must be given before

In the Adverse Effects section, <u>underline</u> indicates most frequent; CAPS indicates life threatening.

pralidoxime but after adequate ventilation has been established.) If patient exhibits cyanosis drug may be administered IM while ventilatory status is stabilized. Atropine may be repeated every 5–60 min until toxic symptoms appear (pulse 140/min) and continued for a minimum of 48 hr.

Adult: 1–2 g, repeated in 1 hr if muscle weakness unrelieved or as a continuous infusion at 500 mg/hr. *Pediatric:* 20–40 mg/kg/dose, may be repeated in 1 hr if muscle weakness unrelieved. With continued exposure/unrelieved symptoms additional doses may be given every 3–8 hr.

Anticholinesterase overdose (neostigmine, pyridostigmine, ambenonium)

Adult: 1 g followed by 250 mg increments every 5 minutes as indicated by symptom improvement/worsening.

CONTRAINDICATIONS/ PRECAUTIONS

Contraindicated in: Hypersensitivity to any component. **Use cautiously in:** Myasthenia gravis (may precipitate myasthenic crisis), renal impairment. **Pregnancy/Lactation:** No well-controlled trials to establish safety. Benefits must outweigh risks. **Pediatrics:** Safety and efficacy has not been established.

PREPARATION

Availability: 1 g emergency kit containing 20 mL sterile water injection, 20 mL syringe, needle, alcohol swab. Hospital package: (6) 20 mL vials containing 1 g pralidoxime without diluent/syringe. Survival

injection: (1) autoinjector containing 600 mg of drug in 2 mL. **Reconstitution:** Each gram is diluted with 20 mL sterile water for injection. **IV Infusion:** Further dilute prescribed dose in 100 mL of compatible IV solution if continuous infusion is required.

STABILITY/STORAGE

Vial: Store at room temperature. **Infusion:** Stable for 24 hr at room temperature.

ADMINISTRATION

General: Not to be administered by continuous/intermittent infusion if pulmonary edema is present. Begin administration within a few hours of poisoning if at all possible. **IV Push:** Give 1 g over 5 min. **Intermittent Infusion:** Prescribed dose to be administered over 15–30 min.

COMPATIBILITY/INCOMPATIBILITY

Data not available.

ADVERSE EFFECTS

CNS: Dizziness, drowsiness, headache. **Ophtho:** Blurred vision, diplopia, impaired accommodation. **CV:** Tachycardia. **Resp:** LARYNGOSPASM, hyperventilation. **GI:** Nausea. **MS:** Muscle rigors, muscle weakness, neuromuscular blockade. **Other:** Rapid IV injection can produce tachycardia, muscle rigidity, and transient neuromuscular blockade.

TOXICITY/OVERDOSE

Signs/Symptoms: Dizziness, headache, blurred vision, diplopia, impaired accommodation, nausea, slight tachycardia. **Treatment:** Mechanical ventilation and airway management. Supportive therapy

P

In the Adverse Effects section, <u>underline</u> indicates most frequent; CAPS indicates life threatening.

431

based on symptoms and emergency resuscitation as required.

DRUG INTERACTIONS
Aminophylline, phenothiazines, reserpine, succinylcholine: Should be avoided in organophosphate poisoning. **Barbiturates, narcotic analgesics, sedative/hypnotics:** Potentiates adverse effects.

NURSING CONSIDERATIONS
Assessment
General:
Continuous monitoring of all vital signs, ECG, respiratory rate, and blood pressure (recommended); intake/output ratio; hydration status; decontamination procedure.
Physical:
Cardiopulmonary status.
Lab Alterations:
Transient elevation of AST (SGOT), ALT (SGPT), CPK (can return to normal levels within 2 weeks).

Intervention/Rationale
Monitor vital signs continuously. ● Assess urinary output hourly. ● Assess lung fields periodically for pending development of pulmonary edema as evidenced by development of jugular venous distention, adventitious sounds, or changes in vital signs. ● If exposure to the skin has occurred clothing must be removed using rubber gloves, and hair and skin washed with sodium bicarbonate or alcohol as close to the time of exposure as possible. ● Notify Poison Control Center for complete information regarding specific effects of insecticide exposure.

Patient/Family Education
Review purpose of the medication and goal of the therapy. Review the need for exposure, clothing removal and destruction, as well as the requirement and rationale for the skin decontamination procedure.

PREDNISOLONE SODIUM PHOSPHATE
(pred-niss'-oh-lone so'-dee-um foss'-fate)
Trade Name(s): Hydeltrasal, Key-Pred SP
Classification(s): Synthetic glucocorticoid
Pregnancy Category: C

PHARMACODYNAMICS/KINETICS
Mechanism of Action: Decreases inflammation primarily by stabilizing leukocyte lysosomal membrane. Suppresses immune response, stimulates marrow production of WBCs, involved in protein, fat, and carbohydrate metabolism. **Onset of Action:** Rapid. **Peak Effect:** 1 hr. **Distribution:** Widely distributed throughout body. **Metabolism/Elimination:** Metabolized by liver and other tissues. Small amount excreted unchanged by the kidneys. Renal clearance is increased as plasma drug levels are increased. **Half-Life:** 115–212 min.

INDICATIONS/DOSAGE

Anti-inflammatory/ immunosuppressant
Adult: 4–60 mg/day dependent on disease being treated. *Pediatric:*

In the Adverse Effects section, <u>underline</u> indicates most frequent; CAPS indicates life threatening.

0.04–0.25 mg/kg one to two times daily.

CONTRAINDICATIONS/ PRECAUTIONS

Contraindicated in: Active infections, except for some types of meningitis, hypersensitivity. **Use cautiously in:** CHF, Cushing's syndrome, diabetes mellitus, emotional instability, GI ulceration, hepatitis, hypertension, myasthenia gravis, metastatic cancer, ocular herpes simplex, osteoporosis, psychotic tendencies, renal disease, tuberculosis. Crosses placenta. Distributed into breast milk. **Pregnancy/Lactation:** No well-controlled trials to establish safety. Benefits must outweigh risks. **Pediatrics:** Chronic use will prevent normal growth and development.

PREPARATION

Availability: 20 mg/mL in 2, 5, and 10 mL vials. **IV Infusion:** Further dilute prescribed dose in 50–1000 mL of compatible IV solution.

STABILITY/STORAGE

Vial: Store at room temperature. Protect from light. Heat labile, must not be autoclaved. **Infusion:** Stable for 24 hr at room temperature.

ADMINISTRATION

IV Push: Single dose is administered over 1 to several minutes at a rate of < 10 mg/min. **Intermittent/Continuous Infusion:** Administer at physician prescribed rate within 24 hr from preparation of admixture.

COMPATIBILITY

Y-site: Heparin, hydrocortisone sodium succinate, potassium chloride, vitamin B with C.

ADVERSE EFFECTS

CNS: Convulsions, depression, euphoria, headache, personality changes, psychoses, restlessness. *Children:* Increased intracranial pressure. **Ophtho:** Cataracts, exophthalmos, glaucoma, increased intraocular pressure. **CV:** Hypertension, cardiac dysrhythmias, CHF. **GI:** Abdominal distention, anorexia, increased appetite, nausea, pancreatitis, ulceration, vomiting. **MS:** Aseptic necrosis of the joints, muscle pain, muscle wasting, osteoporosis, spontaneous fractures. **Derm:** Acne, decreased wound healing, ecchymoses, capillary fragility, hirsutism, hyperpigmentation, impaired wound healing, petechiae. **Endo:** Adrenal suppression, amenorrhea, hyperglycemia, negative nitrogen balance due to catabolism. **Fld/Lytes:** Hypernatremia, hypokalemia, hypokalemic alkalosis, fluid retention (large doses, long-term use). **Hypersens:** Anaphylactoid reactions. **Metab:** Weight loss, weight gain. **Other:** Cushingoid appearance (moon face, buffalo hump), increased susceptibility to infection, masking of signs/symptoms of infection.

TOXICITY/OVERDOSE

Signs/Symptoms: Cushingoid syndrome, decreased spermatazoa, euphoria, fat emboli, fluid/electrolyte imbalance, increased intracranial pressure, menstrual irregularities, protein catabolism with negative nitrogen balance, spontaneous fractures, suppression of growth. **Treatment:** Notify physician with symptom manifestations. Symptomatic/supportive treatment of any side effects.

P

In the Adverse Effects section, <u>underline</u> indicates most frequent; CAPS indicates life threatening.

433

DRUG INTERACTIONS

Alcohol, aspirin, nonsteroidal anti-inflammatory agents: Increase risk of adverse GI effects. **Amphotericin B, diuretics, mezlocillin, piperacillin, ticarcillin:** Increases hypokalemic effects. **Attenuated-virus vaccines:** Enhanced virus replication with potential for severe reactions. **Barbiturates, phenytoin, rifampin:** Decreases corticosteroid effect. **Insulin, oral hypoglycemic agents:** May require increased dosages of prednisolone.

NURSING CONSIDERATIONS

Assessment

General:
Vital signs, intake/output ratio, baseline/daily weight.

Physical:
Cardiopulmonary status, endocrine status, infectious disease status, GI tract.

Lab Alterations:
Evaluate serum calcium, electrolytes, serum, and urine glucose as drug may cause hyperglycemia and electrolyte disturbances. Decreases WBC, potassium, calcium, protein-bound iodine, and thyroxine. Increases serum glucose, sodium, cholesterol, and lipids.

Intervention/Rationale

If drug is ordered daily, administer prior to 9 AM in order to correspond with the body's normal secretion of cortisol. ● Prior to and throughout course of therapy assess patient for signs/symptoms of adrenal insufficiency (hypoglycemia, weight loss, nausea, vomiting, anorexia, lethargy, confusion, and restlessness). ● Monitor intake/output ratio and daily weights for evidence of fluid retention. Observe for

edema and other signs of increased preload. ● May mask usual signs/symptoms of developing infections. ● Observe growth/development patterns for children receiving drug. ● Hematest all stools/vomitus and report positive findings immediately.

Patient/Family Education

Drug may mask signs/symptoms of infection; avoid people with contagious diseases and notify physician of possible infections. Report unusual swelling, weight gain, tiredness, bone pain, bruising, nonhealing wounds, or behavioral changes. Avoid vaccinations without notification and approval of primary physician.

PROCAINAMIDE

(proe-kane′-a-mide)
Trade Name(s): Pronestyl
Classification(s): Antiarrhythmic, Type IA
Pregnancy Category: C

PHARMACODYNAMICS/KINETICS

Mechanism of Action: Decreases membrane permeability of the cell and prevents loss of sodium and potassium ions. Depresses the excitability of cardiac muscle to electrical stimulation and slows the conduction pathway. **Onset of Action:** Immediate. **Peak Effect:** 10–25 min. **Duration of Action:** 3–4 hr. **Therapeutic Serum Level:** 3–10 mcg/mL. **Distribution:** Distributed throughout CSF, liver, spleen, kidneys, lung, muscle, brain, and heart. 14%–23% bound to plasma protein. **Metabolism/Elimination:** Metabolized by

In the Adverse Effects section, <u>underline</u> indicates most frequent; CAPS indicates life threatening.

liver to n-acetylprocainamide (NAPA), an active antiarrhythmic compound. 40%–70% excreted in the urine as unchanged drug. NAPA entirely eliminated by the kidneys. **Half-Life:** 2.5–4.7 hr. NAPA: 6 hr. Prolonged in renal impairment.

INDICATIONS/DOSAGE

Dysrhythmia control

Adult:
Loading Dose: 50–100 mg every 5 min until dysrhythmia is controlled, adverse effects occur, or until a total of 500 mg has been administered, after which a 10 min wait is recommended to allow drug to be distributed before additional doses are given. Range: 200–900 mg generally followed by a maintenance infusion. **Maintenance Dose:** Continuous infusion is to be administered at 1–6 mg/min. Alternatively, a loading dose IV infusion of 500–600 mg may be administered at a constant rate. Followed by a continuous IV infusion of 1–6 mg/min.

Pediatric:
Loading Dose: 2–5 mg/kg not to exceed 100 mg, repeated at intervals of 10–30 min. Not to exceed a **total** of 30 mg/kg/24 hr. **Maintenance Dose:** Followed by a maintenance infusion of 0.02–0.08 mg/kg/min.

CONTRAINDICATIONS/ PRECAUTIONS

Contraindicated in: Complete A-V heart block, second and third degree A-V block, hypersensitivity, systemic lupus erythematosus, Torsades de Pointes. **Use cautiously in:** CHF, myasthenia gravis, patients with marked disturbances of AV conduction or severe cardiac glycoside intoxication, preexisting bone marrow depression or cytopenia, renal and/or hepatic disease. **Pregnancy/Lactation:** No well-controlled trials to establish safety. Benefits must outweigh risks. Crosses placenta. Distributed into breast milk. **Pediatrics:** Safety and efficacy not clearly established.

PREPARATION

Availability: 100 and 500 mg/mL in 2 and 10 mL vials. **Syringe:** Dilute each 100 mg with 10 mL sterile water for injection or compatible IV solution. **IV Infusion:** Further dilute prescribed dose in 50–500 mL compatible IV fluid. Slightly yellow color of solution does not affect potency of drug.

STABILITY/STORAGE

Vial: Store at room temperature. Refrigeration retards oxidation and the associated development of color. **Infusion:** Stable for 24 hr at room temperature after admixture preparation.

ADMINISTRATION

General: Limit IV administration for treatment of serious dysrhythmias in settings capable of continuous ECG and vital sign monitoring. **IV Push:** Usual dose of 20 mg or less over 1 minute. Up to 50 mg may be given direct IV push over 1 minute with **extreme** caution. **Intermittent Infusion: Loading Dose IV Infusion:** Over 30–60 min. **Continuous Infusion: Maintenance Infusion:** Rate of 1–6 mg/min. Use of IV infusion device recommended for safety and accuracy.

P

In the Adverse Effects section, underline indicates most frequent; CAPS indicates life threatening.

COMPATIBILITY
Solution: Sodium chloride solutions, sterile water for injection. **Y-site:** Amiodarone, amrinone, famotidine, heparin, hydrocortisone sodium succinate, potassium chloride, ranitidine, vitamin B complex with C.

INCOMPATIBILITY
Solution: Dextrose solutions (10%–15% loss of drug in 24 hr).

ADVERSE EFFECTS
CNS: SEIZURES, hallucinations, giddiness, mental confusion. **CV:** Hypotension, P-R interval prolongation, VENTRICULAR ASYSTOLE, VENTRICULAR FIBRILLATION, VENTRICULAR TACHYCARDIA. **GI:** Anorexia, bitter taste, nausea, vomiting. **MS:** Joint swelling or pain, weakness. **Derm:** Bruising. **Heme:** AGRANULOCYTOSIS, bleeding, leukopenia, lupus erythematosus-like symptoms, thrombocytopenia. **Hypersens:** Angioneurotic edema, eosinophilia, skin rash. **Other:** Chills, fever, flushing.

TOXICITY/OVERDOSE
Signs/Symptoms: Hypotension, widening of the QRS complex, junctional tachycardia, intraventricular conduction delay, oliguria, lethargy, confusion, nausea, vomiting. **Treatment:** Symptomatic/supportive treatment with continuous ECG and blood pressure monitoring, vasopressor therapy and fluid resuscitation. If toxicity/overdose is severe, hemodialysis may be required. Ventricular pacing may be considered as a prophylactic measure in case of progressing heart block.

DRUG INTERACTIONS
Alcohol: Increases hepatic metabolism of drug. **Anticholinergics, antihypertensive agents, muscle relaxants, neuromuscular blocking agents:** Potentiate additional anticholinergic effects. **Anticholinesterases (neostigmine):** Partial antagonism of therapeutic effects. **Cimetidine:** Reduces renal clearance of procainamide. **Digoxin, quinidine:** Requires lower dosages of both drugs. **Lidocaine:** Additive neurological toxicity (i.e., confusion, seizures). **Other antihypertensives, thiazide diuretics:** May potentiate hypotensive effects.

NURSING CONSIDERATIONS
Assessment
General:
Vital signs, ECG monitoring (recommended), intake/output ratio, baseline/daily weights.
Physical:
Cardiovascular status, neurologic status.
Lab Alterations:
Monitor CBC every 2 weeks during therapy, assess for decreased leukocytes, neutrophils, and platelets. Monitor serum procainamide and NAPA levels periodically. AST (SGOT), ALT (SGPT), LDH, alkaline phosphatase and bilirubin increases. Coombs' test may be positive.

Intervention/Rationale
Blood pressure and ECG should be monitored continuously and the rate of drug administration adjusted accordingly. ● Maintain patient in supine position in order to avoid orthostatic fluctuations. ● Observe for neurological changes such as con-

fusion, drowsiness, dizziness, or seizures. ● Assess fluid status for signs of decreased urination.

Patient/Family Education
Drug may cause dizziness; avoid activities requiring mental alertness until medication response has been determined. Notify physician if soreness of the mouth, throat, or gums, unexplained fever, symptoms of upper respiratory infection, or joint pain/stiffness occurs. Review the goal of drug therapy and the need for cardiac monitoring and frequent or continuous blood pressure assessment.

PROCHLORPERAZINE
(proe-klor-pair'-a-zeen)
Trade Name(s): Compazine, Stemetil ✦
Classification(s): Antiemetic, phenothiazine
Pregnancy Category: Unknown.

PHARMACODYNAMICS/KINETICS
Mechanism of Action: Precise mechanism of action is unknown. Inhibits vomiting by directly affecting the medullary chemoreceptor trigger zone and blocking dopamine receptors. **Onset of Action:** Rapid. **Duration of Action:** 3–4 hr. **Distribution:** Widely distributed throughout body. Increased concentrations in the CNS. 91%–99% bound to plasma proteins. **Metabolism/Elimination:** Metabolized by the liver and GI mucosa. 50% excreted via the kidneys. 50% eliminated via enterohepatic circulation. < 1% excreted as unchanged drug. **Half-Life:** 10–20 hr.

INDICATIONS/DOSAGE

Antiemetic
Adult: 5–10 mg. May be repeated once in 1–2 if necessary for severe nausea/vomiting. **Maximum dose:** 40 mg/24 hr.

Chemotherapy antiemetic
Adult: 20 mg 30 min before and 3 hr after completion of chemotherapy dosage.

Adult surgery/control of nausea and vomiting
Adult: < 40 mg/24 hr.

CONTRAINDICATIONS/ PRECAUTIONS
Contraindicated in: Bone marrow depression, cross-sensitivity with other phenothiazines, hypersensitivity to bisulfites/benzyl alcohol, narrow angle glaucoma, severe liver/cardiac disease. **Use cautiously in:** Central nervous system tumors, diabetes mellitus, elderly/debilitated, epilepsy, intestinal obstruction, prostatic hypertrophy, respiratory distress. **Pregnancy/Lactation:** No well-controlled trials to establish safety. Benefits must outweigh risks. Crosses the placenta. **Pediatrics:** Safety and efficacy for children < 2 years of age or weighing < 9 kg has not been established. Should be avoided in children/adolescents with suspected Reye's syndrome.

PREPARATION
Availability: 5 mg/mL in 2 mL amps, 2 mL disposable syringes, 10 mL multidose vials and 2 and 10 mL vials. **Syringe:** Dilute each 1 mg with 1 mL compatible IV solution. **Infusion:** Further dilute prescribed dose

In the Adverse Effects section, underline indicates most frequent; CAPS indicates life threatening.

437

in not less than 1 L compatible IV solution.

STABILITY/STORAGE
Vial: Store at room temperature in tight, light-resistant containers. **Infusion:** Prepare just prior to use.

ADMINISTRATION
General: Hypotension can occur if given IV push or by rapid infusion. **IV Push:** Do not use bolus injection. Administer diluted drug at < 5 mg/min, not to exceed 10 mg in a single dose. **Intermittent Infusion:** Infuse at physician prescribed rate. Use limited to surgical procedures/anesthesia induction. For surgical use, add 15–30 min prior to anesthesia induction.

COMPATIBILITY
Solution: Dextrose solutions, lactated Ringer's, Ringer's injection, sodium chloride solutions. **Syringe:** Atropine, butorphanol, chlorpromazine, cimetidine, diphenhydramine, droperidol, fentanyl, glycopyrrolate, meperidine, morphine, nalbuphine, ondansetron, pentazocine, perphenazine, promethazine, ranitidine, scopolamine.

INCOMPATIBILITY
Syringe: Dimenhydrinate, midazolam, pentobarbital, thiopental. **Y-site:** Foscarnet.

ADVERSE EFFECTS
CNS: NEUROLEPTIC MALIGNANT SYNDROME, extrapyramidal reactions, hallucinations, hyperthermia, insomnia, sedation, tardive dyskinesia. **Ophtho:** Blurred vision, dry eyes. **CV:** CARDIAC ARREST, CIRCULATORY COLLAPSE, ECG changes, bradycardia, hyperten-

sion, hypotension, postural hypotension, pulmonary edema, syncope, tachycardia. **GI:** Anorexia, constipation, dry mouth, hepatitis, paralytic ileus. **GU:** Pink/reddish-brown discoloration of urine, urinary retention. **Derm:** Pigment changes, photosensitivity. **Endo:** Galactorrhea. **Heme:** AGRANULOCYTOSIS, eosinophilia, leukopenia. **Hypersens:** Allergic reactions, jaundice, rash.

TOXICITY/OVERDOSE
Signs/Symptoms: Blurred vision, cardiac arrest, dizziness, extrapyramidal symptoms, excitement, hypotension, spastic movements, tightness of the throat, tongue discoloration, tongue protrusion, overdosage may result in convulsions, hallucinations, and possibly death. **Treatment:** Discontinue the drug. Treat symptomatically and supportively based on symptom manifestation. Treat extrapyramidal effects with diphenhydramine or benztropine. Epinephrine is contraindicated for hypotension, analeptics (such as doxapram) are to be avoided when treating respiratory depression and unconsciousness. Resuscitate as required.

DRUG INTERACTIONS
Anticholinergics, antidepressants, antiparkinson agents: Increased anticholinergic activity and Parkinson symptoms. **Antihypertensives:** Additive hypotension. **Barbiturates:** Decrease phenothiazine effect. **Epinephrine:** Prochlorperazine blocks alpha-adrenergic receptors causing beta activity to predominate (increased heart rate, vasodilation). **Lithium:** Acute encephalopathy. **Poly-**

In the Adverse Effects section, <u>underline</u> indicates most frequent; CAPS indicates life threatening.

peptide antibiotics: May exacerbate neuromuscular respiratory depression.

NURSING CONSIDERATIONS

Assessment
General:
Vital signs, hypersensitivity reactions.
Physical:
Neuromuscular status, hematopoietic system.
Lab Alterations:
Monitor for decreased WBC, agranulocytosis, possible false-positive or false-negative pregnancy tests, false-positive urine bilirubin test, increased serum prolactin levels.

Intervention/Rationale
Monitor blood pressure, heart rate, and respiratory rate throughout course of dosage adjustment. ● Assess for demonstration of extrapyramidal side effects (muscle spasms and twisting motions, restlessness, pseudoparkinsonism tremors, shuffling gait, drooling). ● To prevent contact dermatitis, avoid getting concentrate or injection solution on hands or clothing. ● Monitor patient for presence of malignant neuroleptic syndrome (fever, respiratory distress, tachycardia, convulsions, hypertension or hypotension, pallor, or tiredness). ● Assess for level of sedation or relief of nausea/vomiting following administration. ● Assess for orthostatic changes when administering via IV route.

Patient/Family Education
Seek assistance or change positions slowly and gradually during and after administration of the drug. Review the need for close monitoring of various blood tests to ascertain and correct adverse effects of the drug. May cause drowsiness; avoid all activities requiring mental alertness until effects of drug can be assessed. Avoid alcohol. Urine may turn a pink to reddish/brown color.

PROMETHAZINE
(proe-meth′-a-zeen)
Trade Name(s): Anergan, Phenazine, Phenergan, Prorex, Prothazine, V-Gan
Classification(s): Antihistamine, antiemetic, sedative/hypnotic
Pregnancy Category: C

PHARMACODYNAMICS/KINETICS
Mechanism of Action: Competitively antagonizes histamine at receptor sites. Inhibits vomiting by affecting the medullary chemoreceptor trigger zone directly. **Onset of Action:** Rapid. **Duration of Action:** 4–6 hr. **Distribution:** Widely distributed throughout the body. Crosses blood–brain barrier. Up to 93% protein bound. **Metabolism/Elimination:** Metabolized by the liver. Metabolites and small amounts of unchanged drug excreted via kidneys. **Half-Life:** 7–15 hr.

INDICATIONS/DOSAGE

Allergic manifestations
Adult: 25 mg. May repeat in 2 hr if symptoms not controlled.

Labor
Adult: 50 mg in the early stages of labor. 25–75 mg may be combined with decreased doses of narcotics.

In the Adverse Effects section, <u>underline</u> indicates most frequent; CAPS indicates life threatening.

439

May be repeated once or twice at 4 hr intervals.

Sedation

Adult: 25–50 mg. Repeat in 4–6 hr as needed. *Pediatric:* 12.5–25.0 mg or 0.5–1.1 mg/kg.

Treatment of acute nausea/vomiting, motion sickness; adjunct to narcotic analgesic in control of postoperative pain

Adult: 12.5–25.0 mg. Should not be administered more frequently than every 4–6 hr. *Pediatric:* 1 mg/kg every 4–6 hr. Not to exceed 50% of the adult dose.

CONTRAINDICATIONS/PRECAUTIONS

Contraindicated in: Bladder neck obstruction, bone marrow depression, coma, hypersensitivity, jaundice, narrow angle glaucoma, prostatic hypertrophy, severe depression. **Use cautiously in:** Children, debilitated, elderly, epilepsy, hypotension. **Pregnancy/Lactation:** Contraindicated in lactation and pregnancy (except for the early stages of labor when labor has clearly been established in a regular progressive pattern). If used within the 2 weeks prior to delivery, may inhibit platelet function in the newborn. **Pediatrics:** Safety and efficacy for children < 2 years has not been established. May cause paradoxical excitation. Use with extreme caution in children with history of sleep apnea, a family history of sudden infant death syndrome (SIDS) or in the presence of Reye's syndrome.

PREPARATION

Availability: 25 mg/mL in 1 mL amps and 10 mL vials. **Syringe:** May dilute each 25 mg with 9 mL sodium chloride. **Never exceed** a final concentration of 25 mg/mL.

STABILITY/STORAGE

Vial: Store at room temperature. Multidose vials may be refrigerated. Protect from light.

ADMINISTRATION

General: Ampule must state "**for IV use**." Do not use if precipitate present. **IV Push:** Not to exceed 25 mg/min.

COMPATIBILITY

Solution: Dextrose solutions, lactated Ringer's, Ringer's injection, sodium chloride solutions. **Syringe:** Atropine, butorphanol, chlorpromazine, cimetidine, diphenhydramine, droperidol, fentanyl, glycopyrrolate, hydromorphone, meperidine, metoclopramide, midazolam, morphine, ranitidine, scopolamine. **Y-site:** Ondansetron.

INCOMPATIBILITY

Syringe: Dimenhydrinate, heparin, phenobarbital, thiopental. **Y-site:** Cefoperazone, foscarnet, heparin.

ADVERSE EFFECTS

CNS: Extrapyramidal reactions, confusion, disorientation, dizziness, excess sedation, hyperexcitability. **Ophtho:** Blurred vision, diplopia. **CV:** Hypertension, hypotension, tachycardia. **GI:** Constipation, dryness of mouth, hepatitis. **MS:** Spastic movements of upper extremities. **Derm:** Photosensitivity. **Hypersens:** Hypersensitivity reactions, rash.

TOXICITY/OVERDOSE

Signs/Symptoms: Cardiac arrest, coma, convulsions, sedation, respiratory depression or deep sleep.

In the Adverse Effects section, underline indicates most frequent; CAPS indicates life threatening.

P

Treatment: Discontinue drug, notify physician. Treatment is symptomatic with fluid resuscitation and vasopressors as required. Epinephrine should not be used as it may decrease blood pressure even further. Hemodialysis is generally not beneficial.

DRUG INTERACTIONS
Alcohol, antianxiety agents, antihistamines, narcotic analgesics, sedative/hypnotics: Additive CNS depression. **Antihistamines, antidepressants, atropine, disopyramide, haloperidol, phenothiazines, quinidine:** Additive anticholinergic effects.

NURSING CONSIDERATIONS
Assessment
General:
Vital signs.
Physical:
GI tract, neurologic/neuromuscular status.
Lab Alterations:
May yield false-positive or false-negative pregnancy tests. May cause false-positive results in allergen skin testing; discontinue at least 72 hr prior to test. Evaluate and follow trend of CBC in order to distinguish development of blood dyscrasias.

Intervention/Rationale
Monitor blood pressure, heart rate, and respiratory rate throughout IV administration. Observe for orthostatic changes. ● Evaluate level of sedation following drug administration. ● If used for antiemetic effect, assess for symptomatic relief of nausea and vomiting. ● Evaluate patient for development of extrapyramidal manifestations (muscle spasms, twisting motions), pseudoparkinson symptoms (drooling, shuffling gait); notify physician. ● Assess need to decrease narcotic/barbiturate dosage by 25%–50% when using concomitantly with promethazine.

Patient/Family Education
May cause drowsiness; avoid engaging in activities requiring mental alertness. Following or during therapy, use sunscreen and cover-up clothing when out of doors in order to prevent photosensitivity reaction of exposed skin. Change positions slowly and gradually and seek assistance with ambulatory activities in order to prevent orthostatic changes. Avoid alcohol and other CNS depressants while taking this drug in order to prevent additional depressant effects. Use of sugarless gum, hard candy, ice chips, or frequent mouth rinses may aid in relieving dry mouth.

PROPIOMAZINE
(proe-pee-oh′-mah-zeen)
Trade Name(s): Largon
Classification(s): Antihistamine, phenothiazine, sedative
Pregnancy Category: C

PHARMACODYNAMICS/KINETICS
Mechanism of Action: Competitively antagonizes histamine at the H-1 receptor site. **Onset of Action:** Rapid. **Metabolism/Elimination:** Extensively metabolized by the liver. **Half-Life:** 7.7 hr.

In the Adverse Effects section, underline indicates most frequent; CAPS indicates life threatening.

441

INDICATIONS/DOSAGE

Obstetrics

Adult: 20–40 mg with 25–75 mg meperidine when labor is definitely established.

Preoperative sedation

Adult: 20–40 mg with 50 mg meperidine. *Pediatric < 27 kg:* 0.55–1.1 mg/kg.

Postoperative sedation

Adult: 10–40 mg alone or in conjunction with 25%–50% of the usual dose of narcotic, every 3–4 hr as required. *Pediatric:* < 27 kg: 0.55–1.1 mg/kg.

Sedation during surgery with local nerve block or spinal

Adult: 10–20 mg.

CONTRAINDICATIONS/ PRECAUTIONS

Contraindicated in: Bone marrow depression, coma, first trimester pregnancy, hypersensitivity, severely depressed states. **Use cautiously in:** Cerebral arteriosclerosis, coronary artery disease, epilepsy, heat exhaustion, hypertension, liver disease, respiratory disorders. **Pregnancy/Lactation:** No well-controlled trials to establish safety. Benefits must outweigh risks.

PREPARATION

Availability: 20 mg/mL in 1 and 2 mL amps, 1 mL Tubex. **Syringe:** Dilute each 20 mg with 9 mL sodium chloride or compatible IV solution.

STABILITY/STORAGE

Vial: Store at room temperature. Protect from light.

ADMINISTRATION

General: Inject IV only into vessels previously undamaged by multiple injections or vascular trauma. Do not allow drug extravasation as severe chemical irritation may result. **IV Push:** Administer each 10 mg or less over 1 min.

COMPATIBILITY

Syringe: Atropine, glycopyrrolate, pentazocine.

INCOMPATIBILITY

Y-site: Barbiturates.

ADVERSE EFFECTS

CNS: Dizziness, drowsiness, extrapyramidal effects. **CV:** Hypotension, mildly elevated blood pressure, tachycardia. **GI:** Dry mouth. **Other:** Thrombophlebitis.

TOXICITY/OVERDOSE

Signs/Symptoms: Extension of adverse effects, extrapyramidal effects. **Treatment:** Discontinue drug if side effects are severe; notify physician. Treat supportively/symptomatically with fluid resuscitation and vasopressor therapy if hypotensive episode occurs. Extrapyramidal effects can be treated with benztropine mesylate or diphenhydramine. Epinephrine is contraindicated for treatment of hypotension.

DRUG INTERACTIONS

Alcohol, anesthetics, barbiturates, CNS depressants, narcotics: Increased CNS depression. **Anticholinergics, antihistamines, antihypertensives, hypnotics, insulin, MAO inhibitors, muscle relaxants, oral hypoglycemics, phenytoin, propra-**

In the Adverse Effects section, <u>underline</u> indicates most frequent; CAPS indicates life threatening.

nolol, rauwolfia alkaloids: May cause additive effects and potentiation of side effects.

NURSING CONSIDERATIONS

Assessment
General:
Vital signs, pain/anxiety management.
Physical:
Neurologic status.

Intervention/Rationale
Monitor blood pressure, heart rate, and respiratory rate and status before administration and between dosages. ● Evaluate level of sedation following drug administration to assess effectiveness of drug and dosage. ● Evaluate patient for development of extrapyramidal manifestations (muscle spasms, twisting motions), pseudoparkinson symptoms (drooling, shuffling gait); notify physician.

Patient/Family Education
May produce drowsiness or dizziness; avoid activities requiring mental alertness. Change positions slowly and gradually to avoid orthostatic changes.

PROPOFOL
(proe'-pah-fal)
Trade Name(s): Diprivan
Classification(s): Anesthetic agent, sedative/hypnotic
Pregnancy Category: B

PHARMACODYNAMICS/KINETICS
Mechanism of Action: Unknown. **Onset of Action:** 40 sec. **Duration of Action:** 1–3 min. **Distribution:** Rapidly and extensively distributed throughout the body. **Metabolism/Elimination:** Metabolized by conjugation in the liver. Eliminated by the kidneys. **Half-Life:** 300–700 min.

INDICATIONS/DOSAGE

Induction
Adult: 2.0–2.5 mg/kg. Usually 40 mg every 10 seconds until induction onset.

Maintenance Infusion: 0.1–0.2 mg/kg/min. **Intermittent Bolus:** Increments 25–50 mg as required by condition and response.

Elderly/debilitated/hypovolemic and/or A.S.A. III or IV patient for anesthesia induction
Adult: (Reduce dosage by approximately 50%.) 1.0–1.5 mg/kg. Usually 20 mg every 10 sec until induction onset according to condition and response.

CONTRAINDICATIONS/PRECAUTIONS
Contraindicated in: Increased intracranial pressure, impaired cerebral circulation, hypersensitivity, whenever general anesthesia is contraindicated. **Use cautiously in:** A.S.A. Class III or IV, debilitated/elderly, hypovolemia. **Pregnancy/Lactation:** No well-controlled trials to establish safety. Benefits must outweigh risks. **Pediatrics:** Safety and efficacy not established.

PREPARATION
Availability: 10 mg/mL in 20 mL amps. **Syringe/Infusion:** Shake vial well before using. Dilute to a con-

P

In the Adverse Effects section, underline indicates most frequent;
CAPS indicates life threatening.

443

centration of less than 2 mg/mL with compatible IV solution.

STABILITY/STORAGE
Vial: Store at room temperature. Refrigeration not recommended. Protect from light. **Infusion:** Stable in glass bottles at room temperature for 8 hr.

ADMINISTRATION
General: When used with general anesthesia for maintenance, supplementation with IV analgesic agents is usually required. Muscle relaxants may also be administered concomitantly. Should be administered only by persons trained in the administration of general anesthesia. Facilities for maintenance of a patent airway, artificial ventilation, and oxygen enrichment as well as circulatory resuscitation must be readily available. Prepare for administration under the strictest of aseptic techniques. Improper preparation/administration have been reported to be associated with septic epidodes. **IV Push:** Single dose every 10 sec until onset of induction is evident. **Intermittent Infusion:** Infuse according to conditions and responses of the patient.

COMPATIBILITY
Solution: Dextrose solutions, lactated Ringer's, Ringer's injection.

ADVERSE EFFECTS
CNS: Headache, dizziness. **CV:** Bradycardia, hypotension, hypertension. **Resp:** Apnea on induction, BRONCHOSPASM, cough. **GI:** Abdominal cramping, nausea, vomiting. **MS:** Jerking, twitching, thrashing, bucking clonic/myoclonic movements. **Other:** Fever, flushing, hiccough, transient local pain may occur during IV injection, tingling, numbness, coldness.

TOXICITY/OVERDOSE
Signs/Symptoms: Overdose is likely to cause cardiorespiratory depression. **Treatment:** Discontinue administration of drug. Treat respiratory depression with artificial ventilation with oxygen, treat cardiovascular depression with vasopressors and anticholinergics.

DRUG INTERACTIONS
CNS depressants, hypnotics, inhalation anesthesia, narcotics, sedatives: Increased CNS depression effects.

NURSING CONSIDERATIONS
Assessment
General:
Vital signs, continuous ECG/respiratory monitoring (recommended), airway management.
Physical:
Cardiopulmonary status.

Intervention/Rationale
Usage should be restricted to personnel who are trained in emergency intubation and airway management. ● Evaluate blood pressure, heart rate, and respiratory rate prior to, throughout, and following administration.

Patient/Family Education
Review the ultimate goal or purpose of the drug.

PROPRANOLOL
(proe-pran'-oh-lole)
Trade Name(s): Inderal
Classification(s): Beta-adrenergic blocking agent, antiarrhythmic, Type II
Pregnancy Category: C

In the Adverse Effects section, <u>underline</u> indicates most frequent; CAPS indicates life threatening.

PHARMACODYNAMICS/KINETICS

Mechanism of Action: Beta-adrenergic blocking agent that inhibits the stimulation of beta-1 (myocardial) and beta-2 (pulmonary, vascular, uterine) receptor sites resulting in decreased oxygen demand by blocking catecholamine induced elevations in heart rate and blood pressure and the force of myocardial contraction. Depresses renin secretion and prevents vasodilation of cerebral arteries. **Onset of Action:** Immediate. **Peak Effect:** 1 min. **Duration of Action:** 4–6 hr. **Distribution:** Widely distributed throughout the body. Crosses blood–brain barrier. 90% bound to plasma protein. **Metabolism/Elimination:** Almost completely metabolized by the liver. < 1% excreted unchanged via kidneys. **Half-Life:** 3.4–6.0 hr.

INDICATIONS/DOSAGE

Treatment of dysrhythmia

Adult: 0.5–3.0 mg administered at 1 mg increments. If no change in rhythm for at least 2 min following initial dose, cycle may be repeated one time. No further drug may be given by any route for a minimum of 4 hr.

CONTRAINDICATIONS/ PRECAUTIONS

Contraindicated in: Allergic rhinitis, asthma, bronchospasm, cardiogenic shock, diabetes mellitus, during ethyl ether anesthesia, heart block > first degree, sinus bradycardia. **Use cautiously in:** CHF, concomitant antihypertensive agents, pheochromocytoma (hazardous to use unless alpha-adrenergic drug is already being used as uncontrolled hypertension could result), respiratory disease, Wolff-Parkinson-White syndrome (may cause severe bradycardia). **Pregnancy/Lactation:** No well-controlled trials to establish safety. Avoid use during the first trimester, use lowest possible dose thereafter if absolutely required. Discontinue 2–3 days prior to delivery if safe. Excreted in breast milk in very low concentrations. **Pediatrics:** Safety and efficacy not established. IV administration not recommended.

PREPARATION

Availability: 1 mg in 1 mL ampules. **Syringe:** Dilution of 1 mg with 9 mL sodium chloride or compatible IV solution.

STABILITY/STORAGE

Vial: Store at room temperature. Protect from light.

ADMINISTRATION

General: Reserve IV administration for life-threatening dysrhythmias or those occurring under anesthesia. **IV Push:** Diluted drug of 1 mg over 10–15 minutes in 0.1–0.2 mg increments.

COMPATIBILITY

Solution: Dextrose solutions, lactated Ringer's, Ringer's injection, sodium chloride solutions. **Syringe:** Benzquinamide, milrinone, potassium chloride, vitamin B complex with C. **Y-site:** Heparin, hydrocortisone, milrinone.

INCOMPATIBILITY

Y-site: Diazoxide.

In the Adverse Effects section, <u>underline</u> indicates most frequent; CAPS indicates life threatening.

ADVERSE EFFECTS

CNS: Confusion, depression, dizziness, drowsiness, fatigue, insomnia, memory loss, mental changes, paresthesia of the hands. **Ophtho:** Blurred vision, visual disturbances. **CV:** BRADYCARDIA, CARDIAC STANDSTILL, PULMONARY EDEMA, chest pain, CHF, edema, hypotension, syncopal attacks, varying degrees of A-V heart block, vertigo. **Resp:** BRONCHOSPASM, LARYNGOSPASM, respiratory distress. **GI:** Abdominal discomfort, constipation, diarrhea, dry mouth, gastric pain, vomiting. **GU:** Dysuria, impotence or decreased libido, nocturia, urinary retention, urinary frequency. **Derm:** Peripheral skin necrosis, skin irritation. **Endo:** Hyperglycemia, hypoglycemia, unstable diabetes mellitus. **Heme:** AGRANULOCYTOSIS, thrombocytopenia purpura. **Hypersens:** ANAPHYLAXIS, pharyngitis, pruritus, rash. **Other:** Facial swelling.

TOXICITY/OVERDOSE

Signs/Symptoms: Bradycardia, hypotension, CHF, cardiogenic shock, intraventricular conduction disturbances, atrioventricular block, pulmonary edema, tachycardia, decreased consciousness, bronchospasm, hypoglycemia, hyperkalemia. **Treatment:** Discontinue drug for manifestation of any side effects. If symptomatic, place patient in a supine position with legs higher than heart level in order to improve blood flow to the brain. Effects can be reversed with dopamine, isoproterenol, or levarterenol. Atropine sulfate can be used to treat bradycardia; cardiac failure can be treated with digoxin and diuretics; hypotension can be treated with epinephrine. Aminophylline may be administered with bronchospasm. Treat other symptoms as needed; resuscitate if required. Temporary pacemaker may be needed to correct heart block.

DRUG INTERACTIONS

Haloperidol: Concomitant use results in severe hypotension. **Lidocaine:** Increased CNS effects with concomitant use. **Nonsteroidal anti-inflammatory agents, salicylates, smoking, sympathomimetics, thyroid hormones:** Decreased beta-adrenergic blocking effects. **Phenobarbital, quinidine, rifampin:** Increased beta-adrenergic blocking effects.

NURSING CONSIDERATIONS

Assessment

General:
Vital signs, continuous ECG/blood pressure monitoring, hemodynamic monitoring (recommended), intake/output ratio, baseline/daily weight.

Physical:
Cardiopulmonary status.

Lab Alterations:
Assess serum glucose levels, especially for known diabetics; observe for the more obscure signs of hypoglycemia. May produce hypoglycemia and interfere with glucose or insulin tolerance tests. May elevate blood urea levels in patients with severe heart disease and impaired renal function. Known to interfere with glaucoma screening test due to false decrease in intraocular pressure. Follow serial chest x-rays for development of symptoms of pulmonary edema.

In the Adverse Effects section, <u>underline</u> indicates most frequent; CAPS indicates life threatening.

Intervention/Rationale
Continuous ECG and blood pressure monitoring is required during IV administration. Monitoring of PWP and CVP is recommended in some patients. ● Discontinue IV administration of drug when a rhythm change is noted. Wait to note the full effect of the drug before additional doses are given. ● When dosage reduction is planned, it should be done gradually in order to avoid rebound angina, MI, or ventricular dysrhythmias. Immediate access to transvenous pacing may be required when administering drug via IV route for treatment of dysrhythmias.

Patient/Family Education
Notify medical personnel if difficulty in breathing occurs, night cough, or swelling or the feeling of tightness of the extremities. Take and record pulse rate; notify physician if slow pulse, dizziness, lightheadedness, confusion, depression, skin rash, fever, sore throat, or unusual bruising or bleeding occurs.

PROTAMINE
(proe´-ta-meen)
Classification(s): Heparin antagonist
Pregnancy Category: C

PHARMACODYNAMICS/KINETICS
Mechanism of Action: Antagonizes the effects of heparin by forming a stable complex. Weak anticoagulant activity when given alone. **Onset of Action:** Rapid. **Peak Effect:** Within 5 min. **Duration:** 2 hr. **Metabolism/Elimination:** Metabolic fate unknown. May be partially metabolized or attacked by fibrinolysin, which may free heparin.

INDICATIONS/DOSAGE

Treatment of heparin sodium or heparin calcium overdosage
Adult: Dosage should be determined by the dose of heparin, its route of administration and time elapsed since administration. See table, this page. A protamine loading dose of 25–50 mg IV push may be given, followed by the remainder of calculated dose by continuous infusion over 8–16 hr (or over the expected duration of the SC duration absorption of heparin).

Neutralization of heparin administered during extracorporeal circulation (*unlabeled use*)
Adult/Pediatric: 1.5 mg protamine for each 100 units of heparin. Alternatively, dosage may be calculated using sequential activated clotting times (ACT) and a dose response

Heparin route	Time elapsed	mg protamine/100 units heparin
IV	few min	1.0–1.5
IV	30–60 min	0.5–0.75
IV	> 2 hr	0.25–0.375
SQ		1.0–1.5

In the Adverse Effects section, underline indicates most frequent; CAPS indicates life threatening.

curve that correlates the results of the coagulation test and the amount of heparin remaining in the body.

CONTRAINDICATIONS/ PRECAUTIONS

Contraindicated in: Hypersensitivity. **Use cautiously in:** Patients with known salmon/fish allergy, vasectomized/infertile males and patients who have received protamine-containing insulin preparations or previous protamine therapy are at risk for hypersensitivity reactions. **Pregnancy/Lactation:** No well-controlled trials to establish safety. Benefits must outweigh risks. **Pediatrics:** Safety and efficacy not established.

PREPARATION

Availability: 10 mg/mL in 5 and 25 mL amps and 5, 10, and 25 mL vials. **Reconstitution:** Add 5 mL sterile water for injection or bacteriostatic water for injection containing 0.9% benzyl alcohol per 50 mg of drug; shake vigorously. Do not use benzyl alcohol in neonates. Results in a 10 mg/mL solution. **Infusion:** Reconstituted solutions are not intended to be diluted further; however, they may be diluted in dextrose or sodium chloride.

STABILITY/STORAGE

Vial: Refrigerate. Stable for 2 weeks at room temperature. **Infusion:** Stable for 24 hr at room temperature.

ADMINISTRATION

IV Push: Give by slow IV injection over 1–3 min. Give no more than 50 mg in any 10 min period. **Continuous Infusion (*unlabeled route*):** May give by continuous infusion via controlled infusion device at rate specified by physician.

COMPATIBILITY

Solution: Dextrose solutions, sodium chloride solutions.

ADVERSE EFFECTS

CV: Bradycardia, <u>hypotension</u>, hypertension. **Resp:** Dyspnea, pulmonary edema. **GI:** Nausea, vomiting. **Derm:** Feeling of warmth (too rapid administration). **Heme:** Heparin rebound with anticoagulation and bleeding. **Hypersens:** ANAPHYLAXIS, angioedema, urticaria.

NURSING CONSIDERATIONS

Assessment
General:
Signs/symptoms of hypersensitivity.
Physical:
Signs/symptoms of bleeding.
Lab Alterations:
Monitor activated partial thromboplastin time (APTT) or activated clotting time (ACT) 5–15 min after administration to evaluate the neutralizing effect of the drug. Perform additional clotting studies in 2–8 hr to assess for the presence of heparin rebound.

Intervention/Rationale
Packed or whole RBCs and fresh frozen plasma may be necessary in cases of severe bleeding. ● Observe for signs/symptoms of anaphylaxis, especially in predisposed patients.

Patient/Family Education
Educate regarding expected therapeutic outcome and adverse effects.

In the Adverse Effects section, <u>underline</u> indicates most frequent; CAPS indicates life threatening.

PROTIRELIN
(pro-tir'-e-lin)
Trade Name(s): Thypinone, Relefact
Classification(s): Diagnostic thyroid function test
Pregnancy Category: Unknown

PHARMACODYNAMICS/KINETICS
Mechanism of Action: Increases release of thyroid-stimulating hormone from the anterior pituitary. **Onset of Action:** Rapid. **Peak Effect:** 20–30 min. **Duration of Action:** 3 hr. **Distribution:** Distributed to anterior pituitary. **Half-Life:** 5 min.

INDICATIONS/DOSAGE

Adjunct in the diagnostic assessment of thyroid function; adjunct to evaluate effectiveness of thyrotropin suppression in patients with goiters; used to detect inhibition of TSH in patients with hyperthyroidism

Adult: Dose range 200–500 mcg. 500 mcg is the optimum dose to give the maximum response. *Pediatric (children 6–16 years of age):* 7 mcg/kg. Maximum dose 500 mcg. *Pediatric (infants and children up to 6 years of age):* Information and experience is limited in this age group. Doses of 7 mcg/kg have been given.

CONTRAINDICATIONS/ PRECAUTIONS
Contraindicated in: None known. **Pregnancy/Lactation:** No well-controlled trials to establish safety. Benefits must outweigh risks. Lactating women have experienced breast enlargement and leakage of milk up to 3 days following administration. Use in lactating women only if clearly needed.

PREPARATION
Availability: 500 mcg/mL in 1 mL amps.

STABILITY/STORAGE
Vial: Store at room temperature.

ADMINISTRATION
IV Push: Give as IV bolus over 15–30 sec with patient supine. Remain supine for 15 min after administration.

COMPATIBILITY/INCOMPATIBILITY
Data not available.

ADVERSE EFFECTS
CNS: <u>Headache</u>, <u>lightheadedness</u>. **CV:** <u>Hypotension</u>. **GI:** <u>Abdominal discomfort</u>, <u>bad taste in mouth</u>, <u>dry mouth</u>, <u>nausea</u>. **GU:** <u>Urge to urinate</u>, <u>breast enlargement and leakage of milk</u>. **Other:** Flushing.

DRUG INTERACTIONS
Aspirin: Inhibited TSH response. **Corticosteroids (pharmacologic doses):** Reduced TSH response. **Levodopa:** Inhibited response to protirelin. **Liothyronine (T_3), levothyroxine (T_4):** Discontinue at least 14 days prior to testing. **Thyroid hormones:** Reduced response to protirelin.

NURSING CONSIDERATIONS
Assessment
General:
Vital signs.
Physical:
GI tract.
Lab Alterations:
Obtain blood sample for TSH determination immediately after administration and a second sample

P

In the Adverse Effects section, <u>underline</u> indicates most frequent; CAPS indicates life threatening.

449

in 30 min. Doses may not differentiate primary hypothyroidism from normal hypothyroidism. Assay methods and therefore results vary with each laboratory performing the test. Elevated serum lipids may interfere with TSH assay.

Intervention/Rationale
Patient should be supine before, during, and after administration. ● Monitor blood pressure for 15 min after administration. ● Evaluate for the presence of nausea/abdominal discomfort.

Patient/Family Education
Educate regarding expected diagnostic outcome and potential side effects.

PYRIDOSTIGMINE
(pye-rid-oh-stig'-meen)
Trade Name(s): Mestinon, Regonol, Rogitine ♥
Classification(s): Antimyasthenic, cholinergic muscle stimulant
Pregnancy Category: C

PHARMACODYNAMICS/KINETICS
Mechanism of Action: Facilitates impulse transmission across myoneural junction through inhibition of acetylcholine destruction by cholinesterase. Increases muscle strength and response to repetitive nerve stimulation by prolonging the duration of action of acetylcholine at the motor end plate. **Onset of Action:** Increased muscle strength seen within 2–5 min. **Duration of Action:** Average 2–3 hr. Varies

with individual patients. Dependent on physical/emotional stress experienced by the patient and severity of the disease. **Distribution:** Distributed to most tissues, with the exception of brain, intestinal wall, fat, and thymus. **Metabolism/Elimination:** Undergoes hydrolysis by cholinesterases. Also is metabolized by enzymes in the liver. Metabolites excreted via urine. **Half-Life:** 2–5 min.

INDICATIONS/DOSAGE

Treatment of myasthenia gravis
Adult: 2 mg (or approximately 1/30 of usual oral dose) every 2–3 hr. Individualize dosage to patient needs and response. Large IV doses should be accompanied by 0.6–1.2 mg atropine sulfate to counteract adverse muscarinic effects. Give myasthenic women in labor 1/30 of usual oral dose 1 hr before completion of the second stage of labor to provide adequate strength during labor and protection to the neonate.

Reversal of the effects of nondepolarizing neuromuscular blocking agents after surgery
Adult: 10–20 mg (range 0.1–0.25 mg/kg). Give with or shortly after 0.6–1.2 mg atropine sulfate IV or 0.2–0.6 mg glycopyrrolate IV.

CONTRAINDICATIONS/ PRECAUTIONS
Contraindicated in: Hypersensitivity, mechanical obstruction of the intestinal or urinary tracts. **Use cautiously in:** Bronchial asthma, bradycardia, cardiac dysrhythmias, epilepsy,

In the Adverse Effects section, <u>underline</u> indicates most frequent; CAPS indicates life threatening.

hyperthyroidism, recent coronary occlusion, peptic ulcer, vagotonia. **Pregnancy/Lactation:** No well-controlled trials to establish safety. Benefits must outweigh risks. Treat neonates (born to myasthenic mothers on anticholinesterase agents) demonstrating transient muscle weakness with IM pyridostigmine. Anticholinesterase may cause uterine irritability and premature labor when given to pregnant women near term. Distribution into breast milk unknown. Potentially serious side effects may occur in breastfed infants. Do not nurse while taking this drug. **Pediatrics:** Safety and efficacy not established.

PREPARATION
Availability: 5 mg/mL in 2 mL amps and 5 mL vials.

STABILITY/STORAGE
Vial: Store at room temperature.

ADMINISTRATION
IV Push: Give slowly IV push.

COMPATIBILITY
Syringe: Glycopyrrolate. **Y-site:** Heparin, hydrocortisone, potassium chloride, vitamin B complex with C.

ADVERSE EFFECTS
CNS: Headache (high doses), syncope. **Ophtho:** Diplopia, miosis, visual changes. **CV:** CARDIAC ARREST, bradycardia, hypotension. **Resp:** RESPIRATORY DEPRESSION/ARREST, BRONCHOSPASM, increased bronchial secretions. **GI:** Abdominal cramps, diarrhea, excessive salivation, increased peristalsis, nausea, vomiting. **MS:** Muscle cramps. **Derm:** Alopecia, skin rash (subsides with discontinuation). **Other:** Excessive sweating, thrombophlebitis.

TOXICITY/OVERDOSE
Signs/Symptoms: Cholinergic crisis (nausea, vomiting, diarrhea, excessive salivation and sweating, increased bronchial secretions, miosis, lacrimation, bradycardia or tachycardia, cardiospasm, bronchospasm, hypotension, incoordination, blurred vision, muscle cramps, weakness, fasciculations, paralysis, agitation, restlessness). Death may result from cardiac arrest, respiratory paralysis, and pulmonary edema. Weakness that begins approximately 1 hr after drug administration suggest overdosage; weakness 3 or more hr after drug administration suggests underdosage or resistance. The muscles first affected by an overdose are those of the neck and of chewing and swallowing, followed by those of the shoulder girdle and upper extremities, and lastly those of the pelvic girdle, extraocular area, and legs. Edrophonium (tensilon) can distinguish between increased symptoms of myasthenia and cholenergic crisis. **Treatment:** Maintain patent airway and adequate ventilation. Administer supplemental oxygen and support ventilation if necessary. Discontinue pyridostigmine. **Antidote(s):** Atropine 1–4 mg with additional doses every 5–30 min if needed (skeletal muscle effects and respiratory paralysis are not alleviated by atropine).

DRUG INTERACTIONS
Aminoglycosides, magnesium: Accentuated neuromuscular blockade/

P

In the Adverse Effects section, <u>underline</u> indicates most frequent; CAPS indicates life threatening.

451

prolonged respiratory depression. **Antiarrhythmics, local and some general anesthetics:** Interference with neuromuscular transmission. **Corticosteroids:** Decreased anticholinesterase effects. **Depolarizing muscle relaxants (succinylcholine, decamethonium):** Prolonged phase I neuromuscular blockade. **Other anticholinesterase drugs:** Symptoms of anticholinesterase overdose (cholinergic crisis) may mimic overdosage (myasthenic weakness).

NURSING CONSIDERATIONS

Assessment
General:
Vital signs (monitor heart rate, respirations, and blood pressure prior to and after administration).
Physical:
Neurologic status, cardiopulmonary status.

Intervention/Rationale
Use in Myasthenia Gravis:
Assess patient for signs/symptoms of cholinergic crisis and myasthenic weakness. Atropine may mask early signs of cholinergic crisis. Individual muscle groups may respond differently to pyridostigmine and one muscle group may be weak while another shows an increase in strength. ● Vital capacity should be routinely measured and trended, especially whenever dose is increased. ● Adequate equipment and facilities for cardiopulmonary resuscitation, cardiac monitoring, and assisted ventilation should be available.

Use for Reversal of the Effects of Non-depolarizing Neuromuscular Blocking Agents after Surgery: Monitor recovery of muscle groups with a peripheral nerve stimulator. Consecutive recovery of the diaphragm and the muscles of the abdomen, glottis, limbs, eyes (levators), and jaw will occur. During the recovery period, observe patient for residual muscle weakness and respiratory distress and assure that the patient has a patent airway.

Patient/Family Education
Call physician/nurse with nausea, diarrhea, excessive sweating and salivary secretions, muscle weakness, severe abdominal pain, irregular heartbeat, or difficulty breathing.

PYRIDOXINE (VITAMIN B$_6$)
(pye-ri-dox′-ine)
Trade Name(s): Beesix
Classification(s): Water-soluble vitamin
Pregnancy Category: A

PHARMACODYNAMICS/KINETICS
Mechanism of Action: Acts as a coenzyme in protein, carbohydrate, and fat metabolism. **Distribution:** Readily absorbed. **Metabolism/Elimination:** Degraded to 4-pyridoxic acid in the liver and then is excreted in urine. **Half-Life:** 15–20 days.

In the Adverse Effects section, <u>underline</u> indicates most frequent; CAPS indicates life threatening.

INDICATIONS/DOSAGE

Pyridoxine deficiency from inadequate diet

Adult: 10–20 mg daily for 3 weeks.

Vitamin B$_6$ dependency syndrome

Adult: Therapeutic dose 600 mg/day and 25–50 mg/day for life.

B$_6$ deficiency due to isoniazid therapy

Adult: Prophylactic dose range of 6–50 mg daily. Treat established neuropathy with 50–300 mg daily.

Acute isoniazid toxicity (treatment of seizure or coma)

Adult: 1–4 g given once. Follow with IM doses.

Treatment of seizures unresponsive to other therapy in pyridoxine-dependent infants exposed to large amounts of B$_6$ in utero

Neonate: 10–100 mg.

CONTRAINDICATIONS/ PRECAUTIONS

Contraindicated in: Hypersensitivity. **Use cautiously in:** Heart disease. **Pregnancy/Lactation:** Pyridoxine requirements are increased during pregnancy and lactation. Pyridoxine-dependent seizures in neonates have developed from the use of large doses during pregnancy. Use doses in excess of RDA with caution in lactating mothers. May inhibit lactation through suppression of prolactin. **Pediatrics:** Safety and efficacy not established.

PREPARATION

Availability: 100 mg/mL in 1, 10, and 30 mL vials.

STABILITY/STORAGE

Vial: Store at room temperature.

ADMINISTRATION

IV Push: Give by slow IV bolus.

COMPATIBILITY

Syringe: Doxapram.

ADVERSE EFFECTS

CNS: Decreased sensation to touch, temperature, and vibration, paresthesia, perioral/foot numbness, sensory neuropathic syndromes, somnolence, unstable gait. **Fld/Lytes:** Low serum folic acid levels.

TOXICITY/OVERDOSE

Signs/Symptoms: Vitamin B$_6$ dependency (adults taking 200 mg/day for 33 days), ataxia, sensory neuropathy (high doses: 500 mg to 2 g daily over extended periods). **Treatment:** Discontinue drug to ablate symptoms. Sensation may return in 6 months.

DRUG INTERACTIONS

Cycloserine, hydralazine, isoniazid, penicillamine, oral contraceptives: Increased pyridoxine requirements. **Levodopa:** Therapeutic effect of levodopa reversed by pyridoxine in doses of more than 5 mg per day. **Phenobarbital:** Decreased serum phenobarbital levels. **Phenytoin:** Decreased serum phenytoin levels.

NURSING CONSIDERATIONS

Assessment
General:
Nutritional assessment.
Physical:
GI tract, neurologic status.

In the Adverse Effects section, underline indicates most frequent; CAPS indicates life threatening.

453

Intervention/Rationale:
Pyridoxine should be given IV to patients who are n.p.o. or who have nausea, vomiting, or malabsorption syndromes. ● Assess for the development of paresthesias, sensory deficits, neuropathies. ● Evaluate dietary requirements following assessment of dietary history.

Patient/Family Education
Inform physician or nurse of previous unusual or allergic reaction to, if pregnant or intending to become pregnant. Eat a well-balanced diet and take vitamins only if nutritional requirements cannot be obtained through dietary means (foods containing pyridoxine are meats, bananas, potatoes, lima beans, whole grain cereals). Amounts of pyridoxine exceeding the recommended daily allowance may result in nerve damage.

QUINIDINE GLUCONATE
(kwin′-i-deen gloo′-kon-ate)
Trade Name(s): Quinidine gluconate
Classification(s): Antiarrhythmic: Type IA
Pregnancy Category: C

PHARMACODYNAMICS/KINETICS
Mechanism of Action: Slows conduction through the AV node, atria, ventricles, and His-Purkinje system. Suppresses automaticity in the His-Purkinje system. Has antimalarial activity. **Onset of Action:** 0.5 hr. **Duration of Action:** 6–8 hr. **Therapeutic Serum Levels:** 2–6 mcg/ml. **Distribution:** Widely and rapidly to all body tissues except brain; concentrated in the heart, liver, kidneys, and skel-

etal muscle. Binds to hemoglobin in erythrocytes. 80% bound to plasma proteins. **Metabolism/Elimination:** Metabolized in the liver. 10%–20% of dose excreted unchanged by the kidneys. Small amounts removed by hemodialysis. Not removed by peritoneal dialysis. **Half-Life:** 6–8 hr (range 3–16 hr).

INDICATIONS/DOSAGE

Suppression and prevention of atrial, AV junctional, and ventricular dysrhythmias
(reserve IV route for critical patients)

Adult: Dose range 500–750 mg. Average dose is 330 mg or less.

Pediatric: 2–10 mg/kg/dose every 3–6 hr as needed (IV route not recommended).

Treatment of severe Plasmodium falciparum malaria when quinine dihydrochloride is not readily available (*unlabeled use*)

Adult: Loading dose of 10 mg/kg infused over 1 hr, followed by continuous infusion of 0.02 mg/kg (20 mcg/kg) per minute for 72 hr or until parasitemia is reduced to less than 1%.

CONTRAINDICATIONS/PRECAUTIONS
Contraindicated in: Cardiac glycoside-induced AV conduction disorders, complete AV block with AV junctional/idioventricular pacemaker, ectopic beats and rhythms due to escape mechanisms, hypersensitivity, intraventricular conduction defects, myasthenia gravis. **Use cautiously in:** Absence of atrial activ-

In the Adverse Effects section, underline indicates most frequent; CAPS indicates life threatening.

ity, asthma, cardiac glycoside toxicity, CHF, extensive myocardial injury, hepatic/renal insufficiency, incomplete AV block, infection with fever, muscle weakness, preexisting hypotension. **Pregnancy/Lactation:** No well-controlled trials to establish safety. Benefits must outweigh risks. Distributed into breast milk. Use with extreme caution in breastfeeding women. **Pediatrics:** Safety and efficacy not established.

PREPARATION
Availability: 80 mg/mL in 10 mL vials. **Syringe/Infusion:** Add 10 mL (800 mg) to 40 mL dextrose. **Vial:** Store at room temperature. **Infusion:** Concentrations of 16 mg/mL are stable for 24 hr at room temperature.

ADMINISTRATION
General: Use IV route only when oral route is not feasible or when rapid therapeutic response is desired. A test dose of 200 mg should be given to assess for intolerance and sensitivity. **IV Push:** Give slowly at a rate of 1 mL/min. **Intermittent Infusion (adult dysrhythmias):** Infuse at initial rate of 16 mg (1 mL) per minute.

COMPATIBILITY
Solution: Dextrose 5%. **Y-site:** Diazepam, milrinone.

INCOMPATIBILITY
Y-site: Furosemide.

ADVERSE EFFECTS
CNS: Apprehension, anxiety, dizziness, headache, syncope, vertigo. **Ophtho:** Blurred vision, diplopia, photophobia, mydriasis. **CV:** ASYS-TOLE, <u>ECG changes</u> (prolonged QT interval, widened QRS complex, flattened T waves), HEART BLOCK, hypotension, increased heart rate, paradoxical rapid ventricular rate, ventricular fibrillation/tachycardia, vascular collapse. **Resp:** RESPIRATORY ARREST, respiratory distress. **GI:** <u>Anorexia</u>, <u>abdominal pain</u>, bitter taste, <u>diarrhea</u>, <u>nausea</u>, vomiting. **Endo:** Hypoglycemia. **Hypersens:** ANAPHYLACTIC SHOCK, thrombocytopenic purpura, exfoliative dermatitis (rare), acute hemolytic anemia, agranulocytosis, hemorrhage, hepatotoxicity, leukopenia, lightheadedness, pruritus, urticaria. **Other:** Fever, systemic lupus erythematosus-like syndrome, tinnitus.

TOXICITY/OVERDOSE
Signs/Symptoms: Absence of P waves, ataxia, apnea, anuria, generalized seizures, irritability, lethargy, prolonged QT interval, respiratory distress, severe hypotension, widened QRS complex, ventricular dysrhythmias. **Treatment:** Symptomatic, monitor blood pressure/ECG, cardiac pacemaker, acidification of urine, IV infusion of sodium lactate may reduce cardiotoxic effects. Do not give CNS depressants. Treat hypotension with metaraminol or norepinephrine after adequate fluid replacement. Peritoneal dialysis is not effective.

DRUG INTERACTIONS
Anticholinergic agents: Additive vagolytic effects. **Atracurium, succinylcholine, tubocurarine:** Potentiation of neuromuscular blockade. **Cimetidine:** Increased pharmacologic effects of quinidine. **Coumarin anticoagulants:** Reduced prothrombin

In the Adverse Effects section, <u>underline</u> indicates most frequent; CAPS indicates life threatening.

455

levels and clotting factor concentrations. **Digoxin:** Increased serum digoxin levels. **Nifedipine:** Decreased serum quinidine levels. **Other antiarrhythmics, phenothiazines, reserpine:** Additive cardiac depressant effects. **Phenobarbital, hydantoins, rifampin:** Reduced quinidine half-life (up to 50%). **Urinary alkalinizers:** Prolonged quinidine half-life. **Verapamil:** Hypertension in patients with IHSS (idiopathic hypertrophic cardiomyopathy).

NURSING CONSIDERATIONS
Assessment
General:
ECG monitoring, vital signs (BP), history of hypersensitivity, signs/symptoms of anaphylaxis.
Physical:
Cardiac status, hematopoietic system.
Lab Alterations:
Monitor CBC, liver, and renal function tests in patients receiving long-term therapy.

Intervention/Rationale
Keep patient supine during infusion to prevent postural hypotension. ● Discontinue drug if blood-dyscrasias or signs of hepatic/renal dysfunction occur. ● Monitor ECG continuously to assess for development of lethal dysrhythmias. Assess blood pressure frequently.
Treatment of dysrhythmias:
Adjust rate of administration so that dysrhythmias are abolished without disturbing the normal heart beat. Discontinue drug if QRS complex widens 25% beyond that seen before injection, P waves disappear, if heart rate falls to 120 beats/minute, if normal sinus rhythm is restored or if severe adverse effects occur.

Eliminate hypokalemia, hypoxia, and acid-base imbalances as causes of dysrhythmias before treatment with quinidine.
Malaria:
Monitor blood pressure, ECG, and plasma quinidine levels closely during therapy. Adjust dose if plasma level exceeds 7 mcg/mL, uncorrected QT interval exceeds 0.16 sec, if QRS widening exceeds 50% of baseline or if clinically significant hypotension unresponsive to fluid administration occurs. Contact CDC Malaria Branch at (404) 488-4046 for instruction on protocol.

Patient/Family Education
Notify physician or nurse if visual disturbances develop, ringing in the ears, headache, dizziness, or severe diarrhea occur.

RANITIDINE
(ra-nit′-ti-deen)
Trade Name(s): Zantac
Classification(s): Histamine H$_2$ antagonist
Pregnancy Category: B

PHARMACODYNAMICS/KINETICS
Mechanism of Action: Histamine H$_2$ antagonist, inhibitor of all phases of gastric secretion. Inhibits secretions caused by histamine, muscarinic agonists, gastrin, food, insulin, caffeine. **Onset of Action:** 15 min. **Peak Effect:** 1–3 hr. **Duration of Action:** 6–8 hr. **Distribution:** Widely distributed. 15% bound to plasma proteins. **Metabolism/Elimination:** Metabolized primarily by the liver. 68%–79% excreted unchanged by the kidneys. Removed by hemodialy-

In the Adverse Effects section, <u>underline</u> indicates most frequent; CAPS indicates life threatening.

sis. **Half-Life:** 2–3 hr. Prolonged in renal impairment.

INDICATIONS/DOSAGE

Short-term treatment of active duodenal or benign gastric ulcer; maintenance therapy for duodenal ulcer; treatment of pathologic GI hypersecretory conditions (Zollinger-Ellison syndrome, postoperative hypersecretion, "short-gut" syndrome); short-term symptomatic relief of gastroesophageal reflux; treatment of recurrent postoperative ulcer (*unlabeled use*); treatment of upper GI bleeding (*unlabeled use*); prevention of acid-aspiration pneumonitis (*unlabeled use*)

Adult: 50 mg every 6–8 hr. Maximum dose 400 mg/day.

CONTRAINDICATIONS/ PRECAUTIONS

Contraindicated in: Hypersensitivity. **Use cautiously in:** Elderly, hepatic dysfunction, renal impairment. **Pregnancy/Lactation:** No well-controlled trials to establish safety. Benefits must outweigh risks. Distributed into breast milk. Do not use in breastfeeding mothers. **Pediatrics:** Safety and efficacy not established in children under age 12.

PREPARATION

Availability: 25 mg/mL in 2, 10, and 40 mL vials and 2 mL syringes. 0.5 mg/mL (preservative free) in 100 mL single dose plastic containers. **Syringe:** Dilute 50 mg in compatible IV solution to a total volume of 20 mL. **Infusion:** Dilute 50 mg in 50–100 mL compatible IV solution. Alternatively, dilute total daily dose in 250 mL compatible IV solution for continuous infusion.

STABILITY/STORAGE

Vial: Store at room temperature. **Infusion:** Stable for 48 hr at room temperature.

ADMINISTRATION

IV Push: Give over 5 min. **Intermittent Infusion:** Infuse over 15–20 min. **Continuous Infusion:** Infuse over 24 hr.

COMPATIBILITY

Solution: Dextrose solutions, fat emulsions, 10%, sodium chloride solutions. **Syringe:** Atropine, dexamethasone, dimenhydrinate, diphenhydramine, dobutamine, dopamine, fentanyl, glycopyrrolate, hydromorphone, isoproterenol, meperidine, metoclopramide, morphine, nalbuphine, oxymorphone, pentazocine, perphenazine, prochlorperazine, promethazine, scopolamine. **Y-site:** Acyclovir, aminophylline, atracurium, bretylium, dobutamine, dopamine, enalaprilat, esmolol, heparin, labetalol, meperidine, morphine, nitroglycerin, ondansetron, pancuronium, procainamide, vecuronium, zidovudine.

INCOMPATIBILITY

Solutions: Dextrose 5%/lactated Ringer's. **Syringe:** Midazolam, pentobarbital, phenobarbital.

ADVERSE EFFECTS

CNS: Agitation, anxiety, <u>headache</u>, reversible mental confusion (elderly, debilitated). **GI:** Abdominal discomfort/pain, constipation, diarrhea, nausea, transient rise in serum transaminase, vomiting. **GU:** Loss of libido, impotence. **Renal:** Transient rise in serum creatinine. **Endo:** Gynecomastia. **Heme:** Reversible granulocytopenia/thrombocy-

R

In the Adverse Effects section, <u>underline</u> indicates most frequent; CAPS indicates life threatening.

457

topenia. **Hypersens:** Rash. **Other:** Transient burning or itching at injection site.

DRUG INTERACTIONS

Diazepam: Decreased pharmacologic effects of diazepam. **Procainamide:** Decreased renal clearance of procainamide. **Theophylline:** Increased plasma theophylline levels. **Warfarin:** Interference with warfarin clearance.

NURSING CONSIDERATIONS

Assessment
Physical:
GI status, neurologic status.
Lab Alterations:
Monitor serum ALT (SGPT) concentrations daily from day 5 of therapy throughout remainder of course in patients receiving doses of 400 mg or more daily for 5 days or longer. Monitor CBC and creatinine periodically during course of therapy. False-positive urine protein with Multistix (use sulfosalicylic acid).

Intervention/Rationale
Assess elderly and debilitated for presence of mental confusion and provide for adequate patient safety. Perform routine abdominal assessment during course of therapy to assess for presence of GI symptoms. Assess abdominal/gastric pain in association with medication schedule. Assess gastric pH every 6 hr and maintain > 4 as per physician order. Hematest stools, vomitus, and nasogastric drainage for the presence of occult blood.

Patient/Family Education
Educate regarding expected therapeutic outcome and potential side effects. Smoking interferes with the action of ranitidine. Inform physician of concomitant drug use, including over-the-counter drugs.

RIFAMPIN
(ri-fam′-pin)
Trade Name(s): Rifadin
Classification(s): Antituberculosis agent
Pregnancy Category: C

PHARMACODYNAMICS/KINETICS

Mechanism of Action: Inhibits bacterial RNA polymerase. **Peak Serum Level:** 1–4 hr. **Distribution:** Distributed throughout body into tissues. Penetrates into CNS. Highly lipid soluble. 80% protein bound. **Metabolism/Elimination:** Extensively metabolized by liver. 50% excreted unchanged in urine. Not removed by hemodialysis. **Half-Life:** 1.17–3.24 hr. Increased in hepatic impairment.

INDICATIONS/DOSAGE

Initial and retreatment of tuberculosis (when drug cannot be taken orally)

Adult: 600 mg once daily. *Pediatric:* 10–20 mg/kg once daily. Not to exceed 600 mg/day.

CONTRAINDICATIONS/ PRECAUTIONS

Contraindicated in: Hypersensitivity. **Use cautiously in:** Hepatic impairment. **Pregnancy/Lactation:** No well-controlled trials to establish safety.

In the Adverse Effects section, underline indicates most frequent; CAPS indicates life threatening.

Crosses placenta. Benefits must outweigh risks. Administration in last few weeks of pregnancy may result in maternal/infant postnatal hemorrhages requiring vitamin K therapy. Excreted in breast milk.

PREPARATION
Availability: 600 mg powder for injection vial. **Reconstitution:** Dilute each 600 mg vial with 10 mL sterile water for injection. Swirl gently. Final concentration 60 mg/mL. **Infusion:** Dilute required dose in 100–500 mL of compatible IV solution.

STABILITY/STORAGE
Vial: Store at controlled room temperature. Reconstituted vial stable for 24 hr at room temperature. **Infusion:** Stable for 24 hr at room temperature.

ADMINISTRATION
General: Administer with at least one other antituberculosis agent. **Intermittent Infusion:** Infuse 100 mL over 30 min or 500 mL over 3 hr.

COMPATIBILITY
Solution: Dextrose solutions, sodium chloride solutions (time dependent).

ADVERSE EFFECTS
CNS: Headache, drowsiness, fatigue, mental confusion, numbness. **Ophtho:** Visual disturbances, exudative conjunctivitis. **CV:** SHOCK, hypotension. **Resp:** Shortness of breath, wheezing. **GI:** Pseudomembranous colitis, elevated liver enzymes, anorexia, nausea, vomiting, diarrhea. **GU:** Hemoglobinuria, hematuria, menstrual disturbances. **Renal:** Acute renal failure, renal insufficiency, increased BUN/creatinine. **MS:** Ataxia, muscular weakness, osteomalacia. **Derm:** Pemphigoid reaction. **Heme:** Increased uric acid, leukopenia, thrombocytopenia, acute hemolytic anemia, eosinophilia. **Hypersens:** Pruritus, rash, urticaria. **Other:** Flu-like syndrome (fever, chills, malaise), edema (face/extremities), flushing, red secretions.

TOXICITY/OVERDOSE
Signs/Symptoms: Extension of adverse effects especially with hepatotoxicity. Rapid increase in direct/total bilirubin levels. **Treatment:** Symptomatic and supportive. Bile drainage may be indicated. Extracorporeal hemodialysis may be beneficial.

DRUG INTERACTIONS
Acetaminophen, anticoagulants, barbiturates, benzodiazepines, beta blockers, corticosteroids, digitoxin, hydantoins, methadone, mexiletine, oral contraceptives, quinidine, theophylline, tocainide, verapamil: Rifampin induces hepatic enzymes resulting in decreased serum levels of these agents. **Digoxin:** Decreased digoxin serum levels. **Halothane:** Hepatotoxicity especially with concurrent INH therapy. **Isoniazid:** Increased hepatotoxicity potential. **Ketoconazole:** Reduced pharmacologic effect of either agent.

NURSING CONSIDERATIONS
Assessment
General:
Vital signs, hypersensitivity reaction.
Physical:
Cardiopulmonary status, neurologic status, GI tract, infectious disease status.

In the Adverse Effects section, <u>underline</u> indicates most frequent; CAPS indicates life threatening.

Lab Alterations:
Monitor baseline and periodic liver enzymes, BUN/serum creatinine, CBC with differential and platelets.

Intervention/Rationale
Evaluate patient for development of hypotension or behavioral changes (somnolence, dizziness, inability to concentrate). ● Evaluate for signs/symptoms of hepatotoxicity and superinfection (pseudomembranous colitis). ● Institute oral therapy as soon as possible. ● Evaluate blood pressure before, during, and following administration.

Patient/Family Education
Educate patient regarding therapeutic outcome and side effects. Drug may cause red-orange discoloration of secretions (saliva, tears, urine, sweat). Avoid use of soft contact lenses during therapy due to lens discoloration. Notify physician/nurse of signs/symptoms of hepatitis (jaundice, nausea/vomiting, malaise, flu-like symptoms) and bleeding (gums, hematuria, melena). Avoid alcohol consumption. Seek assistance with ambulatory activities or those requiring mental alertness.

RITODRINE
(ri′-toe-dreen)
Trade Name(s): Yutopar
Classification(s): Tocolytic, beta-adrenergic agonist
Pregnancy Category: B

PHARMACODYNAMICS/KINETICS
Mechanism of Action: Beta-2-adrenergic stimulant. Inhibits uterine contraction by relaxing uterine muscle. **Onset of Action:** 5 min. **Peak Effect:** 60 min. **Distribution:** 32% bound to plasma proteins. Probably crosses blood–brain barrier. **Metabolism/Elimination:** Conjugated in the liver to inactive metabolites. Excreted primarily unchanged in urine. Removed by hemodialysis. **Half-Life:** 15–17 hr.

INDICATIONS/DOSAGE

Management of preterm labor
Adult: Initial dose 50–100 mcg/min. Gradually increase by 50 mcg/min every 10 min until desired effect is achieved. Effective dosage is usually 150–350 mcg/min. Dosage should be titrated according to patient response, maternal and fetal heart rates, and maternal blood pressure.

CONTRAINDICATIONS/PRECAUTIONS
Contraindicated in: Antepartum hemorrhage demanding immediate delivery, before the 20th week of pregnancy, bronchial asthma already treated by betamimetics or steroids, cardiac dysrhythmias associated with tachycardia or digitalis intoxication, chorioamnionitis, eclampsia/severe preeclampsia, hypovolemia, intrauterine fetal death, maternal cardiac disease, maternal hyperthyroidism, pheochromocytoma, pulmonary hypertension, uncontrolled maternal diabetes mellitus, uncontrolled hypertension. **Use cautiously in:** Presence of migraine headache. **Pregnancy/Lactation:** No well-controlled trials to establish safety before the 20th week of pregnancy. Readily

In the Adverse Effects section, underline indicates most frequent; CAPS indicates life threatening.

crosses the placenta. No evidence of increased fetal risk or abnormalities seen after the 20th week of pregnancy. Follow up in children 2 years postdelivery reveals no evidence of retardation of growth and development but the risk cannot be absolutely excluded. Benefits must outweigh risks.

PREPARATION
Availability: 10 and 15 mg/mL in 5 mL amps and 10 mL vials and syringes. **Infusion:** Dilute 15 mL (150 mg) of drug with 500 mL dextrose 5%. Resultant concentration is 300 mcg/mL. Use sodium chloride containing solutions (sodium chloride, Ringer's injection or Ringer's lactate) only when the use of dextrose is medically undesirable because of the increased risk of pulmonary edema. A more concentrated solution may be used if fluid volume overload is a concern.

STABILITY/STORAGE
Vial: Store at room temperature. **Infusion:** Stable for 48 hr at room temperature.

ADMINISTRATION
General: Should be given only by those personnel educated about the pharmacologic effects of betamimetic therapy and are trained to manage the complications of therapy and pregnancy. **Continuous Infusion:** Continue infusion for at least 12 hr after uterine contractions are eliminated. Must be administered via infusion device.

COMPATIBILITY/INCOMPATIBILITY
Data not available.

ADVERSE EFFECTS
CNS: Anxiety, emotional upset, jitteriness, restlessness, nervousness. **CV:** Dysrhythmias, chest pain/tightness, hypertension, increase in maternal/fetal heart rates, <u>palpitations</u>, sinus bradycardia (drug withdrawal), widening of maternal pulse pressure. **Resp:** PULMONARY EDEMA. **GI:** Nausea, vomiting. **Endo:** Hyperglycemia. **Fld/Lytes:** Hypokalemia.

TOXICITY/OVERDOSE
Signs/Symptoms: Excessive beta-adrenergic stimulation (maternal/fetal tachycardia, palpitations, dysrhythmias, hypotension, nervousness, nausea, vomiting). **Treatment:** Discontinue infusion, removed by hemodialysis. **Antidote(s):** Beta blockers.

DRUG INTERACTIONS
Atropine: Exaggerated systemic hypertension. **Beta-adrenergic blockers:** Inhibition of pharmacologic effects of ritodrine. **Corticosteroids:** May lead to pulmonary edema. **Diazoxide, magnesium sulfate, meperidine, potent general anesthetics:** Potentiated cardiovascular effects of ritodrine. **Sympathomimetic amines:** Additive or potentiated cardiovascular effects.

NURSING CONSIDERATIONS
Assessment
General:
Baseline ECG, maternal vital signs, maternal/fetal monitoring, hydration status, intake/output ratio.
Physical:
Maternal cardiovascular status.
Lab Alterations:
Monitor blood glucose frequently if drug is used for extended period of

R

In the Adverse Effects section, <u>underline</u> indicates most frequent; CAPS indicates life threatening.

461

time, especially in diabetics. Monitor acid-base balance in pregnant diabetics. Monitor electrolytes, especially in those receiving potassium-depleting diuretics.

Intervention/Rationale
Continuously monitor fetal well-being with external or internal monitoring before and during therapy. ● Place patient in left lateral position during administration. Obtain baseline ECG and assessment of cardiovascular status. Closely monitor cardiovascular parameters (maternal/ fetal heart rate, maternal blood pressure) during therapy. ● Monitor hydration status and assess frequently for signs/symptoms of pulmonary edema, discontinue infusion if occurs. Persistent maternal tachycardia may be a sign of impending pulmonary edema. Discontinue if patient complains of chest pain or tightness and obtain stat ECG. ● May resume ambulation within 36–48 hr of discontinuation if contractions do not reoccur. ● Institute oral ritodrine 30 min before termination of IV ritodrine therapy.

Patient/Family Education
Educate regarding potential therapeutic outcome and side effects. Reinforce the signs/symptoms of reoccurrence of preterm labor. Notify nurse if water breaks.

SARGRAMOSTIM
(sar-gram'-o-stim)
Trade Name(s): Leukine, Prokine
Classification(s): Colony stimulating factor
Pregnancy Category: C

PHARMACODYNAMICS/KINETICS
Mechanism of Action: Binds to specific cell surface receptors that support survival, expansion, and differentiation of various hematopoietic cells. Increases the cytotoxicity of monocytes towards various neoplastic cells. **Onset of Action:** 2–4 hr. **Peak Serum Level:** 2–6 hr. **Duration of Action:** 6 days. **Distribution:** Distributed throughout the body specifically into the bone marrow. **Metabolism/Elimination:** Eliminated by kidneys. **Half-Life:** 2 hr.

INDICATIONS/DOSAGE

Myeloid reconstitution after autologous bone marrow transplantation; bone marrow transplantation failure or engraftment delay

Adult: 250 mcg/m^2/day. In myeloid reconstitution, begin 2–4 hr after marrow infusion and ≥ 24 hr after last dose of chemotherapy and 12 hr after radiotherapy; continue for 21 days or until absolute neutrophil count (ANC) exceeds 20,000 cells/m^3. In transplant failure, continue for 14 days and repeat for two courses after 7 days off if engraftment has not occurred. Reduce or discontinue treatment if adverse reaction occurs or evidence of blast cells/disease progression.

CONTRAINDICATIONS/ PRECAUTIONS
Contraindicated in: Hypersensitivity to drug or yeast-derived proteins, excessive leukemic myeloid blasts. **Use cautiously in:** Preexisting cardiac/ lung conditions. **Pregnancy/Lactation:** No well-controlled trials to establish safety. Benefits must out-

In the Adverse Effects section, <u>underline</u> indicates most frequent; CAPS indicates life threatening.

weigh risks. **Pediatrics:** Safety and efficacy not established. No difference in toxicity profile in comparison to adults with same dosage guidelines.

PREPARATION
Availability: 250 and 500 mcg lyophilized powder for injection in single use vial. **Reconstitution:** Dilute with 1 mL sterile water for injection (no preservative). Direct diluent to sides of vial and avoid excess agitation. Discard unused portion. **Infusion:** May dilute in compatible IV solution to a volume sufficient to infuse over at least 2 hr. If concentration < 10 mcg/mL, albumin must be added to prevent adsorption to plastic bag at a final concentration of 1 mg/mL.

STABILITY/STORAGE
Vial: Refrigerate vial. Reconstituted solution stable for 6 hr refrigerated. Discard unused solution. **Infusion:** Store under refrigeration for 6 hr. Prepare just prior to administration.

ADMINISTRATION
General: Do not use inline membrane filter for administration. **Intermittent Infusion:** Infuse over 2 hr.

COMPATIBILITY
Solution: Sodium chloride solutions, sterile water for injection.

INCOMPATIBILITY
Solution: Dextrose solutions.

ADVERSE EFFECTS
CNS: Headache. **CV:** Pericardial effusion, tachycardia, peripheral edema. **Resp:** Dyspnea. **GI:** Anorexia, nausea, stomatitis, vomiting. **MS:** Arthralgia, <u>bone pain</u>, myalgia. **Derm:** Alopecia. **Heme:** Increased WBC, increased platelets. **Hypersens:** Rash. **Other:** SEPSIS, chills, fever.

TOXICITY/OVERDOSE
Signs/Symptoms: Dyspnea, malaise, nausea, fever, rash, sinus tachycardia, headache, chills. **Treatment:** Adverse reactions reported have been reversible by discontinuing therapy. Monitor for increased WBC and improvement in differential. Evaluate respiratory status for need of intervention.

DRUG INTERACTIONS
Corticosteroids, lithium: Potentiate myeloproliferative effects.

NURSING CONSIDERATIONS
Assessment
General:
Vital signs, infectious disease status.
Physical:
Hematopoietic system, cardiopulmonary status.
Lab Alterations:
Obtain baseline/biweekly CBC differential. Evaluate liver function studies upon initiation of therapy and periodically throughout.

Intervention/Rationale
Evaluate blood pressure for the development of transient hypotension. Monitor apical pulse for at least 1 full minute to note development of tachydysrhythmias and consider continuous ECG monitoring if irregular heart rate is noted. Assess heart sounds and lung sounds regularly throughout administration of drug in order to determine any evidence of pleural/pericardial effusion. ● Evaluate

In the Adverse Effects section, <u>underline</u> indicates most frequent; CAPS indicates life threatening.

463

hourly intake/output ratio including signs/symptoms of pending cardiac/pulmonary failure to determine the development of increased preload/afterload. ● Discontinue therapy when absolute neutrophil count reaches 20,000 mm³.

Patient/Family Education
Notify physician/nurse of any signs/symptoms of infection, fever, or bone pain (correlating to the actual administration of the drug). Review expected outcome and potential adverse effects.

SCOPOLAMINE
(scoe-pol′-a-meen)
Classification(s): Anticholinergic, antiemetic, antimuscarinic
Pregnancy Category: C

PHARMACODYNAMICS/KINETICS
Mechanism of Action: Inhibits the muscarinic activity of acetylcholine. Produces CNS depression (may produce paradoxical effect, especially when used in the presence of severe pain). **Onset of Action:** 10 min. **Peak Effect:** 50–80 min. **Duration of Action:** 120 min. **Distribution:** Not fully characterized. Reversibly bound to plasma proteins. Crosses blood–brain barrier. **Metabolism/Elimination:** Not fully determined. Metabolized by the liver. Excreted via the kidneys. **Half-Life:** 8 hr.

INDICATIONS/DOSAGE

Used preoperatively to decrease salivation and respiratory secretions; adjunct to anesthesia for sedation-hypnosis and amnestic effect, antiemetic
Adult: 0.3–0.65 mg. May be repeated three to four times/day. *Pediatric:* 0.006 mg/kg (0.003 mg/lb) or 0.2 mg/m². Maximum dose 0.3 mg.

CONTRAINDICATIONS/PRECAUTIONS
Contraindicated in: Glaucoma (angle-closure), hypersensitivity (patients hypersensitive to belladonna or barbiturates may be sensitive to scopolamine), myasthenia gravis, paralytic ileus, pyloric obstruction, tachycardia secondary to cardiac insufficiency, urinary bladder obstruction. **Use cautiously in:** Elderly, metabolic/hepatic/renal dysfunction. **Pregnancy/Lactation:** No well-controlled trials to establish safety. Benefits must outweigh risks. No teratogenic effects observed in rat studies. Crosses the placenta. **Pediatrics:** Use with caution in infants.

PREPARATION
Availability: 0.3 mg/mL in 1 mL vials. 0.4 mg/mL in 0.5 and 1 mL amps and vials. 0.86 mg/mL in 0.5 mL amps. 1 mg/mL in 1 mL vials. **Syringe:** Dilute with sterile water before injection.

STABILITY/STORAGE
Vial: Store at room temperature. Protect from light.

ADMINISTRATION
General: When given as preoperative medication, give 30–60 min prior to induction of anesthesia. **IV Push:** Give slowly.

COMPATIBILITY
Solution: Sterile water. **Syringe:** Atropine, benzquinamide, butorpha-

nol, chlorpromazine, cimetidine, dimenhydrinate, diphenhydramine, droperidol, fentanyl, glycopyrrolate, hydromorphone, meperidine, metoclopramide, midazolam, morphine, nalbuphine, pentazocine, pentobarbital, perphenazine, prochlorperazine, promethazine, ranitidine, thiopental. **Y-site:** Heparin, hydrocortisone, potassium chloride, vitamin B complex with C.

ADVERSE EFFECTS
CNS: Confusion, CNS stimulation (large doses), dizziness, <u>drowsiness</u>, excitement, headache, insomnia, nervousness. **Ophtho:** Blurred vision, cycloplegia, dilated pupils, increased ocular pressure, mydriasis, photophobia. **CV:** Bradycardia, palpitations, postural hypotension, tachycardia. **Resp:** Nasal congestion. **GI:** Altered taste perception, bloated feeling, constipation, dysphagia, heartburn, nausea, vomiting, <u>xerostomia</u>. **GU:** Impotence, urinary hesitancy/retention. **Hypersens:** ANAPHYLAXIS, rash, urticaria. **Endo:** Suppression of lactation. **Other:** Decreased sweating, flushing.

TOXICITY/OVERDOSE
Signs/Symptoms: Abdominal distention, anxiety, CNS stimulation, circulatory failure, delirium, drowsiness, dry mouth, dysphagia, hypotension, hypertension, psychotic behavior, stupor, respiratory depression, tachycardia, tachypnea, nausea. **Treatment:** Supportive care, assure patent airway, mechanically ventilate if needed, diazepam, short-acting barbiturates, IV sodium thiopental, or chloral hydrate (rectal infusion) may control excitement. **Antidote(s):** Physostigmine 0.2–4.0 mg IV every 1–2 hr up to a total of 6 mg (reverses anticholinergic effects).

DRUG INTERACTIONS
Amantadine, tricyclic antidepressants: Increased anticholinergic side effects (decrease anticholinergic dose). **Atenolol, digoxin:** Increased pharmacological effects by scopolamine. **Phenothiazines:** Decreased antipsychotic effectiveness, increased anticholinergic effects.

NURSING CONSIDERATIONS
Assessment
General:
Vital signs, pain assessment, ECG monitoring (recommended), intake/output ratio.
Physical:
GU tract, mental status.

Intervention/Rationale
Assess for signs/symptoms of urinary retention during therapy. ● Monitor heart rate and blood pressure periodically during therapy. ● In the presence of pain, scopolamine may act as a stimulant and produce delirium—perform pain assessment prior to administration. Give analgesic or sedative concomitantly to avoid scopolamine-induced behavioral changes.

Patient/Family Education
Educate regarding expected therapeutic outcome and side effects. Drug may impair activities requiring mental alertness.

S

In the Adverse Effects section, <u>underline</u> indicates most frequent; CAPS indicates life threatening.

465

SECOBARBITAL
(see-koe-bar'-bi-tal)
Trade Name(s): Seconal
Classification(s): Sedative/
hypnotic, barbiturate
Pregnancy Category: D
Controlled Substance Schedule:
II

PHARMACODYNAMICS/KINETICS
Mechanism of Action: Mechanism of
action not completely known. May
act on the reticular formation system to produce sedation. Depresses the sensory cortex and motor
activity. Produce CNS depression,
ranging from mild sedation to deep
coma and death. **Onset of Action:**
10–15 min. **Duration of Action:** 3–4 hr.
Distribution: Distributed rapidly to all
tissues and fluids. High concentration in brain and liver. Lipid soluble. Crosses blood–brain barrier.
Metabolism/Elimination: Slowly metabolized by the liver. Primarily excreted by the kidneys. Small
amounts excreted in feces and
sweat. **Half-Life:** 15–50 hr.

INDICATIONS/DOSAGE

Preoperative sedation/adjunct to spinal or regional anesthesia
(individualize dose to patient)
Adult: 50–250 mg (dose not to
exceed 250 mg). *Pediatric:*
4–5 mg/kg.

Sedative/hypnotic
Adult: 100–200 mg.

Status epilepticus
Adult: 250–350 mg. Repeat as
needed.

Acute seizures resulting from tetanus
Adult: 5.5 mg/kg. Repeat every
3–4 hr if needed.

Acute episodes of agitated behavior in psychotic patients
Adult: 250 mg. May repeat dose in
5 minutes. Maximum dose 500 mg
(phenothiazines are preferred).

CONTRAINDICATIONS/PRECAUTIONS
Contraindicated in: Hypersensitivity,
manifest or latent porphyria, obstetrical delivery, severe respiratory
distress/respiratory disease with
dyspnea, obstruction, or cor pulmonale. **Use cautiously in:** Acute or
chronic pain, cardiovascular disease, history of drug abuse, liver/
renal impairment, mental depression, suicidal tendencies. **Preg-
nancy/Lactation:** May cause fetal
harm when given to pregnant
women. May cause postpartum
hemorrhage and hemorrhagic disease in newborns. Withdrawal
symptoms may be present in neonates born to women given barbiturates in the last trimester. Benefits
must outweigh risks. Distributed
into breast milk. Discontinue
breastfeeding if infant show signs
of toxicity. **Pediatrics:** May cause irritability, excitability, aggression, or
inappropriate tearfulness in children.

PREPARATION
Availability: 50 mg/mL in 1 and 2 mL
Tubex and 20 mL vials.
Syringe: May be used undiluted or
dilute with sterile water, sodium
chloride injection, or Ringer's injection.

In the Adverse Effects section, <u>underline</u> indicates most frequent;
CAPS indicates life threatening.

STABILITY/STORAGE
Vial/Tubex: Refrigerate, protect from light.

ADMINISTRATION
General: Restrict IV use for when other routes are not feasible. **IV Push:** Give slowly, not to exceed 50 mg per 15 sec. Too rapid administration may cause apnea, respiratory depression, and other pulmonary complications.

COMPATIBILITY
Solution: Ringer's injection, sodium chloride, sterile water.

INCOMPATIBILITY
Syringe: Benzquinamide, cimetidine, glycopyrrolate, pancuronium.

ADVERSE EFFECTS
CNS: Agitation, ataxia, CNS depression, insomnia, lethargy, nightmares, paradoxical excitement, residual sedation, stupor, somnolence, vertigo. **CV:** Bradycardia, hypotension (too rapid administration). **Resp:** APNEA (too rapid administration), LARYNGOSPASM, pharyngospasm, respiratory depression. **GI:** Constipation, diarrhea, epigastric pain, liver damage (chronic use), nausea, vomiting. **Heme:** Agranulocytosis, thrombocytopenia. **Hypersens:** Exfoliative dermatitis, Stevens-Johnson syndrome, angioneurotic edema, skin rashes, serum sickness, morbilliform rash, urticaria.

TOXICITY/OVERDOSE
Signs/Symptoms: CNS and respiratory depression, oliguria, tachycardia, hypotension, hypothermia, coma, shock syndrome. **Treatment:** Supportive, maintain patent airway and use artificial ventilation if necessary. Monitor vital signs and fluid balance.

DRUG INTERACTIONS
Acetaminophen, beta-adrenergic blockers, digitoxin, doxycycline, quinidine, rifampin, tricyclic antidepressants: Decreased effects of these drugs. **Chloramphenicol:** Enhanced chloramphenicol metabolism. **Corticosteroids:** Decreased steroid effects (may require steroid dose adjustment). **Furosemide:** May cause/aggravate orthostatic hypotension. **MAO inhibitors, other CNS depressants:** Additive depressant effects. **Oral anticoagulants:** Decreased anticoagulant response. **Oral contraceptives and estrogens:** Decreased contraceptive and estrogen effect (suggest alternate form of birth control). **Phenytoin:** Unpredictable phenytoin metabolism (monitor phenytoin levels). **Valproic acid:** Decreased barbiturate metabolism, decreased valproic acid half-life.

NURSING CONSIDERATIONS

Assessment
General:
Vital signs, signs/symptoms of hypersensitivity, history of chemical dependency.
Physical:
Cardiopulmonary status, mental status (especially children/elderly), pulmonary status (respiratory depression/barbiturate toxicity/coma).

Intervention/Rationale
Assess respiratory system frequently during therapy. ● Assess for the presence of adverse neurologic symptoms. ● Equipment for

In the Adverse Effects section, <u>underline</u> indicates most frequent;
CAPS indicates life threatening.

467

emergency resuscitation and artificial ventilation should be readily available.

Patient/Family Education
May cause drowsiness/residual sedation or may impair ability to perform activities requiring mental alertness or physical coordination. Provide for patient safety and supervise ambulation following administration. Inform physician if pregnant. Inform physician of sore throat, easy bruising, nosebleed, or petechiae.

SECRETIN
(see'-kri-tin)
Trade Name(s): Secretin-Kabi
Classification(s): In vivo diagnostic aid
Pregnancy Category: Unknown

PHARMACODYNAMICS/KINETICS
Mechanism of Action: Increases volume and bicarbonate content of pancreatic juices. Stimulates gastrin release in patients with Zollinger-Ellison syndrome. **Peak Output:** 30 min. **Duration of Output:** 2 hr. **Half-Life:** 18 min.

INDICATIONS/DOSAGE

Diagnosis of gastrinoma (Zollinger-Ellison syndrome)
Adult: 2 CU/kg.

CONTRAINDICATIONS/PRECAUTIONS
Contraindicated in: Acute pancreatitis (give after attack subsided), hypersensitivity. **Pregnancy/Lactation:** No

well-controlled trials to establish safety. Benefits must outweigh risks.

PREPARATION
Availability: Powder for injection. 75 CU per vial in 10 mL vials. **Reconstitution:** Add 7.5 mL sodium chloride injection immediately prior to use (concentration after dilution is 10 CU/mL). Avoid vigorous shaking.

STABILITY/STORAGE
Vial: Store in freezer. May be stored for 3 weeks in refrigerator. Reconstitute solution just prior to administration.

ADMINISTRATION
General: Draw two blood samples for baseline serum gastrin levels prior to test. Collect postinjection samples for serum gastrin at 1, 2, 5, 10, and 30 min. **IV Push:** Give slowly over 1 min.

COMPATIBILITY/INCOMPATIBILITY
Data not available.

ADVERSE EFFECTS
Hypersens: Allergic reactions from impure preparations and/or repeat injections. **Other:** Thrombophlebitis.

NURSING CONSIDERATIONS
Assessment
General:
Signs/symptoms of hypersensitivity reactions.
Physical:
Pulmonary system.

Intervention/Rationale
Observe for signs/symptoms of allergic reactions and discontinue immediately if any occur. ● Treat anaphylaxis with epinephrine, an-

In the Adverse Effects section, <u>underline</u> indicates most frequent; CAPS indicates life threatening.

tihistamines, corticosteroids, vaso-pressors, and IV fluids. ● Maintain patent airway.

Patient/Family Education
Educate regarding expected diagnostic/therapeutic outcome and adverse reactions.

SINCALIDE
(sin-ka′-lide)
Trade Name(s): Kinevac
Classification(s): In vivo diagnostic aid
Pregnancy Category: Unknown

PHARMACODYNAMICS/KINETICS
Mechanism of Action: Causes contraction of the gallbladder and evacuation of bile in a manner similar to endogenous cholecystokinin. Causes delayed gastric emptying and increased intestinal motility. If given in conjunction with secretin, increases volume of pancreatic secretion, and output of bicarbonate and protein enzymes. **Peak Effect:** 5–15 min.

INDICATIONS/DOSAGE

Causes gallbladder contraction and bile production for diagnostic analysis
Adult: 0.02 mcg/kg (1.4 mcg/70 kg). Give second dose (0.04 mcg/kg) if satisfactory gallbladder contraction does not occur within 15 min.

Use in conjunction with secretin to stimulate pancreatic secretion for analysis of pancreatic fluid and cytology (suspected pancreatic cancer)

Adult: 30 minutes after secretin administration, give sincalide total dose of 0.02 mcg/kg.

CONTRAINDICATIONS/PRECAUTIONS
Contraindicated in: Hypersensitivity. **Pregnancy/Lactation:** No teratogenic or antifertility effects seen in animal studies. No well-controlled trials to establish safety. Benefits must outweigh risks. **Pediatrics:** Safety and efficacy not established.

PREPARATION
Availability: 5 mcg per vial powder for injection. **Reconstitution:** Add 5 mL sterile water for injection to vial. **Infusion:** Dilute 1.4 mL reconstituted solution to 30 mL with sodium chloride injection.

STABILITY/STORAGE
Vial: Store at room temperature. Use diluted solution immediately. Discard unused portion. **Infusion:** Stable at room temperature.

ADMINISTRATION
Gallbladder Contraction: Give over 30–60 sec. X-rays should be taken at 5 min intervals to visualize gallbladder and at 1 min intervals during the first 5 min to visualize cystic duct. **Secretin-Sincalide Test of Pancreatic Function:** Infuse secretin over 30 min. 30 min later, infuse sincalide over 30 min via infusion device at a rate of 1 mL/min.

COMPATIBILITY/INCOMPATIBILITY
Data not available.

ADVERSE EFFECTS
CNS: Dizziness. **GI:** <u>Abdominal discomfort</u>, nausea, urge to defecate. **Other:** Flushing.

NURSING CONSIDERATIONS

Assessment
Physical:
GI tract.

Intervention/Rationale
Assess for adverse reactions and inform physician. ● Evaluate the level of abdominal discomfort.

Patient/Family Education
Educate regarding expected diagnostic/therapeutic outcome and adverse effects.

SODIUM ACETATE
(soe'-dee-um as'-a-tate)
Classification(s): Alkalinizing agent, electrolyte
Pregnancy Category: C

PHARMACODYNAMICS/KINETICS
Mechanism of Action: Provides sodium to the body. Acetate is converted to bicarbonate to provide an alkaline source. **Metabolism/Elimination:** Fully metabolized outside the liver to bicarbonate ions.

INDICATIONS/DOSAGE

Prevention/correction acidosis and/or hyponatremia

Adult: Dosage determined by nutritional needs, assessment of electrolytes, and severity of hyponatremia. Each gram contains 7.3 mEq of sodium and acetate.

CONTRAINDICATIONS/ PRECAUTIONS
Contraindicated in: Metabolic alkalosis, respiratory alkalosis. **Use cautiously in:** Conditions associated with sodium retention. CHF, hypertension, impaired renal function, concomitant corticosteroids, peripheral edema, pulmonary edema. **Pregnancy/Lactation:** No well-controlled trials to establish safety. Benefits must outweigh risks.

PREPARATION
Availability: 2 mEq/mL in 20 and 50 mL vials. **Infusion:** Dosage must be added to a large volume of compatible IV solution.

STABILITY/STORAGE
Vial: Store at room temperature. Protect from excess heat. **Infusion:** Stable at room temperature for 24 hr following preparation.

ADMINISTRATION
General: Rapid or excessive administration may produce alkalosis or hypokalemia. **Intermittent/Continuous Infusion:** Must be diluted. Administer slowly at physician prescribed rate/volume for infusion.

COMPATIBILITY
Solution: Dextrose solutions. **Y-site:** Enalaprilat, esmolol, labetalol.

ADVERSE EFFECTS
CNS: Delirium, dizziness. **CV:** Cardiac dysrhythmias, CHF, hypotension, tachycardia. **GU:** Oliguria. **Fld/Lytes:** Hypernatremia. **Metab:** Alkalosis. **Other:** Fever, headache.

TOXICITY/OVERDOSE
Signs/Symptoms: Hypernatremia with serum sodium levels > 147 mEg/L is the most frequent manifestation. Symptoms include: CHF, delirium, dizziness, edema, fever, flushing, headache, hypotension, oliguria, pulmonary edema, decreased salivation/lacrimation, res-

In the Adverse Effects section, <u>underline</u> indicates most frequent; CAPS indicates life threatening.

piratory arrest, restlessness, swollen tongue, tachycardia, thirst/weakness; alkalosis and fluid/solute overload may occur. **Treatment:** Notify physician of development of side effects. Decrease the rate of the infusion at the first sign of increased preload. Treatment may begin with sodium restriction and/or use of diuretics or dialysis.

NURSING CONSIDERATIONS

Assessment
General:
Vital signs, baseline/daily weight, intake/output ratio.
Physical:
Cardiopulmonary status.
Lab Alterations:
Assess electrolytes before, during, and following therapy.

Intervention/Rationale
Carefully monitor intake/output, daily weights, assess for fluid retention, and development of hypernatremia. ● Evaluate lung fields and vital signs regularly to note symptoms of fluid overload. ● Maintain blood pressure and heart rate prior to, during, and following administration.

Patient/Family Education
Review the expected therapeutic outcome of the drug as well as the potential adverse effects of the therapy.

SODIUM BICARBONATE
(soe′-dee-um bie-kar′-boe-nate)
Classification(s): Alkalinizing agent, electrolyte
Pregnancy Category: C

PHARMACODYNAMICS/KINETICS
Mechanism of Action: Maintains osmotic pressure, raises blood pH. Acts as an alkalizing agent that dissociates to yield bicarbonate ion. Bicarbonate is the primary extracellular buffer in the body. **Onset of Action:** Immediate. **Distribution:** Widely distributed throughout extracellular fluid. **Metabolism/Elimination:** Excreted by the kidneys in the form of sodium and bicarbonate.

INDICATIONS/DOSAGE

Metabolic acidosis
Adult/Pediatric: 2–5 mEq/kg.

Cardiopulmonary resuscitation
Adult: Dose should be determined in accordance with laboratory findings. 1 mEq/kg is the usual dosage. May repeat 50% of the initial dose in 10 min if indicated. *Pediatric/Neonate:* 1–2 mEq/kg. May give repeat doses of 1 mEq/kg every 10 min. Do not administer > 8 mEq/kg/day.

CONTRAINDICATIONS/PRECAUTIONS
Contraindicated in: Excessive chloride loss, hypocalcemia, metabolic alkalosis, respiratory alkalosis. (No contraindications for use in life-threatening emergencies.) **Use cautiously in:** Concomitant corticosteroids, CHF, renal insufficiency, including oliguria/anuria. **Pregnancy/Lactation:** No well-controlled trials to establish safety. Benefits must outweigh risks. **Pediatrics:** Rapid administration in children < 2 years may produce hyperna-

In the Adverse Effects section, underline indicates most frequent; CAPS indicates life threatening.

471

tremia, decreased CSF pressure and possible intracranial hemorrhage.

PREPARATION

Availability: Concentration of 8.4% (1 mEq/mL) in 10 and 50 mL vials. Concentration of 7.5% (0.892 mEq/mL) in 10 and 50 mL vials. Concentration of 4.2% (0.5 mEq/mL) in 10 mL vials. Each gram sodium bicarbonate provides about 12 mEq sodium and bicarbonate ions. **Syringe:** May be given undiluted for resuscitation. **Infusion:** 7.5% and 8.4% concentrations should be diluted with equal amounts of sterile water for injection or compatible IV solution.

STABILITY/STORAGE

Vial: Store at room temperature. **Infusion:** Stable at room temperature for 24 hr.

ADMINISTRATION

General: IV administration can result in fluid/solute overload that can precipitate overhydration, congested states, and pulmonary edema. IV infusion device should be used for safety and accuracy of drug delivery. Confirm patency of peripheral vein. Extravasation can cause chemical cellulitis, necrosis, ulceration, or sloughing of surrounding tissues. Confer with physician regarding use of warm compresses and/or infiltration of site with lidocaine or hyaluronidase. Drug has many incompatibilities and IV line must be carefully cleared with compatible IV solution prior to and following administration to avoid precipitation. **IV Push:** Up to 1 mEq/kg over 1–3 min as appropriate for cardiopulmonary resuscitation. Repeat in 10 minutes as

needed and indicated by pH and PCO_2 **Intermittent Infusion:** *Adult:* Usual rate of administration of diluted drug is 2–5 mEq/kg over 4–8 hr. Do not exceed 50 mEq/hr. *Pediatric < 2 years:* Initially administer 1–2 mEq kg over 1–2 min. Do not exceed a rate of 8 mEq/kg/24 hr. A 4.2% solution is preferred for pediatric use. **Continuous Infusion:** Infuse at physician prescribed rate and in accordance with serum electrolytes/arterial blood gas findings.

COMPATIBILITY

Solution: Dextrose solutions, sodium chloride solutions. **Syringe:** Pentobarbital. **Y-site:** Acyclovir, famotidine, insulin, morphine, potassium chloride, tolazoline, vitamin B complex with C.

INCOMPATIBILITY

Solution: Dextrose 5% in Ringer's lactate. **Syringe:** Glycopyrrolate, metoclopramide, thiopental. **Y-site:** Amrinone, calcium chloride, verapamil.

ADVERSE EFFECTS

Fld/Lytes: Hypernatremia, hypocalcemia, hypokalemia, sodium/water retention. **Metab:** <u>Metabolic alkalosis.</u> **Other:** Chemical cellulitis with extravasation.

TOXICITY/OVERDOSE

Signs/Symptoms: Adverse effects are rare if used cautiously and within guidelines for dosages. Alkalosis, irritability, hyperexcitability, hypokalemia, restlessness, and tetany may develop. **Treatment:** Discontinue drug and notify physician of adverse effects. Hypokalemia can occur with alkalosis; sodium and potassium chloride must be supplemented as a correction mechanism. Hypotonic electrolyte solution may be used to facilitate excretion of bicarbonate via urine.

DRUG INTERACTIONS

Amphetamines, ephedrine, flecainide, mecamylamine, pseudoephedrine, quinine, quinidine: Sodium bicarbonate may potentiate side effects and increase half-life/duration. **Chlorpropamide, lithium, salicylates, tetracyclines:** Sodium bicarbonate increases renal clearance and possibly decreases pharmacologic effect. **Corticosteroids, corticotropin:** Increased potential for sodium retention.

NURSING CONSIDERATIONS

Assessment
General:
Intake/output ratio.
Lab Alterations:
Frequent monitoring of electrolytes/assessment of need for therapy on a continuing basis is required in order to prevent alkalosis. Regular assessment of arterial blood gas measurements is also required for a continuous infusion. Gastric acid secretion test: Antagonizes pentagastrin and histamine with gastric acid secretion test. If possible do not administer during the 24 hr preceding the test.

Intervention/Rationale
May cause fluid retention or overload of solute; evaluate intake/output ratio hourly to determine overload status.

Patient/Family Education
Review purpose of therapy/potential side effects and expected therapeutic outcome.

SODIUM PHOSPHATE
(soe'-dee-um foss'-fate)
Classification(s): Phosphate supplement
Pregnancy Category: C

PHARMACODYNAMICS/KINETICS
Mechanism of Action: Major intracellular anion that participates in providing energy for metabolism of substrates and contributes to metabolic/enzymatic reactions in most organs and tissues. **Metabolism/Elimination:** > 90% is excreted via urine.

INDICATIONS/DOSAGE

Treatment of phosphate depletion
Adult: 10–15 mM/24 hr. *Pediatric:* 1.5–2.0 mM/24 hr. Older children may require up to 15 mM.

CONTRAINDICATIONS/ PRECAUTIONS
Contraindicated in: Hypernatremia, hyperphosphatemia, hypocalcemia. **Use cautiously in:** Adrenal or renal insufficiency, cardiac failure, cirrhosis, edematous or sodium retaining conditions. **Pregnancy/Lactation:** No well-controlled trials to establish safety. Benefits must outweigh risks.

PREPARATION
Availability: 3 mM phosphorus and 4 mEq sodium/mL. 5, 10, 15, 30, and 50 mL vials. **Infusion:** Dilute and thoroughly mix prescribed dose in

In the Adverse Effects section, <u>underline</u> indicates most frequent; CAPS indicates life threatening.

473

large volume of compatible IV solution.

STABILITY/STORAGE
Vial: Store at room temperature. Protect from excessive heat. **Infusion:** Stable at room temperature for 24 hr.

ADMINISTRATION
General: Dosage/rate are dependent on patient needs and overall physical condition as well as concentration of the solution. **Continuous Infusion:** Infuse slowly over at least 4–6 hr in order to avoid phosphate intoxication.

COMPATIBILITY
Solution: Dextrose solutions.

INCOMPATIBILITY
Additive: Solutions containing high calcium concentrations.

ADVERSE EFFECTS
CV: MI, severe hypotension. **Renal:** Nephrotoxicity (associated primarily with hyperparathyroidism). **MS:** Extraskeletal calcification. **Fld/Lytes:** Hypocalcemia, hyperphosphatemia, hypermagnesemia.

TOXICITY/OVERDOSE
Signs/Symptoms: Infusions of high concentrations of phosphorus decrease serum calcium and produce symptoms of hypocalcemic tetany. **Treatment:** Monitor serum calcium levels at regular intervals.

DRUG INTERACTIONS
Glucocorticoids: May result in hypernatremia.

NURSING CONSIDERATIONS

Assessment
General:
Vital signs, intake/output ratio, baseline/daily weights.

Physical:
Neurologic/neuromuscular status associated with electrolyte imbalance.
Lab Alterations:
Monitor renal function studies, including electrolytes, BUN, creatinine, and serum calcium. Alters urinary pH—administration of drug is followed by slight but consistent decrease in urinary pH.

Intervention/Rationale
Assess fluid status and daily weights. ● Monitor for signs/symptoms of hyper/hypophosphatemia, hypomagnesemia, and severe hypotension (anorexia, blood dyscrasia, bone pain, confusion, decreased reflexes).

Patient/Family Education
Review purpose/goals of therapy.

SODIUM THIOSULFATE
(soe'-dee-um thi-o-sul'-fate)
Classification(s): Antidote
Pregnancy Category: C

PHARMACODYNAMICS/KINETICS
Mechanism of Action: Primarily involved in the conversion of cyanide to the nontoxic thiocyanate ion. **Distribution:** Distributed throughout extracellular fluid. **Metabolism/Elimination:** Excreted unchanged via urine. **Half-Life:** 0.65 hr.

INDICATIONS/DOSAGE

Arsenic poisoning
Adult: Initially 1 mL (100 mg), 2 mL (200 mg), 3 mL (300 mg),

In the Adverse Effects section, <u>underline</u> indicates most frequent; CAPS indicates life threatening.

4 mL (400 mg) on successive days. Followed by 5 mL (500 mg) on alternate days as needed.

Cyanide poisoning

Adult: Alone or as an adjunctive therapy with sodium nitrite or amyl nitrite. Following administration of 300 mg IV sodium nitrite, inject 12.5 g of sodium thiosulfate. If necessary, injection of both sodium nitrite and sodium thiosulfate may be repeated at 50% of the initial dose.

CONTRAINDICATIONS/ PRECAUTIONS

Contraindicated in: Hypersensitivity. **Pregnancy/Lactation:** No well-controlled trials to establish safety. Benefits must outweigh risks.

PREPARATION

Availability: 1 g/10 mL and 2.5 g/ 10 mL in 10 and 50 mL vials and 10 mL amps. Cyanide antidote package includes: Sodium nitrite 300 mg/10 mL; sodium thiosulfate 12.5 g/50 mL; amyl nitrite inhalant 0.3 mL; syringes, stomach tube, tourniquet, instructions. **Syringe:** No further dilution required.

STABILITY/STORAGE

Vial: Store at room temperature.

ADMINISTRATION

IV Push: Slow IV use only. 12.5 g or less over approximately 10 min.

COMPATIBILITY/INCOMPATIBILITY

Data not available.

ADVERSE EFFECTS

Hypersens: Allergic manifestations.

NURSING CONSIDERATIONS

Assessment

General:
Vital signs.
Physical:
Respiratory status.

Intervention/Rationale

Assess for level of toxicity. ● Evaluate all vital signs for toxicity manifestations. ● Assess need for emergency airway management and full supportive measures.

Patient/Family Education

Review goals/potential outcomes of drug therapy.

STREPTOKINASE

(strep-toe-kie'-naze)
Trade Name(s): Kabikinase, Streptase
Classification(s): Thrombolytic agent
Pregnancy Category: C

PHARMACODYNAMICS/KINETICS

Mechanism of Action: Acts with plasminogen to produce an activator complex that converts plasminogen to proteolytic enzyme plasmin. Plasmin degrades fibrin clots as well as fibrinogen and other plasma proteins. **Onset of Action:** Immediate. **Peak Effect:** Rapid. **Duration of Action:** 4–12 hr. **Distribution:** Distributed throughout the body. **Metabolism/ Elimination:** Rapidly cleared by antibodies and reticuloendothelial system. Mechanism of elimination is unknown. **Half-Life:** 23 min.

S

In the Adverse Effects section, underline indicates most frequent; CAPS indicates life threatening.

INDICATIONS/DOSAGE

Coronary thrombosis associated with acute transmural MI

Adult: 1.5 million IU.

Treatment of recent or massive vein thrombosis, pulmonary emboli, arterial embolism/thrombosis

Adult:

Loading Dose: 250,000 IU followed by 100,000 IU/hr/24 hr for pulmonary emboli; 72 hr treatment required for recurrent pulmonary emboli/deep vein thrombosis.

Treatment of occluded A-V cannula

Adult: 250,000 IU/2 mL of solution via a controlled infusion device into each occluded limb of the cannula over a 25–35 min period. Clamp cannula limbs for 2 hr, aspirate and follow with flush of saline and reconnect. Observe closely for manifestations of adverse effects while clamped.

CONTRAINDICATIONS/ PRECAUTIONS

Contraindicated in: Active internal bleeding, hypersensitivity, intracranial neoplasm, intracranial or intraspinal surgery, recent (within 2 months) CVA, severe uncontrolled hypertension. **Use cautiously in:** Patients having undergone recent (10 days) major surgery, obstetrical delivery, organ biopsy, trauma, uncontrolled arterial hypertension; recent streptococcal infections; recent streptokinase therapy; subacute bacterial endocarditis. **Pregnancy/Lactation:** No well-controlled trials to establish safety. Benefits must outweigh risks. Exercise cau-

tion when administering drug to nursing women. Crosses the placenta. **Pediatrics:** Safety and efficacy not established.

PREPARATION

Availability: 250,000, 600,000, 750,000 in 5 mL and 6.5 mL vials. 1.5 million IU in 6.5 mL vials and 50 mL infusion bottles. **Reconstitution:** Slowly add 5 mL sodium chloride or 5% dextrose solution to vial or bottle, directing the diluent at the side rather than into drug powder. Roll and tilt gently to reconstitute. Avoid shaking. **Infusion:** Withdraw entire contents of vial slowly/carefully. Further dilute to total volume of 50–500 mL sodium chloride in glass or plastic containers. **Bottle:** Add an additional 40 mL diluent to bottle (total volume: 45 mL). Reconstituted solution may be administered via 0.8 micron or larger pore size filter.

STABILITY/STORAGE

Vial: Store unopened vials at controlled room temperature. Contains no preservatives. Reconstitute immediately before use. **Infusion:** May be used for direct IV administration within 8 hr following reconstitution if refrigerated. Discard unused reconstituted drug.

ADMINISTRATION

General: Volume or syringe infusion pump required. Reconstituted drug will alter drop size and impact correct dosage with drop-size driven machines. **IV Push:** *Coronary Thrombosis:* Give over 60 min. **Intermittent/Continuous Infusion:** *Deep Vein Thrombosis, Pulmonary Emboli:* Loading dose: single dose over

In the Adverse Effects section, underline indicates most frequent; CAPS indicates life threatening.

25–30 min. Maintenance dose: infuse over physician specified time for 24–72 hr.

COMPATIBILITY
Solution: Dextrose solutions, sodium chloride solutions. **Y-site:** Dobutamine, dopamine, heparin, lidocaine, nitroglycerin.

ADVERSE EFFECTS
CNS: Guillain-Barre syndrome, headache. **CV:** Reperfusion dysrhythmias. **MS:** Musculoskeletal pain. **Heme:** <u>Bleeding</u> (minor): superficial, surface. <u>Bleeding</u> (major): internal, severe. **Hypersens:** Angioneurotic edema, BRONCHOSPASM, itching, nausea, urticaria, vasculitis/interstitial nephritis. **Other:** Fever, flushing.

TOXICITY/OVERDOSE
Signs/Symptoms: Bleeding, major/minor, can be considered signs of toxicity. Minor bleeding occurs often at invaded/disturbed sites (i.e., IV sites). Use local measures to control minor bleeding—pressure application for a minimum of 30 minutes followed by a secure pressure dressing. **Treatment:** If uncontrolled bleeding occurs, discontinue infusion and immediately notify physician. If required, replace blood loss and reverse bleeding tendency with fresh whole blood, packed RBCs, cryoprecipitate, or fresh frozen plasma. Aminocaproic acid as an antidote may be considered.

DRUG INTERACTIONS
Anticoagulants, antiplatelet agents (including aspirin, nonsteroidal antiinflammatory agents, dipyridamole): Increase bleeding potential.

NURSING CONSIDERATIONS
Assessment
General:
Vital signs, hemodynamic monitoring, ECG monitoring.
Physical:
Cardiopulmonary status.
Lab Alterations:
Decreased plasminogen/fibrinogen levels, prothrombin time (PT), partial thromboplastin time (PTT), thrombin time (TT). Monitor hemoglobin/hematocrit, platelets, PT, PTT, TT, and CPK prior to the initiation of therapy. Continue monitoring TT and PT every 4 hr throughout administration of the drug. Continually monitor ECG and evaluate ST segment elevation every 15 min for a minimum of 4 hr. Avoid arterial or venipuncture and IM injections if at all possible throughout the course of therapy.

Intervention/Rationale
IV administration decreases blood pressure and peripheral vascular resistance with a corresponding decrease in cardiac output. Carefully monitor blood pressure, peripheral vascular resistance/cardiac output, adjusting therapy according to most recent data. ● Observe patient continuously. Administer drug in hospital setting or under the direction of a physician knowledgeable in its use with immediate access to the required diagnostic and cardiac cath lab facilities.

Patient/Family Education
Review purpose of medication. Emphasize potential for increased bleeding tendencies. Notify nurse/

In the Adverse Effects section, <u>underline</u> indicates most frequent; CAPS indicates life threatening.

477

physician if evidence of frank bleeding is noted. Notify nurse/physician of developing hypersensitivity reactions: difficulty with breathing, itching, flushing, headache, or urticaria.

STREPTOZOCIN

(strep-toe-zoe'-sin)
Trade Name(s): Zanosar
Classification(s): Alkylating agent, antineoplastic
Pregnancy Category: C

PHARMACODYNAMICS/KINETICS
Mechanism of Action: Inhibits DNA synthesis by cross-linking strands of cellular DNA. Interferes with RNA transcription causing imbalance of growth that leads to cellular death. **Distribution:** Rapidly distributed to liver, kidney, intestine, and pancreas. Does not cross blood–brain barrier. **Metabolism/Elimination:** Extensively metabolized in liver. Active drug and metabolites eliminated via kidneys. Approximately 60%–72% of dose can be detected in the urine within 4 hr of administration. **Half-Life:** 35 min (3 min to > 40 hr).

INDICATIONS/DOSAGE

Management of metastatic islet cell carcinoma of pancreas
Adult: Daily dose 500 mg/m^2 for 5 consecutive days every 6 weeks until maximum benefit occurs or until toxicity is noted. Dosage increases are not recommended.
Weekly Dose: Initial dose is 1000 mg/m^2 at weekly intervals for

the first 2 weeks. In subsequent weeks increased drug doses in patients who have not had a therapeutic response and have not experienced significant toxicity. **DO NOT** exceed a single dose of 1500 mg/m^2 BSA.

Patients with creatinine clearance of 10–50 mL/min receive 75% of usual dose; patients with creatinine clearance < 10 mL/min receive 50% usual dose.

CONTRAINDICATIONS/PRECAUTIONS
Contraindicated in: Hypersensitivity. **Use cautiously in:** Active infections, decreased bone marrow activity, hepatic disease, patients with childbearing potential, underlying renal insufficiency. **Pregnancy/Lactation:** No well-controlled trials to establish safety. Benefits must outweigh risks. Has been shown to be teratogenic and abortifacient in animal studies. Milk distribution is not clearly known. **Pediatrics:** Safety and efficacy has not been established.

PREPARATION
Availability: 1 g vials. **Reconstitution:** Each gram vial must be diluted with 9.5 mL sodium chloride or dextrose solution yielding 100 mg/mL. **Exercise caution in the handling and preparation of powder and solution**; use gloves throughout the entire procedure. If powder or solution contacts the skin or mucosa, immediately wash with soap and water. **Infusion:** Solution may be further diluted in 50–250 mL of compatible IV solution.

STABILITY/STORAGE
Vial: Powder for injection should be protected from light and refriger-

In the Adverse Effects section, <u>underline</u> indicates most frequent; CAPS indicates life threatening.

ated. Contains no preservatives; discard unused reconstituted portions within 12 hr. **Infusion:** Following reconstitution, stable for 48 hr at room temperature and 96 hr when refrigerated. Solution is pale gold in color, do not use if dark brown.

ADMINISTRATION

General: IV administration is recommended. Intra-arterial administration increases the possibility that adverse renal effects can develop more rapidly. Handle drug preparation/administration in accordance with institutional guidelines for chemotherapeutic/cytotoxic agents as drug may become a carcinogenic hazard following topical exposure based on various laboratory studies. Drug is a vesicant, carefully assess IV site and assure patency. Discontinue drug with observation of erythema at site or complaints of severe discomfort along vein. **IV Push:** Rapid IV injection in a minimal dilution over 5–15 min. **Intermittent Infusion:** May be administered at physician prescribed rate over 15 minutes to 6 hr via an IV infusion device.

COMPATIBILITY

Solution: Dextrose solutions, sodium chloride solutions.

ADVERSE EFFECTS

CNS: Confusion, depression, lethargy. **GI:** Diarrhea, nausea, vomiting. **GU:** Proteinuria. **Renal:** Nephrotoxicity. **Endo:** Diabetes insipidus, gonadal suppression, hyperglycemia, hypoglycemia (first dose). **Fld/Lytes:** Hypophosphatemia. **Heme:** LEUKOPENIA, THROMBOCY-

TOPENIA, anemia, elevated LDH, AST (SGOT). **Nadir:** 2–3 weeks. **Other:** Fever, phlebitis at IV site.

DRUG INTERACTIONS

Antineoplastic agents: Synergistic myelosuppression. **Nephrotoxic drugs:** Cumulative toxicity. **Phenytoin:** Decreases cytotoxic effects on beta cells of pancreas with concomitant administration.

NURSING CONSIDERATIONS

Assessment
General:
Vital signs, hydration status, intake/output ratio, baseline/daily weight.
Physical:
Renal status, hematopoietic system, GI tract, infectious disease status.
Lab Alterations:
Closely monitor for evidence of hematopoietic, hepatic, or renal toxicity. Assess lab values, including CBC, liver function studies/electrolytes, and serum glucose at regular intervals.

Intervention/Rationale
Assess fluid status and weight daily; evaluate for development of signs/symptoms of diabetes insipidus by careful monitoring of hourly intake/output ratio. Encourage increased oral fluid intake. ● Assess antiemetic requirements with meal schedule in order to optimize caloric and fluid intake of patient. ● Assess urine output and overall fluid status regularly as drug is known to be renal toxic. ● Avoid IM injections and rectal temperatures. ● Observe for development of signs/symptoms of infection.

S

In the Adverse Effects section, underline indicates most frequent; CAPS indicates life threatening.

479

Patient/Family Education
Notify nurse/physician immediately if pain, redness, or discomfort is noted at peripheral IV site. Review side effects of drug. Notify nurse/physician if signs/symptoms of hypoglycemia occur (i.e., anxiety, chills, cold sweats, confusion, cool, pale skin, drowsiness, shakiness, or generalized weakness). Seek physician approval prior to receiving live virus vaccines or chloroquinine. Observe for signs of bleeding or infection. Use a soft toothbrush or electric razor to minimize the tendency for bleeding. Avoid over-the-counter products containing aspirin or ibuprofen.

SUCCINYLCHOLINE
(sux-sin-il-koe′-leen)
Trade Name(s): Anectine, Quelicin, Sucostrin
Classification(s): Depolarizing neuromuscular blocking agent
Pregnancy Category: C

PHARMACODYNAMICS/KINETICS
Mechanism of Action: Prolongs depolarization of the muscle end plate. Causes release of histamines. **Onset of Action:** 30–60 sec. **Peak Effect:** 2–3 min. **Duration of Action:** 10 min. **Distribution:** Widely distributed throughout extracellular fluid. **Metabolism/Elimination:** Rapidly metabolized primarily by plasma pseudocholinesterase. Up to 10% excreted unchanged via urine.

INDICATIONS/DOSAGE

Anesthesia induction for surgical procedures to produce skeletal muscle paralysis

Adult: May repeat doses as needed.
Short Procedures: 0.6 mg/kg over 10–30 sec. (Range: 0.3–1.1 mg/kg.)
Long Procedures: 2.5–4.3 mg/min.
Pediatric: May repeat doses as needed.
Short Procedures: 2 mg/kg for infants and small children. 1 mg/kg for older children/adolescents.

Reduce the intensity of muscle contractions of pharmacologic or electrically induced convulsions; management of patients undergoing mechanical ventilation
Adult:
Prolonged Muscle Relaxation: Initial dose 0.3–1.1 mg/kg. Maintenance dose 0.04–0.07 mg/kg.

CONTRAINDICATIONS/PRECAUTIONS
Contraindicated in: Hypersensitivity to succinylcholine or parabens, penetrating eye injuries, plasma pseudocholinesterase deficiencies. **Use cautiously in:** Elderly/debilitated patients, electrolyte disturbances, fractures/muscle spasms, glaucoma, liver impairment, malignant hyperthermia history, myasthenia gravis/syndrome, patient receiving cardiac glycosides, pulmonary disease, renal impairment. **Pregnancy/Lactation:** May be used to provide muscle relaxation during cesarean section. Should be used only when clearly needed due to potential for residual neuromuscular blockade to fetus. Crosses placenta in small amounts. **Pediatrics:** Neonates/children have an increased risk of malignant hyperthermia. Continuous infusion of drug is contraindicated.

In the Adverse Effects section, <u>underline</u> indicates most frequent; CAPS indicates life threatening.

PREPARATION

Availability: 20 mg/mL, 50 mg/mL, 100 mg/mL in 10 and 20 mL vials. Powder for injection 100 mg/vial. Powder for infusion 500 mg or 1 g/vial. **Infusion:** Use only freshly prepared solution. Incompatible with alkaline solutions (will precipitate if mixed or administered simultaneously). Do not mix in same syringe or administer simultaneously via same needle with solutions of short-acting barbiturates.

STABILITY/STORAGE

Vial: Should be refrigerated to minimize loss of potency. Stable at room temperature for up to 14 days after opening multidose vial. Unreconstituted powder for injection stable indefinitely at room temperature when stored in an unopened container. **Infusion:** Following reconstitution of powder with sodium chloride or dextrose solution to a concentration of 1–2 mg/mL, stable for 4 weeks at 5° C or 1 week at 25° C. Does not contain preservatives; it is recommended that use occur within 24 hr and unused portion be discarded.

ADMINISTRATION

General: *Test Dose:* Given to evaluate patients' ability to metabolize drug. **Dose:** 0.1 mg/kg may be administered to spontaneously breathing patients after anesthesia has been induced. If patient metabolizes normally, respiratory depression seldom occurs and if it does, it usually disappears within 5 minutes. Usually administered IV with individualized dosage. May be given IM to infants and older children or adults when a suitable vein is not immediately accessible. To avoid patient distress administer after a state of unconsciousness has been induced. **IV Push:** Over 10–30 sec. **Intermittent Infusion:** Administer loading and maintenance dose at appropriate intervals to maintain required degree of relaxation. **Continuous Infusion:** Solutions contain 0.1%–0.2% (1–2 mg/mL). Administer 1 mg/mL IV solution at 0.5–10.0 mg/min to obtain desired level of relaxation. The 0.2% (2 mg/mL) solution is used to prevent circulatory overload.

COMPATIBILITY

Solution: Dextrose solutions, lactated Ringer's, Ringer's injection, sodium chloride solutions.

INCOMPATIBILITY

Syringe/Y-site: Barbiturates.

ADVERSE EFFECTS

Ophtho: Increased intraocular pressure. **CV:** CARDIAC ARREST, bradycardia, dysrhythmia, hypertension, hypotension. **Resp:** APNEA, BRONCHOSPASM. **GI:** Excess salivation. **GU:** Myoglobinuria. **MS:** Initial muscle fasciculation that may result in postoperative pain. **Fld/Lytes:** Hyperkalemia. **Heme:** Myoglobinemia. **Hypersens:** Rash. **Other:** MALIGNANT HYPERTHERMIA.

TOXICITY/OVERDOSE

Signs/Symptoms: Cardiac dysrhythmias, hyperthermia, malignant hyperthermic crisis, prolonged period of apnea with progression to phase II neuromuscular block. **Treatment:** Discontinue drug with appearance of major side effects. Maintain con-

In the Adverse Effects section, underline indicates most frequent; CAPS indicates life threatening.

481

trolled ventilation. Reverse neuromuscular blockade with anticholinesterase drugs following return of muscle twitching. Atropine sulfate can be used to treat bradycardia. Malignant hyperthermia crisis can be symptomatically treated with cooling measures, restoration of fluid/electrolyte balance. Dantrolene may be required.

DRUG INTERACTIONS
Beta-adrenergic blocking agents, cimetidine, cyclophosphamide, furosemide, kanamycin, lidocaine, magnesium salts, neomycin, quinidine, quinine: Concurrent use potentiates neuromuscular blocking effects. **Cholinesterase inhibitors:** Concurrent administration/exposure decreases pseudocholinesterase activity and increases the degree of paralysis. **Procaine:** Concomitant use results in prolonged apnea.

NURSING CONSIDERATIONS
Assessment
General:
Vital signs, continuous ECG, blood pressure, and respiratory monitoring.
Physical:
Cardiopulmonary status, neuromuscular status.

Intervention/Rationale
Evaluate respiratory status throughout administration of the drug. Emergency airway management, equipment, and skilled medical personnel must be available for immediate intervention. ● Continuously monitor ECG, heart rate, blood pressure throughout period of drug usage. Be prepared to iden-

tify and rapidly treat dysrhythmias and hypotension. ● Observe for signs/symptoms of potential malignant hyperthermic crisis: tachycardia, tachypnea, hypercarbia, jaw muscle spasm, hyperthermia. ● Assess neuromuscular response with peripheral nerve stimulator during intraoperative phase. ● Monitor respirations closely until fully recovered from neuromuscular blockade as evidenced by tests of muscle strength (hand grasp, head lift, ability to cough).

Patient/Family Education
Postoperative muscle stiffness is to be expected and will subside presently. Impaired communication will resolve following recovery from drug.

SUFENTANIL
(soo-fen′-ta-nil)
Trade Name(s): Sufenta
Classification(s): Narcotic agonist analgesic
Pregnancy Category: C (D for prolonged use or use of high doses at term)
Controlled Substance Schedule: II

PHARMACODYNAMICS/KINETICS
Mechanism of Action: Binds with opiate receptors at various sites in CNS, altering perception of and emotional response to pain via an unknown mechanism. **Onset of Action:** Within 1–3 min. **Duration of Action:** 5 min. **Distribution:** Does not readily penetrate adipose tissue. **Metabolism/Elimination:** Primarily metabo-

lized by liver. Lesser amounts in the small intestine. Eliminated via kidneys. **Half-Life:** 2.5 hr (increased with the use of cardiopulmonary bypass).

INDICATIONS/DOSAGE

Individualize dosages. In obese patients (> 20% above ideal body weight), calculate dosage based on lean body weight. Reduce dosage in elderly/debilitated.

Adjunct to general anesthesia

Adult: 1–8 mcg/kg administered with nitrous oxide and oxygen. **Maintenance Dose:** 10–50 mcg for stress or lightening of analgesia.

Primary anesthetic

Adult: 8–30 mcg/kg. Administered with 100% oxygen and muscle relaxation. Produces sleep at doses > 8 mcg/kg. Dosages up to 25 mcg/kg release catecholamines. 25–30 mcg/kg blocks sympathetic response including catecholamine release. **Maintenance Dose:** 25–50 mcg for stress and lightening of anesthesia.
Pediatric: < 12 years: **Induction/ Maintenance Dose:** 10–25 mcg/kg with 100% oxygen. Supplemental doses of 25–50 mcg are recommended for maintenance.

CONTRAINDICATIONS/ PRECAUTIONS

Contraindicated in: During labor/delivery of preterm infants, hypersensitivity. **Use cautiously in:** Acute abdominal conditions, asthma, chronic obstructive lung disease, elderly, debilitated, renal/hepatic dysfunction, suppressed cough reflex. **Pregnancy/Lactation:** No well-controlled trials to establish safety. Benefits must outweigh risks. Crosses the placenta. May produce depression of the respiratory tract of the fetus requiring resuscitation on delivery. Lab studies have demonstrated embryocidal effects in animals. Appears in breast milk. Some clinicians recommend a 4–6 hr wait before initiating breastfeeding after receiving drug. **Pediatrics:** Safety and efficacy for children < 2 years undergoing cardiovascular surgery has been documented in a limited number of cases.

PREPARATION

Availability: 50 mcg/mL in 1, 2, and 5 mL amps.

STABILITY/STORAGE

Vial: Store at room temperature. Contains no preservatives. Discard unused portions after opening.

ADMINISTRATION

IV Push: Administer slowly by direct IV push.

COMPATIBILITY/INCOMPATIBILITY

Data not available.

ADVERSE EFFECTS

CNS: Dizziness, euphoria, light-headedness, <u>sedation</u>. **Ophtho:** Blurred vision. **CV:** CARDIAC ARREST, SHOCK, circulatory depression, hypertension, hypotension. **Resp:** APNEA, RESPIRATORY ARREST, respiratory depression. **GI:** <u>Dry mouth</u>, nausea, vomiting. **MS:** Thoracic muscle rigidity. **Hypersens:** Erythema, pruritus. **Other:** Chills, sweating, wheal and flare over vein may occur with IV injection.

S

In the Adverse Effects section, <u>underline</u> indicates most frequent; CAPS indicates life threatening.

483

TOXICITY/OVERDOSE

Signs/Symptoms: Apnea, circulatory collapse, convulsions, cardiopulmonary arrest and death may occur, hypotension, bradycardia, pulmonary edema or shock are serious overdose symptoms, less severe reactions include CNS depression, miosis and respiratory depression.
Treatment: Maintain adequate ventilation via mechanical means. Administer narcotic antagonists as indicated. Treat symptomatically and supportively to reverse manifestations.

DRUG INTERACTIONS

Alcohol, antidepressants, antihistamines, sedatives: Additive CNS depression. **Benzodiazepines:** Increased risk of hypotension. **Neuromuscular blocking agents:** Dose-dependent increase in heart rate during anesthesia induction.

NURSING CONSIDERATIONS

Assessment
General:
Continuous blood pressure, ECG, respiratory monitoring, pain control.
Physical:
Cardiopulmonary status.

Intervention/Rationale
Assess respiratory rate, depth, and pattern throughout administration of drug. Respiratory depressive effects outlast analgesic effects. ● Monitor postoperative narcotic dosages, consider decreasing dosages by 25%–33% of the usual recommended dose. ● Continuous ECG, blood pressure monitoring throughout administration period.

Plan interventions to correct dysrhythmias, hypotension, hypertension. ● Carefully assess special risk patients (elderly/debilitated patients sensitive to CNS depression including those with acute alcoholism, Addison's disease, cardiovascular disease, cerebral arteriosclerosis, convulsive disorders, delirium tremens, fever, kyphoscoliosis, myxedema, prostatic hypertrophy, recent GI or GU surgery, toxic psychoses, ulcerative colitis, urethral stricture) for potentiation of depressant effects.

Patient/Family Education
May cause drowsiness or dizziness in the postoperative phase of recovery. Seek assistance with ambulatory activities. Change positions slowly and gradually in order to prevent orthostatic shifts in blood pressure. Avoid alcohol or CNS depressants for 24 hr following drug administration because of increased potential for respiratory depression.

TERBUTALINE

(ter-byoo′-ta-leen)
Trade Name(s): Brethine, Bricanyl
Classification(s): Bronchodilator, tocolytic agent
Pregnancy Category: B

PHARMACODYNAMICS/KINETICS

Mechanism of Action: Beta-2 adrenergic agonist whose primary effect is the relaxation of smooth muscle of the bronchial tree, uterus, and peripheral vasculature. Responsible for the accumulation of cyclic ade-

In the Adverse Effects section, <u>underline</u> indicates most frequent; CAPS indicates life threatening.

nosine monophosphate at receptor sites. **Distribution:** Distributed throughout the body. **Metabolism/ Elimination:** Partially metabolized in liver. 60% excreted unchanged in urine. 3% excreted in feces via bile. **Half-Life:** 2–5 hr (may be prolonged with repeat doses).

INDICATIONS/DOSAGE

Arrest of preterm labor (*unlabeled use*)

Adult: 10 mcg/min. Titrate upward to a maximum dose of 80 mcg/min.

CONTRAINDICATIONS/ PRECAUTIONS

Contraindicated in: Hypersensitivity. **Use cautiously in:** Cardiac disease, diabetes mellitus, history of seizures, hypertension, hyperthyroidism, ketoacidosis. **Pregnancy/Lactation:** Serious adverse reactions including pulmonary edema, hypoglycemia, transient hypokalemia have occurred during premature labor administration. Hypoglycemia has also been reported in neonates born to women treated with this drug during labor. Use cautiously in breastfeeding women. **Pediatrics:** Not recommended for children less than 12 years.

PREPARATION

Availability: 1 mg/mL in 2 mL amps with 1 mL fill. **Infusion:** Dilute in compatible IV solution as per physician specified volume.

STABILITY/STORAGE

Vial: Store at room temperature. Protect from light. Do not use if discolored. **Infusion:** Stable at room temperature for 7 days.

ADMINISTRATION

General: Evaluate change to oral dosage form when the patient is contraction free for 4–8 hr on the minimum effective IV dosage. Use of infusion device is required to assure accuracy and safety of medication delivery. **Intermittent/Continuous Infusion:** Begin infusion at 10 mcg/min, increase by 5 mcg every 10 min to a **maximum** of 80 mcg/min until contractions cease. Begin tapering dosage by 5 mcg increments following a period of 30–60 min of contraction free time. Maintain IV dosage at minimal effective dose for 4–8 hr after contractions have completely ceased.

COMPATIBILITY

Solution: Dextrose solutions, sodium chloride solutions. **Syringe:** Doxapram.

ADVERSE EFFECTS

CNS: Anxiety, headache, insomnia, <u>nervousness</u>, <u>restlessness</u>, <u>tremor</u>. **CV:** <u>PULMONARY EDEMA</u>, angina, dysrhythmias, hypertension, <u>palpitations</u>. **GI:** Nausea, vomiting. **Endo:** Hyperglycemia, hypoglycemia. **Fld/ Lytes:** Hypokalemia.

TOXICITY/OVERDOSE

Signs/Symptoms: Observe for signs/ symptoms of dysrhythmias and pending development of pulmonary edema. **Treatment:** Symptomatic/supportive treatment is required including ventilatory support, diuretics, and afterload reducers.

DRUG INTERACTIONS

Adrenergic agents: Additive adrenergic effects. **MAO inhibitors:** Concomitant use may lead to hypertensive

In the Adverse Effects section, <u>underline</u> indicates most frequent; CAPS indicates life threatening.

485

crisis. **Sympathomimetic agents:** Additive adverse cardiovascular effects.

NURSING CONSIDERATIONS

Assessment

General:
Continuous monitoring of maternal blood pressure, heart rate, and respiratory rate. Continuous fetal monitoring. Continuous monitoring of contractions and labor progression. Intake/output ratio.

Physical:
Cardiopulmonary status.

Lab Alterations:
Evaluate serum glucose and potassium periodically. Observe for signs/symptoms of hypoglycemia, to include anxiety, cold sweats, nervousness, poor concentration, weakness. Hypokalemia symptoms: dysrhythmias, fatigue, weakness.

Intervention/Rationale
Continuous monitoring of maternal blood pressure, heart rate, frequency/duration of contractions, as well as fetal heart rate, is required throughout administration of this drug. ● Observe development of adverse effects including anxiety, headache, tachycardia, and tremor. ● Assess lung sounds at least every 4 hr, monitor intake/output ratio hourly, note development of jugular venous distention, dyspnea, frothy sputum, increased respiratory rate—all signs/symptoms of propensity for pulmonary edema.

Patient/Family Education
Review the potential outcome of drug therapy, including potential adverse effects. If labor contractions resume notify nurse/physician immediately.

TERIPARATIDE
(ter-a-par′-a-tide)
Trade Name(s): Parathar
Classification(s): In vivo diagnostic aid
Pregnancy Category: C

PHARMACODYNAMICS/KINETICS
Mechanism of Action: Initial effect on bone is to promote an increased rate of release of calcium from bone into blood through stimulation of adenylate cyclase in the involved organ.

INDICATIONS/DOSAGE

Diagnostic agent for hypoparathyroidism or pseudohypoparathyroidism in hypocalcemic patients

Adult: 200 units. *Pediatric:* > 3 years: 3 units/kg. Maximum dosage 200 units

---

CONTRAINDICATIONS/ PRECAUTIONS
Contraindicated in: Hypersensitivity. **Use cautiously in:** Borderline hypercalcemic patients. **Pregnancy/Lactation:** No well-controlled trials to establish safety. Benefits must outweigh risks. Percentage of drug excretion in breast milk is unknown. Exercise caution when administering drug to breastfeeding women. **Pediatrics:** Limited data available. Has been used in children 3 years and older without untoward effects.

In the Adverse Effects section, <u>underline</u> indicates most frequent; CAPS indicates life threatening.

PREPARATION
Availability: 200 units hPTH activity in 10 mL vials with 10 mL diluent.
Reconstitution: Reconstitute by adding 10 mL of provided diluent to 10 mL vial.

STABILITY/STORAGE
Vial: Store at room temperature. Use reconstituted solution within 4 hr after preparation. Discard unused portion.

ADMINISTRATION
IV Push: Give 10 mL of drug over 10 min.

ADVERSE EFFECTS
CV: Hypertension. **GI:** Abdominal cramps, diarrhea, metallic taste, nausea, urge to defecate. **Fld/Lytes:** Hypocalcemia, hypocalcemic convulsions. **Hypersens:** ANAPHYLAXIS, systemic allergic reactions. **Other:** Pain at injection site, tingling of extremities.

TOXICITY/OVERDOSE
Signs/Symptoms: Repeated doses > 500 units may cause hypercalcemia. If hypercalcemia occurs discontinue drug immediately and notify physician. **Treatment:** Increase hydration orally and intravenously.

NURSING CONSIDERATIONS
Assessment
General:
Vital signs.
Lab Alterations:
Monitor serum calcium levels throughout therapy. Obtain baseline electrolytes and monitor as needed.

Intervention/Rationale
Monitor patient for development of any hypersensitivity reaction. ● Assess blood pressure for hypertension associated with administration of drug.

Patient/Family Education
Review purpose of drug and expected adverse effects. Note possible tingling of extremities and metallic taste in the mouth that can accompany administration of the drug; report positive findings to physician/nurse. Fasting state must be maintained prior to the test and 200 mL of water/hr for 2 hr prior to the study, continuing throughout the study, will be required. Urine specimens will be collected at specific intervals throughout testing.

THEOPHYLLINE
(thee-off'-i-lin)
Classification(s): Bronchodilator
Pregnancy Category: C

PHARMACODYNAMICS/KINETICS
Mechanism of Action: Directly relaxes smooth muscle of respiratory tract. Central respiratory stimulation. **Onset of Action:** Within minutes. **Peak Effect:** 30 min. **Therapeutic Serum Levels:** 10–20 mcg/mL. **Distribution:** Readily distributed throughout extracellular fluids and body tissue. Does not distribute into fatty tissue. 60% protein bound. **Metabolism/Elimination:** Metabolized by the liver. Approximately 80% excreted by the kidneys as metabolites and 15% excreted unchanged. Removed by hemodialysis. **Half-Life: *Adult Nonsmokers:*** 7–9 hr. **Adult Smokers:** 4–5 hr. **Children:** 3–5 hr. **Neonates:** 20–30 hr.

In the Adverse Effects section, underline indicates most frequent;
CAPS indicates life threatening.

487

INDICATIONS/DOSAGE

Symptomatic treatment of asthma, reversible bronchospasm associated with bronchitis or emphysema, status asthmaticus refractory to epinephrine

Adjust dose based on serum levels. *Adult:* Dosages based on lean body weight. Smokers may need higher doses. **Loading Dose:** 6 mg/kg. **Maintenance Infusion: Healthy, Nonsmokers:** 0.5–0.7 mg/kg/hr in first 12 hr, then 0.1–0.5 mg/kg/hr. **Elderly/Cor Pulmonale:** 0.6 mg/kg/hr in first 12 hr, then 0.3 mg/kg/hr. **CHF/Liver Disease:** 0.5 mg/kg/hr in first 12 hr, then 0.1–0.2 mg/kg/hr.
Pediatric: Dosages based on lean body weight. **Loading Dose:** 6 mg/kg. Not recommended for infants under 6 months. **Maintenance Infusion: 6 months to 9 years:** 1.2 mg/kg/hr in first 12 hr, then 1.0 mg/kg/hr thereafter. **9–16 years:** 1.0 mg/kg/hr in first 12 hr, then 0.8 mg/kg/hr there(after.)
Neonate (*unlabeled use*): Dosages based on lean body weight. **Loading Dose:** 6 mg/kg. Not recommended for infants under 6 months. **Maintenance Infusion:** 0.2 mg/kg/hr.

Periodic apnea in Cheyne-Stokes respiration (*unlabeled use*).
Adult: 200–400 mg.

Apnea and bradycardia of prematurity (*unlabeled use*)
Neonate: 1 mg/kg for each 2 mcg/mL serum theophylline level desired, to maintain serum concentrations between 3–5 mcg/mL. Alternate dosage 1 mg/kg every 12 hr.

Cystic Fibrosis (*unlabeled use*)
Pediatric: 10–12 mg/kg/day.

CONTRAINDICATIONS/PRECAUTIONS

Contraindicated in: Hypersensitivity to ethylenediamine or xanthine, uncontrolled seizure disorder. **Use cautiously in:** Acute MI, CHF (may have prolonged half-life), cor pulmonale, elderly, hyperthyroidism, neonates, peptic ulcer, renal or hepatic disease, severe cardiac disease, severe hypertension, severe hypoxemia. **Pregnancy/Lactation:** No well-controlled trials to establish safety. Crosses placenta. Benefits must outweigh risks. Readily distributes into breast milk. **Pediatrics:** Use cautiously in children under the age of 6 months.

PREPARATION

Availability: 200 mg premixed container of 50 and 100 mL. 400 mg premixed container in 100, 250, 500, and 1000 mL. 800 mg premixed container in 250, 500, and 1000 mL. **Infusion:** Administer as premixed infusion or further dilute to physician specified volume.

STABILITY/STORAGE

Vial: Store at room temperature. **Infusion:** Stable for 24 hr at room temperature.

ADMINISTRATION

General: Slow administration—not to exceed 25 mg/min to avoid hypotension, syncope, dysrhythmias, or death. Administer via infusion device to monitor accuracy of dos-

In the Adverse Effects section, <u>underline</u> indicates most frequent; CAPS indicates life threatening.

age. **Intermittent Infusion:** Infuse over at least 20–30 min. **Continuous Infusion:** Infuse at physician specified rate.

COMPATIBILITY

Solution: Amino acids 4.25%/dextrose 25%, dextrose solutions, lactated Ringer's, Ringer's solutions, sodium chloride solutions. **Syringe:** Heparin, metoclopramide, pentobarbital, thiopental. **Y-site:** Amrinone, atracurium, cimetidine, enalaprilat, esmolol, famotidine, foscarnet, heparin, hydrocortisone, labetalol, morphine, netilmicin, pancuronium, potassium chloride, ranitidine, tolazoline, vecuronium, vitamin B complex with C.

INCOMPATIBILITY

Syringe: Doxapram. **Y-site:** Amiodarone, dobutamine, hetastarch, hydralazine, ondansetron.

ADVERSE EFFECTS

CNS: Seizures, dizziness, headache, insomnia, <u>irritability</u>, reflex hyperexcitability, <u>restlessness</u>, severe depression. **CV:** CIRCULATORY FAILURE, VENTRICULAR DYSRHYTHMIAS, extrasystoles, hypotension, <u>palpitations</u>, <u>sinus tachycardia</u>. **GI:** <u>Abdominal cramps</u>, <u>anorexia</u>, diarrhea, <u>epigastric pain</u>, hematemesis, increased AST (SGOT), <u>nausea</u>, <u>vomiting</u>. **GU:** Urinary retention (in males with prostate enlargement). **Renal:** Dehydration, diuresis, proteinuria. **Endo:** Hyperglycemia. **Hypersens:** Exfoliative dermatitis, rash. **Other:** Flushing.

TOXICITY/OVERDOSE

Signs/Symptoms: Agitation, anorexia, cardiac arrest, headache, insomnia, irritability, muscle fasciculations, nausea, nervousness, tachycardia, tachypnea, ventricular dysrhythmias, vomiting. Tonic/clonic seizures may occur without other preceding symptoms. Toxicity may occur with serum levels > 20 mcg/mL. May result in death. **Treatment:** Overall treatment is supportive. Mild symptoms—drug may be continued at reduced rate of administration. Discontinue drug for more serious symptoms. Maintain adequate hydration and electrolyte balance. Seizures may be refractory to anticonvulsants. Hemodialysis or charcoal hemoperfusion may be beneficial.

DRUG INTERACTIONS

Aminoglutethimide, barbiturates, carbamazepine, charcoal, cigarettes/marijuana, hydantoins, isoniazid, ketoconazole, loop diuretics, rifampin, sulfinpyrazone, sympathomimetics: Decreased theophylline levels. **Allopurinol, beta blockers, calcium channel blockers, carbamazepine, cimetidine, corticosteroids, disulfiram, ephedrine, influenza vaccine, interferon, isoniazid, loop diuretics, mexiletine, oral contraceptives, quinolones, ranitidine, thiabendazole, thyroid hormone:** Increased theophylline levels. **Digitalis:** Enhanced digitalis sensitivity and toxicity. **Halothane:** Cardiac dysrhythmias. **Ketamine:** Seizures (toxicity). **Lithium carbonate:** Increased lithium excretion and reduction of lithium effect. **Nondepolarizing muscle relaxants:** Resistance to or reversal of neuromuscular-

In the Adverse Effects section, <u>underline</u> indicates most frequent; CAPS indicates life threatening.

489

blockade. **Propofol:** Theophylline antagonizes sedative effects.

NURSING CONSIDERATIONS

Assessment
General:
Vital signs (every 15 min for first hour), intake/output ratio.
Physical:
Pulmonary status.
Lab Alterations:
False-positive elevations of serum uric acid. Monitor serum theophylline levels.

Intervention/Rationale
Monitor intake/output ratio for an increase in diuresis or fluid volume overload. ● Elevated/toxic levels may cause excessive nausea, vomiting, tremors, palpitations. ● Monitor ABGs and electrolytes (when given for Cheyne-Stokes respiration).

Patient/Family Education
Notify physician/nurse if side effects develop or if condition worsens during therapy. Avoid smoking. Minimize intake of xanthine-containing foods or beverages (colas, coffee, chocolate).

THIAMINE
(thye'-a-min)
Trade Name(s): Biamine
Classification(s): Water-soluble vitamin
Pregnancy Category: A

PHARMACODYNAMICS/KINETICS
Mechanism of Action: Combines with ATP in the liver, kidneys and leukocytes to form thiamine diphosphate, a coenzyme in carbohydrate metabolism. **Distribution:** Widely distributed to all body tissues. **Metabolism/Elimination:** Metabolized by the liver. Excreted primarily unchanged by the kidneys. After large doses, thiamine and metabolites are excreted after tissue stores are saturated.

INDICATIONS/DOSAGE

Treatment of thiamine deficiency (beriberi, pellagra); malabsorption syndromes; prevention of Wernicke's encephalopathy; dietary supplement in patients with alcoholism, GI disease, and cirrhosis

Adult: 5–100 mg 1–3 times a day.
Pediatric: 10–25 mg daily.

CONTRAINDICATIONS/PRECAUTIONS
Contraindicated in: Hypersensitivity.
Use cautiously in: Renal impairment.
Pregnancy/Lactation: Safe for use in pregnant and lactating women. Follow RDA guidelines.

PREPARATION
Availability: 100 mg/mL in 1 mL amps/syringes and 1, 2, 10, and 30 mL vials. 200 mg/mL in 30 mL vials. **Syringe:** No further dilution required. **Infusion:** Further dilute in physician specified volume of compatible IV solution.

STABILITY/STORAGE
Vial: Store at room temperature. **Infusion:** Stable for 24 hr at room temperature.

ADMINISTRATION
General: IV route of administration should only be used if other routes are not feasible. Give intradermal test dose for patients suspected of

In the Adverse Effects section, <u>underline</u> indicates most frequent; CAPS indicates life threatening.

hypersensitivity. **IV Push:** Give each 100 mg over at least 5 min. **Intermittent/Continuous Infusion:** Infuse over physician specified time.

COMPATIBILITY
Solution: Dextrose solutions, lactated Ringer's, Ringer's injection, sodium chloride solutions. **Syringe:** Doxapram. **Y-site:** Famotidine.

ADVERSE EFFECTS
CNS: Restlessness. **CV:** DEATH, hypotension, vascular collapse. **Resp:** Pulmonary edema, RESPIRATORY DISTRESS, cyanosis. **GI:** Nausea. **Hypersens:** Angioedema, throat tightness, urticaria. **Other:** Feeling of warmth, pain at injection site, sweating.

DRUG INTERACTIONS
Neuromuscular blocking agents: Enhanced neuromuscular blockade.

NURSING CONSIDERATIONS
Assessment
General:
Nutritional assessment, vital signs, anaphylaxis.
Physical:
Cardiopulmonary status.

Intervention/Rationale
Monitor blood pressure before and after dose. ● Assess for signs/symptoms of CHF/pulmonary edema and respiratory distress. ● Assess for development of anaphylactic reactions. ● Evaluate nutritional needs based on dietary history.

Patient/Family Education
Inform physician/nurse of previous unusual or allergic reaction to thiamine. Eat a well-balanced diet and take vitamins only if nutritional requirements cannot be achieved through dietary means.

THIOPENTAL
(thye-oh-pen'-tal)
Trade Name(s): Pentothal
Classification(s): Anesthetic, barbiturate
Pregnancy Category: C
Controlled Substance Schedule: III

PHARMACODYNAMICS/KINETICS
Mechanism of Action: Depresses the CNS. Produces hypnosis and anesthesia without analgesia. Short-acting barbiturate. **Onset of Action:** Hypnosis within 30–40 sec. Anesthesia within 1 min. **Duration of Action:** 20–30 min. **Distribution:** Highly lipid soluble. Quickly crosses blood–brain barrier and then rapidly distributes to other tissues (first to liver, kidneys, heart, then muscle, and fatty tissues). **Metabolism/ Elimination:** Metabolized largely by the liver to mostly inactive metabolites. Minimally excreted by the kidneys. **Half-Life:** 3–8 hr.

INDICATIONS/DOSAGE

Provides anesthesia in combination with muscle relaxants and/or analgesics, primarily during short procedures

Adult: 50–75 mg (2–3 mL of 2.5% solution) at intervals of 20–40 sec. Additional doses of 25–50 mg can be given as necessary. *Pediatric:* Initial dose 3–5 mg/kg, followed by 1 mg/kg as needed.

Treatment of convulsive states

Adult: 75–125 mg (3–5 mL of 2.5% solution) as soon as possible after

In the Adverse Effects section, <u>underline</u> indicates most frequent; CAPS indicates life threatening.

491

the onset of convulsion. Maximum dose 250 mg.

CONTRAINDICATIONS/ PRECAUTIONS

Contraindicated in: Hypersensitivity, latent/manifest porphyria, status asthmaticus. **Use cautiously in:** Addison's disease, asthma, hepatic/renal dysfunction, hypotension, increased blood urea, increased intracranial pressure, myasthenia gravis, myxedema, severe cardiac disease, shock, severe anemia. **Pregnancy/Lactation:** No well-controlled trials to establish safety. Benefits must outweigh risks. Small amounts distributed into breast milk. Use with caution or discontinue breastfeeding.

PREPARATION

Availability: 250, 400, and 500 mg syringes and 500 mg, 1 g vials with diluent. 1 g (2.5%), 2.5 g (2%), 2.5 g (2.5%), 5 g (2%), and 5 g (2.5%) kits. **Syringe:** Dilute each 500 mg with 20 mL sterile water for injection to make a 2.5% solution. Prepared solutions should be used promptly. **Infusion:** Dilute in physician specified volume of compatible IV solution.

STABILITY/STORAGE

Vial: Store undiluted solutions at room temperature. Use diluted solutions promptly and discard unused portions.

ADMINISTRATION

General: Should be given by or in the presence of a physician or by those personnel educated to intubate and manage the complications of anesthetic agents. Give test dose of 25–75 mg to assess tolerance or sensitivity. **IV Push:** Give each 25 mg slowly over 1 minute to avoid respiratory depression. Assure patency of vein. Extravasation may cause tissue necrosis and sloughing. Inadvertent intra-arterial injection may cause arteritis, vasospasm, thrombosis, and gangrene. **Infusion:** May be given as an infusion when used as a primary anesthetic agent. Give at rate prescribed by physician.

COMPATIBILITY

Solution: Dextrose 5%, sodium chloride solutions.

INCOMPATIBILITY

Solution: Dextrose 10%, lactated Ringer's, Ringer's injection.

ADVERSE EFFECTS

CNS: Anxiety, emergency delirium, headache, prolonged somnolence/recovery, restlessness. **CV:** PERIPHERAL VASCULAR COLLAPSE, CIRCULATORY DEPRESSION, dysrhythmias, hypotension, myocardial depression. **Resp:** APNEA, BRONCHOSPASM, respiratory depression, coughing, dyspnea, sneezing. **GI:** Abdominal pain, nausea, vomiting. **MS:** Skeletal muscle hyperactivity. **Hypersens:** ANAPHYLAXIS, rash. **Other:** Pain at injection site, shivering, thrombophlebitis, tissue sloughing (extravasation), hiccoughs.

TOXICITY/OVERDOSE

Signs/Symptoms: Occur from too rapid or repeated injection: Severe hypotension, shock, apnea, laryngospasm, respiratory depression. **Treatment:** Discontinue drug, maintain or establish patent airway, ad-

In the Adverse Effects section, <u>underline</u> indicates most frequent; CAPS indicates life threatening.

minister oxygen or mechanically ventilate if necessary.

DRUG INTERACTIONS
CNS depressants: Additive CNS and respiratory depression. **Furosemide:** Aggravated orthostatic hypotension. **Sulfisoxazole IV:** Altered pharmacological effects of thiopental (decrease dose, give more frequently).

NURSING CONSIDERATIONS
Assessment
General:
Vital signs, ECG monitoring (recommended).
Physical:
Cardiopulmonary status.

Intervention Rationale
Monitor blood pressure, heart rate, ECG, and respirations before, periodically during, and after administration. ● Assess for signs/symptoms of respiratory distress and maintain patent airway. ● Assure patency of IV site and avoid extravasation or intra-arterial injection. ● Use narcotics preoperatively for analgesia and anticholinergics for control of secretions.

Patient/Family Education
Psychomotor impairment may persist for up to 24 hr following administration. Avoid driving or other activities requiring mental alertness for 24 hr. Avoid other CNS depressants, including alcohol, for 24 hr after receiving drug.

THIOTEPA
(thye-oh-tep′-a)
Classification(s): Antineoplastic agent, alkylating agent
Pregnancy Category: Unknown

PHARMACODYNAMICS/KINETICS
Mechanism of Action: Blocks the synthesis and use of purine nucleotides. Disrupts protein, DNA, and RNA synthesis. **Distribution:** Incorporated into the DNA and RNA of bone marrow cells. Does not cross blood–brain barrier. **Metabolism/Elimination:** Rapidly and extensively metabolized in the liver and other tissues. Excreted via urine primarily as metabolites. **Half-Life:** 11 hr.

INDICATIONS/DOSAGE

Adenocarcinoma of the breast or ovary; treatment of superficial carcinoma of the bladder
Adult: 0.3–0.4 mg/kg at 1–4 week intervals. Alternately, 0.2 mg/kg or 6 mg/m^2 daily for 4–5 days at intervals of 2–4 weeks. Base dose on clinical and hematologic response and patient tolerance.

CONTRAINDICATIONS/PRECAUTIONS
Contraindicated in: Existing or recent chicken pox exposure, hypersensitivity, herpes zoster. **Use cautiously in:** Preexisting hepatic, renal, or bone marrow damage (reduce dose and closely monitor hepatic, renal, and hematopoietic function), previous radiation or cytotoxic therapy, presence of infection/sepsis, tumor invasion of bone marrow. **Pregnancy/Lactation:** Has terato-

T

In the Adverse Effects section, underline indicates most frequent; CAPS indicates life threatening.

493

genic effects. Do not use in pregnancy unless benefits clearly outweigh risks to fetus.

PREPARATION
Availability: Powder for injection 15 mg/vial. **Reconstitution:** Add 1.5 mL sterile water for injection to 15 mg vials to make a concentration of 10 mg/mL of solution. Solution should be clear to slightly opaque. **Infusion:** Add reconstituted solution to physician specified volume of compatible IV solution.

STABILITY/STORAGE
Vial: Store in refrigerator. Protect from light. Reconstituted solutions stable for 5 days refrigerated. Do not use solutions that are grossly opaque or precipitated after reconstitution. **Infusion:** Stable for 24 hr refrigerated.

ADMINISTRATION
General: Give only under the supervision of a physician experienced in therapy with cytotoxic agents. Handle with care according to institutional guidelines for the handling of chemotherapeutic/cytotoxic agents. **IV Push:** May be given rapidly. **Continuous Infusion:** Give via infusion device at physician specified rate.

COMPATIBILITY
Solution: Dextrose solutions, lactated Ringer's, Ringer's injection, sodium chloride solutions.

ADVERSE EFFECTS
CNS: Dizziness, headache. **GI:** Anorexia, nausea, vomiting. **GU:** Amenorrhea, interference with spermatogenesis. **Derm:** Alopecia (rare). **Heme:** PANCYTOPENIA, anemia, leukopenia, thrombocytopenia.

Nadir: 10–14 days. **Hypersens:** Hives, rash (rare). **Other:** Febrile reactions, pain/burning at injection site, tissue necrosis/sloughing (extravasation).

TOXICITY/OVERDOSE
Signs/Symptoms: Hematopoietic toxicity. **Treatment:** Discontinue drug if WBC count falls to 3000/mm³ or less or if platelet count falls to 150,000/mm³.

DRUG INTERACTIONS
Bone marrow depressant agents, radiation therapy: Additive hematopoietic depression. **Succinylcholine:** Prolonged apnea after succinylcholine.

NURSING CONSIDERATIONS
Assessment
General:
Infectious disease status, hypersensitivity reaction.
Physical:
Hematopoietic system, GI tract.
Lab Alterations:
Monitor hematologic status closely, with CBC and differential and platelet count at least weekly during therapy and for at least 3 weeks after the completion of therapy (nadir of leukocytes usually occurs 10–14 days after initiation of therapy but may be delayed up to 1 month). Monitor BUN, hemoglobin/hematocrit, ALT (SGPT), AST (SGOT), serum bilirubin, serum creatinine, uric acid, and LDH periodically during therapy.

Intervention/Rationale
Assess for the presence of nausea or vomiting and administer antiemetics accordingly. ● Monitor for bleeding. Hematest stools, vomitus, and nasogastric drainage. ● Avoid

In the Adverse Effects section, <u>underline</u> indicates most frequent; CAPS indicates life threatening.

rectal temperatures and IM injections. ● Monitor for sign/symptoms of superinfection.

Patient/Family Education
Notify physician of fever, chills, bleeding, sore throat, or signs of infection during therapy and up to 1 month after completion. Avoid crowded environments and persons with known infections. Perform good oral care with a soft toothbrush and alcohol-free mouthwash. Use electric razor. Do not drink alcohol or take over-the-counter medications containing aspirin or ibuprofen. Advise of potential for hair loss and explore feelings and coping methods.

TICARCILLIN
(tye-kar-sil'-in)
Trade Name(s): Ticar
Classification(s): Antibiotic-extended spectrum penicillin
Pregnancy Category: B

PHARMACODYNAMICS/KINETICS
Mechanism of Action: Bactericidal, binds to enzymes in cytoplasmic membranes and interferes with cell-wall synthesis/cell division. **Peak Serum Level:** 30 min to 2 hr. **Distribution:** Widely distributed. 45%–65% bound to serum proteins. Minimally distributed into CSF. **Metabolism/Elimination:** Metabolized by hydrolysis in the liver. Excreted primarily by the kidneys and minimally in feces via bile. Removed by hemodialysis. **Half-Life:** 1.5 hr. Renal impairment 13.5–16.2 hr.

INDICATIONS/DOSAGE

Treatment of infections caused by susceptible gram-negative aerobic bacilli and mixed aerobic-anaerobic bacterial infections

(including infections of the urinary and respiratory tract, blood, skin and skin-structures, bone and joint, inner abdomen, and gynecological structures)
Adult: 150–300 mg/kg/day in divided doses every 4–6 hr. Usual dose 3 g every 4–6 hr. Seriously ill patients should receive the higher doses.
Pediatric:
Children ≥ 40 kg: May give usual adult dose.
Children Older than 1 Month < 40 kg: 50–200 mg/kg/day in divided doses every 4–8 hr. Treat serious infections with 200–300 mg/kg/day every 4–6 hr.
Neonate:
< 2 kg and < 7 days old: 75 mg/kg every 12 hr (150 mg/kg/day). **< 2 kg and > 7 days old:** 75 mg/kg every 8 hr (225 mg/kg/day). **> 2 kg and < 7 days old:** 75 mg/kg every 8 hr (225 mg/kg/day). **> 2 kg and > 7 days old:** 100 mg/kg every 8 hr (300 mg/kg/day).

Empiric anti-infective treatment in febrile granulocytopenic patients
Adult: 4 g every 4 hr. Alternatively, 300 mg/kg/day IV in divided doses every 6 hr.

CONTRAINDICATIONS/PRECAUTIONS
Contraindicated in: Hypersensitivity to penicillins or cephalosporins. **Use cautiously in:** Renal impairment, history of allergies, hay fever/hy-

T

In the Adverse Effects section, underline indicates most frequent; CAPS indicates life threatening.

495

persensitivity, severe liver disease. **Pregnancy/Lactation:** No well-controlled trials to establish safety. Benefits must outweigh risks. Teratogenic to pregnant mice when given in human-equivalent doses. Distributed into breast milk. Use with caution in breastfeeding women.

PREPARATION

Availability: Powder for injection in 1, 3, 6, 20, and 30 g vials. 3 g piggyback bottles or Add-Vantage vials. Contains 5.2 mEq sodium/g. **Reconstitution:** Dilute each gram with 4 mL compatible IV solution. Resultant concentration is 200 mg/mL. In neonates, do not reconstitute with bacteriostatic water for injection containing benzyl alcohol as preservative. **Infusion:** Further dilute reconstituted solution to a concentration of 10–100 mg/mL. Add 30, 60, or 100 mL compatible IV solution to 3 g piggyback vials. Reconstitute Add-Vantage vials according to manufacturer's directions.

STABILITY/STORAGE

Vial: Store at room temperature. Stable for 7 days refrigerated. **Infusion:** Stable for 24 hr at room temperature and 7 days (sodium chloride) or 3 days (D_5W) refrigerated.

ADMINISTRATION

Intermittent Infusion: Give over at least 30 min.

COMPATIBILITY

Solution: Dextrose solutions, sodium chloride solutions. **Y-site:** Ondansetron.

INCOMPATIBILITY

Syringe: Doxapram. **Y-site:** Acyclovir, cyclophosphamide, famotidine, hydromorphone, magnesium sulfate, meperidine, morphine, perphenazine, verapamil.

ADVERSE EFFECTS

CNS: Seizures, hallucinations, lethargy, neurotoxicity, neuromuscular irritability. **CV:** CHF. **GI:** Pseudomembranous colitis, <u>diarrhea</u>, nausea. **Fld/Lytes:** Hypokalemia, hypernatremia. **Heme:** Anemia, bleeding, leukopenia, granulocytopenia, thrombocytopenia, transient neutropenia. **Hypersens:** ANAPHYLAXIS, myocarditis, rash, urticaria. **Other:** Pain at injection site, superinfection, thrombophlebitis.

DRUG INTERACTIONS

Aminoglycosides: Inactivation of aminoglycoside. **Bacteriostatic antibiotics (erythromycin, tetracycline):** Diminished bactericidal effect of penicillins. **Beta-adrenergic blockers:** Increased risk/severity of anaphylactic reactions. **Chloramphenicol:** Decreased penicillin effect, increased chloramphenicol half-life. **Heparin, oral anticoagulants:** Altered coagulation/increased risk of bleeding. **Probenecid:** Prolonged penicillin blood levels.

NURSING CONSIDERATIONS

Assessment

General:

Infectious disease status, history and signs/symptoms of hypersensitivity.

Physical:

Cardiac status, hematopoietic system.

In the Adverse Effects section, <u>underline</u> indicates most frequent; CAPS indicates life threatening.

Lab Alterations:

Monitor serum electrolytes, periodically evaluate renal, hepatic, and hematologic systems with long-term use. False-positive/negative urinary protein results (use Albustix, Albutest, or Multistix only).

Intervention/Rationale

Obtain specimens for culture and sensitivity before therapy is initiated (first dose may be given while awaiting results). Assess patient for signs and symptoms of infection prior to, during, and at completion of therapy. ● Question patient about prior use of penicillins or cephalosporins and allergic or hypersensitivity reactions prior to initiation of therapy. Observe closely for signs and symptoms of anaphylaxis. Hypersensitivity reactions may be immediate and severe in penicillin-sensitive patients with a history of allergy, asthma, hay fever, or urticaria. ● Assess for signs and symptoms of CHF due to high sodium content of drug, periodically during therapy. ● Discontinue therapy and call physician if bleeding occurs. ● Assess for signs and symptoms of superinfection or bacterial or fungal overgrowth, especially in elderly, debilitated, or immunosuppressed. ● If concurrently given with aminoglycosides, administer in separate infusions as far apart as possible.

Patient/Family Education

Notify physician if skin rash, itching, hives, severe diarrhea, or signs of superinfection occurs.

TICARCILLIN-CLAVULANATE

(tye-kar-sil′-in klav-yoo-la′-nate)
Trade Name(s): Timentin
Classification(s): Antibiotic-extended spectrum penicillin
Pregnancy Category: B

PHARMACODYNAMICS/KINETICS

Mechanism of Action: Bactericidal. Binds to enzymes in cytoplasmic membranes and interferes with cell-wall synthesis and cell division. Clavulanic acid has a high affinity for beta-lactamases that generally inactivate ticarcillin. **Peak Level:** 30 min to 2 hr. **Distribution:** Widely distributed. 45%–65% bound to serum proteins. Minimally distributed into CSF. **Metabolism/Elimination:** Ticarcillin and clavulanic acid are both removed by hemodialysis. *Ticarcillin:* Metabolized by hydrolysis in the liver. Excreted primarily by the kidneys and minimally in feces via bile. *Clavulanic acid:* Extensively metabolized in the liver and excreted by the kidneys. **Half-Life:** Ticarcillin 1.5 hr. Clavulanate 1.1–1.5 hr. Prolonged in renal impairment.

INDICATIONS/DOSAGE

Treatment of infections caused by susceptible beta-lactamase-producing strains of susceptible organisms

(including infections of the lower respiratory tract, skin and skin-structure, urinary tract, bone and

In the Adverse Effects section, <u>underline</u> indicates most frequent;
CAPS indicates life threatening.

497

joint, blood and gynecological structures).

Adult/Pediatric (> 12 years and > 60 kg): 200–300 mg/kg/day in divided doses every 4–6 hr (based on ticarcillin content). *Pediatric (15 months to 12 years)*: 207–310 mg/kg/day (based on ticarcillin content) in divided doses every 4–6 hr.

CONTRAINDICATIONS/ PRECAUTIONS

Contraindicated in: Hypersensitivity to penicillins or cephalosporins. **Use cautiously in:** Renal impairment (reduce dose), history of allergies, hay fever/hypersensitivity, severe liver disease. **Pregnancy/Lactation:** No well-controlled trials to established safety. Benefits must outweigh risks. Reproduction studies in rats reveal no harm to fetus. Distributed into breast milk. Use with caution in breastfeeding women. **Pediatrics:** Safety and efficacy not established for children under the age of 12. Has been used in a limited number of children under this age without adverse effects.

PREPARATION

Availability: Powder for injection 3.1 g vial (3 g ticarcillin and 100 mg clavulanic acid). Contains 4.75 mEq sodium/g. **Reconstitution:** Add 13 mL sterile water or sodium chloride for injection to 3.1 g vial to provide solutions containing 200 mg ticarcillin/mL and 6.7 mg clavulanic acid/mL. Shake vial until dissolved. **Infusion:** Dilute reconstituted solutions with 50–100 mL compatible IV solution.

STABILITY/STORAGE

Vial: Store at room temperature. Stable for 6 hr at room temperature or 72 hr refrigerated after reconstitution. **Infusion:** Stable for 24 hr at room temperature. Stable 3 days (D_5W) and 4 days (NSS) refrigerated.

ADMINISTRATION

General: If given through Y-site, discontinue primary solution until infusion is complete. Administer separately from aminoglycosides or other anti-infective agents. **Intermittent Infusion:** Infuse over at least 30 min.

COMPATIBILITY

Solution: Dextrose solutions, sodium chloride solutions, sterile water for injection. **Y-site:** Cyclophosphamide, famotidine, meperidine, morphine, ondansetron, perphenazine.

ADVERSE EFFECTS

CNS: Seizures, headache, hallucinations. **Ophtho:** Blurred vision. **GI:** Pseudomembranous colitis, <u>diarrhea</u>, flatulence, nausea, transient increases in AST (SGOT), ALT (SGPT), alkaline phosphatase, LDH, and bilirubin, vomiting. **Fld/Lytes:** Hypokalemia, hypernatremia. **Heme:** Anemia, bleeding, eosinophilia, leukopenia, granulocytopenia, positive direct antiglobulin (Coombs' test), thrombocytopenia, transient neutropenia. **Hypersens:** ANAPHYLAXIS, BRONCHOSPASM, myocarditis, pruritus, wheezing. **Other:** Pain at injection site, superinfection, thrombophlebitis.

In the Adverse Effects section, <u>underline</u> indicates most frequent; CAPS indicates life threatening.

DRUG INTERACTIONS
Aminoglycosides: Inactivation of aminoglycosides. **Bacteriostatic antibiotics (erythromycin, tetracycline):** Diminished bactericidal effect of penicillins. **Beta-adrenergic blockers:** Increased risk and severity of anaphylactic reactions. **Chloramphenicol:** Decreased penicillin effect, increased chloramphenicol half-life. **Heparin, oral anticoagulants:** Altered coagulation/increased risk of bleeding. **Probenecid:** Prolonged penicillin blood levels.

NURSING CONSIDERATIONS
Assessment
General:
Infectious disease status, history or signs/symptoms of hypersensitivity.
Physical:
Cardiac status, GI tract.
Lab Alterations:
Monitor serum electrolytes. Periodically evaluate renal, hepatic, and hematologic systems with long-term use. Causes false-positive/negative urinary protein results (use Albustix, Albutest, or Multistix only). Positive direct antiglobulin (Coombs' test caused by clavulanic acid).

Intervention/Rationale
Obtain specimens for culture and sensitivity before therapy is initiated (first dose may be given while awaiting results). ● Assess patient for signs and symptoms of infection prior to, during, and at completion of therapy. Question patient about prior use of penicillins or cephalosporins and allergic or hypersensitivity reactions prior to initiation of therapy. Observe closely for signs and symptoms of anaphylaxis. Hypersensitivity reactions may be immediate and severe in penicillin-sensitive patients with a history of allergy, asthma, hay fever, or urticaria. ● Periodically assess for signs/symptoms of CHF due to high sodium content of drug. ● Assess for signs and symptoms of superinfection or bacterial or fungal overgrowth, especially in elderly, debilitated, or immunosuppressed. ● If concurrently given with aminoglycosides, administer in separate infusions as far apart as possible. ● Discontinue therapy and call physician if bleeding occurs. Observe quality, frequency, and odor of stools and report frequent/foul smelling stool to physician.

Patient/Family Education
Notify physician if skin rash, itching, hives, severe diarrhea, or signs of superinfection occurs.

TOBRAMYCIN
(toe-bra-mye'-sin)
Trade Name(s): Nebcin
Classification(s): Aminoglycoside antibiotic
Pregnancy Category: D

PHARMACODYNAMICS/KINETICS
Mechanism of Action: Bactericidal. Blocks bacterial protein synthesis. Exhibits some neuromuscular blocking action. **Peak Serum Level:** Within 30 min of infusion completion. **Therapeutic Serum Levels:** Peak 4–8 mcg/mL. Trough < 2 mcg/mL. **Distribution:** Widely distributed in extracellular fluids. Lower serum

In the Adverse Effects section, <u>underline</u> indicates most frequent; CAPS indicates life threatening.

499

concentrations result in expanded extracellular fluid volume. **Metabolism/Elimination:** Excreted unchanged via glomerular filtration in kidneys. **Half-Life:** 2.0–2.5 hr. Prolonged in renal impairment (up to 24–60 hr).

INDICATIONS/DOSAGE

Treatment of gram-negative organisms/combination therapy in severe immunocompromised patients

Dosage interval may need to be adjusted in renal impairment. Adjust dosage based on serum levels.

Adult: Load 2 mg/kg followed by 3 mg/kg/day in divided doses every 8 hr. Not to exceed 5 mg/kg/day. *Pediatric:* 6.0–7.5 mg/kg/day in divided doses every 6–8 hr. *Neonate:* 7.5 mg/kg/day in divided doses every 6–8 hr. Premature ≤ 1 week: 5 mg/kg/day in divided doses every 12 hr.

CONTRAINDICATIONS/ PRECAUTIONS

Contraindicated in: Known hypersensitivity. **Use cautiously in:** Neuromuscular disorders (myasthenia gravis, Parkinson's disease, infant botulism). Newborns of mothers receiving high doses of magnesium sulfate. Concurrent administration of neuromuscular blocking agents. **Pregnancy/Lactation:** No well-controlled trials to establish safety. Benefits must outweigh risks. Crosses placenta. **Pediatrics:** Caution in premature infants/neonates due to renal immaturity and prolonged half-life.

PREPARATION

Availability: 10 mg/mL in 2 mL vials. 40 mg/mL in 1.5, 2 mL vials. 1.2 g powder for injection vials. **Infusion: Adults:** Further dilute in 50–200 mL of compatible IV solution. **Pediatrics:** Further dilute in compatible solution to a volume sufficient to infuse over 20–30 min.

STABILITY/STORAGE

Vial: Store at room temperature. **Infusion:** Stable for 24 hr at room temperature and 4 days refrigerated.

ADMINISTRATION

General: Avoid rapid bolus administration. Schedule first maintenance dose at a dosing interval apart from loading dose. Administer additional dose after hemodialysis. Schedule dosing of penicillins and aminoglycosides as far apart as possible to prevent inactivation of aminoglycosides. **Intermittent Infusion:** Infuse over at least 30–60 min.

COMPATIBILITY

Solution: Amino acids, dextrose solutions, Ringer's injection, sodium chloride solutions. **Syringe:** Doxapram, clindamycin, penicillin sodium. **Y-site:** Acyclovir, ciprofloxacin, enalaprilat, esmolol, famotidine, foscarnet, furosemide, hydromorphone, labetalol, magnesium sulfate, meperidine, morphine, tolazoline, zidovudine.

INCOMPATIBILITY

Solution: Fat emulsion. **Syringe:** Ampicillin, heparin. **Y-site:** Furosemide, heparin, hetastarch, mezlocillin.

ADVERSE EFFECTS

CNS: Convulsions, confusion, disorientation, neuromuscular block-

In the Adverse Effects section, <u>underline</u> indicates most frequent; CAPS indicates life threatening.

ade, lethargy, depression, headache, numbness, nystagmus, pseudotumor cerebri. **CV:** Hypertension, hypotension, palpitations. **Resp:** Respiratory depression, pulmonary fibrosis. **GI:** Anorexia, hepatic necrosis, hepatomegaly, increased bilirubin/LDH/transaminase, nausea, salivation, stomatitis, vomiting. **GU:** Casts, hematuria. **Renal:** Azotemia, increased BUN/serum creatinine, oliguria, proteinuria. **MS:** Arthralgia. **Fld/Lytes:** Hyperkalemia, hypomagnesemia. **Heme:** Agranulocytosis (transient), anemia (transient), eosinophilia, leukocytosis, leukopenia, pancytopenia, reticulocyte count alterations, thrombocytopenia. **Hypersens:** Angioneurotic edema, exfoliative dermatitis, purpura, rash, urticaria. **Other:** Fever, ototoxicity (deafness, dizziness, tinnitus, vertigo).

TOXICITY/OVERDOSE

Signs/Symptoms: Increased serum levels with associated nephrotoxicity and ototoxicty (tinnitus, high frequency hearing loss). **Treatment:** Removed by peritoneal/hemodialysis. Hemodialysis is more efficient. Exchange transfusions may be used in neonates. **Antidote(s):** Ticarcillin (12–20 g/day) may be given to promote complex formation with aminoglycosides to lower elevated serum levels.

DRUG INTERACTIONS

Amphotericin B, bacitracin, cephalothin, cisplatin, methoxyflurane, potent diuretics, vancomycin: Increased potential for nephrotoxicity, neurotoxicity, ototoxicity. **Anesthetics, anticholinesterase agents, citrate anticoagulated blood, metocurine, neuromuscular blocking agents, pancuronium, succinylcholine, tubocurarine:** Increased neuromuscular blockade/respiratory paralysis. **Beta lactam antibiotics (penicillins, cephalosporins) especially ticarcillin:** Inactivation of aminoglycosides. **Cephalosporins, penicillins:** Synergism against gram negative and enterococci.

NURSING CONSIDERATIONS

Assessment
General:
Maintain adequate hydration. Superinfection/infectious disease status.
Physical:
CN VIII (acoustic) evaluation, renal function.
Lab Alterations:
Measure peak/trough levels. Beta lactam antibiotic (penicillins, cephalosporins) may cause in vitro inactivation of gentamicin.

Intervention/Rationale
Assess BUN and serum creatinine/creatinine clearance to determine presence of renal toxicity. Adequate hydration recommended to prevent renal toxicity. ● Antibiotic use may cause overgrowth of resistant organisms; observe for (fever, change in vital signs, increased WBC, vaginal infection/discharge). ● Draw peak serum levels 30 min after the infusion is complete and trough 30 min prior to the next dose. ● CN VIII evaluation important to assess presence of ototoxicity.

Patient/Family Education
Increase oral fluid intake in order to minimize chemical irritation of

In the Adverse Effects section, underline indicates most frequent; CAPS indicates life threatening.

501

kidneys. Notify physician/nurse if tinnitus, vertigo, or hearing loss is noted.

TOLAZOLINE
(tole-as'-oh-leen)
Trade Name(s): Priscoline
Classification(s): Antihypertensive-vasodilating agent
Pregnancy Category: C

PHARMACODYNAMICS/KINETICS
Mechanism of Action: Causes peripheral vasodilation and decreases peripheral vascular resistance by direct relaxation of vascular smooth muscle. Reduces pulmonary arterial pressure. Has some alpha-adrenergic blocking properties. **Onset of Action:** Within 30 min. **Peak Effect:** 30–60 min. **Metabolism/Elimination:** Concentrated in the liver and excreted largely unchanged by the kidneys. **Half-Life:** 3–10 hr (neonates).

INDICATIONS/DOSAGE

Persistent pulmonary hypertension of the newborn
Neonate: 1–2 mg/kg as initial bolus, followed by infusion of 1–2 mg/kg hr.

Adjunctive therapy in the treatment of peripheral vasospastic disorders associated with acrocyanosis, arteriosclerosis obliterans, thromboangitis obliterans (Berger's disease), diabetic arteriosclerosis, gangrene, frostbite, and scleroderma (*unlabeled use*)

Adult: 10–50 mg four times daily. Begin with lower dose and increase gradually until optimum dose is attained (evidenced by appearance of flushing).

CONTRAINDICATIONS/PRECAUTIONS
Contraindicated in: Hypersensitivity, coronary artery disease, following cerebrovascular accident. **Use cautiously in:** Mitral stenosis, peptic ulcer. **Pregnancy/Lactation:** No well-controlled trials to establish safety. Benefits must outweigh risks.

PREPARATION
Availability: 25 mg/mL in 4 mL amps. **Infusion:** Dilute in physician specified volume of compatible IV solution.

STABILITY/STORAGE
Vial: Store at room temperature. Protect from light. **Infusion:** Stable for 24 hr at room temperature.

ADMINISTRATION
General: In treatment of pulmonary hypertension in the newborn, there is little experience with infusions lasting longer than 36–48 hr. **IV Push:** Give initial bolus slowly over 10 min. **Continuous Infusion:** Administer via infusion device.

COMPATIBILITY
Solution: Dextrose solutions, lactated Ringer's, Ringer's injection, sodium chloride solutions. **Y-site:** Aminophylline, ampicillin, calcium gluconate, cefotaxime, cimetidine, dobutamine, dopamine, furosemide, gentamicin, phytonadione, sodium bicarbonate, tobramycin, vancomycin.

T

In the Adverse Effects section, <u>underline</u> indicates most frequent; CAPS indicates life threatening.

INCOMPATIBILITY
Y-site: Indomethacin.

ADVERSE EFFECTS
CV: Dysrhythmias, edema, hypotension, hypertension, tachycardia. **Resp:** Pulmonary hemorrhage. **GI:** Hepatitis, diarrhea, GI hemorrhage, nausea, vomiting. **GU:** Hematuria, oliguria. **Derm:** Increased pilomotor activity with tingling or chilliness. **Heme:** Leukopenia, thrombocytopenia. **Hypersens:** Rash. **Other:** Flushing.

TOXICITY/OVERDOSE
Signs/Symptoms: Increased pilomotor activity, peripheral vasodilation/skin flushing, hypotension (rare), shock (rare). **Treatment:** Place in Trendelenburg position and give IV fluids to treat hypotension. Do not use epinephrine (large doses of tolazoline may cause epinephrine reversal/further reduction in blood pressure followed by exaggerated rebound).

DRUG INTERACTIONS
Epinephrine: Epinephrine reversal with large doses.

NURSING CONSIDERATIONS
Assessment
General:
Vital signs (monitor blood pressure, heart rate, and ECG continuously). Monitor pulmonary artery pressure periodically (neonates treated for pulmonary hypertension).
Physical:
GI tract, hematopoietic system, cardiopulmonary status.
Lab Alterations:
Monitor arterial blood gases and electrolytes periodically during therapy.

Intervention/Rationale
Wean from tolazoline and give potassium and chloride if metabolic acidosis develops. ● Monitor gastric aspirate for presence of blood (drug stimulates gastric secretions and may activate stress ulcers). Pretreatment with antacids may prevent GI bleeding. ● Assess for bleeding, bruising, petechiae, or blood in urine or stools periodically during therapy.

Patient/Family Education
Pulmonary Hypertension in Neonate:
Explain rationale of therapy to parents, provide emotional support, and answer questions.
Treatment of Peripheral Vasospastic Disorders:
Educate regarding potential therapeutic outcomes and side effects.

TRANEXAMIC ACID
(tran'-x-a-mic a-cid)
Trade Name(s): Cyklokapron
Classification(s): Systemic hemostatic agent
Pregnancy Category: B

PHARMACODYNAMICS/KINETICS
Mechanism of Action: Competitive inhibitor of plasminogen activation. Actions similar to aminocaproic acid. **Distribution:** Widely distributed. Rapidly distributed into joint fluid and synovial membranes. Crosses blood–brain barrier. **Metabolism/Elimination:** Minimally metabolized.

In the Adverse Effects section, underline indicates most frequent; CAPS indicates life threatening.

503

Excreted by the kidneys. **Half-Life:** 2 hr.

INDICATIONS/DOSAGE

Used in hemophilia patients to reduce or prevent hemorrhage and to reduce the need for replacement therapy during and following tooth extraction

Adult/Pediatric: 10 mg/kg before surgery followed by oral dose postoperatively. Alternate: 10 mg/kg three to four times daily for patients unable to take oral therapy. Reduce dose in renal impairment.

CONTRAINDICATIONS/ PRECAUTIONS

Contraindicated in: Acquired defective color vision, subarachnoid hemorrhage. **Pregnancy/Lactation:** No well-controlled trials to establish safety. Benefits must outweigh risks. Animal reproductive studies reveal no adverse effects on the fetus.

PREPARATION

Availability: 100 mg/mL in 10 mL amps. **Infusion:** Dilute in physician specified amount of compatible IV solution. Prepare and use the same day. Do not mix with blood. Heparin may be added to solution.

ADMINISTRATION

IV Push: Give slowly (1 mL/min) to avoid hypotension.

STABILITY/STORAGE

Vial: Store at room temperature.

COMPATIBILITY/INCOMPATIBILITY

Data not available.

ADVERSE EFFECTS

CNS: Giddiness. **Ophtho:** Visual abnormalities. **CV:** Hypotension (too rapid injection). **GI:** Diarrhea, nausea, vomiting (dose related).

NURSING CONSIDERATIONS

Assessment
General:
Vital signs (blood pressure).
Physical:
GI tract, ophthalmologic exam.

Intervention/Rationale
Monitor for the presence of diarrhea, nausea, or vomiting and report to physician. ● Complete ophthalmologic examination should be done before and at regular intervals in patients receiving repeated treatment or for duration of more than 2–3 days.

Patient/Family Education
Educate regarding therapeutic outcome and potential side effects. Report changes in visual acuity or color vision.

TRIMETHAPHAN
(trye-meth´-a-fan)
Trade Name(s): Arfonad
Classification(s): Antihypertensive, ganglionic blocker
Pregnancy Category: Unknown

PHARMACODYNAMICS/KINETICS

Mechanism of Action: Short-acting ganglionic blocking agent. Blocks transmission in autonomic sympathetic and parasympathetic ganglia. Causes peripheral vasodilation and

In the Adverse Effects section, underline indicates most frequent; CAPS indicates life threatening.

liberation of histamine. **Onset of Action:** Almost immediate. **Duration of Action:** BP returns to pretreatment level within 10 min after discontinuation. **Metabolism/Elimination:** May be metabolized by pseudocholinesterase. Excreted by the kidneys.

INDICATIONS/DOSAGE

Controlled hypotension during surgery

Adult: 0.3–6.0 mg/min (average dose 3–4 mg/min). *Pediatric:* 50–150 mcg/kg/min.

Blood pressure reduction in severe hypertension and hypertensive emergencies

Adult: 0.5–2.0 mg/min.

CONTRAINDICATIONS/PRECAUTIONS

Contraindicated in: Anemia, asphyxia, hypersensitivity, hypovolemia, respiratory insufficiency, shock. **Use cautiously in:** Addison's disease, arteriosclerosis, cardiac disease, children, conditions where fluid/blood replacement is impossible, degenerative disease of CNS, debilitated, diabetes mellitus, elderly, glaucoma, hepatic/renal disease, history of allergies/hay fever, concomitant corticosteroids. **Pregnancy/Lactation:** Avoid use during pregnancy. Crosses the placenta. Decreases fetal GI motility and results in meconium ileus. Induced hypotension may cause serious adverse effects in the fetus. **Pediatrics:** Use with extreme caution.

PREPARATION

Availability: 50 mg/mL in 10 mL amps. **Infusion:** Dilute 500 mg (10 mL) in 500 mL of 5% dextrose.

STABILITY/STORAGE

Vial: Refrigerate. Stable for 14 days at room temperature. **Infusion:** Prepare just prior to using and discard unused portion. Stable at room temperature for 24 hr.

ADMINISTRATION

General: Give via infusion device and titrate per physician's order. *Controlled hypotension during surgery:* Should be given only by personnel educated in this technique who are prepared to handle potential complications. Position patient with head up to avoid cerebral anoxia. Titrate drug to reduce bleeding after patient is anesthetized and discontinue prior to wound closure to allow normalization of blood pressure. Do not decrease systolic blood pressure below 60 mmHg. *Severe hypertension/hypertensive emergencies:* Gradually increase infusion until desired blood pressure is achieved. Do not lower blood pressure to more than ⅔ of pretreatment level.

COMPATIBILITY

Solution: Dextrose solutions, sodium chloride solutions. **Y-site:** Heparin, hydrocortisone, potassium chloride, vitamin B complex with C.

ADVERSE EFFECTS

CNS: Restlessness. **Ophtho:** Mydriasis. **CV:** Orthostatic hypotension, precipitation of angina, tachycardia. **Resp:** APNEA, RESPIRATORY ARREST (large doses). **GI:** Anorexia, dry mouth, nausea, vomiting.

In the Adverse Effects section, <u>underline</u> indicates most frequent; CAPS indicates life threatening.

GU: Urinary retention. **Endo:** Prevents surgically induced blood glucose elevations. **Fld/Lytes:** Hypokalemia (slight). **Hypersens:** Itching, urticaria. **Other:** Histamine release (history of allergies, hay fever).

TOXICITY/OVERDOSE
Signs/Symptoms: Severe hypotension. **Treatment:** Discontinue drug or decrease dose. IV fluids. Vasopressor agents may be used if blood pressure does not rebound within 10 minutes (use phenylephrine or mephentermine initially; reserve epinephrine for refractory cases).

DRUG INTERACTIONS
Anesthetic agents: Additive hypotensive effects. **Neuromuscular blocking agents:** Potentiation of neuromuscular blockade.

NURSING CONSIDERATIONS
Assessment
General:
Monitor ECG, blood pressure, and respirations continuously.
Physical:
Cardiopulmonary/vascular status.

Intervention/Rationale
Reverse excessive hypotension by lowering patient's head or elevating the lower extremities. ● Have adequate facilities/equipment and personnel available to handle emergencies that may arise during therapy. ● Assess IV site and vein for histamine-type reaction.
Controlled hypotension during surgery:
Continuously monitor circulation. Maintain adequate coronary and cerebral perfusion. Drug causes mydriasis, which cannot be used as an indication of anoxia or depth of anesthesia.
Management of severe hypertension and hypertensive emergencies:
Monitor respiratory status, especially with large doses.

Patient/Family Education
Educate regarding expected therapeutic outcome and side effects. Remain supine during and immediately after to prevent orthostatic hypotension.

TRIMETHOPRIM-SULFAMETHOXAZOLE
(trye-meth′-o-prim sulf-a-meth′-ox-a-zole)
Trade Name(s): Bactrim IV, Septra IV
Classification(s): Antibiotic
Pregnancy Category: C

PHARMACODYNAMICS/KINETICS
Mechanism of Action: Bactericidal. Prevents folic acid formation and reduces folates essential to growth of organism. **Distribution:** Widely distributed, including CSF and bronchial secretions. 40%–70% bound to plasma proteins. **Metabolism/Elimination:** Metabolized in the liver. Rapidly excreted primarily in urine. Small amounts excreted in bile. **Half-Life:** 8–11 hr (trimethoprim). 10–13 hr (sulfamethoxazole).

INDICATIONS/DOSAGE
Dosage based on trimethoprim component. Adjust dose/interval in renal impairment.

In the Adverse Effects section, <u>underline</u> indicates most frequent; CAPS indicates life threatening.

Severe urinary tract infections or shigellosis

Adult/Pediatric (older than 2 months): 8–10 mg/kg/day in two to four divided doses every 6–12 hr for 5–14 days. Maximum dose of trimethoprim 960 mg/day.

Treatment of *Pneumocystis carinii*

Adult/Pediatric (older than 2 months): 15–20 mg/kg/day in three to four divided doses every 6–8 hr for 14–21 days.

CONTRAINDICATIONS/ PRECAUTIONS

Contraindicated in: Creatinine clearance less than 15 mL/min, group A beta-hemolytic streptococcal pharyngitis, hypersensitivity, megaloblastic anemia secondary to folate deficiency. **Use cautiously in:** Folate or glucose-6-phosphate-dehydrogenase (G6PD) deficiency, impaired renal/hepatic function, severe allergy/bronchial asthma. **Pregnancy/ Lactation:** No well-controlled trials to establish safety. Benefits must outweigh risks. Animal studies reveal teratogenicity, cleft palate, and increase in fetal loss. May interfere with folic acid metabolism. Distributed into breast milk. **Pediatrics:** Safety and efficacy not established in children younger than 2 months of age. Safety and efficacy of repeated courses of therapy in children younger than 2 years (except with documented *P. carinii*) has not been fully determined. Do not use in children with mental retardation associated with fragile X chromosome.

PREPARATION

Availability: 80 mg trimethoprim and 400 mg sulfamethoxazole per 5 mL in 5, 10, 20, and 30 mL amps/vials, and 5 and 10 mL Add-Vantage vials. **Infusion:** Dilute each 5 mL of drug with 125 mL 5% dextrose. May add 5 mL of drug to 75 mL of dextrose in patients requiring fluid restriction. Reconstitute Add-Vantage vials according to manufacturer's instructions.

STABILITY/STORAGE

Vial: Store at room temperature. **Infusion:** Stable at room temperature for 24 hr in glass bottles. Do not refrigerate. Do not use solutions that precipitate after mixing or that are cloudy.

ADMINISTRATION

General: Avoid rapid or direct IV injection. **Intermittent Infusion:** Infuse over 60–90 min.

COMPATIBILITY

Solution: Dextrose solutions, sodium chloride (time dependent). **Syringe:** Heparin. **Y-site:** Acyclovir, atracurium, cyclophosphamide, enalaprilat, esmolol, hydromorphone, labetalol, magnesium sulfate, meperidine, morphine, pancuronium, perphenazine, vecuronium, zidovudine.

INCOMPATIBILITY

Y-site: Foscarnet.

ADVERSE EFFECTS

CNS: Aseptic meningitis, convulsions, ataxia, hallucinations, headache, mental depression. **GI:** Pseudomembranous colitis, <u>anorexia</u>, diarrhea, elevated serum transaminase/bilirubin, glossitis, hepatitis, <u>nausea</u>, pancreatitis, sto-

In the Adverse Effects section, <u>underline</u> indicates most frequent; CAPS indicates life threatening.

507

matitis, <u>vomiting</u>. **Renal:** Elevated serum creatinine/BUN, renal failure. **Heme:** Bone marrow depression. **Hypersens:** ANAPHYLAXIS, <u>allergic skin reactions</u>, <u>exfoliative dermatitis</u>, Stevens-Johnson syndrome, allergic myocarditis, erythema multiforme, <u>generalized skin eruptions</u>, photosensitivity, serum sickness, systemic lupus erythematosus, <u>urticaria</u>. **Other:** Pain/irritation at injection site, peripheral neuritis, periarteritis nodosa.

TOXICITY/OVERDOSE

Signs/Symptoms: Decreased motor activity, loss of righting reflex, tremors/convulsions, respiratory depression. **Treatment:** Supportive measures. Acidifying urine increases renal elimination. Monitor blood chemistries and blood counts. Hemodialysis only moderately effective.

DRUG INTERACTIONS

Cyclosporine: Decreased cyclosporine therapeutic effects, increased nephrotoxicity. **Methotrexate:** Potentiation of bone marrow depression. **Phenytoin:** Prolonged phenytoin half-life. **Sulfonylureas:** Increased hypoglycemic response. **Thiazide diuretics:** Increased incidence of thrombocytopenia purpura in elderly. **Warfarin:** Prolonged prothrombin time.

NURSING CONSIDERATIONS

Assessment

General:
Infectious disease status, signs/symptoms of hypersensitivity.

Physical:
Hematopoietic system, skin assessment.
Lab Alterations:
Monitor CBC with differential and platelet count before and periodically during therapy. Obtain urinalysis and microscopic urine analysis, especially in those with impaired renal function.

Intervention/Rationale

Obtain specimens for culture and sensitivity (first dose may be given while awaiting results). ● Discontinue drug at first sign of rash or bone marrow depression. ● Treat bone marrow depression with leucovorin. ● Closely monitor patients with AIDS for adverse reactions (higher incidence of side effects, especially fever, dermatologic, and hematologic reactions). ● Elderly are especially prone to decreased platelet counts, severe adverse dermatologic reactions, and generalized bone marrow depression.

Patient/Family Education

Report fever, sore throat, pallor, jaundice, or purpura. Maintain adequate fluid intake.

TROMETHAMINE

(troe-meth′-a-meen)
Trade Name(s): Tham, Tham-E
Classification(s): Alkalinizing agent, electrolyte
Pregnancy Category: C

PHARMACODYNAMICS/KINETICS

Mechanism of Action: Tromethamine is a highly alkaline, sodium free organic amine that acts as a proton (hydrogen ion) acceptor to prevent/correct acidosis. By combining with hydrogen ions from acid anions, it forms bicarbonate and a cationic buffer with salts excreted in urine. Also acts as a weak osmotic diuretic, increasing urine flow, pH, and excretion acids, CO_2, and electrolytes. **Metabolism/Elimination:** Not significantly metabolized. Rapidly excreted in urine as bicarbonate form at rate dependent on infusion rate—greater than 75% in 8 hr, 25% within 3 days.

INDICATIONS/DOSAGE

Prevention and correction of metabolic acidosis

Dosage depends on severity and progression of acidosis. Dosage should be the least amount to raise the blood pH to within normal limits (7.35–7.45). Do not administer longer than 24 hr unless life-threatening situation.

Adult/Pediatric: General guideline: wgt(kg) × base deficit (mEq/L) × 1.1 equals dose (mL). NOTE: Do NOT multiply by 1.1 if Tham-E is used.

Acidosis during cardiac bypass surgery

Adult/Pediatric:

Tham: Average dose: 9 mL/kg (2.7 mEq/kg). Total single dose 500 mL (150 mEq) is adequate. Up to 1000 mL may be needed in severe cases. **Tham-E:** Average dose: 300 mg (8.3 mEq/kg). Average total dose 694 mL (25 g). Up to 500 mg/kg may be needed in severe cases.

Treatment of metabolic acidosis in neonatal respiratory distress syndrome refractory to ventilation/bicarbonate) (*unlabeled use*)

Neonates: 1–2 mEq/kg/dose. Alternate dosage wgt (kg) × base deficit (mEq/L) × 1.1 equals dose (mL). NOTE: Do NOT multiply by 1.1 if Tham-E is used.

CONTRAINDICATIONS/ PRECAUTIONS

Contraindicated in: Anuria, uremia. **Use cautiously in:** Renal impairment, respiratory depression. **Pregnancy/ Lactation:** Contraindicated in pregnancy except in life-threatening situations. No well-controlled trials to establish safety. Benefits must outweigh risks. **Pediatrics:** Severe hemorrhagic liver necrosis has occurred in neonates. Hypoglycemia may occur in premature/full-term neonates.

PREPARATION

Availability: Tham: 18 g (150 mEq) per 500 mL (0.3 M), 500 mL. Tham-E: 36 g (45 mEq) per 150 mL, 150 mL powder for injection. Tham-E contains sodium 30 mEq/L, potassium 5 mEq/L, chloride 35 mEq/L; total osmolarity 367 mOsm/L. 1 mEq equals 1 mmol equals 120 mg. **Infusion:** Use undiluted injection. 0.3 M solution may be administered as Tham or by adding 150 mL Tham-E to 1000 mL sterile water for injection in glass bottles.

STABILITY/STORAGE

Vial: Store at room temperature. **Infusion:** Discard solutions 24 hr after preparation. Stable at room temperature. Highly alkaline solutions may erode glass.

T

In the Adverse Effects section, <u>underline</u> indicates most frequent; CAPS indicates life threatening.

509

ADMINISTRATION

General: Avoid extravasation. Assess IV site frequently. Administer as slow IV infusion or via pump-oxygenator. Use largest antecubital vein via large needle or indwelling catheter. If extravasation causes vasospasm, local infiltration of phentolamine or 1% procaine with hyaluronidase. **Intermittent/Continuous Infusion:** Total dose should be infused over at least 1 hr. Individual doses should not exceed 500 mg/kg. Avoid infusion via umbilical vein unless catheter has traversed the ductus venosus.

COMPATIBILITY/INCOMPATIBILITY

Data not available.

ADVERSE EFFECTS

Resp: RESPIRATORY DEPRESSION. **GI:** HEMORRHAGIC HEPATIC NECROSIS (neonates). **Endo:** Transient depression blood glucose. **Fld/Lytes:** Hyperkalemia (in renal impairment), hypervolemia. **Metab:** Metabolic alkalosis. **Other:** Fever, local infection, venous thrombosis/phlebitis.

TOXICITY/OVERDOSE

Signs/Symptoms: Alkalosis, overhydration, solute overload, prolonged hypoglycemia. **Treatment:** Discontinue infusion. Symptomatic and supportive.

NURSING CONSIDERATIONS

Assessment
General:
Vital signs.
Physical:
Pulmonary status, GI tract.
Lab Alterations:
Determine blood pH, carbon dioxide tension, bicarbonate, glucose, electrolyte concentrations before, during, and after administration. Evaluate liver enzymes periodically.

Intervention/Rationale
Monitor vital signs, especially in patients predisposed to respiratory depression. If respiratory acidosis is present, mechanical ventilation must be initiated. ● Monitor patient for signs/symptoms of hepatic dysfunction (jaundice, ascites).

Patient/Family Education
Educate the patient/family regarding the critical nature of the drug to correct the patient's blood pH.

TUBOCURARINE
(too-boh-cure′-r-een)
Trade Name(s): Tubarine ♣
Classification(s): Nondepolarizing neuromuscular blocking agent
Pregnancy Category: C

PHARMACODYNAMICS/KINETICS

Mechanism of Action: Causes partial paralysis by interfering with neural transmission at myoneural junction. Prevents acetylcholine from binding to receptors at muscle end plate. **Onset of Action:** Rapid. **Peak Effect:** 6 min. **Duration of Action:** 25–90 minutes. Maximum effect 35–60 min. **Distribution:** Rapidly distributed into extracellular fluid and site of action of motor end plate myoneural junction. 50% bound to plasma proteins. **Metabolism/Elimination:** 1% hepatically metabolized. 11% (active drug and metabolite) excreted

In the Adverse Effects section, <u>underline</u> indicates most frequent; CAPS indicates life threatening.

in bile. 30%–43% excreted unchanged in urine. **Half-Life:** 2 hr.

INDICATIONS/DOSAGE

Adjunct to anesthesia to induce skeletal muscle relaxation; to facilitate mechanical ventilation

Individualize dosage based on patient response. Reduce dosage with concurrent inhalation anesthetics or in renal impairment. Administer in incremental doses.

Adult: Initially, 3 mg less than calculated dose. 0.1–0.2 mg/kg for limb paresis; 0.4–0.5 mg/kg for abdominal relaxation; 0.5–0.6 mg/kg for endotracheal intubation. Repeat incremental doses in 40–60 minutes as required in prolonged procedures. In surgery, 6–9 mg when incision is made and 3.0–4.5 mg if required in 3–5 minutes; give 3 mg (0.15 mg/kg) supplemental doses in prolonged operations. *Pediatric:* Initially 0.2–0.4 mg/kg (up to 0.6 mg/kg). 0.04–0.2 mg/kg as needed to maintain paralysis. *Neonate:* Initially 0.3 mg/kg. 0.15 mg/kg/dose as needed to maintain paralysis.

To reduce intensity of muscle contractions in pharmacologic/electrical induced convulsions

Adult: 0.165 mg/kg as a sustained 1.0–1.5 min injection just before therapy. Initially, 3 mg less than calculated dose.

Diagnostic agent for myasthenia gravis

(when other tests inconclusive)

Adult: 0.004–0.033 mg/kg. Terminate test in 2–3 min in neostigmine.

CONTRAINDICATIONS/ PRECAUTIONS

Contraindicated in: Hypersensitivity, patients in whom histamine release is life threatening. **Use cautiously in:** Elderly, myasthenia gravis, renal impairment, patients sensitive to sodium bisulfite, respiratory depression, impaired pulmonary, hepatic, cardiovascular, or endocrine function. **Pregnancy/Lactation:** No well-controlled trials to establish safety. Benefits must outweigh risks. Prolonged doses may cause fetal contractures. **Pediatrics:** Premature infants may be more sensitive to effects. Reduce dosage in prematurity, acidosis, hypothermia, halothane use.

PREPARATION

Availability: 3 mg/mL (20 units) in 5 mL syringes, 10 mL, and 20 mL vials. Abbott/Squibb/Marsam products contain benzyl alcohol 9 mg as preservative (should not be used in neonates). **Syringe:** No further dilution required.

STABILITY/STORAGE

Vial: Store at room temperature. **Infusion:** Stable in PVC plastic bags for 24 hr.

ADMINISTRATION

General: Unconsciousness must be established prior to administration to prevent patient distress. Administer only by trained personnel with the ability to provide ventilatory support. **IV Push:** Give over 1.0–1.5 min. Avoid rapid administration.

T

In the Adverse Effects section, underline indicates most frequent; CAPS indicates life threatening.

511

COMPATIBILITY

Solution: Dextrose solutions, lactated Ringer's, sodium chloride solutions. **Syringe:** Pentobarbital, thiopental (if 1:19 ratio).

ADVERSE EFFECTS

CNS: <u>Prolonged paralysis</u>, <u>skeletal muscle weakness</u>. **CV:** CARDIAC ARREST, CARDIAC DYSRHYTHMIAS, hypotension, bradycardia. **Resp:** APNEA, <u>RESPIRATORY DEPRESSION</u>. **GI:** Excess salivation. **MS:** <u>Prolonged neuromuscular blockade</u>. **Hypersens:** ANAPHYLAXIS.

TOXICITY/OVERDOSE

Signs/Symptoms: Extended skeletal muscle weakness, decreased respiratory status, prolonged apnea, low tidal volume, cardiovascular collapse, sudden histamine release. **Treatment:** Symptomatic and supportive. Assess residual neuromuscular blockade with peripheral nerve stimulator. **Antidote(s):** Pyridostigmine, neostigmine, or edrophonium in conjunction with atropine or glycopyrrolate will antagonize tubocurarine action. Concurrent administration of other neuromuscular blockers or impaired renal/hepatic function may not allow complete reversal.

DRUG INTERACTIONS

Acetylcholine, anticholinesterases, potassium: Antagonize tubocurarine. **Aminoglycosides, bacitracin, clindamycin, inhalation anesthetics** (halothane, ether, cycloproprane, fluroxene, isoflurane, penthrane, methoxyflurane, enflurane): Increased duration and intensity of neuromuscular blockade. **Amphotericin B, corticosteroids, diuretics (loop/thiazide), carbonic anhydrase inhibitors:** Increased sensitivity to blockade. **Calcium, diazepam, lidocaine, lithium, magnesium, MAO inhibitors, propranolol, quinine:** Potentiates action of tubocurarine. **Depolarizing muscle relaxants:** Synergistic effects.

NURSING CONSIDERATIONS

Assessment

General:
Vital signs, ECG (recommended), continuous monitoring of respiratory rate.

Physical:
Cardiopulmonary status, neuromuscular status.

Lab Alterations:
In tetanus patients, continuous administration interferes with detection of catecholamines in urine assayed fluorimetrically.

Intervention/Rationale

Produces apnea (use cautiously in patients with cardiovascular disease, severe electrolyte disorders, bronchogenic cancer, and neuromuscular diseases). Maintain patent airway. ● Monitor response to drug during intraoperative period by use of a peripheral nerve stimulator. Assess postoperatively for presence of any residual muscle weakness. Evaluate hand grip, head lift, and ability to cough in order to ascertain full recovery from residual effects of drug. ● Correct electrolyte deficiencies prior to surgery. ● Assess status of corneas; consider lubrication as needed. ● Assess need for sedation; obtain order and administer during use of paralytic agent. ● Monitor blood pressure, respiratory status, and ECG before and during administration.

Patient/Family Education
Discuss the rationale for hand grip, head lift, and cough demonstration in the immediate postoperative phase in order to assure patient cooperation. Inform patient and family that consciousness is unaffected by drug. Explain side effects to patient and family. Continue to explain procedures and therapies to patient unless sedation is administered.

UREA
(yoor-e′-a)
Trade Name(s): Ureaphil
Classification(s): Osmotic diuretic
Pregnancy Category: C

PHARMACODYNAMICS/KINETICS
Mechanism of Action: Osmotic effect causes water to be drawn from cells of the brain and the CSF into blood resulting in decreased intracranial pressure and cerebral edema. Induces diuresis by increasing osmotic pressure of glomerular filtrate so that tubular reabsorption of water/solutes decreases. **Onset of Action:** 30–45 min. **Peak Effect:** 1 hr. **Duration of Action:** 5–6 hr. **Distribution:** Distributed to extracellular and intracellular fluids including lymph, bile, CSF, and blood in equal concentrations. Passes readily into the eye. High concentrations in kidneys. **Metabolism/Elimination:** Hydrolyzed in GI tract by bacterial urease to ammonia and CO_2 that may be resynthesized to urea. Excreted by kidneys.

INDICATIONS/DOSAGE

Individualize dosage based on condition and requirements.

Reduce intracranial pressure (in cerebral edema) and intraocular pressure
Adult: 1.0–1.5 g/kg. Not to exceed 120 g/day. *Pediatric:* 0.5–1.5 g/kg. Up to 2 years, 0.1 g/kg may be adequate. Not to exceed 120 g/day.

Rapid correction of hyponatremia in syndrome of inappropriate antidiuretic hormone (SIADH) (*unlabeled use*)
Adult: 80 g infused over 6 hr as 30%.

Acute sickle cell crisis (*unlabeled use*)
Adult: Administer sufficient 30% solution to elevate BUN 150–200 mg% until pain subsides. Alternate dosage 6 g/kg as 15% in 10% invert sugar over 12–16 hr at 4.5 mL/kg/hr.

CONTRAINDICATIONS/ PRECAUTIONS
Contraindicated in: Active intracranial bleed, frank liver failure, marked dehydration, severely impaired renal function. **Use cautiously in:** Liver impairment, renal impairment. **Pregnancy/Lactation:** No well-controlled trials to establish safety. Crosses placenta. Benefits must outweigh risks. Distributed into breast milk.

PREPARATION
Availability: 40 g per 150 mL single dose container. **Reconstitution:** Disso-

In the Adverse Effects section, <u>underline</u> indicates most frequent; CAPS indicates life threatening.

513

lution will occur more quickly if diluent warmed to 50° C immediately prior to mixing. 30%: add 105 mL D_5W or $D_{10}W$ to 40 g bottle; final concentration 300 mg/mL, 135 mL volume. 40%–50%: add sufficient volume D_5W to 80 g (two bottles) to make 150–200 mL of 50% (500 mg/mL) or 40% (400 mg/mL), respectively. **Infusion:** Cool solution to body temperature before administration.

STABILITY/STORAGE
Vial: Store at room temperature. **Infusion:** Prepare just prior to administration. Stable for 24 hr at room temperature. Discard after 24 hr.

ADMINISTRATION
General: Administer by slow IV infusion. Do not stop infusion abruptly. Assess IV site frequently. Avoid extravasation; administer via large extremity veins. Avoid lower extremity veins in elderly. An indwelling catheter should be in place to facilitate emptying bladder and measuring urine output. **Intraocular Surgery:** Administer 1–2 hr preoperatively. **Intracranial Surgery:** Administer ⅔ of dose during time dura exposed; infuse remainder at controlled rate. **Intermittent/Continuous Infusion:** Administer over 1.0–2.5 hr. Not to exceed 4 mL/min. An iso-osmotic dextrose or invert sugar should be administered concurrently to prevent hemolysis. Do not administer through same administration set as blood.

COMPATIBILITY
Solution: Dextrose 5% and 10%, invert sugar 10%.

ADVERSE EFFECTS
CNS: Agitated, confusional state, disorientation, <u>headache</u>, syncope. **CV:** CIRCULATORY COLLAPSE, CHF. **Resp:** Pulmonary edema. **GI:** Nausea, vomiting. **Fld/Lytes:** Hypervolemia. **Other:** Fever, localized infection, phlebitis, thrombosis.

TOXICITY/OVERDOSE
Signs/Symptoms: Unusually elevated BUN levels. **Treatment:** Discontinue infusion, symptomatic and supportive therapy.

DRUG INTERACTIONS
Lithium: Increased renal excretion lithium; decreased lithium effects.

NURSING CONSIDERATIONS
Assessment
General:
Vital signs, intracranial pressure, intake/output ratio.
Physical:
Cardiopulmonary status, hydration status.
Lab Alterations:
Monitor serum electrolytes, BUN, and serum creatinine.

Intervention/Rationale
Assess for signs/symptoms of CHF/pulmonary edema. Monitor intake/output hourly for development of fluid overload. ● Assess for signs/symptoms of increased intracranial pressure (confusion, decreased level of consciousness, changes in mental status, Cushings triad).

Patient/Family Education
Notify physician/nurse if IV site becomes painful or swollen.

In the Adverse Effects section, <u>underline</u> indicates most frequent;
CAPS indicates life threatening.

UROKINASE

(yoor-oh-kye'-nase)
Trade Name(s): Abbokinase,
Abbokinase Open-Cath
Classification(s): Thrombolytic
agent
Pregnancy Category: B

PHARMACODYNAMICS/KINETICS

Mechanism of Action: Directly converts plasminogen to plasmin, which degrades fibrin clots and fibrinogen. **Onset of Action:** Immediate. **Peak Effect:** Rapid. **Duration of Action:** Up to 12–24 hr. **Metabolism/Elimination:** Rapid clearance by liver. Small amounts eliminated via urine and bile. **Half-Life:** 10–20 min. Increased in severe hepatic impairment.

INDICATIONS/DOSAGE

Pulmonary emboli

Adult/Pediatric: 4400 IU/kg as priming dose. Followed by 4400 IU/kg/hr for 12 hr.

Coronary artery thrombosis

Adult/Pediatric: 6000 IU/min (4 mL/min) intracoronary for up to 2 hr (average total dose 500,000 IU). Continue until artery is maximally open (usually 15–30 min after initial opening or until 2 hr).

IV catheter clearance

Adult/Pediatric: Inject amount of 5000 IU/mL (1.0–1.8 mL) equal to internal volume of catheter. A second dose may be needed for resistant thrombi.

CONTRAINDICATIONS/PRECAUTIONS

Contraindicated in: Active internal bleeding, hypersensitivity, intracranial neoplasm, intracranial/intraspinal surgery, recent (within 2 months) cerebrovascular accident. **Use cautiously in:** Age ≥ 75 years, cerebrovascular disease, diabetic hemorrhagic retinopathy, hemostatic defects, organ biopsy, obstetrical delivery, pregnancy, previous puncture of noncompressible vessels, recent (within 10 days) serious GI bleeding/major surgery, recent trauma including CPR, septic thrombophlebitis or occluded AV cannula at infected sites, severe uncontrolled arterial hypertension or likely left heart thrombus, subacute bacterial endocarditis. **Pregnancy/Lactation:** Safety for use has not been established. Benefits must outweigh risks. Exercise caution in breastfeeding patients. **Pediatrics:** Safety and efficacy has not been established in children.

PREPARATION

Availability: 250,000 IU/5 mL vial. Open Cath: 5000 IU and 9000 IU Univials. **Reconstitution:** Use sterile water for injection only. Roll/tilt vial gently. Do not shake. **Infusion/Intracoronary Use:** Dilute each 250,000 IU with 5 mL sterile water for final concentration of 50,000 IU/mL (clear/slightly straw colored solution). **Catheter Clearance:** Open Cath: Dilute each vial by activating plunger to mix diluent with drug for final concentration of 5000 IU/mL of clear/colorless solution. 250,000 IU vial: Dilute with 5.2 mL sterile water, withdraw 1 mL and

In the Adverse Effects section, <u>underline</u> indicates most frequent; CAPS indicates life threatening.

515

add to 9 mL sterile water for final concentration 5000 IU/mL. **Syringe:** No further dilution required. **Infusion:** Further dilute total dose to 200 mL with dextrose 5% or 0.9% sodium chloride.

Intracoronary: Further dilute 750,000 IU (three vials) in 500 mL dextrose 5% for a final concentration of 1500 IU/mL.

STABILITY/STORAGE

Vial: Store vial in refrigerator. Unreconstituted Open-Cath may be stored at room temperature or refrigerated. Reconstituted solutions should be used immediately after preparation (stable for 24 hr refrigerated/room temperature). Open-Cath may be stored for 24 hr at room temperature after reconstitution. Presence of thin filaments does not alter potency or adverse effect potential. **Infusion:** Stable for 24 hr at room temperature.

ADMINISTRATION

General: 0.45 micron or smaller cellulose membrane filter may be used prior to administration. **Intermittent/ Continuous Infusion:** Use continuous infusion device capable of delivering 195 mL total volume. Infuse priming dose at 90 mL/min over 10 minutes. Follow at rate of 15 mL/ min for 12 hr. Flush tubing following completion for any remaining drug by using volume of D_5W or NSS equal to tubing; pump flush solution through tubing at rate of 15 mL/hr. At end of infusion, heparin infusion should begin after thrombin time is less than twice normal (approximately 3–4 hr). **Intracoronary:** Prior to infusion, give heparin bolus. Begin administra-

tion at 4 mL/min for up to 2 hr. Continue until artery maximally opened. Continue heparin after artery has opened. **Catheter Clearance:** Instruct patient to exhale and hold breath whenever catheter is not connected to tubing or syringe to prevent air from entering. Disconnect IV tubing and attach 10 mL syringe, gently attempt to aspirate blood. If aspiration is impossible, connect 1 mL tuberculin syringe containing urokinase and slowly, gently inject equal volume of catheter. Remove 1 mL syringe and connect 5 mL syringe. Wait at least 5 min. Repeat aspiration attempts every 5 min. If catheter is not open within 30 min, cap catheter and allow urokinase to remain 30–60 min before next aspiration attempt. A second injection may be needed. When patent, aspirate and remove 4–5 mL blood, then replace syringe with 10 mL syringe filled with 0.9% sodium chloride injection. Gently irrigate catheter with this solution. Remove syringe and reconnect to IV tubing. Ineffective for catheter clearance related to substances other than blood clots. Avoid excessive pressure.

COMPATIBILITY

Solution: Dextrose solutions, sodium chloride solutions. **Syringe:** Heparin.

ADVERSE EFFECTS

CV: Reperfusion atrial/ventricular dysrhythmias. **Heme:** <u>BLEEDING</u> (minor/major), <u>bruising</u>, <u>hematoma</u>, HEMORRHAGE, moderate decrease hematocrit. **Hypersens:** ANAPHYLAXIS, BRONCHOSPASM, rash. **Other:** Fever.

In the Adverse Effects section, <u>underline</u> indicates most frequent; CAPS indicates life threatening.

TOXICITY/OVERDOSE

Signs/Symptoms: Severe bleeding/hemorrhage. **Treatment:** Discontinue treatment, plasma volume expanders other than dextran, packed RBCs if needed. **Antidote(s):** For rapid reversal, aminocaproic acid or antifibrinolytic may be considered.

DRUG INTERACTIONS

Anticoagulants, antiplatelets (aspirin, dipyridamole, NSAIDs): Increased bleeding.

NURSING CONSIDERATIONS

Assessment

General:
Continuous ECG monitoring, vital signs.
Physical:
Cardiopulmonary status, hematopoietic system.
Lab Alterations:
Monitor hemoglobin/hematocrit, platelet count, thrombin time, activated partial thromboplastin time, prothrombin time, and fibrinogen prior to therapy and 4 hr after initiation.

Intervention/Rationale

Monitor all potential bleeding sites for hematoma formation and bleeding (bleeding occurs most at vascular access sites). Avoid IM injections and nonessential handling of patient. Avoid arterial punctures unless absolutely necessary (use brachial or radial artery), and if done, apply pressure for at least 30 min, followed by application of pressure dressing and frequent inspection of site. ● Monitor ECG during therapy for reperfusion-related atrial and/or ventricular dysrhythmias. Monitor blood pressure periodically during therapy. ● Discontinue heparin prior to urokinase and until thrombin time less than twice normal. During infusion, decreased plasminogen/fibrinogen and increased FDP indicate lysis of thrombi. ● Monitor vital signs and clinical response at least every 4 hr. Avoid taking blood pressure in lower extremities when deep vein thrombosis (DVT) is present.

Patient/Family Education

Educate regarding potential therapeutic outcome and side effects, especially bleeding potential.

VANCOMYCIN

(van-koe-mye′-sin)
Trade Name(s): Vancocin, Vancoled
Classification(s): Antibiotic
Pregnancy Category: C

PHARMACODYNAMICS/KINETICS

Mechanism of Action: Bactericidal. Interferes with bacterial cell wall synthesis in multiplying organisms. Inhibits RNA synthesis and bacterial cytoplasmic membranes. **Peak Serum Level:** Up to 2 hr after administration. **Therapeutic Serum Levels:** Peak 25–40 mcg/mL. Trough 5–10 mcg/mL. **Distribution:** With inflammation, penetrates pleural fluid, pericardial fluid, ascitic fluid, synovial fluid, bile. Low concentration in meninges. 50%–60% protein bound especially albumin. **Metabolism/Elimination:** Eliminated primarily by kidneys in urine via glomerular filtration. **Half-Life:** 4–8 hr

In the Adverse Effects section, underline indicates most frequent; CAPS indicates life threatening.

517

(adults), 2–3 hr (children), 7.5 days anuria.

INDICATIONS/DOSAGE

Treatment of severe gram-positive infections including staphylococcal and streptococcal infections (in combination with aminoglycosides)

Adjust dose based on serum levels. Adjust dosage interval in renal impairment. Hemodialysis patients: 15 mg/kg once; administer subsequent doses when serum levels within desired therapeutic range.

Adult: 500 mg every 6 hr or 1 g every 12 hr. Initial doses should not exceed 2 g/day. *Pediatric:* 10 mg/kg every 6 hr. Up to 15 mg/kg every 6 hr in serious infections. *Neonate:* Load 15 mg/kg. Maintenance: < 1 month old: 10 mg/kg every 12 hr. > 1 month old: 10 mg/kg every 8 hr.

Prophylaxis of bacterial endocarditis in penicillin-allergic patients in dental/upper respiratory tract surgery/instrumentation and GI/GU surgery/instrumentation (with aminoglycosides)

Adult/Pediatric (> 27 kg): 1 g 1 hr prior to procedure. May repeat in 8–12 hr if high risk patients. *Pediatric (< 27 kg):* 20 mg/kg 1 hr prior to procedure. May repeat in 8–12 hr if high risk patients.

CONTRAINDICATIONS/PRECAUTIONS

Contraindicated in: Known hypersensitivity. **Use cautiously in:** Previous hearing loss, renal impairment. **Pregnancy/Lactation:** No well-controlled trials to establish safety.

Benefits must outweigh risks. Readily crosses placenta. **Pediatrics:** Use with caution in premature/full-term neonates since renal function not fully developed.

PREPARATION

Availability: 500 mg and 1 g vials. 10 g bulk vials. **Reconstitution:** Dilute each 500 mg with 10 mL sterile water for injection. **Infusion:** Further dilute each 500 mg in at least 100 mL compatible IV solution for a maximum concentration of 5 mg/mL.

STABILITY/STORAGE

Vial: Store at room temperature. Reconstituted solution stable for 14 days refrigerated/room temperature. **Infusion:** Stable for 14 days refrigerated/room temperature.

ADMINISTRATION

General: Avoid bolus administration. **Intermittent Infusion:** Infuse over 30–60 min. Not to exceed 15 mg/min. **Continuous Infusion:** Infuse total daily dose in volume of fluid sufficient for 24 hr administration.

COMPATIBILITY

Solution: Dextrose solutions, lactated Ringer's, sodium chloride solutions. **Y-site:** Acyclovir, atracurium, cyclophosphamide, enalaprilat, esmolol, hydromorphone, labetalol, magnesium sulfate, meperidine, morphine, ondansetron, pancuronium, perphenazine, tolazoline, vecuronium, zidovudine.

INCOMPATIBILITY

Syringe: Heparin. **Y-site:** Aztreonam, foscarnet.

ADVERSE EFFECTS

CNS: Dizziness, vertigo. **CV:** CARDIAC ARREST, hypotension (with

In the Adverse Effects section, <u>underline</u> indicates most frequent; CAPS indicates life threatening.

rapid infusion). **Resp:** Dyspnea, wheezing. **GI:** Nausea. **Renal:** Nephrotoxicity. **Heme:** Eosinophilia, reversible neutropenia, thrombocytopenia. **Hypersens:** ANAPHYLACTOID REACTIONS, macular rash, pruritus, red man syndrome (rapid decrease in blood pressure and maculopapular rash), urticaria. **Other:** Chills, fever, ototoxicity, thrombophlebitis.

TOXICITY/OVERDOSE
Signs/Symptoms: Rapid administration causes red man syndrome, hypotension, and cardiac arrest. **Treatment:** Symptomatic and supportive.

DRUG INTERACTIONS
Amikacin, amphotericin B, bacitracin, cisplatin, colistin, gentamicin, kanamycin, neomycin, netilmicin, polymyxin B, streptomycin, tobramycin: Increased risk of neurotoxicity and nephrotoxicity. **Anesthetic agents:** Erythema and histamine-like flushing in children. **Loop diuretics, thiazide diuretics:** Increased potential for ototoxicity.

NURSING CONSIDERATIONS
Assessment
General:
Blood pressure, heart rate, intake/output ratio, hypersensitivity reaction, infectious disease status.
Physical:
Baseline auditory function, renal function.
Lab Alterations:
Measure peak/trough serum levels. Monitor serum creatinine.

Intervention/Rationale
Obtain cultures for sensitivity prior to first dose. May give first dose before results are available. ● Main-

tain adequate hydration to avoid nephrotoxicity. ● Assess for red man syndrome. ● Assess baseline auditory function. ● Draw peak serum level 60 min after infusion is complete and trough 30 min prior to next dose.

Patient/Family Education
Increase oral fluid intake in order to minimize chemical irritation of kidneys. Notify physician/nurse if tinnitus, vertigo, or hearing loss occurs. Inform patient of the need for several weeks of therapy for certain serious infections despite feeling well.

VASOPRESSIN
(vay-soe-press'-in)
Trade Name(s): Pitressin synthetic, Pressyn ✤
Classification(s): Antidiuretic hormone, vasopressor
Pregnancy Category: C

PHARMACODYNAMICS/KINETICS
Mechanism of Action: Increases water reabsorption by renal tubules resulting in concentrated urine. Stimulates contraction of smooth muscle with resultant vasoconstriction. **Duration of Action:** 30–60 min. **Distribution:** Distributed throughout extracellular fluid. **Metabolism/Elimination:** Rapidly destroyed by liver and kidneys. 5%–15% total dose appears in urine. **Half-Life:** 10–20 min.

INDICATIONS/DOSAGE

Treatment of acute GI hemorrhage
Adult:
Individualize dosage based on patient condition and response.

In the Adverse Effects section, <u>underline</u> indicates most frequent;
CAPS indicates life threatening.
519

Intravenous: 0.2–0.4 units/min initially; increase as needed to control bleeding up to 0.9 units/min. **Intra-arterial:** 0.1–0.5 units/min initially; increase as needed to control bleeding up to 0.9 units/min. After 24 hr, taper to patient's response; may be continued up to 3–14 days.

CONTRAINDICATIONS/ PRECAUTIONS

Contraindicated in: Anaphylaxis or hypersensitivity to vasopressin/ components. **Use cautiously in:** Asthma, epilepsy, heart failure, migraine, renal disease, vascular disease. **Pregnancy/Lactation:** No well-controlled trials to establish safety. Benefits must outweigh risks.

PREPARATION

Availability: (Aqueous) 20 pressor units/mL in 0.5 and 1 mL amps. **Infusion:** Dilute desired dose in volume of compatible diluent for a final concentration 0.1–1.0 unit/mL.

STABILITY/STORAGE

Vial: Store at room temperature. **Infusion:** Prepare just prior to administration. Stable for 24 hr at room temperature.

ADMINISTRATION

General: For safe and accurate administration, use infusion control device. Administer only under supervision of physician familiar with drug's effects. **Intra-arterial Infusion:** Infuse via superior mesenteric artery, inferior mesenteric artery, splenic/celiac axis. Assess catheter placement by angiography. After 20–30 min, vasoconstrictive and clotting response should be assessed by angiography. **Continuous Infusion:** Preferred route of administration. Infuse via peripheral vein at physician specified rate and assess site frequently.

COMPATIBILITY

Solution: Dextrose solutions, sodium chloride solutions.

ADVERSE EFFECTS

CNS: <u>Head pounding</u>, tremor, vertigo. **CV:** CARDIAC ARREST, circulatory collapse, bradycardia, circumoral pallor, coronary insufficiency, coronary thrombosis, dysrhythmias, increased blood pressure, MYOCARDIAL INFARCTION, peripheral emboli, peripheral vascular collapse. **GI:** Abdominal cramps, diarrhea, flatulence, intestinal hyperactivity, nausea, reversible ischemic colitis, vomiting. **GU:** Uterine cramps. **Hypersens:** ANAPHYLAXIS, angioedema, bronchoconstriction, urticaria, wheezing. **Other:** Fever, sweating.

TOXICITY/OVERDOSE

Signs/Symptoms: Water intoxication, increased potential of cardiovascular effects. **Treatment:** Discontinue drug, symptomatic and supportive.

DRUG INTERACTIONS

Alcohol, demeclocycline, epinephrine (high dose), heparin, lithium: Blocks antidiuretic effect. **Carbamazepine, chlorpropamide, clofibrate, fludrocortisone, phenformin, tricyclic antidepressants, urea:** Potentiates antidiuretic response. **Ganglionic blocking agents:** Marked increase in sensitivity to pressor effects.

In the Adverse Effects section, <u>underline</u> indicates most frequent; CAPS indicates life threatening.

NURSING CONSIDERATIONS

Assessment
General:
ECG (recommended), intake/output ratio.
Physical:
Cardiovascular status, signs/symptoms of water intoxication.
Lab Alterations:
Monitor serum electrolytes during therapy.

Intervention/Rationale
Monitor signs/symptoms of water intoxication (drowsiness, listlessness, headache, anuria, confusion, weight gain). ● Monitor ECG for cardiac effects including development of chest pain and dysrhythmias.
Intra-arterial Infusion:
Monitor portal pressures and hepatic wedge pressure during angiography.

Patient/Family Education
Notify physician of any signs of allergic reaction, confusion/dizziness, or excess GI effects.

VECURONIUM
(ve-kure-oh′-nee-yum)
Trade Name(s): Norcuron
Classification(s): Nondepolarizing neuromuscular blocking agent
Pregnancy Category: C

PHARMACODYNAMICS/KINETICS
Mechanism of Action: Causes partial paralysis by interfering with neural transmission at myoneural junction. Prevents acetylcholine from binding to receptors at muscle end plate. **Onset of Action:** 1 min. **Peak Effect:** 3–5 min. **Duration of Action:** 25–40 min. Recovery time 45–65 min. Prolonged in cirrhosis/cholestasis. **Distribution:** Unknown. Rapidly distributes into extracellular spaces. 60%–90% protein bound. **Metabolism/Elimination:** Metabolized by liver to one metabolite present in urine and bile. Primarily excreted as unchanged drug and metabolites via biliary elimination in feces. **Half-Life:** 65–75 min. 35–45 min in late pregnancy.

INDICATIONS/DOSAGE

Individualize dosage based on patient response. Reduce dosage with concurrent inhalation anesthetic agents.

Adjunct to anesthesia to induce skeletal muscle relaxation; to facilitate mechanical ventilation and endotracheal intubation

Adult/Pediatric (10–17 years):
Initial Dose: 0.08–0.1 mg/kg/dose. If administered ≥ 5 minutes after start of inhalation agents, reduce initial dose by 15%. If prior succinylcholine administered, reduce initial dose to 0.04–0.06 mg/kg/dose with inhalation or 0.05–0.06 mg/kg/dose with balanced anesthesia. **Maintenance Dose:** Intermittent injection: After 25–40 min, may increase to 0.01–0.015 mg/kg/dose in prolonged surgical procedures with balanced anesthesia or 0.008–0.012 mg/kg with inhalation anesthetics. Additional doses may be administered if needed at 12–15 min intervals with balanced anesthesia or slightly longer under inhalation anesthesia. If less frequent

In the Adverse Effects section, underline indicates most frequent;
CAPS indicates life threatening.

521

administration is needed, use higher maintenance doses. Burn patients may develop resistance requiring dosage increase.

Pediatric (*1–10 years*): Slightly higher initial doses and more frequent maintenance dose administration may be needed. 7 weeks old to less than 1 year old are moderately more sensitive and take 1.5 times longer to recover.

Continuous infusion maintenance (for prolonged surgical procedures)

Adult: After 25–40 min and spontaneous recovery is evident, initially 1 mcg/kg/min and adjusted to maintain 90% blockade. 0.8–1.2 mcg/kg/min are usually adequate to maintain blockade. Reduce dosage in patients receiving general anesthetics; 25%–60% reduction in dosage in patients receiving enflurane and isoflurane.

CONTRAINDICATIONS/ PRECAUTIONS

Contraindicated in: Hypersensitivity. **Use cautiously in:** Anephric patients, cardiovascular disease, edematous states, electrolyte imbalance, elderly, hepatic impairment, myasthenia gravis, neuromuscular disease, patients with history of malignant hyperthermia. **Pregnancy/Lactation:** No well-controlled trials to establish safety. Benefits must outweigh risks. Administration during cesarean section achieves umbilical vein levels but without adverse effects noted. Minimal placenta transfer. **Pediatrics:** Infants less than 1 year old are more sensitive. Not recommended for use in neonates.

PREPARATION

Availability: 10 mg powder for injection in 5 and 10 mL vials with/without diluent. Diluent contains bacteriostatic water with 0.9% benzyl alcohol. **Reconstitution:** Reconstitute each 10 mg with 5 mL diluent, bacteriostatic water for injection or sterile water for injection for final concentration of 2 mg/mL. **Syringe:** No further dilution required. **Infusion:** Dilute to desired concentration in compatible IV solution for a final concentration 0.1–0.2 mg/mL.

STABILITY/STORAGE

Vial: Store at room temperature. Stable for 24 hr after reconstitution at room temperature/refrigerated. Use within 8 hr if sterile water for injection is used. Discard unused portion. If reconstituted with bacteriostatic water, stable for 5 days room temperature/refrigerated. Protect from light. **Infusion:** Prepare just prior to administration. Stable for 24 hr.

ADMINISTRATION

General: Intradermal test dose (0.005–0.02 mg/kg) may be given to monitor response in neuromuscular disease patients. Unconsciousness must be established prior to administration to prevent patient distress. Administer only by trained personnel with the ability to provide ventilatory support. Dosage reduction should occur with concurrent inhalation anesthetic administration. **IV Push:** Administer by rapid direct IV push. If patient has history of histamine reactions, administer slowly over at least 1–2 min to observe for reaction. **Continuous Infusion:** Administer via infu-

In the Adverse Effects section, <u>underline</u> indicates most frequent; CAPS indicates life threatening.

sion device at physician prescribed rate to monitor accuracy of dosage.

COMPATIBILITY

Solution: Dextrose solutions, lactated Ringer's, sodium chloride solutions, sterile water for injection. **Y-site:** Aminophylline, cefazolin, cefuroxime, cimetidine, dobutamine, dopamine, epinephrine, esmolol, fentanyl, gentamicin, heparin, hydrocortisone, isoproterenol, lorazepam, midazolam, morphine, nitroglycerin, rantidine, sodium nitroprusside, trimethoprim-sulfamethoxazole, vancomycin.

INCOMPATIBILITY

Syringe: Alkaline solutions, barbiturates. **Y-site:** Diazepam.

ADVERSE EFFECTS

CNS: <u>Prolonged paralysis</u>, <u>skeletal muscle weakness</u>. **CV:** Increased cardiac output, heart rate, mean arterial pressure. **Resp:** APNEA, <u>RESPIRATORY INSUFFICIENCY</u>. **Hypersens:** Histamine release reactions (test dose in patients with history of histamine hypersensitivity).

TOXICITY/OVERDOSE

Signs/Symptoms: Prolonged skeletal muscle relaxation, respiratory depression. **Treatment:** Symptomatic/supportive treatment. **Antidote(s):** Pyridostigmine, neostigmine, or edrophonium in conjunction with atropine or glycopyrrolate will antagonize vecuronium action. Concurrent administration of other neuromuscular blockers may not allow complete reversal.

DRUG INTERACTIONS

Aminoglycosides, bacitracin, clindamycin, inhalation anesthetics (enflurane, halothane, isoflurane), lincomycin, magnesium sulfate, neuromuscular blocking agents (metocurine, tubocurarine), quinidine, quinine, polymyxin B, succinylcholine, tetracycline: Increased neuromuscular blockade and prolonged paralysis.

NURSING CONSIDERATIONS

Assessment

General:
Vital signs, ECG (recommended), continuous monitoring of respiratory rate, hypersensitivity reaction.
Physical:
Cardiopulmonary status, neuromuscular status.

Intervention/Rationale

Produces apnea (use cautiously in patients with cardiovascular disease, severe electrolyte disorders, bronchogenic cancer, and neuromuscular diseases). Maintain patent airway. ● Monitor response to drug during intraoperative period by use of a peripheral nerve stimulator. Assess postoperatively for presence of any residual muscle weakness. Evaluate hand grip, head lift, and ability to cough in order to ascertain full recovery from residual effects of drug. ● Assess status of corneas; consider lubrication as needed. ● Assess need for sedation; obtain order and administer during use of paralytic agent. ● Monitor blood pressure, respiratory status, and ECG before and during administration. ● Observe for signs/symptoms of histamine reaction with initial dose or test dose (bronchospasm, flushing, redness, hypotension, tachycardia).

In the Adverse Effects section, <u>underline</u> indicates most frequent; CAPS indicates life threatening.

523

Patient/Family Education

Discuss the rationale for hand grip, head lift, and cough demonstration in the immediate postoperative phase in order to assure patient cooperation. Inform patient and family that consciousness is unaffected by drug. Explain side effects to patient and family. Continue to explain procedures and therapies to patient unless sedation is administered.

VERAPAMIL

(ver-ap′-a-mil)
Trade Name(s): Isoptin
Classification(s): Calcium channel blocker
Pregnancy Category: C

PHARMACODYNAMICS/KINETICS

Mechanism of Action: Inhibits movement of calcium ions across the cell membrane resulting in depression of mechanical contraction (myocardial and smooth muscle), depression of automaticity and conduction velocity. **Onset of Action:** Immediate. **Peak Effect:** Hemodynamic 3–5 min. AV node 1–2 min. **Duration of Action:** Hemodynamic 10–20 min. AV Node 30–60 min (up to 6 hr). **Therapeutic Serum Levels:** 80–300 ng/mL (not routinely monitored). **Distribution:** Distributed throughout body. Crosses into CNS. 90% protein bound. **Metabolism/Elimination:** Rapid and complete metabolism by the liver primarily to norverapamil, an active metabolite. Excreted by the kidneys as active metabolite, 3%–4% unchanged drug. Hemodialysis does not affect clearance. **Half-Life:** 3–

7 hr. Prolonged in elderly/hepatic cirrhosis.

INDICATIONS/DOSAGE

Treatment of supraventricular tachy-dysrhythmias; temporary control of rapid ventricular rate in atrial flutter/fibrillation

Reduce repeat doses in renal/hepatic impairment.

Adult: Initially 5–10 mg (0.075–0.15 mg/kg). Repeat 10 mg (0.15 mg/kg) in 15–30 min if no response from initial dose.
Continuous Infusion (*unlabeled use*): Initially 5–10 mg bolus (0.075–0.15 mg/kg) followed by 2.5–5.0 mcg/kg/min or 5 mg/hr.

Pediatric (1–15 years): Initially 2–5 mg (0.1–0.3 mg/kg). Not to exceed 5 mg/initial dose. Repeat dose in 15–30 minutes if no response from initial dose. Not to exceed 10 mg.

Pediatric (< 1 year)/Neonate: Initially 0.75–2.0 mg (0.1–0.2 mg/kg). Not to exceed 5 mg/initial dose. Repeat in 30 min if no response from initial dose.

CONTRAINDICATIONS/ PRECAUTIONS

Contraindicated in: Atrial flutter/fibrillation with accessory bypass tract, cardiogenic shock, severe CHF unless secondary to supraventricular tachycardia (SVT), severe left ventricular dysfunction, within a few hours of IV beta blockers. **Use cautiously in:** Duchenne muscular dystrophy, elderly, hepatic/renal impairment, patients receiving antihypertensive agents, supratentorial tumors. **Pregnancy/Lactation:** No well-controlled trials to establish safety. Teratogenicity has been reported in animals; no adverse effects in humans. Crosses placenta and appears in umbilical vein blood. Benefits must outweigh risks. Excreted into breast milk. Consider discontinuation of breast-feeding. **Pediatrics:** Safety and efficacy not established; however, seems to be safe in limited usage. Severe hemodynamic effects have been noted. Patients < 6 months may not respond.

PREPARATION

Availability: 5 mg/2mL in 2 and 4 mL amps, vials, syringes. **Syringe:** No further dilution required. May dilute to 0.5 mg/mL in compatible solution. **Infusion:** Not recommended for infusion. Further dilute to 0.4 mg/mL or as prescribed by physician in compatible IV solution.

STABILITY/STORAGE

Vial: Store at room temperature. Protect from light. Discard unused portion. **Infusion:** Use not recommended. Prepare just prior to administration. Stable for 24 hr at room temperature. Protect from light.

ADMINISTRATION

General: Continuous ECG and blood pressure monitoring. **IV Push:** Administer as direct slow IV push over at least 2 minutes (over at least 3 minutes in elderly patients). **Continuous Infusion:** Administer at physician prescribed rate.

COMPATIBILITY

Solution: Dextrose solutions, lactated Ringer's, Ringer's injection, sodium chloride solutions. **Syringe:** Heparin, milrinone. **Y-site:** Amrinone, dobutamine, dopamine, famotidine, hydralazine, methicillin, milrinone, penicillin G potassium, piperacillin, ticarcillin.

INCOMPATIBILITY

Y-site: Albumin, ampicillin, mezlocillin, nafcillin, oxacillin, sodium bicarbonate.

ADVERSE EFFECTS

CNS: Seizures, asthenia, dizziness, headache, mental depression, sleepiness, vertigo. **Ophtho:** Rotary nystagmus. **CV:** ASYSTOLE, CARDIOVASCULAR COLLAPSE, VENTRICULAR FIBRILLATION, atrial fibrillation/flutter, AV block/dissociation, bradycardia, bundle branch block, congestive heart failure, <u>hypotension</u>, palpitations. **Resp:** Pulmonary edema, dyspnea, shortness of breath. **GI:** Abdominal discomfort, <u>constipation</u>, dry mouth, hepatotoxicity (chronic therapy), nausea. **MS:** Muscle fatigue. **Derm:** Dermatitis. **Fld/Lytes:** Peripheral edema. **Hypersens:** BRONCHOSPASM/LARYNGOSPASM, rash. **Other:** Diaphoresis.

TOXICITY/OVERDOSE

Signs/Symptoms: Extension of adverse effects. **Treatment:** Symptomatic and supportive therapy. **Antidote(s):** In hypertrophic cardiomyopathy, beta agonist and IV calcium. In clinically significant hypotension, IV calcium or vasopressor (isoproterenol, norepinephrine) (except in hypertrophic cardiomyopathy, use alpha agonists such as metaraminol, methoxamine, phenylephrine). In bradycardia or fixed second/third degree

In the Adverse Effects section, <u>underline</u> indicates most frequent; CAPS indicates life threatening.

525

AV block, use IV atropine, isoproterenol, calcium, norepinephrine.

DRUG INTERACTIONS
Antihypertensive agents: Increased
hypotension. **Barbiturates:** Decreased verapamil bioavailability.
Beta blockers: Increased verapamil
adverse effects. **Calcium salts:** Decreased clinical effects/toxicity of
verapamil. **Carbamazepine, digitoxin,
digoxin:** Verapamil increases serum
levels. **Cyclosporine (cya):** Increased
cya serum levels; verapamil may be
nephroprotective if given prior to
cya. **Dantrolene IV:** Increased cardiovascular collapse incidence. **Disopyramide:** Additive effects and left
ventricular impairment. **Etomidate:**
Increased anesthetic effect. **Fentanyl:** Increased severe hypotension
or fluid volume required. **Lithium:**
Decreased serum lithium level.
Nondepolarizing muscle relaxants: Increased muscle relaxation and prolonged respiratory depression. **Prazosin:** Increased prazosin serum
level and postural hypotension.
Quinidine: Increased hypotension,
bradycardia, ventricular tachycardia, AV block, pulmonary edema.
Sulfinpyrazone: Increased verapamil
clearance. **Theophylline:** Increased
theophylline effect/toxicity. **Vitamin
D:** Decreased verapamil efficacy.

NURSING CONSIDERATIONS

Assessment
General:
Vital signs, continuous ECG moni-
toring.
Physical:
Cardiopulmonary status.
Lab Alterations:
Monitor serum creatinine during
therapy.

Intervention/Rationale
Continuous ECG monitoring required during administration. Rapid
treatment of extrasystoles and AV
block may be required. Emergency
equipment, pacemaker, and defibrillator must be readily available. ● Evaluate renal function to
avoid metabolite accumulation and
toxicity.

Patient/Family Education
Educate regarding side effects and
expected therapeutic outcome of
drug. Seek assistance with ambulatory activities.

VIDARABINE
(vye-dare′-a-been)
Trade Name(s): Vira-A
Classification(s): Antiviral agent
Pregnancy Category: C

PHARMACODYNAMICS/KINETICS
Mechanism of Action: Unknown. Selective inhibitor of DNA polymerase causing inhibition of viral
replication. **Distribution:** Rapidly
distributed into body tissues and
fluids as well as CNS. Protein
bound 20%–30% parent, 0%–3%
Ara-Hx. **Metabolism/Elimination:** Rapidly deaminated to active metabolite, arabinosyl hypoxanthine (Ara-
Hx). Excreted by the kidneys as
active metabolite, 1%–3% unchanged drug. **Half-Life:** 1.5 hr.
Ara-Hx 3.3 hr.

INDICATIONS/DOSAGE

**Herpes simplex (HSV), encephalitis;
herpes zoster infections in immunocompromised states; varicella-zoster**

In the Adverse Effects section, underline indicates most frequent;
CAPS indicates life threatening.

infections in immunocompromised states (*unlabeled use*)

Adult/Pediatric/Neonate: 15 mg/kg/day for 10 days. Up to 30 mg/kg/day. Reduce dosage in renal/hepatic impairment. If creatinine clearance < 10 mL/min, reduce dosage by 25%.

CONTRAINDICATIONS/PRECAUTIONS
Contraindicated in: Hypersensitivity. **Use cautiously in:** Imparied renal/hepatic function. Patients susceptible to fluid overload or cerebral edema. **Pregnancy/Lactation:** No well-controlled trials to establish safety. Benefits must outweigh risks. Teratogenicity has been reported in animals.

PREPARATION
Availability: 200 mg/mL (as monohydrate) in 5 mL vials. Equivalent to 187.4 mg vidarabine. **Infusion:** Shake vial well to suspend drug. Prewarming IV solution to 35–40° C may be helpful for solubilizing. Dilute each 1 mg drug with at least 2.2 mL. Each 450 mg must be diluted in at least 1000 mL compatible IV solution. Not to exceed final concentration of 0.7 mg/mL. Agitate admixture until clear. In neonates, add 1 mL drug to 9 mL sodium chloride or sterile water for 20 mg/mL; further dilute in volume of compatible solution not to exceed final concentration of 1 mg/2.2 mL.

STABILITY/STORAGE
Vial: Store at room temperature. **Infusion:** Prepare just prior to administration and use within 48 hr. Stable for 2 weeks at room temperature. Do not refrigerate.

ADMINISTRATION
General: Administer by slow IV infusion. **Continuous Infusion:** ≤ 0.45 micron inline filter must be used. Administer total daily dose over 12–24 hr. Greater than 1000 mL may be required for total dose.

COMPATIBILITY
Solution: Dextrose solutions, sodium chloride solutions.

INCOMPATIBILITY
Solution: Blood products, protein containing solutions.

ADVERSE EFFECTS
CNS: Ataxia, confusion, dizziness, hallucinations. headache, malaise, METABOLIC ENCEPHALOPATHY, psychosis, tremor **GI:** <u>Anorexia</u>, <u>diarrhea</u>, elevation of AST and total bilirubin, hematemesis, <u>nausea</u>, <u>vomiting</u>. **Heme:** Decreased hemoglobin, hematocrit, platelet count, reticulocyte count, WBC count. **Hypersens:** Pruritus, rash. **Other:** Pain at injection site, <u>weight loss</u>.

TOXICITY/OVERDOSE
Signs/Symptoms: Doses > 20 mg/kg/day cause bone marrow depression with thrombocytopenia and leukopenia. **Treatment:** Discontinue treatment. Symptomatic and supportive therapy.

DRUG INTERACTIONS
Allopurinol: Increased vidarabine serum levels/adverse effect potential.

NURSING CONSIDERATIONS
Assessment
General:
Intake/output ratio.

In the Adverse Effects section, <u>underline</u> indicates most frequent; CAPS indicates life threatening.

527

Physical:
GI tract, hematopoietic system, neurologic status.
Lab Alterations:
Monitor hematologic profile (hemoglobin, hematocrit, WBC, platelets), liver and renal function.

Intervention/Rationale
Large volumes of fluid are required. Observe for signs/symptoms of fluid overload, cerebral edema, or other adverse effects. ● Treatment should be discontinued if brain biopsy is negative for HSV in cell culture.

Patient/Family Education
Explain the reason for therapy and potential side effects.

VINBLASTINE
(vin-blass'-teen)
Trade Name(s): Alkaban-AQ, Velban, Velbe ♣, Velsar
Classification(s): Antineoplastic agent, vinca alkaloid
Pregnancy Category: D

PHARMACODYNAMICS/KINETICS
Mechanism of Action: Unknown. Periwinkle aklaloid that arrests mitotic division at metaphase. Reversibly binds to microtubule and spindle proteins in the S phase. **Peak Serum Level:** Immediate. **Duration of Action:** 1 week. **Distribution:** Rapidly and widely distributed throughout the body including platelets and leukocyte fractions. 75% bound to plasma proteins. **Metabolism/Elimination:** Extensive hepatic metabolism to an active metabolite with greater activity than parent compound. Primarily excreted via biliary tract slowly. **Half-Life:** 24.8 hr. Increased in hepatic impairment.

INDICATIONS/DOSAGE

Combination therapy as palliative treatment for Hodgkin's disease, lymphocytic lymphoma, histiocytic lymphoma, mycosis fungoides, advanced testicular carcinoma, Kaposi sarcoma, Letterer-Siwe disease, choriocarcinoma, unresponsive breast cancer

Individualize subsequent doses based on clinical hematologic response and tolerance. Reduce dosage 50% if direct serum bilirubin is > 3 mg/dL. Reduce dosage in patients with recent radiation exposure (single dose should not usually exceed 5.5 mg/m^2).

Adult: Initially 3.7 mg/m^2. At weekly intervals, increase the dose in increments of 1.8 mg/m^2 until the desired response occurs, the leukocyte count reaches 3000/mm^3, or a maximum weekly dose of 18.5 mg/m^2. Optimum weekly dose is usually 5.5–7.4 mg/m^2. When leukopenia occurs, do not administer the next dose until the leukocytes are 4000/mm^3. Once the dosage that produces a leukocyte count ≤ 3000/mm^3 is determined, a maintenance dose of 1.8 mg/m^2 **less than this amount** should be given at weekly intervals. Continue therapy for at least 4–6 weeks. *Pediatric:* Initially 2.5 mg/m^2. At weekly intervals, increase the dose in increments of 1.25 mg/m^2 until the desired response occurs, the leukocyte count reaches 3000/mm^3, or a maximum weekly dose of 12.5 mg/m^2. When leukopenia occurs, do not administer the next dose until the leukocytes are 4000/mm^3. Once the dosage that produces a leukocyte count ≤ 3000/mm^3 is determined, a maintenance dose of 1.25 mg/m^2 **less than this amount** should be given at weekly intervals. Continue therapy for at least 4–6 weeks.

CONTRAINDICATIONS/PRECAUTIONS

Contraindicated in: Hypersensitivity, leukopenia, presence of bacterial infection, significant granulocytopenia unless result of disease being treated. **Use cautiously in:** Hepatic impairment. **Pregnancy/Lactation:** Causes fetal harm. Benefits must outweigh risks. Women of childbearing age should be instructed to use contraceptives. Patients becoming pregnant during therapy should be apprised of the risks to the fetus.

PREPARATION

Availability: 10 mg powder for injection vial. 1 mg/mL in 10 mL vials (contains 0.9% benzyl alcohol). **Reconstitution:** Dilute 10 mg vial with 10 mL sodium chloride for a final concentration 1 mg/mL. **Syringe:** No further dilution required. **Infusion:** Dilute to desired concentration in compatible IV solution. Do not add to solutions that would change the pH outside of 3.5–5.0 range. Do not dilute in large volumes of fluid (i.e., ≥100 mL).

STABILITY/STORAGE

Vial: Store in refrigerator. Stable at room temperature for 1 month. If reconstituted with bacteriostatic diluent, stable for 30 days refrigerated. Discard unused portions if preservative-free diluent used. Protect from light.

ADMINISTRATION

General: Prepare and handle solution according to institutional guidelines for the handling of chemotherapeutic/cytotoxic substances. Avoid extravasation—discontinue administration immediately and change IV site (inject hyaluronidase locally and apply moderate heat to disperse drug and minimize discomfort) as per physician's order. Must be administered into tubing of running IV solution or directly into vein. Do not administer for long periods (i.e., 30–60 min). Do not inject intrathecally. Do not inject into extremity with impaired or potentially impaired circulation. Avoid eye contamination—wash eyes immediately. In the event of a spill, sodium hypochlorite 5% (household bleach) should be added to inactivate the drug. **IV Push:** Administer directly into vein over at least 1 min. **Intermittent Infusion:** Administer over physician prescribed time interval.

COMPATIBILITY

Solution: Dextrose solutions, lactated Ringer's, sodium chloride solutions. **Syringe:** Bleomycin, cisplatin, cyclophosphamide, droperidol, fluorouracil, leucovorin calcium, methotrexate, metoclopramide, mitomycin, vincristine. **Y-site:** Bleomycin, cisplatin, cyclophosphamide, doxorubicin, droperidol, fluorouracil, heparin, leucovorin calcium, methotrexate, metoclopramide, mitomycin, ondansetron, vincristine.

In the Adverse Effects section, underline indicates most frequent; CAPS indicates life threatening.

529

INCOMPATIBILITY
Syringe/Y-site: Furosemide.

ADVERSE EFFECTS
CNS: Cerebrovascular accident, convulsions, digit numbness, dizziness, headache, loss of deep tendon reflex, mental depression, neurotoxicity, paresthesia, peripheral neuritis. **CV:** MI, hypertension. **GI:** Abdominal pain, anorexia, constipation, diarrhea, hemorrhagic enterocolitis, <u>nausea</u>, pharyngitis, rectal bleed, recurrent peptic ulcer bleed, vesiculation of mouth, <u>vomiting</u>. **Derm:** <u>Alopecia</u>, epilation, skin vesiculation. **Fld/Lytes:** Syndrome of inappropriate antidiuretic hormone (SIADH). **Heme:** <u>LEUKOPENIA</u>, thrombocytopenia, anemia. **Nadir:** 7–10 days. **Other:** Bone/jaw pain, fever, malaise, thrombophlebitis, tumor site pain, weakness.

TOXICITY/OVERDOSE
Signs/Symptoms: Exaggerated adverse effects, especially hematologic and neurologic. **Treatment:** Symptomatic and supportive. Prevent SIADH by use of diuretic and fluid restriction; seizures with anticonvulsant; ileus with cathartics.

DRUG INTERACTIONS
Immunosuppressants: Increased bone marrow suppression. **Mitomycin:** Acute pulmonary reactions may occur. **Phenytoin:** Decreased phenytoin levels.

NURSING CONSIDERATIONS
Assessment
General:
Vital signs, intake/output ratio, hypersensitivity reactions.

Physical:
Neurologic status, GI tract, infectious disease status, hematopoietic system.
Lab Alterations:
Assess CBC with differential and platelet count, BUN, serum creatinine, uric acid, and liver function prior to and throughout course of therapy.

Intervention/Rationale
Assess patient for any signs of neurotoxicity. ● Assess for development of fever, chills, or other signs of infection and notify physician immediately. ● Maintain adequate hydration during therapy. ● Assess patient for development of bleeding (bleeding gums, easy bruising, hematest positive stools/urine/vomitus). ● Avoid intramuscular injections and rectal temperatures. ● If nausea becomes a problem, antiemetics may be administered 0.5 hr prior to administration. ● Monitor for signs of acute shortness of breath especially in combination with mitomycin. ● Monitor blood pressure, heart rate, and respiratory rate prior to, throughout, and following administration.

Patient/Family Education
Observe for signs of infection (fever, sore throat, fatigue) or bleeding (melena, hematuria, nosebleeds, easy bruising). Take and record oral temperature daily and report persistent elevation to physician. Use a soft toothbrush and electric razor to minimize bleeding tendency. Avoid crowded environments and persons with known infections. Use reliable contraception throughout the duration of therapy

In the Adverse Effects section, <u>underline</u> indicates most frequent; CAPS indicates life threatening.

and 4 months following due to potential teratogenic and mutagenic effects of drug. Seek physician approval prior to receiving live virus vaccinations. Avoid over-the-counter products containing aspirin or ibuprofen due to increased potential for bleeding. Report dizziness, unusual fatigue, or shortness of breath (drug may cause anemia). Scalp hair will regrow to pretreatment extent even with continued treatment.

VINCRISTINE

(vin-kriss'-teen)
Trade Name(s): Oncovin, Vincasar PFS
Classification(s): Antineoplastic agent, vinca alkaloid
Pregnancy Category: D

PHARMACODYNAMICS/KINETICS
Mechanism of Action: Unknown. Periwinkle alkaloid. Arrests mitotic division at metaphase. Reversibly binds to microtubule and spindle proteins in the S phase. **Peak Serum Level:** Immediate. **Duration of Action:** 1 week. **Distribution:** Rapidly and widely distributed throughout the body. Poor CNS penetration. Tightly and reversibly bound in tissues. **Metabolism/Elimination:** Extensive hepatic metabolism. Drug and metabolites excreted in feces via biliary tract; 30% within 24 hr, 70% within 72 hr. 10% excreted in urine. **Half-Life:** 85 hr (19–155 hr). Increased in hepatic impairment.

INDICATIONS/DOSAGE

Combination therapy in acute leukemia, Hodgkin/nonHodgkin malignant lymphoma, rhabdomyosarcoma, neuroblastoma, Wilm's tumor

Individualize subsequent doses based on clinical hematologic response and tolerance. Reduce dosage 50% if direct serum bilirubin > 3 mg/dL.

Adult: 1.4 mg/m^2 weekly. Not to exceed 2 mg/dose.

Pediatric: 2 mg/m^2 weekly. Not to exceed 2 mg/dose. If ≤ 10 kg or < 1 m^2, 0.05 mg/kg once a week.

CONTRAINDICATIONS/ PRECAUTIONS
Contraindicated in: Patients with demyelinating Charcot-Marie-Tooth syndrome, hypersensitivity. **Use cautiously in:** Decreased WBCs, infections, neurologic impairment, hepatic impairment, preexisting neuromuscular disease. **Pregnancy/ Lactation:** Causes fetal harm. Benefits must outweigh risks. Women of childbearing age should be instructed to use contraceptives. Patients becoming pregnant during therapy should be apprised of the risks to the fetus.

PREPARATION
Availability: 1 mg/mL in 1, 2, and 5 mL vials. **Syringe:** No further dilution required. **Infusion:** Dilute to desired concentration in compatible IV solution. Do not add to solutions that would change the pH outside of 3.5–5.5 range.

STABILITY/STORAGE
Vial: Store in refrigerator. Stable at room temperature for 1 month. **Infusion:** Stable for 21 days at room temperature/refrigeration.

In the Adverse Effects section, underline indicates most frequent;
CAPS indicates life threatening.

531

ADMINISTRATION

General: Prepare and handle solution according to institutional guidelines for the handling of chemotherapeutic/cytotoxic substances. Avoid extravasation—discontinue administration immediately and change IV site (inject hyaluronidase locally and apply moderate heat to disperse drug and minimize discomfort) as per physician's order. Must be administered into tubing of running IV solution or directly into vein. Do not administer intrathecally. If patient receives radiation therapy, do not give through same radiation ports that include liver. Avoid eye contamination—wash eyes immediately. In the event of a spill, add sodium hypochlorite 5% (household bleach) to spill to inactivate drug. **IV Push:** Administer directly into vein over at least 1 minute. **Intermittent/Continuous Infusion:** Administer over physician prescribed time interval.

COMPATIBILITY

Solution: Dextrose solutions, lactated Ringer's, sodium chloride solution. **Syringe:** Bleomycin, cisplatin, cyclophosphamide, doxapram, doxorubicin, droperidol, fluorouracil, heparin, leucovorin calcium, methotrexate, metoclopramide, mitomycin, vinblastine. **Y-site:** Bleomycin, cisplatin, cyclophosphamide, doxorubicin, droperidol, fluorouracil, heparin, leucovorin calcium, methotrexate, metoclopramide, mitomycin, ondansetron, vinblastine.

INCOMPATIBILITY

Syringe/Y-site: Furosemide.

ADVERSE EFFECTS

CNS: Convulsions, ataxia, cranial nerve deficits, especially extraocular and laryngeal, footdrop, headache, <u>neuritic pain</u>, paralysis, paresthesia, sensory loss. **Ophtho:** Blindness, diplopia, optic atrophy, photophobia, ptosis, transient cortical blindness. **CV:** Hypertension, hypotension. **Resp:** BRONCHOSPASM, acute shortness of breath. **GI:** Abdominal cramps, anorexia, <u>constipation</u>, diarrhea, intestinal necrosis, nausea, oral ulceration, paralytic ileus, vomiting. **GU:** Dysuria, polyuria, urinary retention. **MS:** Myalgias, loss deep tendon reflex, muscle wasting. **Derm:** <u>Alopecia</u>. **Fld/Lytes:** Hyponatremia, syndrome of inappropriate antidiuretic hormone. **Heme:** MYELOSUPPRESSION, leukopenia, thrombocytopenia, anemia. *Nadir:* 7–10 days. **Hypersens:** ANAPHYLAXIS, rash. **Other:** Fever, weight loss.

TOXICITY/OVERDOSE

Signs/Symptoms: Exaggerated adverse effects, especially neurologic and hematologic. **Treatment:** Symptomatic and supportive treatment. Prevent SIADH by use of diuretic and fluid restriction; seizures with anticonvulsant; ileus with cathartics. **Antidote(s):** In addition to supportive measures, folinic acid 100 mg IV every 3 hr for 24 hr and then every 6 hr for at least 48 hr as per physician order.

DRUG INTERACTIONS

Digoxin: Decreased digoxin levels and renal excretion. **L-asparaginase:** Reduces hepatic clearance of vincristine (administer vincristine

12–24 hr before). **Mitomycin:** Acute pulmonary reactions may occur. **Phenytoin:** Decreased phenytoin levels.

NURSING CONSIDERATIONS
Assessment
General:
Vital signs, intake/output ratio, hypersensitivity reactions.
Physical:
Neurologic status, GI tract, infectious disease status, hematopoietic system.
Lab Alterations:
Assess CBC with differential and platelet count, BUN, serum creatinine, uric acid, and liver function prior to and throughout course of therapy.

Intervention/Rationale
Assess patient for any signs of neurotoxicity. ● Assess for development of fever, chills, or other signs of infection and notify physician immediately. ● Maintain adequate hydration during therapy. ● Assess patient for development of bleeding (bleeding gums, easy bruising, hematest positive stools/urine/ vomitus). ● Avoid intramuscular injections and rectal temperatures. ● If nausea becomes a problem, antiemetics may be administered 0.5 hr prior to administration. ● Monitor for signs of acute shortness of breath especially in combination with mitomycin. ● Monitor blood pressure, heart rate, and respiratory rate prior to, throughout, and following administration.

Patient/Family Education
Observe for signs of infection (fever, sore throat, fatigue) or bleeding (melena, hematuria, nosebleeds, easy bruising). Take and record oral temperature daily and report persistent elevation to physician. Use a soft toothbrush and electric razor to minimize bleeding tendency. Avoid crowded environments and persons with known infections. Use reliable contraception throughout the duration of therapy and 4 months following due to potential teratogenic and mutagenic effects of drug. Seek physician approval prior to receiving live virus vaccinations. Avoid over-the-counter products containing aspirin or ibuprofen due to increased potential for bleeding. Report dizziness, unusual fatigue, or shortness of breath (drug may cause anemia). Scalp hair will regrow to pretreatment extent even with continued treatment.

WARFARIN
(war'-fa-rin)
Trade Name(s): Coumadin
Classification(s): Anticoagulant
Pregnancy Category: Unknown

PHARMACODYNAMICS/KINETICS
Mechanism of Action: Interference with hepatic synthesis of vitamin K-dependent clotting factors, II, VII, IX, X. **Peak Effect:** 1.5–3.0 days. **Duration of Action:** 2–5 days. **Distribution:** Highly bound (> 99%) to plasma proteins. **Metabolism/Elimination:** Metabolized by hepatic microsomal enzymes to inactive metabolites. Excreted primarily in urine and feces. **Half-Life:** 1.5–2.5 days.

INDICATIONS/DOSAGE

Prophylaxis and treatment of venous thrombosis; treatment of

In the Adverse Effects section, underline indicates most frequent; CAPS indicates life threatening.

533

atrial fibrillation with embolization; prophylaxis and treatment of pulmonary embolism; adjunct in treatment of coronary occlusion

Individualize dosage based on prothrombin time.

Adult: 10–15 mg daily for 2–5 days. Alternate dosage 40–60 mg as single dose. Maintenance doses should be based on prothrombin response with ranges of 2–10 mg. Use lower initial doses of 20–30 mg for elderly or debilitated patients. *Pediatric:* 0.05–0.34 mg/kg/dose daily. Not to exceed adult dosage. Adjust dose based on prothrombin time.

CONTRAINDICATIONS/ PRECAUTIONS

Contraindicated in: Acute nephritis, aneurysm, ascorbic acid deficiency, blood dyscrasias, cerebrovascular hemorrhage, eclampsia/pre-eclampsia, hemophilia, hemorrhagic tendencies, hepatic insufficiency, pericardial effusion, pregnancy, recent surgery of the eye, CNS, or regional lumbar block anesthesia, subacute bacterial endocarditis, threatened abortion, thrombocytopenic purpura, uncontrolled/malignant hypertension, visceral carcinoma. **Use cautiously in:** Active tuberculosis, antibiotic altered intestinal flora, hypertension, history of ulcerative disease of GI tract, indwelling catheters, major surgery, menstruation, polycythemia vera, postpartum renal insufficiency, severe diabetes, trauma, vasculitis. **Pregnancy/Lactation:** Anticoagulants cross the placenta. Fetal hemorrhage, spontaneous abortion, stillbirth, congenital

malformations, CNS defects, and prematurity have been reported. If patient should become pregnant, the risks should be discussed. Appears in breast milk; there is limited data as to the risks. **Pediatrics:** Infants < 12 months may require doses at/near high end of range. Anticoagulation may be difficult to maintain in < 5 years old.

PREPARATION

Availability: 50 mg vial with 2 mL diluent. **Reconstitution:** Dilute with 2 mL diluent or sterile water for injection for a final concentration of 25 mg/mL. **Syringe:** Withdraw desired dose into syringe.

STABILITY/STORAGE

Vial: Store at room temperature. Use immediately after reconstitution.

ADMINISTRATION

IV Push: Administer by direct IV push.

COMPATIBILITY

Solution: Ringer's injection, sodium chloride solutions. **Syringe:** Heparin.

INCOMPATIBILITY

Solution: Dextrose solutions, lactated Ringer's.

ADVERSE EFFECTS

CNS: Compressive neuropathy. **GI:** Hepatitis, hepatotoxicity, abdominal cramping, anorexia, diarrhea, jaundice, nausea, retroperitoneal hematoma, vomiting. **GU:** Priapism, red-orange urine. **Renal:** Nephropathy. **Derm:** Alopecia, dermatitis, gangrene/necrosis. **Heme:** AGRANULOCYTOSIS, eosinophilia, HEMORRHAGE, leukopenia. **Hypersens:**

In the Adverse Effects section, <u>underline</u> indicates most frequent; CAPS indicates life threatening.

Delayed hypersensitivity, urticaria. **Other:** Fever, purple toe syndrome.

TOXICITY/OVERDOSE
Signs/Symptoms: Microscopic hematuria, excessive menstrual bleeding, petechiae, prolonged bleeding. **Treatment:** Discontinue therapy, symptomatic/supportive therapy. **Antidote(s):** Vitamin K (subsequent control of PT may be difficult).

DRUG INTERACTIONS
Acetaminophen, anabolic steroids, clofibrate, danazol, erythromycin, gemfibrizol, glucagon, influenza vaccine, ketoconazole, propranolol, ranitidine, sulindac, thyroid drugs: Enhanced anticoagulant effects. **Adrenal corticosteroids, indomethacin, oxyphenbutazone, phenylbutazone, potassium, salicylates:** Increased bleeding tendency because of ulcerogenic potential. **Alcohol, allopurinol, amiodarone, chloramphenicol, cimetidine, disulfiram, methylphenidate, metrondiazole, phenylbutazone, propoxyphene, sulfinpyrazone, sulfonamide, trimethoprim-sulfamethoxazole:** Enhanced anticoagulant effects by metabolism inhibition. **Antimetabolites, quinidine, quinine, salicylates:** Increased bleeding tendency due to inhibition of procoagulant factors. **Barbiturates, carbamazepine, glutethimide, griseofulvin, nafcillin, phenytoin, rifampin:** Decreased anticoagulant effect due to enzyme induction. **Cephalosporins, dipyridamole, indomethacin, oxyphenbutazone, penicillin, phenylbutazone, salicylates, sulfinpyrazone:** Increased bleeding tendency due to platelet aggregation inhibition. **Chloral hydrate, clofibrate, diazoxide, ethacrynic acid, miconazole, nalidixic acid, phenylbutazone, salicylates, sulfonamides, sulfonylureas, triclofos:** Enhanced anticoagulant effects by anticoagulant displacement. **Estrogens, oral contraceptives, vitamin K:** Decreased anticoagulant effect due to increased procoagulant factors. **Ethchlorvynol, spironolactone, sucralfate:** Decreased anticoagulant effect. **Oral antibiotics:** Enhanced anticoagulant effects by decreased vitamin K. **Phenytoin, oral sulfonylureas:** Anticoagulants increase activity and toxicity by competitive inhibition microsomal enzymes. **Streptokinase, urokinase:** Concurrent use not recommended.

NURSING CONSIDERATIONS
Assessment
Physical:
Hematopoietic system, GI tract.
Lab Alterations:
Red discoloration of urine may interfere with lab tests. Monitor prothrombin time (PT) daily during initiation of therapy or dosage adjustment. Once patient is stabilized, monitor PT every 4–6 weeks.

Intervention/Rationale
Assess patient for unusual bleeding (easy bruising, hematuria, occult blood in stools, or tarry stools). ● Venipuncture/injections may require prolonged application of site pressure to prevent bleeding and/or hematoma formation. ● Hematest stools/vomitus/urine for presence of occult blood.

Patient/Family Education
Do not take any other medication unless recommended by physician. Notify physician of unusual bleed-

In the Adverse Effects section, <u>underline</u> indicates most frequent; CAPS indicates life threatening.

535

ing, bruising, red urine, or black tarry stools or diarrhea. Instruct patient as to the importance of frequent blood tests.

ZIDOVUDINE (AZIDOTHYMIDINE, AZT)

(zy-doe'-vu-deen)
Trade Name(s): Retrovir
Classification(s): Antiviral agent
Pregnancy Category: C

PHARMACODYNAMICS/KINETICS

Mechanism of Action: Converted by cellular kinases to zidovudine triphosphate, which interferes with HIV viral RNA-dependent DNA polymerase (reverse transcriptase) resulting in inhibition of viral replication. Also active against some mammalian retroviruses as well as Epstein-Barr virus. **Distribution:** Limited information. Seems to be widely distributed. Distributes into CSF. 34%–38% protein bound. **Metabolism/Elimination:** Rapidly hepatically metabolized to inactive metabolite. Active drug and metabolite cleared by glomerular filtration and tubular secretion by kidneys. **Half-Life:** 1.1 hr.

INDICATIONS/DOSAGE

Management of patients with symptomatic HIV infection who have a history of cytologically confirmed *Pneumocystis carinii* pneumonia or absolute CD$_4$ lymphocyte count of < 200/mm^3

Adult: 1–2 mg/kg every 4 hr. Begin oral therapy as soon as possible. 100 mg orally equals 1 mg/kg

IV. Pediatric (unlabeled use): 100 mg/m^2 every 6 hr.

CONTRAINDICATIONS/PRECAUTIONS

Contraindicated in: Severe hypersensitivity reactions. **Use cautiously in:** Bone marrow depression, hepatic/renal impairment. **Pregnancy/Lactation:** No well-controlled trials to establish safety. Benefits must outweigh risks. Crosses placenta. Unknown if excreted in breast milk; discontinue breastfeeding during administration. **Pediatrics:** Safety and efficacy has not been established in children < 12 years old. However, it has been administered without unusual adverse effects. Data is limited in < 3 months. Clearance may be reduced in < 1 month. Confirmatory tests must determine if HIV antibody test is positive due to maternal antibodies.

PREPARATION

Availability: 10 mg/mL in 20 mL single use vial. **Infusion:** Dilute dose in dextrose 5%. Final concentration should not exceed 4 mg/mL.

STABILITY/STORAGE

Vial: Store at room temperature. Protect from light. **Infusion:** Stable for 24 hr at room temperature and 48 hr refrigerated. Should be used within 8 hr if stored at room temperature and 24 hr if refrigerated.

ADMINISTRATION

General: Infuse at a constant rate. Avoid rapid administration. **Intermittent Infusion:** Infuse over 1 hr.

COMPATIBILITY

Solution: Dextrose 5%. **Y-site:** Acyclovir, amikacin, amphotericin B, az-

In the Adverse Effects section, <u>underline</u> indicates most frequent; CAPS indicates life threatening.

treonam, ceftazidime, ceftriaxone, cimetidine, clindamycin, dexamethasone, dobutamine, dopamine, erythromycin lactobionate, gentamicin, heparin, imipenem/cilastatin, lorazepam, metoclopramide, morphine, nafcillin, ondansetron, oxacillin, pentamidine, phenylephrine, piperacillin, potassium chloride, ranitidine, tobramycin, trimethoprim-sulfamethoxazole, trimetrexate, vancomycin.

ADVERSE EFFECTS

CNS: Seizures, agitation, anxiety, <u>asthenia</u>, confusion, depression, <u>headache</u>, hyperalgesia, insomnia, malaise, manic syndrome, restlessness, somnolence, tremor, vertigo. **Ophtho:** Amblyopia, photophobia. **Resp:** Cough, dyspnea, pharyngitis, rhinitis, sinusitis. **GI:** <u>Abdominal pain</u>, anorexia, <u>diarrhea</u>, increased liver function test, <u>nausea</u>, vomiting. **GU:** Dysuria, polyuria, urinary frequency/hesitancy. **MS:** Necrotizing myopathy, arthralgia, back pain, muscle spasm, myalgia. **Derm:** Acne, pigmentation finger/toenails. **Heme:** <u>Anemia</u>, MYELOSUPPRESSION, <u>granulocytopenia</u>, lymphadenopathy, thrombocytopenia. **Hypersens:** Pruritus, rash, urticaria. **Other:** Chills, diaphoresis, epistaxis, fever, flu-like syndrome.

TOXICITY/OVERDOSE

Signs/Symptoms: Spontaneous or induced nausea/vomiting. Transient hematologic changes. **Treatment:** Symptomatic/supportive. Hemodialysis has little effect on active drug removal; metabolite removal is increased.

DRUG INTERACTIONS

Acetaminophen, aspirin, indomethacin, probenecid: Reduced renal excretion of zidovudine by inhibition of glucuronidation. **Acyclovir:** Increased neurotoxicity. **Amphotericin B, dapsone, doxorubicin, flucytosine, interferon, pentamidine, vinblastine, vincristine:** Increased nephrotoxic, cytotoxic, and bone marrow suppression potential. **Nucleoside antivirals (DDI, DDC), ribavirin:** Increased hematologic toxicity. **Phenytoin:** Decreased phenytoin serum levels.

NURSING CONSIDERATIONS

Assessment

General:
Vital signs.

Physical:
GI tract, neurologic status, infectious disease status.

Lab Alterations:
Monitor baseline and periodic CBC with differential and platelet count.

Intervention/Rationale

Evaluate patient for signs/symptoms of neurologic dysfunction (confusion, headache, seizures, somnolence). ● Hematest stools/vomitus/drainage for presence of occult blood. ● Evaluate for presence of opportunistic infections (excess diarrhea, difficulty breathing). ● Monitor blood pressure, heart rate, and respiratory rate prior to, throughout, and following administration.

Patient/Family Education

Drug is not a cure for HIV infections. Contact physician if any change in health. Notify physician/nurse of fever, excessive weight loss, significant bleeding. Avoid taking other medications, including nonprescription drugs, without consulting physician. Prevention of further disease transmission is necessary.

In the Adverse Effects section, <u>underline</u> indicates most frequent; CAPS indicates life threatening.

Z

REFERENCES

Barnhart ER (publ). *Physician's Desk Reference.* Oradell, NJ, Medical Economics Data; 1992.

Benitz WE. *The Pediatric Drug Handbook,* 2nd ed. Chicago, Yearbook Medical Publishers; 1988.

Compendium of Pharmaceuticals and Specialties, 27th ed. Ottawa, Ontario, Canada, Canadian Pharmaceutical Association; 1992.

Ford DC. *Guidelines for Administration of Intravenous Medications to Pediatric Patients,* 3rd ed. Bethesda, MD, American Society of Hospital Pharmacists; 1988.

Gilman AG. *Goodman and Gilman's: The Pharmacological Basis of Therapeutics,* 8th ed. Elmsford, NY, Pergamon Press; 1990.

King JC. *Guide to Parenteral Admixtures.* St. Louis, Pacemarq; 1991.

Mason N. Preparing intravenous paraldehyde. *Hosp Ther* 1989; 14(3):22,24–25.

McEvoy GK (ed). *AHFS Drug Information 1992.* Bethesda, MD, American Society of Hospital Pharmacists; 1992.

Olin BR (ed). *Facts and Comparisons.* St. Louis, Facts and Comparisons; 1992.

Taketomo CK. *Pediatric Dosage Handbook.* Hudson, Ohio, Lexi-Comp; 1992.

Trissel LA. *Handbook of Injectable Drugs,* 6th ed. Bethesda, MD, American Society of Hospital Pharmacists; 1990.

Trissel LA. *Supplement to Handbook on Injectable Drugs,* 6th ed. Bethesda, MD, American Society of Hospital Pharmacists; 1991.

USPDI 1992, 12th ed. Rockville, MD, United States Pharmacopeial Convention; 1992.

APPENDICES

◆ APPENDIX A. FDA PREGNANCY CATEGORIES

The FDA has identified five categories describing the potential for fetal abnormalities secondary to drug administration during pregnancy. Consideration of risk versus benefit should always be made since most agents have not been extensively studied in controlled clinical trials in pregnant women. Those agents categorized as "X" should not be used since these are clearly documented as having a teratogenic effect.

Category A
Adequate studies in pregnant women have not shown fetal injury in the first trimester and no evidence in the last two trimesters.

Category B
Adequate studies in pregnant women have not shown fetal injury in the first trimester and no evidence in the last two trimesters; however, animal studies have shown a potential adverse effect.

Category C
Animal studies have shown fetal injury; however, no adequate studies in humans have been conducted. Benefits of use must outweigh risks of fetal injury.

Category D
Potential human fetal injury risk has been shown; however, benefits of use may be acceptable despite potential risk.

Category X
Animal and human studies indicate significant fetal injury risk. The risk of injury clearly outweighs benefit of use.

◆ APPENDIX B   CONTROLLED SUBSTANCE DEA SCHEDULES

The Controlled Substances Act of 1970 regulates manufacturing, distribution, and dispensing of drugs that have abuse potential. The Drug Enforcement Administration (DEA) of the US Department of Justice is the chief federal agency responsible for enforcement.

Drugs under the Controlled Substance Act are categorized based on their abuse potential and physical/psychological dependence.

Schedule I

High abuse potential; no accepted medical use (Examples: heroin, LSD).

Schedule II

High abuse potential with significant dependence potential (Examples: amphetamines, narcotics, some barbiturates, dronabinol).

Schedule III

Less abuse potential than schedule II with moderate dependence potential (Examples: sedatives, some narcotics).

Schedule IV

Less abuse potential than schedule III with limited dependence potential (Examples: some sedatives/antianxiety agents, nonnarcotic analgesics).

Schedule V

Limited abuse potential. Limited quantities may be purchased without a prescription but with proper documentation by the pharmacy. (Examples: small amounts of narcotics present as antitussives/antidiarrheals).

♦ APPENDIX C   WORK PRACTICE GUIDELINES FOR PERSONNEL DEALING WITH CYTOTOXIC (ANTINEOPLASTIC) DRUGS*

Current practices in the preparation, storage, administration and disposal of the widely used group of antineoplastic (anti-new growth; anticancer) drugs, also called cytotoxic drugs (CDs) because they are toxic to cells, may expose nurses, pharmacists, physicians and other health care workers to high environmental levels of these drugs. Several sets of work practice guidelines have been issued by various professional bodies in the United States and in foreign institutions. These guidelines are addressed to persons who have a broad spectrum of qualifications and experience and are issued by OSHA as a means of protection for health care providers. The risks to workers handling CDs are a combined result of the drugs' inherent toxicity and the extent to which workers are directly exposed to CDs on their job. The main routes of exposure are through the *inhalation* of drug dusts or droplets, *absorption* through the skin, and *ingestion* through contact with contaminated food or cigarettes. Opportunity for exposure may occur at many points in the handling of these drugs.

Environmental Protection for Preparation Areas

CDs are usually prepared in the pharmacy in large oncology centers, but may be prepared by physicians or nurses in smaller institutions, often in patient care or staff areas, which may be poorly ventilated. Many CDs must be dissolved, transferred from one container to another or manipulated before they can be administered to a patient. Even if care is taken, opportunity for absorption through inhalation or direct skin contact may occur.

A horizontal-air-flow, clean work bench is often used to provide an aseptic environment for the preparation of an injectable drug. Because this unit provides a flow of filtered air originating at the back of the work space and exiting towards the employee using the unit, it provides protection for the drugs but increases the likelihood of exposure to the preparer of the drugs and other personnel who may be in the room. Thus, CLASS II vertical flow containment hoods (Biological Safety Cabinets) provide the appropriate protection required. Type A Biological Safety Cabinets are a minimal requirement. Type A hoods that are vented are actually preferred.

Disposal of Drugs/Contaminated Equipment

Materials used in the preparation and administration of CDs, such as gloves, gowns, syringes, or vials, present a possible source of exposure or injury to all health care workers, even those not directly involved with preparation/administration. The use of properly labeled, sealed, and covered containers, handled only by trained and protected personnel, should

* *OSHA Instruction PUB 8-1.1.* Office of Occupational Medicine, US Department of Labor. January 29, 1986.

be routine. Spills also represent a potential hazard and all employees should be familiar with appropriate spill procedures for their own safety.

Personal Protective Equipment

Surgical latex gloves are less permeable to many CDs than the polyvinyl-chloride gloves previously recommended. Latex gloves should be used for drug preparation unless the manufacturer stipulates that some other glove provides better protection. Powdered gloves should *never* be used. A protective disposable gown made of lint-free, low-permeability fabric with a closed front, long sleeves, and elastic or knit-closed cuffs must be worn with the cuffs tucked under the gloves. Gowns/gloves should not be worn outside of the preparation area.

A Biological Safety Cabinet (BSC) is essential for the preparation of CDs but where one is not available, a respirator with a high efficiency filter provides the best protection until a BSC is installed.

Surgical masks *do not* protect against the breathing of aerosols. A plastic face shield or splash goggles should be worn if a BSC is not in use. An eyewash fountain should also be available.

Drug Preparation Equipment

Work with CDs must be carried out in a BSC on a disposable, plastic-backed paper liner, which should be changed at least daily. Syringes and IV sets with luer-lock fittings should always be used and syringes should always be large enough so that they need never be more than 75% full. The use of large-bore needles will ensure that high-pressure syringing of the solutions is avoided. Drug administration sets should be attached and primed within the hood before the drug is added to the fluid to obviate the need to prime the set in a less well-controlled area and to ensure that any fluid that escapes during priming contains no drug. All syringes and needles used during the course of preparation should be placed in a puncture-proof container for disposal without being crushed, clipped, or capped.

Drug Administration Practices

Hands should be washed before putting on gloves. Contaminated gowns/gloves should be changed immediately. Infusion sets/pumps that have luer-lock fittings should be watched for leakage during administration. A plastic-backed absorbent pad should be placed under the tubing during administration to catch any leakage. The line should be bled into a gauze inside a sealable bag to remove air. Syringes, IV bottles/bags and pumps should be wiped clean of any drug contamination with an alcohol wipe. Needles/syringes should not be capped, crushed, or clipped, but should be placed in a CD disposal container along with all other contaminated material. All gauze and alcohol wipes must be put in an appropriate container for toxic waste disposal.

Caring for Patients Receiving Cytotoxic Drugs

Personnel dealing with blood, vomitus, or excreta from patients receiving CDs in the last 48 hours should wear surgical latex gloves and disposable gowns, which should be discarded after each use. No protective equipment is necessary for ordinary patient contact for employees not dealing with drug administration or bodily secretions.

Linen contaminated with blood, vomitus, or excreta from a patient receiving CDs up to 48 hours before should be placed in a specially marked laundry bag and then placed in a labeled impervious bag. Laundry personnel should wear surgical latex gloves and disposable gowns when handling this contaminated linen.

Treatment of Spills

Spills and breakage should be cleaned up immediately by a properly trained person. Broken glass should be carefully removed. A spill should be identified with a warning sign so that other persons in the area will not be contaminated.

Spills of less than 5 mL or 5 g outside of a hood should be cleaned up by personnel wearing gowns and double surgical latex gloves and eye protection. Liquids should be wiped with absorbent gauze pads; solids should be wiped with wet absorbent gauze pads. The spill area should be cleaned (three times) using a detergent solution followed by clean water. Any broken glass fragments should be placed in a small cardboard or plastic container and then into a CD disposal bag, along with the used absorbent pads and any noncleanable contaminated items.

For spills more than 5 mL or 5 g, limit spread by gently covering with absorbent sheets or spill-control pads or pillows or, if a powder is involved, with damp cloths or towels. Be sure not to generate aerosols. Access to spill areas should be restricted. Protective apparel should be used, with the addition of a respirator when there is danger of airborne powder or an aerosol being generated. All contaminated surfaces should be thoroughly cleaned with detergent solution and then wiped with clean water. All contaminated absorbents and other materials should be disposed of in the CD disposal bag.

Personnel Contamination

Overt contamination of gowns/gloves or direct skin or eye contact should be treated as follows:

1. Immediate removal of the gloves and gown
2. Wash the affected skin area immediately with soap (not germicidal cleaner) and water. For eye exposure, immediately flood the affected eye with water or isotonic eyewash designated for that purpose for at least 5 minutes.
3. Obtain medical attention immediately

Training and Information Dissemination

All personnel involved in any aspect of the handling of CDs (shipping–receiving personnel, physicians, nurses, pharmacists, housekeepers, employees involved in the transport/storage of drugs) must receive an orientation on CDs, including their known risks, relevant techniques/procedures for their handling, the proper use of protective equipment and materials, spill procedures, and medical policies (including those dealing with pregnancy and with staff actively trying to conceive children).

Pregnancy

On the basis of the available evidence, it seems reasonable to assure that if appropriate procedures are followed and proper equipment and protection are provided, reproductive hazards will be reduced.

1. Employees should be fully informed of the potential reproductive hazard and, if they so request, staff members who are pregnant or breastfeeding should be transferred to comparable duties that do not involve CDs.
2. A similar policy covering male or female personnel who are actively trying to conceive a child should be established.

INDEX

Nomogram for calculating the body surface area of adults: Place [a straightedge from] the patient's height in the left column to the weight in the right [column. The inter-] section point in the center column is the body surface area. (Fr[om the formula of] DuBois and DuBois: Arch Int Med. *1916; 17:863.* Reproduced wit[h permission from] Lentner C (ed): Geigy Scientific Tables, 8th ed. Basle, Switzerland: [publisher] *1981; vol 1, p 227.*)

HEIGHT   **BODY SURFACE AREA**   **WE[IGHT]**